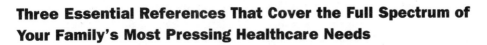

The Source Families Turn To for Authoritative Guidance on Drugs, Health, and Nutrition

Three Essential References That Cover the Full Spectrum of Your Family's Most Pressing Healthcare Needs

Here are the fast, accurate answers your family deserves—brought to you by the publishers of *Physicians' Desk Reference*, the professional reference that doctors have relied on for fully half a century. Keep the complete set on hand for ready reference:

■ The PDR® Family Guide to Prescription Drugs®
■ The PDR® Family Guide to Women's Health and Prescription Drugs™
■ The PDR® Family Guide to Nutrition and Health™

Save 20% off cover price! Only $19.95 each...with shipping and handling FREE.
Send this postpaid card today, or for fastest service call toll-free: 1-800-331-0072 (To fax your order, dial 1-201-573-4956)

Yes! Send me another copy or the other books checked below at the special price of $19.95 each. I understand that shipping and handling are free. NJ residents add 6% tax; in IA add 5%, in GA add 4%, in FL add 6%.

___ Copies of The PDR® Family Guide to Prescription Drugs®
___ Copies of The PDR® Family Guide to Women's Health and Prescription Drugs™
___ Copies of The PDR® Family Guide to Nutrition and Health™

Name

Address

City   State

Zip   Phone (   )

Charge ☐ MasterCard   ☐ Visa   ☐ American Express   ☐ Discover

Number   Expiration

FX5008-FX10

Only prepaid orders are accepted. Allow 3 weeks for delivery.

Three Vital Volumes
to Safeguard Your Family's Health

■ The PDR® Family Guide to Prescription Drugs®

The official facts on all the nation's most frequently prescribed medications, plus
23 fact-filled chapters on common medical conditions and their treatment. Covers side effects,
dangerous interactions, standard dosage, signs of overdose, and much more. Newly updated,
with over 900 pages and a full-color drug identification guide.

■ The PDR® Family Guide to Women's Health and Prescription Drugs™

With over 40 chapters on every aspect of health, fertility, and family planning,
this comprehensive resource brings all the latest medical facts together in a single frank,
sensitive, easy-to-read reference. Includes a 300-page guide to women's medications
and a full-color drug identification guide.

■ The PDR® Family Guide to Nutrition and Health™

Finally, a realistic, medically proven way of upgrading your family's diet without
needless denial. Covers weight-loss, heart-health, cancer prevention, stress, energy, fitness,
and more—with easy, practical steps you can take at every stage of life, from infancy
through retirement. Includes a complete guide to nutritional supplements and drugs,
a comprehensive fat and calorie counter, a full-color drug identification guide, and more.

NO POSTAGE
NECESSARY
IF MAILED
IN THE
UNITED STATES

BUSINESS REPLY MAIL

FIRST CLASS MAIL   PERMIT NO. 35   MONTVALE, NJ

POSTAGE WILL BE PAID BY ADDRESSEE

ATTN: FAMILY GUIDE ORDER DEPARTMENT
MEDICAL ECONOMICS
P.O. Box 430
Montvale, NJ 07645-9875

We need your help...

Thank you for your interest in The PDR® Family Guide to Nutrition and Health™. We sincerely hope that this edition meets your needs; and we want to make sure that future editions are even better. To help us improve the book, your advice is crucial; so please take a moment to tell us what features you'd like to see added or revised. By completing and returning this brief questionnaire, you will be registering to receive product information on new drugs. We will do our best to implement your suggestions.

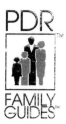

PDR™
FAMILY GUIDES™

1. Why did you purchase this book?

_____
_____
_____

2. What do you LIKE most about this book?

_____
_____
_____

3. What do you DISLIKE most about this book?

_____
_____

4. What would you like added to the book?

_____
_____
_____

5. We are considering publishing other books What subjects are of most interest to you?

_____
_____
_____

6. Are you interested in an update that will include new drugs? ☐ Yes ☐ No

7. How did you hear about this book?

☐ friend   ☐ pharmacist   ☐ saw in store
☐ relative   ☐ advertising   ☐ other
☐ doctor   ☐ mailer _____

8. What other healthcare and drug reference books do you own?

_____

And just a few more questions.

9. Please check: ☐ Male   ☐ Female

10. How many medications do you take daily?
   1   2   3   4   5   6   7   8   9   10 or more

11. In which of these age groups do you fall?

☐ 19 and under   ☐ 50-59
☐ 20-29   ☐ 60-69
☐ 30-39   ☐ 70 and over
☐ 40-49

12. Which of the following best describes your formal education level?

☐ Some high school   ☐ Some college
☐ High school   ☐ College
                     ☐ Graduate School or more

13. Which of the following best describes your family's income?

☐ less than $19,999   ☐ $50,000-$59,999
☐ $20,000-$29,999   ☐ $60,000-$69,999
☐ $30,000-$39,999   ☐ $70,000-$79,000
☐ $40,000-$49,999   ☐ over $80,000

Name _____

Address _____

City _____ State _____ Zip _____

Phone _____

Thank you,

MEDICAL ECONOMICS
Five Paragon Drive
Montvale, New Jersey 07645-1742

N951

IIII

What Experts Are Saying about The PDR® Family Guide to Nutrition and Health™

"Covers important information about vitamins, nutrients, antioxidants, diet, cancer, and eating disorders.... Contains all the information needed for a healthy diet."

SONIA CAPRIO, MD
Assistant Professor of Pediatrics
Yale University

"Contains something for everyone.... This timely publication will be a useful and informative addition to every home library."

ANDREA SCHNEIDER, RD
Consultant Dietitian
Irvington, NY

"Provides critical information on diet and nutrition in a very understandable manner.... While the information was developed for family use, health professionals will find it useful for instructing their patients."

PAUL F. ENGSTROM, MD
Senior Vice President for Population Science
Fox Chase Cancer Center
Philadelphia, PA

"Comprehensive, easy-to-understand.... Sorts out fact from fantasy in a lucid, interesting style."

STEPHEN BRUNTON, MD
Clinical Professor, Department of
Family Medicine
University of California Irvine

"Indispensable for anyone who wishes to maximize the beneficial impact of nutrition on health."

PAUL MISKOVITZ, MD
Clinical Associate Professor of Medicine
Cornell University Medical College

Other Books and Services from Medical Economics

The PDR® Family Guide to Prescription Drugs®

For up-to-the-minute information on all your prescription medications, turn to this vital home reference. Presents all the key facts in a convenient, easy-to-read format. Covers leading pediatric medicines, allergy remedies, pain medications, anticonvulsants, blood pressure medications, heart medicines, skin products, and more. To order, call toll-free 1-800-331-0072.

The PDR® Family Guide to Women's Health and Prescription Drugs™

For a frank, in-depth look at all of a woman's unique health concerns, add this PDR® Family Guide to your home health library. From menstrual problems to menopause, you'll find the latest information on a full range of gynecological infections and disorders, plus up-to-the-minute facts on AIDS-prevention, recovery from rape, contraceptive technology, osteoporosis, heart disease, diet, cancer, and more. To order, call toll-free 1-800-331-0072.

Professional References

Physicians' Desk Reference®
PDR For Nonprescription Drugs®
PDR For Ophthalmology®
PDR Guide to Drug Interactions•Side
  Effects•Indications™
PDR Generics™
PDR® Medical Dictionary™
Pocket PDR™ (Handheld Electronic Database)
PDR Library on CD-ROM™
PDR Drug Interactions/Side Effects/Indications
  Diskettes™

Medical Device Register™
Breast Implant Problem Reports™
Directory of Healthcare Group Purchasing
  Organizations™
Directory of Hospital Personnel™
Directory of U.S. Nursing Homes and Nursing Home
  Chains™
HMO/PPO Directory™
Product Development Directory™
Product SOS™ (FDA Problem Reports)
Surgeons' Reference for Minimally Invasive Surgery
  Products™

Red Book® (Pharmaceutical Prices)
MicREData
The Red Book® Database

THE PDR® FAMILY GUIDE TO

NUTRITION

AND HEALTH™

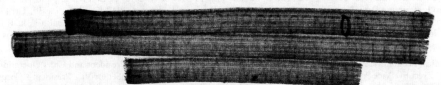

MEDICAL ECONOMICS   **MONTVALE, NEW JERSEY**

Publisher's Note

The drug information contained in this book is based on product labeling published in Physicians' Desk Reference®, supplemented with facts from other sources the publisher believes reliable. While diligent efforts have been made to assure the accuracy of this information, the book does not list every possible action, adverse reaction, interaction, and precaution; and all information is presented without guarantees by the authors, consultants, and publisher, who disclaim all liability in connection with its use.

This book is intended only as a reference for use in an ongoing partnership between doctor and patient in the vigilant management of the patient's health. It is not a substitute for a doctor's professional judgment, and serves only as a reminder of concerns that may need discussion. All readers are urged to consult with a physician before beginning or discontinuing use of any prescription drug or undertaking any form of self-treatment.

Brand names listed in this book are intended to represent only the more commonly used products. Inclusion of a brand name does not signify endorsement of the product, absence of a name does not imply a criticism or rejection of the product. The publisher is not advocating the use of any product described in this book, does not warrant or guarantee any of these products, and has not performed any independent analysis in connection with the product information contained herein.

ISBN: 1-56363-135-0 (Medical Economics Company)

Manufactured in the United States of America

10 9 8 7 6 5 4 3 2 1

Bulk copy inquiries are invited. Contact the Trade Sales Department at 1-800-442-6657

Contents

Part 1: Your Diet's Impact on Health

Section I. Reality Check: The Facts Versus the Fads

Section II. Keeping Your Weight in Check

Section III. Food and Your Heart

Section IV. Cancer: Foods that Could Cause It—or Fend It Off

Section V. Fine-Tuning Your Diet For the Stages of Your Life

The PDR® Family Guide to Nutrition and Health™

Editor-in-Chief: David W. Sifton
Product Manager: Karen B. Sperber
Director of Professional Services: Mukesh Mehta, R Ph
Art Director: Robert Hartman

Assistant Editors: Ann Ben Larbi; Paula Benus; Beret R. Erway; Jayne Jacobson; Michael Jahn; Libby Machol; Thelma Perrin; Alice Z. Weiss

Writers: Brenda L. Becker; Lynn H. Buechler; Paul L. Cerrato, RD; Kris Hallam; Ami Havens; Randi Henderson; Jayne Jacobson; Judith K. Ludwig; Virginia M. Mason; Eileen McCaffrey; Sara Altshul O'Donnell; Marie Powers; Marcia Ringel; Ronni Sandroff

Illustrations: Christopher Wikoff, MAMS

Managing Pharmaceutical Editor: Marion Gray, R Ph

Pharmaceutical Consultants: Nancy Jacoby, R Ph; Kathryn M. Martin, PharmD

Editorial Production: Vice President of Production: Steven R. Andreazza; Contracts and Support Services Director: Marjorie Duffy; Director of Production: Carrie Williams; Production Managers: Kimberly Hiller-Vivas, Tara L. Walsh; Electronic Publishing Coordinator: Joanne M. Pearson; Electronic Publishing Designer: Kevin J. Leckner; Digital Photography: Shawn W. Cahill, Frank J. McElroy, III

Drug Information Services Group

President and Chief Operating Officer: Thomas F. Rice

Director of Product Management: Stephen B. Greenberg

Trade Sales Manager: Robin B. Bartlett; Trade Sales Account Executive: Bill Gaffney; Direct Marketing Manager: Robert W. Chapman; Marketing Communications Manager: Maryann Malorgio; Director of Corporate Communications: Gregory J. Thomas; Manager, Database Administration: Lynne Handler; Manager, Electronic Publishing: David Levy, Fulfillment Manager: Roni LaVine; Administrative Assistants: Linda Levine, Sandra Loeffler, Martina Murtagh, Helene Wattman

Board of Medical Consultants

Chair:
Audrey Cross, JD, PhD
Associate Clinical Professor of Nutrition,
School of Public Health
Columbia University, New York, NY

David Alberts, MD
Professor of Medicine and Pharmacology
Director, Cancer Prevention and Control,
Arizona Cancer Center
University of Arizona College of Medicine,Tucson, AZ

Susan Schukar Berdy, MD
Instructor in Clinical Medicine
Washington University School of Medicine,
St. Louis, MO

Marc A. Clachko, MD
Associate Director, Department of Obstetrics and
Gynecology
Hackensack Medical Center, Hackensack, NJ

Andrea Dmitruk, RD
Coordinator of Clinical Nutritional Services,
Department of Food and Nutrition
The New York Hospital—Cornell Medical Center,
New York, NY

Karen Reznik Dolins, MS, RD
Nutrition Consultant
Private Practice, Scarsdale, NY

Naomi K. Fukagawa, MD, PhD
Assistant Professor and Associate Program Director,
The Clinical Research Center
The Rockefeller University, New York, NY

Richard A. Galbraith, MD, PhD
Medical Director
The Rockefeller University, New York, NY

Yvonne Padgett Hiott
Senior Managing Editor
American Health Consultants, Atlanta, GA

Victoria Kaprielian Johnson, MD
Department of Community and Family Medicine
Duke University Medical Center, Durham, NC

Jerry Levine, MD
Chief, Infectious Diseases
Hackensack Medical Center, Hackensack, NJ

Louise Merriman, RD
Associate Director, Department of Food and Nutrition
The New York Hospital—Cornell Medical Center,
New York, NY

Frank L. Meyskens, Jr., MD
Professor of Medicine
University of California, Irvine

Sylvia A. Moore, PhD, RD
Professor of Family Medicine,
School of Human Medicine
University of Wyoming, Cheyenne, WY

Gwendolyn C. Murphy, RD, PhD
Pediatric Nutritionist, Pediatric Department
Duke University Medical Center, Durham, NC

Lynda Olender, RN, MA, CNSN
Clinical Nurse Specialist, Nutrition Support
VA Medical Center, Brooklyn, NY

Irwin H. Rosenberg, MD
Professor of Medicine and Nutrition
Tufts University, Boston, MA

Daniel A. Sugarman, PhD
Professor, Department of Psychology
William Paterson College, Wayne, NJ

Annette Warpeha-Adams, RD
Nutrition Consultant
Private and Corporate Practice, New York, NY

Shelley Weinstock, PhD
Assistant Professor, Department of Chemisty
and Biochemistry
Montclair State University, Montclair, NJ

David Wilson
Vice President and Publisher
American Health Consultants, Atlanta, GA

Foreword

Nutrition is a confused and contentious field, full of potential benefits, but very short on certainties. Experts are now convinced that the right dietary choices can improve health and protect from disease—yet few can agree on the precise course to take in every circumstance.

Fads come and go in nutrition with breathtaking speed. Today's "fact" is often tomorrow's delusion; and were we to take each conflicting claim and warning seriously, we would surely wind up eating nothing at all! The purpose of this book is to winnow out enduring principles of good nutrition from the passing fancies that often obscure the facts, charting a reasonable, practical course that improves your odds of good health without imposing needless dietary demands.

This is a surprisingly difficult feat to accomplish. In nutrition, even the most obvious fact can be the object of bitter debate; and for each scientist advocating a course of action there's another who rejects it. Is too much fat bad for you? Most experts say Yes; but you'll still find reputable authorities who question the benefit of a low-fat diet. Are vitamins and minerals good for you? Virtually everyone agrees that they are; yet many dedicated nutritionists hotly oppose vitamin supplements, recommending dietary sources instead.

Often these arguments ignore the realities of everyday life. Though there may be no iron-clad, scientifically proven guarantee that cutting down on fat will spare you from heart disease, there's still no question that we currently get much more fat than we need. And while it's undeniably true that food is the best source of vitamins, it's also a fact that many of us cannot—or will not—eat enough of the foods that supply them.

Should we then reject supplements, and do without the extra vitamins entirely? Or take the supplements for what they're worth, recognizing that we're missing out on the other nutrients that good food supplies?

In this book we take the latter position. For those who've decided to take supplements, we identify the maximum safe amounts, the potential benefits, and the possible drawbacks. For those who prefer the dietary route, we list the richest sources and the amounts typically needed. And for both sides, we endeavor to set sensible guidelines that exclude the totally useless (or even harmful) supplements and "health foods" that abound in today's marketplace, waiting to separate the unwary from their dollars.

Recognizing that few people are willing to subsist on a diet of black-strap molasses, brown rice, and Brussels sprouts, we've also tried to strike a practical balance between health and enjoyment. For instance, though too much fat is bad, a certain amount is mandatory. Therefore, it's not only unnecessary, but even unwise to give up every fat-laden dish you enjoy. All you need to do is aim for moderation. To help, we've tried to portray not only the current consensus on what's ideal, but also on what's acceptable, so that you'll have a shot at a healthier diet, even if you can't stomach nutritional perfection.

In keeping with this pragmatic approach, we've also tried to address certain health concerns that seem only tenuously related to nutrition. For instance, while scientists are still unable to explain the cause of many types of arthritis, for some people, a change in diet has in fact proven helpful. We don't know why this so: there's no cause-and-effect explanation and no guarantee that what works for one person will work for the next. Still, we've included the more reliable of the reports in this area, on the chance that they could prove helpful for some people until better answers are known.

Moderation, balance, practicality, and consensus: these are the watchwords of this book; and holding to them really can improve your odds of good health. On the other hand, you'll find few, if any, instant cures outlined in these pages. Unfortunately, they simply don't exist. For instance, we'd love to tell you about a diet that cures cancer; but the best that science can do right now is alert us to some foods that cut our cancer risk. That's not the answer we're all looking for, but it's more than we knew a few years ago—and in the long run, just as life-saving.

The goal of this book is to provide the tools you need to improve your diet —and your health—with ordinary, enjoyable food available from the nearest supermarket. The book includes some new ways of cooking and suggests a variety of interesting new ingredients; but there's no need to subject your family to anything they don't like. Keep experimenting. See what works for you. A healthy diet doesn't have to be horrible—in fact, it can be absolutely delicious. Bon appetit!

Audrey Cross, JD, PhD
Associate Clinical Professor of Nutrition
School of Public Health
Columbia University, New York, NY

How to Use this Book

This is a book for real people with genuine appetites. It's for those of us with a natural concern for our health, and a healthy skepticism about nutritionists' all-too-often contradictory claims. It's designed for use as a practical, everyday reference, a source you can turn to for quick, reliable answers to the common questions that are bound to crop up just about every time your family sits down to eat.

Like a cookbook or a dictionary, this book is designed to let you zero in on a specific problem, get the information you need, and lay the book aside until the next question comes up. Are you concerned about heart disease? High blood pressure? Infections...cancer...stress? We've included special chapters on all these problems and more. Whether your planning meals for a baby, the kids, or your grandparents, there's detailed information on nutritional needs at every stage of life. And, of course, if you need to know more about a specific vitamin, mineral, or nutritional medication, you'll find a full description ready at hand.

To make all these facts as accessible as possible, we've divided the book into five major parts.

Part One, Your Diet's Impact on Health

This part of the book explores the specific goals that people have in mind when they decide it's time to improve their diets. It's divided into six sections that deal with the questions that come up most frequently whenever the conversation turns to nutrition.

Reality Check: The Facts Versus the Fads

This introductory section offers a general overview of what's really known about nutrition today. It tells how to judge the blizzard of research reports that fill the media, what to make of those often exaggerated health-food claims, and how to pick a sensible diet plan from the scores of contenders flooding the market.

Keeping Your Weight in Check

This section is devoted entirely to weight loss and fitness. In it, you'll find the current thinking on establishing your ideal healthy weight, a more detailed examination of popular weight-reduction plans, a crucial chapter on the right strategy for keeping weight off, and important advice on what to do when worry over weight gets completely out of hand.

Food and Your Heart

The need to cut back on fat and cholesterol is probably the best known watchword in modern nutrition; and this third section of the book is designed to help you put the low-fat craze into proper perspective. There's valuable information here, too, on salt, blood pressure, and what you really need to do about it.

Cancer: Foods That Could Cause It— Or Fend It Off

During the past 20 years, cancer scares have been prime grist for the headline writers' mill. Section Four sorts out the real dangers from the many false alarms. Perhaps more importantly, it spotlights the many foods with potentially protective qualities, as well as recommending dietary measures targeted at specific cancer risks.

Fine-Tuning Your Diet for the Stages of Your Life

From birth through old age, our nutritional requirements are constantly changing—often moderately, sometimes drastically. Section Five sets down the key requirements for each age group. In it, you'll find crucial advice on fat restriction for babies and kids, the surprising need for calcium after reaching adulthood, the way menopause can affect your dietary requirements, and the many nutritional demands of our senior years.

Special Problems, Special Diets

Section Six rounds out the first part of the book with detailed recommendations for a variety of health problems, ranging from allergies and arthritis to stress and the ravages of smoking. Whether you're concerned about diabetes, brittle bones, infection, or below-par immunity, you'll find sensible nutritional guidelines waiting for you here.

Part Two,
Keeping the Fun in Your Food

In recent years, dire warnings about everything from egg rolls to tacos have become so common that many people now approach the dinner table with nothing short of trepidation. Conflicting and exaggerated headlines have left us afraid to eat almost anything but skim milk and fortified cereal.

This is no way to live, and there's no good reason for it. The chapters in this part of the book sketch out the dietary tactics that will make your meals healthy and enjoyable. Included are in-depth guides to "junk food" and fast food, restaurant dining, and the many ethnic cuisines that are becoming so popular today. There's also a cornucopia of tips for "nutritionally correct" cooking at home, a complete guide to the creative use of herbs and spices, and nutritional ratings of all the most popular cookbooks. You'll even find examples of the fresh and exciting recipes you can use to keep the healthiest meal plan bursting with flavor.

Part Three, Nutrition, A to Z

For quick reference when you want information on a specific vitamin, mineral, or supplement, this handy section presents all details you need, including recommended allowances for every age group, maximum safe dosage, signs of overdosage, effects of deficiency, best dietary sources, and each substance's role in good health. The entries are listed alphabetically by the most frequently used names, and are cross-referenced by other common names.

Part Four, Medications in Nutrition

Only a few decades ago, when you developed a digestive or metabolic disorder, the best the doctor could do was advise a special diet. Today physicians have a variety of powerful medications at their disposal for everything from ulcers and colitis to heartburn and high cholesterol. This unique section of *The PDR Family Guide to Nutrition and Health* provides you with complete information on these and other drugs related to your nutritional status, including "diet pills," antacids, vitamin/mineral supplements, and medications commonly prescribed for anorexia.

These potent medicines often work wonders; but they are not without their risks. For certain people, at certain times, some drugs can cause problems. And for all people, misusing a medication is an invitation to trouble. The purpose of this section is to alert you to those times and those conditions which should make you wary, and to help you use all of your medications safely and effectively.

The information in this part of the book is not a substitute for a visit to the doctor. Only a doctor can weigh all the diverse aspects of your condition and choose the treatment most likely to meet your needs. What we hope this information can do, however, is help you sort out the facts and questions that deserve further discussion. Your doctor, after all, can respond only to the problems and concerns you mention. And a seemingly unimportant question could turn out to be a crucial aspect of your particular case.

Most prescription products have two names — a generic chemical name and a manufacturer's brand name. Both are listed alphabetically in this section, with a profile of the drug appearing under the more familiar of the two. In most instances, that means the brand name. In a few cases — such as insulin, for example — the generic name heads the profile. In either case, the drug's other name gives you a cross-reference to the profile.

If there is more than one brand of a drug, you'll usually find the profile under the name that's most frequently prescribed. For example, information on the cholesterol-lowering drug gemfibrozil can be found in the profile of Lopid, the nation's leading brand. Another brand of gemfibrozil, called Gemcor, is cross-referenced to the Lopid entry.

The drug profiles begin with correct pronunciation of the name, followed by the other brand and generic names for the drug. The information that follows these names is divided into 10 sections. Here's what you'll find in each.

Why is this drug prescribed?

This section provides an overview of the major diseases and disorders for which the drug is generally given. It names each basic problem, but does not go into technical details. For instance, the information here will confirm that a particular drug is used to fight, say, heartburn. The section does not, however, attempt to explain all the conditions, such as gastroesophageal reflux disorder, that may lie at the root of the problem.

Most important fact about this drug

Highlighted here is one key point — out of the dozens found in a typical profile — that is especially worthwhile to remember. We've placed it here for the sake of emphasis. Never regard this section as a definitive summary of the drug.

How should you take this medication?

Some drugs should never be taken with meals. Others must be. This section details such special instructions including how and when to take the medication, and any dietary restrictions that may apply. Also found here is advice on what to do when you forget a dose, and any special storage requirements that apply.

What side effects may occur?

Shown here are the potential side effects that the manufacturer has highlighted in the drug's FDA-approved product labeling. Virtually any drug will occasionally cause an unwanted reaction. However, even the most common of these reactions is generally seen in only a small minority of patients. For that reason, presence of a long list of possible side effects does not mean that the drug is unusually dangerous or trouble-prone. In fact, your odds of experiencing even one of these effects are typically very low. Not listed are the few side effects that can be detected only by a physician or analysis in a laboratory.

Why should this drug not be prescribed?

A few drugs are known to be harmful under certain specific conditions, which are detailed here — the most common being hypersensitivity to the drug itself. If you think one of these restrictions applies to you, you should alert your doctor immediately. If you're correct, he or she may decide to use an alternative treatment.

Special warnings about this medication

This cautionary information is presented as a double check. If it includes any problems or conditions that your doctor may be unaware of, be sure to bring them to his or her attention. Chances are that no change in treatment will be called for; but it's worth making sure. In any event, do not take this information as a signal to change your dosage or discontinue the drug without consulting your doctor. Such a change might well do more harm than good.

Possible food and drug interactions when taking this medication

In this section you'll find a list of specific drugs — and types of drugs — that have been known to interact with the medicine being profiled. Generally, the list includes a few examples of each type. However, it is far from inclusive. If you're not certain whether a medication you're taking falls into one of these categories, be sure to check with your doctor or pharmacist.

Remember, too, that the chances of an interaction — and its intensity if one occurs— vary from person to person. In many cases, the benefits of the two medicines may outweigh the results of an interaction. Don't stop taking either drug without first consulting your doctor.

Special information
if you are pregnant or breastfeeding

Very few medicines have been definitively proved safe for use during pregnancy. On the other hand, only a handful are known to be inevitably harmful. Most drugs fall in-between, in a gray area where no harm has been reported, but neither has safety been conclusively proved. With many of these drugs, the small theoretical risk they pose may be overshadowed by your need for treatment. This section will tell you whether a drug has been confirmed safe, is known to be dangerous, or is part of that large group about which scientists are not really sure.

Recommended dosage

Shown here are excerpts of the dosage guidelines your doctor uses. They generally present a range of doses recommended for typical cases, and sometimes include a recommended maximum. The information is presented as a convenient double-check in case you suspect a misunderstanding or a typographical error on your prescription label. It is not useful for determining an exact dosage yourself. The dose that's best for you depends on numerous factors — such as your age, weight, physical condition, and response to the drug — that can be properly evaluated only by your doctor.

Overdosage

As another safety measure, this section lists, when available, the signs of an overdose. If the symptoms listed in this section lead you to suspect an overdose, your best response is to seek emergency medical attention immediately.

Part Five,
Lists, Tables, and Guides

For quick reference, you'll find a number of useful tables and directories near the end of the book. They range from a detailed list of fat and cholesterol counts to an index of medications for specific nutritional and digestive problems. Here's a brief look at each.

Fat, Cholesterol, and Calorie Counter

For many people, cutting back on fat is still the single most pressing dietary concern; here you'll find a comprehensive table giving the fat content of all the most common foods. It shows both the actual amount of fat in a typical serving and the share of total calories accounted for by fat. Since everybody's goal should be to get no more than 30 percent of their calories from fat, this table allows you to immediately pick out the foods that help you meet that goal—and the ones that will make it harder. For people who are watching their weight, the total number of calories in a serving is also included. For those with a cholesterol problem, that figure is listed too.

How to Read the "Nutrition Facts" Label

Exactly what is a "% Daily Value"? The brief overview of the standard food label tells what each section can mean for you. You'll be surprised at the amount of really helpful information you can find on this label once you've learned how to decipher it.

How to Keep Your Food Safe

In this short review, you'll find all the guidelines dietitians recommend for maximum hygiene in the kitchen, plus a valuable quick-reference table that tells which infections a food may harbor, what the symptoms are, and how to treat the problem.

Safe Medication Use

Certain precautions are in order whenever you take a prescription drug—or even use a nutritional supplement. This brief section summarizes the points to remember when taking, storing, and disposing of drugs. Included are pointers on what to ask when visiting the doctor or going to the pharmacy.

Special Terms in Nutrition and Health

What's a "nitrosamine"? Where can you find a "phytochemical"? Turn to this section for plain-English definitions of some of the more technical terms you're likely to encounter when reading articles about nutrition today.

Nutrition Directory

Today more than ever, there are a host of reliable sources for further information on nutrition and many specific health problems. A few of the major ones can be found in this brief directory.

Disease and Disorder Index

This special index enables you to quickly identify drugs available for a particular medical condition. Arranged alphabetically by ailment, it lists all the medications profiled in the book.

General Index

Found at the very end of the book, this index directs you to every key topic mentioned in Parts One and Two. Also included are the vitamins, minerals, supplements, and prescription drugs profiled in Parts Three and Four.

Product Identification Guide

It's wise to keep all your prescription medications in their original bottles or vials. However, if they do somehow get mixed up, you may find this section helpful for sorting them out. It includes actual-size photographs of the leading products discussed in the book, organized alphabetically by brand name. Manufacturers occasionally change the color and shape of a product, so if a prescription does not match the photo shown here, check with your pharmacist before assuming there's been a mistake.

An End to Needless Worry and Confusion

The goal of this book is help you focus on what really matters in nutrition so that you can make meaningful changes that really will improve your health and the quality of your life without useless hardship or unnecessary expense. Although there is often fervent disagreement among nutritionists, we've sought to present the mainstream consensus on all the questions with the greatest impact on your health.

Still, even the best general consensus is no substitute for a professional evaluation of your unique, individual health problems, should any arise. Self-treatment can take you only so far, no matter how well informed it may be. If you have a disorder—or think you're developing one—don't hesitate to check with your doctor. The answer may be simpler than you think.

Naomi K. Fukagawa, MD, PhD
Assistant Professor and Associate
Program Director,
The Clinical Research Center,
The Rockefeller University, New York, NY

Richard A. Galbraith, MD, PhD
Medical Director
The Rockefeller University, New York, NY

Drug Identification Guide

AXID

NIZATIDINE
ELI LILLY

150 MG

300 MG

AZULFIDINE EN-TABS

SULFASALAZINE
KABI

500 MG

BENTYL

DICYCLOMINE HCL
MARION MERRELL DOW

10 MG

20 MG

CALCIUM RICH ROLAIDS

ANTACID
WARNER-LAMBERT

CHEWABLE

CALTRATE 600

CALCIUM
LEDERLE

600 MG

CARAFATE

SUCRALFATE
MARION MERRELL DOW

1 GM

CENTRUM

**MULTIVITAMIN/
MULTIMINERAL
SUPPLEMENT**
LEDERLE

CENTRUM SILVER

**MULTIVITAMIN/
MULTIMINERAL
SUPPLEMENT**
LEDERLE

COLACE

DOCUSATE SODIUM
ROBERTS

50 MG

100 MG

COLBENEMID

PROBENECID/ COLCHICINE
MERCK

0.5 GM/0.5 MG

DIABINESE

CHLORPROPAMIDE
PFIZER

100 MG

250 MG

DONNATAL

**BELLADONNA ALKALOIDS/
PHENOBARBITAL**
A. H. ROBINS

DONNATAL EXTENTABS

**BELLADONNA ALKALOIDS/
PHENOBARBITAL**
A. H. ROBINS

FASTIN

PHENTERMINE HCL
SMITHKLINE BEECHAM

30 MG

GAVISCON

ANTACID
SMITHKLINE BEECHAM

CHEWABLE

GAVISCON EXTRA
STRENGTH

ANTACID
SMITHKLINE BEECHAM

CHEWABLE

GAVISCON-2

ANTACID
SMITHKLINE BEECHAM

CHEWABLE

GELUSIL

ANTACID/ANTI-GAS
WARNER-WELLCOME

CHEWABLE

GLUCOTROL

GLIPIZIDE
PRATT

5 MG

10 MG

IONAMIN

PHENTERMINE RESIN
FISONS

15 MG

30 MG

KAON-CL 10

POTASSIUM CHLORIDE
SAVAGE LABORATORIES

750 MG

K-DUR

POTASSIUM CHLORIDE
KEY

10 MEQ

20 MEQ

KLOR-CON 8

POTASSIUM CHLORIDE
UPSHER-SMITH

8 MEQ

KLOR-CON 10

POTASSIUM CHLORIDE
UPSHER-SMITH

10 MEQ

LESCOL

FLUVASTATIN SODIUM
SANDOZ

20 MG

40 MG

LEVSIN

HYOSCYAMINE SULFATE
SCHWARZ

0.125 MG

LEVSIN/SL

HYOSCYAMINE SULFATE
SCHWARZ

0.125 MG

LEVSIN TIMECAPS

HYOSCYAMINE SULFATE
SCHWARZ

0.375 MG
EXTENDED-RELEASE

LIBRAX

**CHLORDIAZEPOXIDE HCL/
CLIDINIUM BROMIDE**
ROCHE

5 MG/2.5 MG

LOPID

GEMFIBROZIL
PARKE-DAVIS

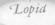

600 MG

LORELCO

PROBUCOL
MARION MERRELL DOW

250 MG

500 MG

LURIDE SF LOZI-TABS

FLUORIDE
COLGATE-HOYT

1 MG
CHEWABLE

MAALOX ANTACID

ANTACID
CIBA

MAALOX ANTACID PLUS
ANTI-GAS

ANTACID/ANTI-GAS
CIBA

CHEWABLE

EXTRA STRENGTH
MAALOX ANTACID PLUS
ANTI-GAS

ANTACID
CIBA

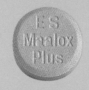

CHEWABLE

MATERNA

VITAMINS, PRENATAL
LEDERLE

MEVACOR

LOVASTATIN
MERCK

10 MG

20 MG

40 MG

MICRO-K EXTENCAPS

POTASSIUM CHLORIDE
A. H. ROBINS

8MEQ

MICRO-K 10 EXTENCAPS

POTASSIUM CHLORIDE
A. H. ROBINS

10 MEQ

MICRONASE

GLYBURIDE
UPJOHN

1.25 MG   2.5 MG

5 MG

MYLANTA

ANTACID/ANTI-GAS
J&J MERCK

CHEWABLE

MYLANTA DOUBLE
STRENGTH

ANTACID/ANTI-GAS
J&J MERCK

CHEWABLE

MYLANTA GELCAPS

ANTACID
J&J MERCK

MYLANTA SOOTHING
LOZENGES

ANTACID
J&J MERCK

NATALINS

VITAMINS, PRENATAL
BRISTOL-MYERS SQUIBB

NATALINS RX

VITAMINS, PRENATAL
BRISTOL-MYERS SQUIBB

NICOLAR

NIACIN
RHONE-POULENC RORER

500 MG

OBY-CAP

PHENTERMINE HCL
RICHWOOD

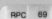

30 MG

ORINASE

TOLBUTAMIDE
UPJOHN

250 MG

500 MG

PAXIL

PAROXETINE HCL
SMITHKLINE BEECHAM

20 MG

30 MG

PEPCID

FAMOTIDINE
MERCK

20 MG 40 MG

POLY-VI-FLOR

SODIUM FLUORIDE/ MULTIVITAMINS
MEAD JOHNSON

0.5 MG
CHEWABLE

1 MG
CHEWABLE

PONDIMIN

FENFLURAMINE HCL
A.H ROBINS

20 MG

PRAVACHOL

PRAVASTATIN SODIUM
BRISTOL-MYERS SQUIBB

10 MG 20 MG

PRILOSEC

OMEPRAZOLE
MERCK

20 MG

PROPULSID

CISAPRIDE
JANSSEN

10 MG

PROZAC

FLUOXETINE HCL
DISTA PRODUCTS

10 MG

20 MG

SLOW-K

POTASSIUM CHLORIDE
SUMMIT

8 MEQ

STUARTNATAL PLUS

VITAMINS, PRENATAL
WYETH-AYERST

TAGAMET

CIMETIDINE
SMITHKLINE BEECHAM

200 MG 300 MG

400 MG

800 MG

TENUATE

DIETHYLPROPION HCL
MARION MERRELL DOW

25 MG

TENUATE DOSPAN

DIETHYLPROPION HCL
MARION MERRELL DOW

75 MG

THERAGRAN

MULTIVITAMIN/ MULTIMINERAL SUPPLEMENT
BRISTOL-MEYERS SQUIBB

THERAGRAN-M

MULTIVITAMIN/ MULTIMINERAL SUPPLEMENT
BRISTOL-MEYERS SQUIBB

THERAGRAN STRESS FORMULA

MULTIVITAMIN/ MULTIMINERAL SUPPLEMENT
BRISTOL-MEYERS SQUIBB

TOLINASE

TOLAZAMIDE
UPJOHN

100 MG 250 MG

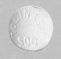

500 MG

TUMS

ANTACID
SMITHKLINE BEECHAM

CHEWABLE

TUMS E-X

ANTACID
SMITHKLINE BEECHAM

CHEWABLE

TUMS ULTRA

ANTACID
SMITHKLINE BEECHAM

CHEWABLE

VI-DAYLIN

MULTIVITAMIN
ABBOTT LABORATORIES

CHEWABLE

VI-DAYLIN PLUS IRON

MULTIVITAMIN/IRON
ABBOTT LABORATORIES

12 MG
CHEWABLE

ZANTAC

RANITIDINE HCL
GLAXO

150 MG

300 MG

ZANTAC EFFERDOSE

RANITIDINE HCL
GLAXO

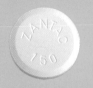

150 MG

ZANTAC GELDOSE

RANITIDINE HCL
GLAXO

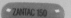

150 MG

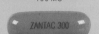

300 MG

ZOCOR

SIMVASTATIN
MERCK

5 MG 10 MG

20 MG 40 MG

ZYLOPRIM

ALLOPURINOL
BURROUGHS WELLCOME

100 MG 300 MG

PART ONE

Your Diet's Impact on Health

Section One

Reality Check: The Facts Versus the Fads

CHAPTER 1

What's Really Important in Nutrition?

Not all that many years ago, nutrition experts told us to avoid fattening sugar and starch. Now they're telling us to *load up* on starch, but never, never eat fat. What, you might well ask, is going on here? And why should anyone bother paying attention?

The self-appointed "food police" can turn any meal into a minefield. We're told to avoid Chinese, give up guacamole, eat our popcorn dry. But here's the good news about all of this: *None of it is invariably true.* If you talk to an authentic nutritionist, you'll find that there's plenty of stuff you can eat at the Peking Garden, and a way to have your buttered popcorn too.

Despite the confusion, we really do know more about nutrition today than ever before—and the basic facts turn out to be surprisingly simple. Moderation and balance are crucial. Everything else is a detail. The rest of this chapter—and this book—is given over to those details, sorting out what really matters in nutrition, and highlighting ways to upgrade your diet for a healthier life.

Proven Facts

The government has incorporated most of the nutritional facts we're sure of into two excellent tools—the new food labels and the Food Guide Pyramid. The food labels are designed to pinpoint what's really important for most Americans. Experts now agree that most of us eat too much fat, saturated fat, cholesterol, sodium, and sugar, and not enough starch and fiber—and these are what you'll find highlighted on the labels.

These nutrients have been singled out not only because they are problem areas, but also because they are the focus of some of the strongest evidence available on the way food affects our health. We are as certain as science can be, for example, that, for many people, a high-fat, high-cholesterol diet can lead to heart disease and stroke. The nearby

DAILY VALUES: WHAT THE GOVERNMENT NOW RECOMMENDS

In setting these amounts, the U.S. Food and Drug Administration assumed an average diet of 2,000 calories a day.

Ingredient	Amount
fat	65 grams
saturated fatty acids	20 grams
cholesterol	300 milligrams
total carbohydrate	300 grams
fiber	25 grams
sodium	2,400 milligrams
potassium	3,500 milligrams
protein	50 grams
vitamin A	5,000 International Units
vitamin C	60 milligrams
thiamin	1.5 milligrams
riboflavin	1.7 milligrams
niacin	20 milligrams
calcium	1.0 gram
iron	18 milligrams
vitamin D	400 International Units
vitamin E	30 International Units
vitamin B_6	2.0 milligrams
folic acid	0.4 milligrams
vitamin B_{12}	6 micrograms
phosphorus	1.0 gram
iodine	150 micrograms
magnesium	400 milligrams
zinc	15 milligrams
copper	2 milligrams
biotin	0.3 milligrams
pantothenic acid	10 milligrams

Source: *FDA Consumer*

box, "Certain enough to be allowed on food labels," lists health claims with enough evidence behind them for the U. S. Food and Drug Administration (FDA) to allow them on labels.

Values for vitamin B, D, E, and other nutrients are not required on labels any more—not because they're unimportant, but because the FDA believes that most of us get enough of them. By eliminating unneeded information like this, the FDA made room for more of the facts that can make a real difference.

As part of the new labeling, the government for the first time has set recommended Daily Values (DVs) for many of the nutrients considered most important (see the table nearby). It has also adopted the rule of thumb that about 60 percent of our food should be carbohydrates (bread, rice, pasta, fruits, and vegetables are mostly carbohydrates), 30 percent fat (including 10 percent saturated fat), and 10 percent protein. By law, food labels now tell you not only how many grams of fat a serving has, for example, but how much of your Daily Value of carbohydrates, fat, and protein it delivers. A food that packs 50 percent of your recommended daily fat allotment in one serving, for example, should give you pause. You don't have to pass it up—but you may want to compensate for it by loading the rest of your menu with especially low-fat options.

The Food Guide Pyramid, issued by the U.S. Department of Agriculture, translates the 60 percent carbohydrates, 30 percent fat,

THE FOOD GUIDE PYRAMID

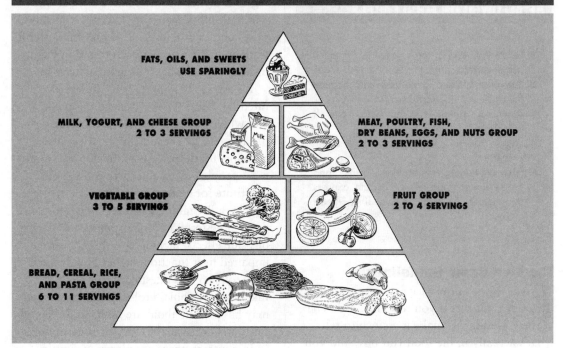

FATS, OILS, AND SWEETS
USE SPARINGLY

MILK, YOGURT, AND CHEESE GROUP
2 TO 3 SERVINGS

MEAT, POULTRY, FISH,
DRY BEANS, EGGS, AND NUTS GROUP
2 TO 3 SERVINGS

VEGETABLE GROUP
3 TO 5 SERVINGS

FRUIT GROUP
2 TO 4 SERVINGS

BREAD, CEREAL, RICE,
AND PASTA GROUP
6 TO 11 SERVINGS

10 percent protein guideline into servings of specific types of food. The biggest difference between the pyramid and its predecessor, the Basic Four Food Groups, is that meat is no longer the centerpiece of a meal. Instead, rice, pasta, or other grains, along with fruits and vegetables, are supposed to account for the bulk of our food. This is because grains, fruits, and vegetables are high in fiber, carbohydrates, and needed vitamins and minerals, and gratifyingly low in fat. Meat has not been banished from a healthy diet, but most of us eat far more of it than we actually need, while short-changing ourselves on grains, fruits, and vegetables.

The pyramid was released in 1992, and polls indicate that most Americans are aware of it. The polls also show that we don't follow it. An August 1994 survey of 372 house-holds by Parade magazine found that those questioned ate an average of 3.4 servings from the grain group per day, although the pyramid calls for 6 to 11. Other reports show that, from day to day, most of us eat about half of the 2 to 4 servings of fruit and the 3 to 5 servings of vegetables the pyramid recommends. Many of us go all day without eating any fruits or vegetables. And, despite everything we've been told, most of us still eat too much meat, too many dairy products, and excessive amounts of all the other things the experts warn against.

CERTAIN ENOUGH TO BE ALLOWED ON FOOD LABELS

- Excessive intake of fat is linked to increased risk of certain cancers
- Saturated fat and cholesterol can increase the likelihood of heart disease
- A generous supply of calcium helps stave off osteoporosis (thinning bones)
- Salt or sodium can aggravate high blood pressure
- Fiber-containing vegetables, fruits, and grains lower your risk of certain cancers and—especially with soluble fiber—heart disease

The Five Basic Guidelines

Ironically, it's now easier than ever to up-grade your diet if you're so inclined. The new food labels make it a cinch to tell what's actually in the food you buy; and you don't have to calculate each ingredient to the last calorie. Instead, just keep these five general guidelines firmly in mind.

1. Cut Back on Fat and Cholesterol

The experts recommend that we get *no more, and preferably less,* than 30 percent of our calories from fat. That 30 percent includes 10 percent from saturated fat and 10 percent from polyunsaturated fat. We also should limit cholesterol to 300 milligrams a day. Right now, most of us get 35 percent to 40 percent of our calories from fat.

In susceptible people (and there's currently no way to tell whether or not you're suscep-tible), fat is conclusively linked to heart dis-ease and perhaps to cancer as well (for infor-mation about the possible cancer link, see

the "Promising Theories" section below). A high-fat diet is also associated with stroke and high blood pressure. Excessive fat intake raises cholesterol levels, and high cholesterol leads to the clogged arteries found in victims of heart disease, heart attack, and stroke.

It's especially important to eat less satu-rated fat. Meat (both red meat and poultry) and whole milk are the two main sources of saturated fat for most of us. Meat also accounts for 30 percent of the cholesterol in most people's diets, and there is no good substitute for cutting down on cholesterol. Niacin, a B vitamin, has been shown to re-duce cholesterol; but it has potentially danger-ous side effects, including flushing, rashes, impaired liver function, higher blood sugar, and stomach and intestinal problems. Likewise, the cholesterol-lowering drugs you may have heard about are reserved for serious cases and are available only by prescription.

In contrast, there are plenty of simple, relatively painless ways to cut the fat in your cooking. Here are five tips from *Consumer Reports on Health.*

Don't use fat as a flavoring. Let's face it—fat is tasty, and a pat of butter or margarine on your bread or vegetables may not seem like much. But nutritionists warn that these little extras add up quickly. As a substitute for butter or margarine, try baking garlic in the oven for 1 hour with a little bit of olive oil,

FIVE RULES TO REMEMBER

- Cut back on fat and cholesterol
- Cut the calories (if you're overweight)
- Slow down on the salt
- Boost your carbohydrates (starches)
- Don't worry about protein

PAINLESS WAYS TO CUT FAT

INSTEAD OF	fat grams	GO FOR	fat grams
Bacon and eggs	37	Pancakes with syrup	6
Tuna salad sandwich	16	Turkey breast sandwich with mustard	7
Cheeseburger	30	Bagel with lox and low-fat cream cheese	10
French fries	20	Oven-fried potatoes	8
Cream-of-chicken soup	18	Chicken noodle soup	6
Potato chips	18	Pretzels	2
Alfredo sauce	10	Tomato sauce	1
Sautéed vegetables	14	Steamed vegetables	0
Ice cream	18	Sorbet	0
Apple pie	16	Four fig bars	4

Researched by Peter Jaret. Adapted from HEALTH, © 1995.

then using it on bread or pasta. It comes out with a spreadable consistency. Herbs or lemon juice can season vegetables. If you must use fat, try olive oil instead of butter.

Eat less meat. Reducing or eliminating meat from recipes such as spaghetti sauce greatly lowers their fat content. Try using vegetables and herbs in casseroles and other combination recipes where you might once have used meat. Let pasta, rice, and fruits and vegetables step in as the mainstays of your meal. A serving of meat should be no more than 3 ounces—the size of a deck of cards or a woman's palm. Remember that the pyramid recommends only 2 to 3 servings a day from a group that includes eggs, beans, nuts, poultry, and fish along with meat.

Thin out the meat you do eat. Buy leaner cuts of meat, trim the fat, eat poultry without skin, eat smaller portions, and don't fry.

Substitute low-fat or non-fat versions of fatty foods. This means using skim milk instead of whole milk, low-fat or non-fat yogurt, and choices from the array of low-fat or non-fat mayonnaises, salad dressings, and other foods. See the box on "Painless Ways to Cut Fat" for additional ideas.

GIVEAWAYS TO FATTY FOODS

Alfredo	Crispy
Au gratin	En croute
Batter-dipped	Escalloped
Bearnaise	Flaky
Bechamel	Hollandaise
Beurre blanc	Mornay
Breaded	Parmigiana
	Tempura

Source: *Environmental Nutrition,* September 1992.

FAT AND CHOLESTEROL CONTENT: A SAMPLER OF COMMON FOODS

For more counts, see the "Fat, Cholesterol, and Calorie Counter" at the end of the book.

	Amount	Total Fat (grams)	Cholesterol (milligrams)
Beef			
flank, trimmed, braised	3 ounces	11.8	60.9
ground, lean, broiled	3 ounces	15.9	74.6
salami	1 slice	5.9	18.6
bologna	1 slice	8.1	16.6
hot dog	1	14.3	30.5
pot pie, 9-in diam.	1/3 pie	30.0	42.0
Pork			
chop, loin, lean, broiled	3 ounces	9.6	85.2
ham, cured, roasted	3 ounces	7.7	50.6
sausage, fresh, cooked	3 ounces	25.2	66.0
Lamb			
leg, lean, roasted	3 ounces	7.0	76.3
Chicken			
roasted, with skin	3 ounces	11.6	75.0
roasted, skinless	3 ounces	6.3	75.8
fried (breaded) breast	5.6 ounces	18.0	119.0
roll, light meat	1 ounce slice	2.0	14.0
Turkey			
light meat, with skin	3 ounces	3.9	81.4
dark meat, with skin	3 ounces	6.1	100.3
Seafood			
haddock, baked	3 ounces	0.8	63.0
pink salmon, canned	3 ounces	5.0	34.0
flounder fillet, baked	3 ounces	1.3	57.8

	Amount	Total Fat (grams)	Cholesterol (milligrams)
Seafood, continued:			
shrimp, boiled	1 large	trace	10.8
oysters, raw	1 cup	4.0	120.0
tuna in oil, chunk light	3 ounces	7.0	55.0
tuna in water, solid white	3 ounces	1.0	48.0
trout, broiled	3 ounces	9.0	71.0
Milk			
whole	1 cup	8.2	33.0
2% fat	1 cup	4.7	18.0
1% fat	1 cup	2.6	10.0
light cream	1/4 cup	11.6	40.0
whipped topping, pressurized	1 Tbsp.	1.0	0
Cheese			
blue	1 ounce	8.2	21.0
cheddar	1 ounce	9.4	30.0
Swiss	1 ounce	7.1	26.0
American	1 ounce	8.9	27.0
cottage, 1% fat	4 ounces	1.0	5.0
cottage, 2% fat	4 ounces	2.0	9.0
Eggs			
scrambled	1 large	8.0	282.0
fried	1 large	9.0	278.0
Fats			
butter	1 Tbsp.	11.0	31.0
vegetable-oil margarine	1 Tbsp.	11.0	0.0

Replace fatty foods with produce. Try snacking on apples, grapes, carrots, and other fruits and vegetables instead of fat-filled chips and sweets. This not only cuts down on fat, but boosts your intake of many valuable nutrients.

You can also hold down fat by watching for certain code words on packages and menus (see "Giveaways to Fatty Foods" box nearby). Remember, though, that you can't always rely on labels saying "low-fat," "diet," or "sugar-free" when eating out. Laboratory analysis of 10 frozen desserts

WHAT COUNTS AS A SERVING

Breads, Cereals, Rice, and Pasta
1 slice of bread
1/2 cup of cooked rice or pasta
1/2 cup of cooked cereal
1 ounce of ready-to-eat cereal

Vegetables
1/2 cup of chopped raw or cooked vegetables
1 cup of leafy raw vegetables

Fruits
1 piece of fruit or melon wedge
3/4 cup of juice
1/2 cup of canned fruit
1/4 cup of dried fruit

Milk, Yogurt, and Cheese
1 cup of milk or yogurt
1-1/2 to 2 ounces of cheese

Meat, Poultry, Fish, Dry Beans, Eggs, and Nuts
2-1/2 to 3 ounces of cooked lean meat, poultry, or fish

Count 1/2 cup of cooked beans, or 1 egg, or 2 tablespoons of peanut butter as 1 ounce of lean meat (about 1/3 serving)

Source: FDA Consumer

billed as low-fat, low-calorie in New York establishments revealed that most packed as many calories as ice cream. One exception was Haagen-Dazs frozen vanilla yogurt, which had 88 calories and 0.2 grams of fat in a 5-ounce cup. To make matters worse, advertised calories are often based on a 4-ounce serving, while the "small" size you buy varies from 5 to 11.3 fluid ounces.

The only conclusive way to determine how much fat you're really eating is to keep a daily diary of everything (yes, everything) you eat, then check labels to count fat grams and percent of Daily Values.

2. Cut the Calories (If You're Overweight)
Partly because so many of us eat more fat than we need, excess weight is relatively common in the U.S. Too many extra pounds increase your chances of developing high blood pressure and, therefore, of having a stroke. Being overweight is associated with the higher cholesterol levels that can lead to heart disease. And obesity is a factor in type II diabetes—the kind that usually develops in adulthood. (To learn your ideal weight, see Chapter 5, "Setting a Healthy Goal.")

How much you need to eat depends on your gender, age, and activity. Men need more than women, younger people need more than older adults, and active people need more than the inactive. The Daily Value information on food labels is based on a relatively modest 2,000-calorie diet unless otherwise specified.

When adding up your calories based on food labels, be careful about the definition of a serving. The FDA's idea of a serving is surprisingly small and may not match yours.

(Does your spaghetti dinner usually amount to half a cup?) See "What Counts as a Serving" for the official numbers. It may be worth measuring what you actually eat for a few days to see how closely it mirrors the printed serving sizes.

If you are cutting back on fat, this will automatically help you cut calories. One gram of fat packs about 9 calories, more than double the 4 calories in a gram of protein or carbohydrates. A regular exercise program will also help. What you burn, as well as what you eat, affects how much weight actually stays on you. Finally, there's the old stand-by:

Hold the sugar. Mom and your dentist were right—sugar is mostly empty calories that fill you up, leaving less room for food with other nutrients. And sticky sweets *can* rot your teeth, though the sugar in beverages won't. So, when the FDA recommends getting 60 percent of our calories from carbohydrates, they are really talking about the complex carbohydrates in starch, not the simple ones in sugars.

Adding a teaspoon of sugar to your coffee or tea isn't a problem for most of us. All table sweeteners combined contribute less than a fifth of our daily intake. The major sources of sugar to keep in mind include:

- Soft drinks—25%
- Packaged foods, dressings, and other—21%
- Table sugar, jams, syrups—18%
- Baked goods—13%
- Ice cream, dairy—10%
- Breakfast cereals—5%
- Candy—2%

The Sugar Association says that, when you add it up, more than half the sugar we eat comes from processed foods—another reason (along with sodium), to favor fresh products.

When you do buy processed foods, watch the labels. Sugar can pop up in the oddest places—ketchup (11 percent sugar), salad dressing, frozen pizza, and nondairy creamer, for example. Don't be fooled by sugar's disguises on labels, either—your body sees most sweeteners as basically identical. Sucrose, fructose, dextrose, honey, raw sugar, "sweetened with fruit juice" all mean the same thing. And remember that the natural fructose in fruit does count towards your total sugar intake.

Sugary foods may seem like quick energy boosters, but the initial burst is followed by a slump. Complex carbohydrates work more slowly but are a better choice for longer-lasting energy.

3. Slow Down on the Salt

The FDA recommends that we get 2,400 milligrams a day of sodium, about the amount in 1 teaspoon of salt. But by one estimate, men actually eat 4,000 milligrams, or 2 teaspoons per day, while women get 3,000 milligrams a day, or one-and-a-third teaspoons daily.

Reducing the sodium you take in can be tougher than you'd expect, because 75 percent of the sodium we eat is hidden in processed foods. Only 15 percent of most people's sodium intake comes from the salt shaker; about 10 percent is found naturally in food. Sodium also is not necessarily where your taste buds would lead you to believe. McDonald's french fries have less salt than any McDonald's sandwich, biscuit, or Danish. Some salad dressings have 200 milligrams of sodium per tablespoon.

To get your sodium intake down, you'll need to cut back on most brands of frozen

WHAT ABOUT ALCOHOL?

Recent studies suggesting health benefits from moderate drinking have caused a bit of a stir. Alcohol apparently raises levels of "good" HDL cholesterol (the type that helps keep arteries clear) and may help prevent blood clots, thus reducing the likelihood of heart disease. However, evidence of an actual protective effect is still considered inconclusive. For example, one large, long-term study revealed that men who had one or two drinks a week had a lower death rate than both heavy drinkers and those who did not drink at all, but experts say that this could be due to other factors not evaluated in the investigation. Also, some of the other studies showing reduced heart disease with moderate drinking did not measure complicating factors that could have affected the results, such as whether or not the people in the study smoked.

On the other hand, the harmful effects of heavy drinking are quite certain. People who have one to three drinks a day run a 60 percent higher risk of developing oral cancer than do nondrinkers. Heavy drinkers are also at higher risk for larynx and esophageal cancer. Given these facts, doctors continue to warn against anything more than moderate drinking, if you drink at all. Moderate drinking is one drink or less daily for women and two or less for men. One drink is a glass (5 ounces) of wine, a can (12 ounces) of beer, 1.5 ounces of liquor or spirits (80 proof).

dinners or pizza (Healthy Choice is one exception); processed meats like hot dogs or bacon; processed American-style cheese; canned or dried soup; salad dressings; and canned meats, beans, vegetables, and tomato sauce. Restaurant food and fast food are also notoriously high in sodium. It's a tall order. Choosing fresh rather than canned foods, and looking for items labeled "less sodium," "sodium-free," or "light-in-sodium," can go

a long way. Also, avoid foods with a "high-sodium" label—they pack 20 percent of the recommended daily value in one serving.

Instead of seasoning food with salt, try cooking with herbs, spices, and lemon juice, to broaden your palate's taste sensations. Try recipes in cookbooks or magazines that emphasize healthy (low-fat, low-calorie, low-sodium) meals (see Part 2 of this book for suggestions). Stop cooking with salt, or add only half the amount specified in the recipe—chances are you won't notice the difference. And move gradually to lower-sodium products and cooking, so your taste buds can adjust.

The reason for all the concern over sodium is its link with high blood pressure. In certain "sodium-sensitive" individuals, too much salt can cause a sustained increase in blood pressure, and since there's no way of telling in advance whether you're among the sensitive ones, cutting back on salt is the only completely safe course. If you do develop high blood pressure, your chance of heart disease goes up. Optimal blood pressure is less than 120/80; high is 140/90; and anything above *optimal* raises the risk of heart disease. About 4 out of 5 people aged 35 or older have blood pressure above optimal levels; and even if your pressure is low now, it's likely to increase with age. On average, the first number in the blood pressure measurement goes up 15 points between the ages of 25 and 55. If everyone lowered salt intake by 1 teaspoon a day, the thinking goes, the average increase with age could be pared back to 6 points.

High blood pressure isn't the only problem with too much sodium. Because it causes your body to lose calcium, it can raise your chances of developing osteoporosis, the brittle-bones disease of old age. Losing calcium is all right if you eat enough to compensate, but most of us don't.

4. Boost Your Carbohydrates

Getting more carbohydrates (the complex kind) means eating more bread, pasta, rice, and other grains as well as extra fruits and vegetables. The goal is to make carbohydrates 60 percent of your calories, compared with the 20 to 25 percent that most of us get today. Just as eating less fat and sodium can help cut the odds of heart disease and high blood pressure, eating more fiber-containing grains, fruits, and vegetables can help lower your chances of getting cancer and heart disease.

The facts about fiber. Fiber is found in fruits, vegetables, and grains, and you should get 25 grams of it per day. The new food labels tell you how many grams of fiber a serving contains. However, because testing is not always accurate, some nutritional experts estimate that the amount on the label is often 5 to 25 percent higher than the actual content. What about unlabeled produce? The nearby box gives the numbers for some of our favorite fruits and vegetables. Juice counts as a serving of a fruit or vegetable, but won't provide fiber. (Remember that only 100 percent pure juice counts—some products are mostly sweetened water.) Whole grains give you more fiber than refined products from which the fiber-containing husk is removed.

Fiber reduces your risk of the top two killers in this country—cancer and, in the case of soluble fiber, heart disease. Diets lacking in insoluble fiber have been linked to colon cancer. Diets high in fruit, vegetables, and fiber have been shown to reduce your chances of developing precancerous colon polyps. Try to get your fiber from food rather than supplements: Some benefits of a

FINDING FIBER IN THE PRODUCE SECTION

Fruits & Juices	Fiber (grams)
Apple (1) or Pear (1)*	4
Apricots, dried (1/3 cup)	4
Blueberries, raw (1 cup)	4
Figs, dried (2)	4
Apple, without skin (1)	3
Banana (1)* or Orange (1)*	3
Cherries (1 cup)1 or Prunes, dried (5)	3
Strawberries (1 cup)*	3
Grapefruit (1/2)	2
Grapes (1-1/2 cup) or Plums (2)	2
Nectarine (1)* or Peach (1)	2
Cantaloupe (1 cup)	1
Orange juice (1 cup)	1
Watermelon (2 cup)	1

Vegetables	Fiber (grams)
(Serving size: 1/2 cup, cooked.)	
Green peas	4
Potato, baked, with skin (1)*	4
Sweet potato, baked, with skin (1)	4
Carrots	3
Asparagus or Broccoli	2
Cabbage1 or Spinach1	2
Carrots, raw, or Corn kernels	2
Cauliflower or Green beans	2
Lettuce, romaine (1-1/2 cup)	2
Celery, raw, or Green pepper, raw	1
Lettuce, iceberg (1-1/2 cup)	1
Mushrooms, raw (1 cup)	1
Tomato, fresh, raw (1/2)	1
Cucumber, sliced, raw	0

Copyright 1994, CSPI. Reprinted from *Nutrition Action Healthletter* (1875 Connecticut Ave., N.W., Suite 300, Washington, D.C. 20009-5728. $24.00 for 10 issues).

high fiber diet come from the sources as well as the fiber itself.

Even with fiber, it is possible to get too much of a good thing. Fiber scoops up minerals such as calcium, iron, and zinc on its way out of the gastrointestinal tract, making it potentially unhealthy for people at risk of osteoporosis and iron deficiency. Additionally, eating too much fiber without drinking enough liquid can clog your intestines.

Fiber added to food, especially breads, is sometimes really cellulose, an altered substance not like whole foods. Cellulose is rarely listed on the label, but the presence of added soy fiber or vegetable fiber should arouse suspicion. Cellulose may fight constipation but it's not as effective as an equal amount of wheat bran. To avoid cellulose, stick to whole wheat bread.

Added benefits from fruits and vegetables. In addition to boosting your fiber and carbohydrate intake, increasing the fruits and vegetables in your diet may possibly lower your risk of lung, prostate, bladder, esophageal, and stomach cancers—or so some researchers believe. Choose fresh fruits and vegetables, if possible, to avoid the sugar and salt that may lurk in frozen and canned products. If you can't find fresh, look for products without— or with little—added sugar, heavy syrup, sweetened fruit juice, or sodium. Aim for a variety of fruits and vegetables, not just the same few all the time. That will help ensure that you get the nutrients you need—you may be surprised by some of the intriguing new flavors you discover.

5. Don't Worry about Protein

You can probably get by with less of this nutrient. The average American eats twice the amount needed. For most of us, there's no danger in eating too much protein itself—but a problem arises when it crowds out other foods with nutrients we need. People with diabetes are an exception to this rule—they should not exceed the recommended value for protein (50 grams per day). Pregnant women and nursing mothers need more protein—as much as 60 and 65 grams per day, respectively.

If you're concerned about the fat in your diet, you might want to consider getting more of your protein from vegetable sources such as beans and nuts, rather than fattier meats, eggs, and dairy products.

Promising Theories

Many of the nutrition stories you see in the media are based on research that is, at best, inconclusive. The best of these stories contain important ideas for which evidence is accumulating, but for which there is not yet absolute proof. Some of these theories will eventually be confirmed; others will quietly disappear. In judging them, it's important to remember that even in science, "proof" is a relative term. It simply means that many carefully planned studies have supported the idea. Theories that are promising rather than proven generally have fewer studies to back them up, or have some studies that contradict others. (See the box on "When to Believe a Media Report," for details.) Here are some of today's theories most likely to become tomorrow's facts.

Is the "Mediterranean Diet" Better than the USDA Food Pyramid?

As eminent an authority as the chairman of Harvard University's nutrition department says Yes, and he's not alone. The Harvard School of Public Health, the European office

WHICH PYRAMID FOR YOU?

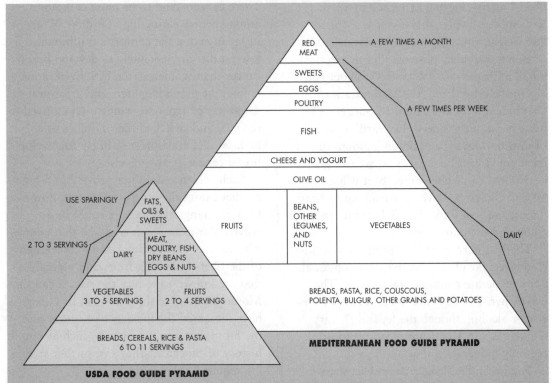

RED MEAT ———— A FEW TIMES A MONTH

SWEETS

EGGS

POULTRY ———— A FEW TIMES PER WEEK

FISH

CHEESE AND YOGURT

OLIVE OIL

USE SPARINGLY

FATS, OILS & SWEETS

FRUITS

BEANS, OTHER LEGUMES, AND NUTS

VEGETABLES

DAILY

2 TO 3 SERVINGS

DAIRY

MEAT, POULTRY, FISH, DRY BEANS EGGS & NUTS

VEGETABLES 3 TO 5 SERVINGS

FRUITS 2 TO 4 SERVINGS

BREADS, PASTA, RICE, COUSCOUS, POLENTA, BULGUR, OTHER GRAINS AND POTATOES

BREADS, CEREALS, RICE & PASTA 6 TO 11 SERVINGS

MEDITERRANEAN FOOD GUIDE PYRAMID

USDA FOOD GUIDE PYRAMID

Some experts have gone a step beyond the government and endorsed a nutrition plan called the "Mediterranean Diet," which comes complete with its own food pyramid. This plan shifts the emphasis further away from meat, focusing on fish, beans, nuts, cheese, and yogurt as alternative sources of protein. Small amounts of wine, considered good for the heart, are optional. Regular exercise is mandatory.

Adapted from *Tree Nuts, Health, and the Mediterranean Diet, A Summary Report;* page 53; Oldways Preservation & Exchange Trust, 1994

of the World Health Organization, and Oldways Preservation & Exchange Trust, a nutrition think tank, also endorse the Mediterranean Diet as a tasty, nutritionally superior alternative to the USDA pyramid.

The Mediterranean Diet is similar to—but more detailed than—the pyramid. It focuses on lowering animal fat, rather than all fat. It recommends little or no red meat (a few times a month), compared with the 2 to 3 servings a day from the catch-all "meat group" compiled by the USDA. It also puts

vegetable protein (such as that in beans and nuts) into a separate category from meat. These differences yield a diet with less saturated fat than the government pyramid (7 to 8 percent of calories), but more fat overall (35 percent of calories).

In the Mediterranean Diet, vegetable fat in the form of olive oil is actually recommended in certain quantities. The reason: Olive oil and other monounsaturated fats increase "good," artery-clearing HDL cholesterol, but not "bad," artery-clogging LDL cholesterol. Remember, however, that if you're trying to lose weight, you still need to limit your intake of all fats, including olive oil. (For more on oils, see Chapter 10, "What to Do about Fat.")

On the other hand, the Mediterranean Diet includes no more than 16 ounces of red meat per *month*. Indeed, Harvard's chairman of nutrition says the optimum amount of red meat could well be zero, as (a) we can get its nutritional value elsewhere, (b) it is high in fat and cholesterol, which are linked to heart disease, and (c) some data link red meat to colon and prostate cancer.

The Mediterranean Diet program also includes regular physical activity and optional, daily moderate consumption of wine. The USDA pyramid does not address either exercise or alcohol, though the federal Dietary Guidelines for Americans recommend drinking only moderately, if at all.

Interest in the Mediterranean Diet stems from observations more than 30 years ago that people on the Greek island of Crete got 40 percent of their calories from fat but were only about one twentieth as likely to die of heart disease as Americans. A key difference was that much of the fat came from olive oil rather than meat. Despite their high-fat diet, the people of Crete actually took in less cholesterol-raising saturated fat than did Americans.

Today, it's generally agreed that the Mediterranean Diet won't hurt you, and some nutritional authorities say it's healthier than the USDA pyramid approach. It can be tasty, too. Spain, southern Italy, Greece, and the Provençal region of France, the historical havens of Mediterranean cooking, are well known for their culinary delights.

Is Fat Intake Linked to Breast, Colon, Lung, Prostate, and Bladder Cancer?

These cancers tend to be more common among people eating high-fat diets. Women in Japan eating the country's traditional low-fat diet are less likely to develop breast cancer than women in the U.S. Even more telling, the granddaughters and great-granddaughters of Japanese women who moved to the U.S. and switched their families to a high-fat diet are almost as likely to develop breast cancer as anyone else.

Such evidence does not prove that a high-fat diet causes these types of cancer, however, because many other factors could be involved. For example, it could be that people who eat lots of fat simply don't get enough of the fiber-containing fruits and vegetables that are known to reduce the risk of cancer. Moreover, most of the studies in this area have measured the incidence of cancer and the fat in diet, but not factors, such as family history of cancer. As they say, further studies are required.

Is Alcohol Linked to Breast, Pancreatic, and Colon Cancer?

No firm relationship between drinking and these cancers has been established yet. However, some evidence points to such a link.

Is Red Meat Linked to Colon and Prostate Cancer?

Several large, long-term studies have found that colon cancer—or the colon polyps that often precede cancer—is much more common among people who eat red meat

TIP-OFFS OF NUTRITIONAL HYPE

Much of what we see and hear about nutrition is at best exaggerated, and at worst deliberately misleading. Here are a few clues that what you're hearing is hype.

Hype is most common in areas where:

■ **There's a product to sell and a profit to make.**

■ **There are no acknowledged experts.** Although there are plenty of experts in nutrition, most people don't know who they are. This creates an opening for impostors and charletons. Moreover, most doctors don't know enough about how food affects our health—60 percent of medical school graduates don't learn enough about nutrition, according to the Association of American Medical Colleges.

■ **The experts don't know the answer, so there's a void to fill.**

■ **The true answers are difficult or take a long time.** This is why losing weight, cutting fat, slowing aging, and curing arthritis, cancer, and AIDS are common targets for food hype. Ask lots of questions, for example, about a diet or weight-loss regimen promising that you'll take off 10 pounds in the week or two before your beach vacation. Most legitimate authorities advise that it's safest to lose no more than a pound or two a week—and half a pound to a pound is even better.

Be suspicious if:

■ **The claim sounds too good to be true.** It usually is. Diet and supplements may alleviate disease, but they rarely cure it. Bad nutrition contributes to conditions like heart disease and cancer, but changing your diet is not a quick cure-all.

■ **Testimonials rather than research are used to support claims.** One person's experience, as compelling as it may be, is just that—it may apply only to that individual. A myriad of factors may be responsible for any change in health; and only careful research can sift out the effect of nutrition from other factors, such as exercise, smoking, and heredity.

frequently. And a similar, long-term study has found that prostate cancer is more than twice as common in the men who eat the greatest amounts of red meat. This research doesn't prove that red meat is the *cause* of colon and prostate cancer. After all, most meat-eaters don't get either disease. Still, it appears that cutting down on red meat improves your odds of escaping those diseases.

Can Grilling Meat at Very High Temperatures Create Cancer-Causing Compounds?

Some research says Yes; but the practical significance of this—if any—is still unknown. For details, see Chapter 13, "Cut Back on These Foods to Cut Your Cancer Risk."

Is Plant Protein Better than Animal Protein?

Maybe. If nothing else, switching from animal sources (red meat, poultry, fish, and dairy products) to plant sources (beans, grains, and nuts) will lower your fat and cholesterol intake. Americans get twice the protein they need as it is, and two-thirds of that comes from animal sources. Switching even half of your meat intake to plant protein can cut your cholesterol levels—by 13 percent in one study. That's important, because if your cholesterol is more than 200,

WHEN TO BELIEVE A MEDIA REPORT

How many times have you given up trying to figure out what's healthy because the experts can't make up their minds? A few months—or years—of stuffing down oatmeal or oat-bran muffins in what turned out to be a vain hope of lowering cholesterol could turn anybody sour on science.

The problem is not that researchers or the media are lying, or that they really don't know *anything*. It's just that a single, limited study is often ballyhooed as if it were the final answer. Unfortunately, the standards of good science require many types of studies to agree before something can be considered a certainty. Much of the research so prominently reported in the media is just one step along the way, not conclusive evidence. Unfortunately, that part of the news doesn't make the headlines.

Here are some questions to ask before believing the next "bulletin" from the laboratory:

Is it an animal study? Ideas are usually tried out on animals before they are tested in people, both to ensure safety and to find out if the concept is worth the extra cost of a human study. Evidence from animal studies is important. But what happens in a lab rat, for example, may have no relevance to you and me. Findings from animal studies are clues, not facts.

Is it a test-tube experiment? Like results from an animal study, the findings from test-tube ("in vitro") research may have no bearing on what happens to people. Like animal studies, test-tube work is a way of testing the safety and validity of an idea before trying it in people.

Is it a population study? Population studies do involve people, but they too have limitations. Here's how population studies usually are conducted: If an investigator thinks that factor A (for example, fat in the diet) plays a role in development of disease B (breast cancer), he will count the number of cases in a large group and measure the amount of fat consumed by women who did, and did not, develop the disease. If those who did not

develop breast cancer ate much less fat than those who did, this finding lends support to the scientist's theory. The flaw in most such studies is that they fail to account for the many other factors that could be at work, such as heredity, smoking, and use of birth-control pills. Ultimately, this type of finding is a clue, not a fact.

Is it a real-time study? This type of research, called a prospective study, assembles a group of people with specific characteristics, measures certain things about them, then tracks changes in them over a period of time. A retrospective study, on the other hand, involves searching through records for characteristics and changes after the fact. Because accuracy will be greater if you know in advance which change to track, a prospective study is viewed as more reliable than a retrospective one that relies on records made for a totally different purpose. However, retrospective studies often serve to point the direction a more definitive prospective study should take.

Did it use a placebo? A placebo, or dummy pill, contains no active ingredient, yet can make some people get better if they think it might be real. This is the famous placebo effect, and it helps scientists sort out how much of an effect is really caused by a medicine and how much is in people's minds. Placebo-control, as this technique is called, is one sign of a reliable study. Unfortunately, it's not practical in many studies, where a fake could be detected or the test involves withholding a substance rather than giving one. And if the real pill turns out to be a life-saver, ethics demand that the study be halted.

How many people were studied? The fewer the people in a study, the more likely that the findings are due to special circumstances or chance. Smaller studies are performed before larger ones to ensure the safety of the therapy being tested and to find out whether the cost of a large study is justified. This does not mean that 10-person studies are worthless—just that they are not definitive.

How long did the study go on? All other factors being equal, longer studies are better than short ones. This is because it may take a long time for dietary changes or drugs to make a difference. Cancer and heart disease, for example, develop over a long period of time, and, researchers often don't know how long it will take for a change in diet or a drug to have its effect. On the other hand, a change in, say, blood pressure that's seen after a few months could be just temporary. The only way to know for sure is to follow people for a longer period of time.

Did the scientists allow for other possibilities? Many factors besides diet can influence development of a problem like heart disease or cancer, including smoking, exercise, heredity, and age. If there is a placebo group in the study, one way to account for these factors is to make sure that the placebo and treatment groups both include, for example, the same percentage of smokers. If one group then suffers an increase in disease, it can't be blamed on smoking.

Is this a new "discovery," or do other studies back it up? No matter how carefully the research is done, scientists almost never regard a single study as definitive proof. It's the whole body of evidence that counts. One study could be a fluke—its findings could be due to a mistake, or to some unrecognized characteristic of the people evaluated. Usually, many studies—and at least a few different types of studies—must support a point before researchers view the finding as definitive.

every 1 percent drop could diminish your heart disease risk by 2 percent. One caution: most research in this area uses soy protein. Wheat, rice, or other plant foods might not have the same effect. Also, the best results have been found in Italy and Switzerland, where other factors may be at work.

Is Salt Linked to Stomach Cancer?

Stomach cancer is rare in the U.S., but deadly when it strikes—and some evidence seems to show that avoiding very salty food can help reduce risk. Salt intake is higher among people with stomach cancer; and some research suggests that salt-cured, pickled, or nitrite-preserved foods may be responsible for the higher rates of stomach and esophageal cancer found in countries where these foods are common. The risk in the U.S. diet, however, appears to be small.

Where the Experts Disagree

Although we learn more about nutrition every year, there are still areas where the experts still don't have an answer. Sometimes this is due to conflicting research, sometimes to conflicts in interpretation. Here's a quick look at three of today's biggest controversies.

Are Recommended Daily Allowances too Low?

Some nutritionists believe they are—at least in some cases. For example, older people may need more of certain minerals to counterbalance the decline in immunity that can come with age (see Chapter 27 for more on this.) Likewise, many authorities feel that the RDA for calcium is too low to prevent the weakened bones of osteoporosis, especially in those at risk for the problem. Other ex-

WHAT TO LOOK FOR ON LABELS

The new food labels make it easy to see whether a product is "nutritionally correct." The most important things to look for are the ones most prominently displayed: fat, saturated fat, cholesterol, sodium, calories, and fiber. (Remember though, that the FDA allows manufacturers a 20 percent margin of error in the labeled amounts.)

If you're watching specific ingredients, you'll find them listed in the order of their amount. An ingredient not among the first three probably isn't included in significant proportions.

Be careful to check serving sizes, too. If cereal A lists serving size as half a cup and cereal B says it's two-thirds of a cup, then you can't do a head-to-head comparison of nutrient content without some math. Also compare the serving size to what you really eat. If you pour yourself a cup of cereal every morning, and the label gives calories for half-a-cup, remember to double it, however painful that is. Fortunately, serving sizes have been somewhat standardized on the new labels.

Look for health claims because in order to carry them, the food must meet stringent requirements for fat, saturated fat, cholesterol, and sodium, providing no more than 20 percent of the Daily Value for each. For example, even though whole milk is high in calcium, its labeling can't make a claim about preventing osteoporosis, because it's too high in fat.

A number of common advertising buzzwords now have strict definitions. Here's what the FDA assures us they mean:

Fiber and soluble fiber. To carry a claim that it contains fiber that reduces heart disease, a product must be high in soluble fiber (at least 0.6 grams per serving). Labels don't have to list soluble fiber, so this is one way you can find out if it's there. Manufacturers can only make health claims for foods containing naturally occurring fiber.

"Free," "without," "no," "zero." To use these words on food labels in connection with fat, saturated fat, cholesterol, sodium, sugars, and calories, the food must contain zero or a trivial amount of each. For example, fat-free means a serving contains less than half a gram of fat, which is insignificant even if you eat several servings. The FDA can't require zero because fat can't be measured below a certain level.

"Lean." On meat, poultry, and seafood, this word means less than 10 grams of fat, less than 4 grams of saturated fat, and less than 95 milligrams of cholesterol per serving and per 100 grams.

"Extra lean." Meat, poultry, and seafood bearing this phrase must contain less than 5 grams of fat, less than 2 grams of saturated fat, and less than 95 milligrams of cholesterol per serving and per 100 grams.

"95 percent fat free." This means that the food contains 5 grams or less of fat per 100 grams of the food.

"High," "rich in," "excellent source of." Foods using these words in connection with any nutrient must contain at least 20% of the recommended Daily Value for that nutrient per serving.

"Good source of". This means one serving contains 10 to 19 percent of the Daily Value for that nutrient.

"Light," "lite." These favorites can mean one of two things: (1) a nutritionally altered product containing one-third fewer calories or half the fat of the "real" food (eg, mayonnaise); or (2) the sodium content of a low-calorie, low-fat food has been reduced by 50 percent. These terms can still be used to describe color and texture if it's made clear what "light" refers to.

"Low cholesterol." This means the product contains no more than 20 milligrams of cholesterol per serving, or no more than 2 grams of saturated fat per serving. No matter how low the cholesterol, a product can't make a cholesterol claim if there's more than 2 grams of saturated fat in a serving.

perts believe the RDA is too low for vitamin E and folic acid.

Part of the controversy centers around the purpose of the RDAs. Originally established to prevent acute deficiency diseases, RDAs are now intended to reflect what a majority (80 percent) of the population needs to stay in good health. Neither then nor now do they indicate the optimum amounts needed to forestall chronic disease.

Some nutritional experts argue that they should; and in their latest release, they do in fact move in that direction. For instance, the RDA for calcium is now 1,200 milligrams per day up to age 24, not just to age 18, in order to prevent osteoporosis later in life.

Still, for most vitamins and minerals, the RDA is generally all you need unless you have a specific health problem or condition. In some cases, exceeding the RDA can hurt you. So it's best to follow it unless a doctor, or dietitian, advises you otherwise. The new Daily Values system does include some nutrients for which there is no RDA; but when one exists, the Daily Value is usually the same.

Does Sodium Cause High Blood Pressure?

Some experts insist that response to sodium varies from one person to the next. According to some estimates, extra sodium increases blood pressure in about 5 to 15 percent of the population, and in 25 to 60 percent of those with high blood pressure. Sensitivity to sodium increases with age. Other authorities believe that sodium does affect blood pressure in most of us, though more in some than others.

To add to the confusion, experts disagree over the interpretation of what information we have available. Some say that research has not conclusively demonstrated a direct, strong link between sodium and high blood pressure. They suggest that large, sustained reductions in sodium are needed to affect blood pressure, or that not everyone's blood pressure benefits from cutting sodium intake. Others, looking at the same studies, say they confirm the link.

If there is this much controversy, why does the government recommend limiting sodium? For starters, no one really knows how many people are sensitive to sodium's blood pressure-elevating effects, nor is there any way of telling who's sensitive and who's not. Since almost all of us eat far more than required, cutting back won't hurt, and could help reduce the risk of heart disease.

Does Fish Oil Help the Heart?

Hotly disputed research suggests that the omega-3 fatty acids in fish lower cholesterol levels, perhaps by reducing the amount of cholesterol manufactured by the body.

Less controversial is fish oil's ability to increase the time it takes blood to clot. This may reduce the chance of a clot, blocking an artery and causing a heart attack, but it can also increase your risk of bleeding, bruising, and anemia. Accordingly, moderate amounts of fish oil are considered healthy, while the large quantities found in fish oil capsules should never be taken without medical supervision. Though the capsules have been shown to reduce triglyceride (blood fat) levels and are prescribed for that reason, they have not been shown to reduce "bad" LDL cholesterol.

Correcting Some Common Misconceptions

Nutrition is a vast area, often vulnerable to oversimplification and misinterpretation. And, once enshrined by the media, the resulting half-truths and outright errors take on a life of their own.

YOUR INCENTIVES

			CHANGE DIET		
		REDUCE FATS	CONTROL CALORIES	INCREASE STARCH AND FIBERS	REDUCE SODIUM	CONTROL ALCOHOL
REDUCE RISK	HEART DISEASE	👍	👍		👍	
	CANCER	👍	👍	👍		👍
	STROKE	👍	👍		👍	👍
	DIABETES	👍	👍	👍		
	GASTROINTESTINAL DISEASES	👍	👍	👍		👍

Adapted from: McGinnis JM and Nestle M: The Surgeon General's Report on Nutrition and Health: Policy implications and implementation strategies. Am J Clin Nutr 49:23, 1989, p 26.

Here is the truth about some of the misconceptions still making the rounds today.

Protein Does Not Promote Osteoporosis

Eating more protein, plant or animal, does pull more calcium from the body, but not as much as once was thought. Additionally, your body may adapt and stop losing calcium at some point. A 1980 study found less osteoporosis among vegetarians, but more recent studies have failed to confirm that.

Too Much Protein Does Not Cause Kidney Disease

There is no direct evidence of a problem here. Kidney disease is rare in this country despite our high protein intake. Only diabetics need to limit protein to the level specified in the RDAs (50 grams per day).

Too Much Protein Does Not Cause Cancer

There is little evidence that animal protein increases the risk of cancer. Researchers, including those at Dana-Farber Cancer Institute in Boston, have been unable to verify a strong link between protein and breast, colon, or kidney cancer. Researchers at Cornell University did find that feeding rats more protein, especially animal protein, made them more likely to develop liver cancer when given a substance known to cause the disease. But this could be unique to the cancer-causing substance used in the study, and to liver cancer, which is rare in the U.S. despite our high-protein diet. Most experts agree that this finding does not justify changing your diet.

Oat Bran Does Not Lower Cholesterol

There is a kernel of truth to oat bran's cholesterol-lowering powers. Early studies did find that oatmeal or foods containing oat bran could lower cholesterol. In 1990, however, researchers failed to verify these findings in a study done on a group of young women. Analysis of data from several previous studies then revealed that oat bran lowers cholesterol by so small a percentage (5 percent or less) that its effects are insignificant for most of us.

Cutting your intake of saturated fat and cholesterol is clearly a more effective way of reducing your risk of heart disease. This doesn't mean it's bad to eat oat bran or oatmeal—grains provide fiber and should form the basis of our diet. It's just that oats won't have a major effect on your cholesterol.

Starchy Foods Are Not Fattening

It used to be conventional wisdom that dieting meant cutting down on starch—bread, potatoes, pasta, and rice. Now, for most people these foods are considered the basis of any good diet, including weight-loss programs. Starch has the same number of calories as protein—4 per gram—and many fewer than fat, which has 9 calories per gram.

Most starchy foods are nearly fat-free, as long as you forgo toppings like sour cream on potatoes or Alfredo sauce on pasta. The body uses more energy processing starch than it needs to burn fat; so starch not only gives you less fat and fewer calories than fatty foods, but also makes the body burn more calories—a good combination. In some overweight people with a problem called "insulin resistance," excess carbohydrates do tend to add extra pounds. But for most of us, they remain the best source of needed energy.

What a "Balanced Diet" Means Today

Following the current guidelines for healthy nutrition doesn't doom you to life with a calculator. The theoretical target is 60 percent carbohydrates, 30 percent fat, and 10 percent protein, but in daily life that simply means going heavier on fruits, vegetables, and grains, lighter on meat and dairy, and very light on oils, salad dressings, mayonnaise, and sweets.

A balanced diet means just that—balance. You don't have to make sure every food, or even every meal, is exactly 30 percent fat—just balance a rich restaurant meal with a light vegetable-and-rice dinner the next day. Healthy eating does not have to mean giving up foods you like, feeling guilty when you have a big meal, or viewing every decision about what to eat as inherently "good" or "bad"—all or nothing. You *can* eat ice cream or chocolate cake—just watch how much, and how often, you do it. Here's the bottom line on today's balanced diet and how it differs from what most of us are used to.

Less meat

All the experts agree: Eat less meat. How much less? For most of us there's so much room for improvement that it really doesn't matter. Though statistics show that we are eating less red meat, most of us have switched to white meat rather than grains, fruits, and vegetables. We're also still eating too much fat—34 percent of calories from fat, instead of the recommended 30 percent, and 12 percent from saturated fat, rather than the recommended 10 percent, according to one estimate.

Fewer Eggs and Dairy Products

These foods are out of favor for the same reason as meat: many are high in fat and cholesterol, and most of us eat too much of them. You don't have to cut back severely, however. Switching to low-fat or skim versions will go a long way towards balancing you diet with little pain. Moderation is the key. Avoid having eggs and bacon every day, but don't hesitate to have an omelet on the weekend.

More Fruits, Vegetables, and Grains

Low in fat, full of fiber, these are the foods we don't get nearly enough of. Even if your fat intake is low, you probably need more rice, pasta, whole-grain bread, fruits, and vegetables.

Gain Without Pain

With so much evidence that a diet low in fat and high in fiber, fruits, and vegetables can help fend off the top two killers of Americans—heart disease and cancer—making a few sacrifices in your diet seems well worth the effort. Surprisingly, those sacrifices are much smaller and easier than you'd expect.

As the title of Dr. Dean Ornish's popular book announces, you really can "eat more, weigh less." It's all in *what* you eat. Cutting way back on high-calorie fat leaves room in your diet for more food than before—with no increase in total calories. And trimming the fat shouldn't leave you hungry, either. Your body is designed to signal you when carbohydrates drop, but not when fat intake goes down. On an "eat more, weigh less" diet, you'll get plenty of carbohydrates to keep you feeling full.

Big benefits can come from minor changes. One small study at the University of Washington in Seattle showed that switching to skim milk from whole milk for 6 weeks reduced total cholesterol by 7 percent and "bad" (LDL) cholesterol by 11 percent without diminishing "good" HDL cholesterol. In a study at a Harvard University–affiliated hospital, women lost an average of 5 percent of their weight by making seven simple changes, including substituting skim for whole milk, non-fat frozen yogurt for ice cream, and fruit spread for margarine or butter.

Take advantage of foods reformulated as low-fat, low-calorie, and low-cholesterol. They can be a boon if you absolutely cannot pass up certain favorite dishes. They can also help you get past the mental block that healthy eating has to mean cutting out what you like. Just remember not to view the "fat-free" label as a license to eat extra amounts, or "reward" yourself for foregoing one fatty food by gobbling up another.

Keep fruits, vegetables, and grains ready to eat in the house. Don't bring home as much meat and fatty food from the supermarket. If it's not in the refrigerator when you get home for the day, you probably won't run back out to buy it.

Above all, be patient with yourself. An overnight make-over isn't all that important, as long as you keep making progress. If you eat a 10 ounce piece of meat for dinner every night, try cutting back to 8 ounces, then 6 ounces, gradually filling in with pasta, rice, vegetables, and fruit. Don't let yourself go hungry. If it takes you a few years to get down to the USDA's recommended 3 ounce serving, that's better than never making it at all. □

CHAPTER 2

Basic Questions: Vitamins, Minerals, Fiber, and More

Should you really be taking vitamin supplements? How about megadosing? Or increasing your antioxidants? And how do protein, carbohydrates, and fiber fit in? Our knowledge about nutrition is growing on an almost daily basis. Though there's still much disagreement among the experts on the exact amount of nutrients the average person needs, the broad picture is coming into sharper and sharper focus. Here's a brief overview of the basic building blocks of nutrition, and the dietary guidelines authorities recommend today.

Vitamins and Minerals: Which Do What?

Vitamins and minerals are almost always mentioned in the same breath, but there *are* differences between the two. Vitamins are complex molecules that keep the body's chemical mechanisms in gear. They contribute to the storage and release of energy (metabolism) and maintain the bones, blood, and nerves. Minerals are inorganic substances in body tissues and fluids that trigger or prevent the production of enzymes and hormones, govern certain of their activities, and serve as raw material for structures such as the bones. Everyday, your body uses up some or all of the vitamins and minerals that keep it going. So each day, you need to replenish your supply, remembering that each vitamin and mineral has specific and necessary properties.

Vitamins. You can find detailed information on each vitamin in Part 3 of this book (Nutrition, A to Z), but just to give you a quick idea of how important each one is: Vitamin A contributes to growth and reproduction, vision, normal function of the nervous system, and development and maintenance of body tissues (including skin and bone). The B vitamins build red blood cells, guide body metabolism, maintain the protective covering of the nervous system, and boost the body's use of proteins, fats, and carbohydrates.

Vitamin C heals wounds; contributes to the formation of cells, tissues, teeth, and bones; and boosts the immune system. Vitamin E helps to protect the outer membranes of the body's cells from damage. By protecting white blood cells, vitamin E also helps the immune system fight off threats of disease. Vitamin K promotes blood clotting in wounds.

Minerals. Minerals perform equally varied functions. About 20 minerals play major roles in the body. Even those that are needed in tiny (called "trace") amounts pack tremendous force and fend off serious illness. The "macrominerals," needed in larger amounts, are calcium, chlorine, magnesium, phosphorus, potassium, sodium, and sulfur. "Microminerals," needed in trace amounts, include chromium, copper, fluorine, iodine, iron, manganese, molybdenum, nickel, selenium, silicon, tin, vanadium, and zinc.

Iodine keeps the thyroid gland working. Copper is a component of many enzymes needed for metabolism. Iron transports oxygen to cells throughout the body. Phosphorus and calcium build teeth and bones. Potassium maintains the fluid balance inside cells, helps the muscles contract, and assists the transmission of messages by the nerves. It also keeps the heart and kidneys working properly. Zinc keeps enzymes working and helps metabolize proteins.

How they interrelate. Besides acting directly on the body, vitamins and minerals empower each other. Vitamin C helps the body absorb iron, for example, and vitamin D does the same for calcium and phosphorus. The interrelationships are so complex that only a regular, wide sampling can provide everything your body needs. The body can supply only two vitamins itself: D and K. Vitamin K is synthesized by bacteria in the intestine. Vitamin D is created by the skin when it's exposed to sunlight. All the others must be supplied to the body from outside sources. (For the foods that pack the richest supplies, see the box on "Best Dietary Sources of Major Vitamins and Minerals.")

Vitamins That Wash Away, Vitamins That Build Up

Vitamins fall into two categories, depending on the substance that transports them in the body.

Water-soluble vitamins are stored and carried by the water that permeates every part of the body. Because water is constantly being lost in the urine, sweat, and other body fluids, most of these vitamins must be replaced daily. The water-soluble vitamins are vitamin C and the many B-complex vitamins, including thiamin (B_1), riboflavin (B_2), niacin (B_3), pyridoxine (B_6), folacin (folic acid), cyanocobalamin (B_{12}), biotin, and pantothenic acid. Not all will be discussed in this chapter.

Fat-soluble vitamins—A (retinol), D (calciferol), E (d-alpha- tocopherol), and K (menaquinone)—are transported by the fats in the bloodstream. Because the body stores fat much more readily than water, a temporary interruption in the supply of these vitamins is less damaging than a lack of water-soluble vitamins. By the same token, however, excessive intake of these vitamins can quickly build up toxic levels in your system.

BEST DIETARY SOURCES OF MAJOR VITAMINS AND MINERALS

Vitamins

Vitamin A (retinol)
Milk
Egg yolks
Liver and other organ meats

Beta-carotene
Yellow and orange vegetables
  (carrots, sweet potatoes, squash)
Dark green leafy vegetables
  (broccoli, spinach, asparagus)
Yellow and orange fruits (cantaloupes, apricots)

Vitamin B$_1$ (thiamin)
Poultry
Fish
Whole grains
Legumes
Nuts
Liver

Vitamin B$_2$ (riboflavin)
Dairy products (milk, cheese, yogurt)
Dark green leafy vegetables
Whole grains
Eggs
Organ meats

Vitamin B$_3$ (niacin)
Whole grains
Legumes
Poultry
Fish
Red meat

Vitamin B$_6$ (pyridoxine)
Meat
Fish
Poultry
Dried beans
Bananas
Potatoes
Raisins and dried figs, dates, and prunes
Yeast
Whole grains
Green vegetables

Vitamin B$_{12}$ (cyanocobalamin)
Meat
Fish
Poultry
Dairy products
Eggs

Folic Acid (a B-complex vitamin)
Dark green leafy vegetables
Liver
Dried beans
Seeds
Citrus fruits and juice
Soybeans and other legumes
Wheat germ
Whole grains

Vitamin C (ascorbic acid)
Yellow, orange, and red fruits
Dark green leafy vegetables
Potatoes

Vitamin D (calciferol)
Liver
Egg yolks
Fortified milk
Oily fish with bones (sardines, salmon)
Vitamin E (tocopherol)
Polyunsaturated vegetable oils
Dark green leafy vegetables
Wheat germ
Whole grains
Dried beans
Liver
Nuts
Seeds

Vitamin K (menaquinone)
Liver
Dark green leafy vegetables
Vegetable oils
Egg yolks

BEST DIETARY SOURCES OF MAJOR VITAMINS AND MINERALS

Minerals

Calcium
Low-fat dairy products
Oily fish with bones (sardines, salmon)
Dark green leafy vegetables
Tofu
Sesame seeds

Chromium
Yeast
Oysters
Potatoes
Liver
Cheese
Beef
Whole grains

Copper
Legumes
Oysters
Raisins
Whole grains
Dried fruits
Organ meats
Iodine
Seafood
Iodized salt

Iron
Red meat
Spinach
Eggs
Whole grains
Dark green leafy vegetables
Beets
Raisins
Dried beans

Magnesium
Nuts and seeds
Bran
Whole grains
Dark green leafy vegetables
Seafood
Legumes
Milk

Phosphorus
Red meat
Poultry
Fish
Eggs
Dark green leafy vegetables
Dairy products
Whole grains
Legumes
Nuts

Potassium
Bananas
Apricots
Potatoes
Lima beans
Milk and dairy products
Poultry
Avocados
Mushrooms
Citrus fruits and juices

Selenium
Whole-grain cereals
Meat
Poultry
Fish
Dairy products

Zinc
Oysters and other seafood
Lean meats
Whole grains
Wheat germ
Bran
Legumes
Nuts and seeds
Herring
Milk
Egg yolks
Liver

The Antioxidants: Theory and Fact

Some of the most familiar old stand-bys among the vitamins and minerals are suddenly taking on exciting new roles as scientists mount intensive investigations of their antioxidant properties. Whether these "souped-up" embodiments of vitamins and minerals can actually prevent chronic illness or weaken its effects remains to be proved, but evidence is growing all the time.

Many highly respected researchers take antioxidants very seriously. Dr. Dean Ornish's Life Choice diet for reversing heart disease, for example, is deliberately low in oxidants and high in antioxidants to help the body remove them. Common diseases and conditions that certain vitamins and minerals may prevent or improve include high blood pressure, heart disease, diabetes, and cancer.

How antioxidants work. Floating in the bloodstream are molecules of unstable oxygen called free radicals. During the normal breakdown of food, these molecules have been stripped of an electron. When the free radical fills its "electron deficiency" by locking onto another molecule, oxidation (like burning) occurs. Free radicals kill bacteria, fight inflammation, and keep the smooth muscles well-toned so they can regulate the blood vessels and organs. But when too many free radicals are circulating at once, some grab electrons from places where the electron ought to stay, such as the genetic material (DNA) in a cell.

The harmful effects of excessive free radicals range from cosmetic to life-threatening. They can break down skin tissue, making it look older than it is. They can injure the lenses of the eyes, leading to cataracts. And they can make it harder for cells to repair themselves, increasing the risk of cancer, heart disease, and other chronic disorders.

Antioxidants come to the rescue by scavenging excess free radicals before they can cause trouble. The body contains its own antioxidants, but not enough to fight off the huge amount of free radicals that assault the body daily from a variety of sources, including air pollution, stress, cigarette smoke, too much sun, electromagnetic fields, lack of exercise, and high-fat diets.

What antioxidants do. At least 25 studies of tens of thousands of people are now under way to verify the effects of antioxidants on health. So far, benefits have been documented in over 200 published articles (though other studies have shown little or no results).

Beta-carotene is a "provitamin" that becomes vitamin A in the body as needed. Its benefits have been known for at least a decade. In the laboratory, beta-carotene has shown promise in preventing cancers of the breast, lung, stomach, and cervix.

Vitamin E has been credited with lowering the risk of heart disease, the number one killer in America, by reducing the build-up of LDL ("bad") cholesterol inside blood vessels. Vitamin E may also help prevent prostate and colon cancers.

Vitamin C enhances the immune system by enabling white blood cells to break down bacteria, and may prevent nitrates and nitrites from being converted into cancer-causing compounds called nitrosamines. Although no absolute proof exists, vitamin C may also protect against cancers of the breast, cervix, and gastrointestinal system. And, of course, many people believe in the fabled power of vitamin C to relieve colds and sore throats, though most scientists still say more proof is needed.

Selenium, which isn't accepted as an antioxidant by all experts, must be ingested in very small amounts to avoid tissue damage. This mineral is found in food and water (especially seafood, meat, poultry, and grain). The precise amount depends on the levels of selenium in the soil in which the food was grown or through which the water flowed.

Finally, there's glutathione, a substance built from amino acids, that acts as one of the body's major antioxidants. Glutathione supplements are now available in most health food stores.

The New Phytochemical Cancer Fighters: What's Known Today

A few years ago, researchers in cancer prevention began to concentrate in a big way on a new group of chemicals found in plants (phytochemicals). In the fields, phytochemicals keep bugs away and protect against too much sun. For people, they may be science's newest key to controlling cancer and other diseases.

Whether phytochemicals are the magic elixirs they seem to be has yet to be proved. Meanwhile, what's being discovered about them suggests that they apparently can provide the body with numerous ways to prevent cancer and even zap cancer cells before they can develop or spread. They're especially powerful in the epithelial cells that line body organs (the lung, bladder, cervix,

THE POTENT CRUCIFEROUS VEGETABLES

These vegetables, collectively named for the cross shape within their flowers, are among the biggest stars in the nutritional line-up for the many healthful roles they play. As long as you don't cook them beyond recognition, they'll serve you well in any form, including cole slaw and sauerkraut.

Bok choy	Kale
(Chinese cabbage)	Kohlrabi
Broccoli	Mustard greens
Brussels sprouts	Rutabagas
Cabbage	Turnip greens
Cauliflower	Turnips
Collard greens	Watercress
Horseradish	

mouth, larynx, throat, esophagus, stomach, pancreas, colon, and rectum).

A huge project by the National Cancer Institute is expected to show exciting results. In the research spotlight are the chemical components of a vast number of foods, including garlic, licorice root, citrus fruits, soybeans, celery, barley, ginger root, hot peppers, and green tea.

The leading phytochemicals today.

P-coumaric acid and chlorogenic acid, found in tomatoes, carrots, strawberries, pineapples, and other fruits and vegetables, remove nitric oxide from cells before it can combine with chemicals called amines to create the damaging nitrosamines involved in cancer cell formation.

Sulforaphane, a compound contained in cruciferous vegetables (see the box on "The Potent Cruciferous Vegetables"), has prevented breast cancer in laboratory animals. The compound seems to make certain enzymes in breast cells go into action, locating cancer-causing substances and attaching those substances to molecules that escort them out of the cell. Allyl sulfides, found in garlic and onions, also mobilize enzymes that defuse carcinogenic chemicals. Allylic sulfides may also reduce the risk of heart disease by inhibiting cholesterol formation.

Indole-3-carbinol seems to repress the formation of cancer-causing estrogens in the breast. Other indoles found in cruciferous vegetables apparently stimulate enzymes that break down cancer-causing substances into harmless ones, especially useful against cancers of the stomach and intestine. Cruciferous vegetables also contain phenethyl isothiocyanate, which has inhibited lung cancer in mice and rats.

Flavonoids, various substances that interfere with hormones that promote cancer, are found in tomatoes, peppers, yams, soybeans, carrots, and many other foods. Limonene, found in citrus fruits, encourages the production of enzymes that may help obliterate potential carcinogens.

Other phytochemicals work to deprive tumors of their blood supply, protect the DNA inside cells, get in the way of cancer-causing hormones that are trying to become attached to the cell—and might well do a lot of other things that researchers haven't discovered yet. When new discoveries are confirmed, expect to see ads for "designer foods" crammed with extra phytochemicals. Food companies have to be careful, though. Like vitamins and minerals, phytochemicals may be toxic in large amounts. Right now, the best way to get phytochemicals, says registered dietician Mona Sutnick, Ed.D, a consultant in Philadelphia, "is to eat generous amounts of fruits and vegetables and dried beans."

Vitamins and Minerals as Medications

Plenty of Americans must believe in the power of vitamins, since we spend $4.4 billion on them every year. In a 1993 poll conducted for the American Dietetic Association and Weight Watchers, more than half of the women surveyed, especially those over age 30, said they took at least one type of mineral or vitamin supplement.

The idea of swallowing pills to replace a decent diet, however, makes most dietitians frown. If you do take vitamins, you have to regard them as supplements—not substitutes—for healthy food. Although their own research is confirming the beneficial effects of many vitamins, the experts refuse to recommend them in pill form, fearing that people will forsake regular food, with all the other irreplaceable nutrients it provides.

However, most people already have less than ideal diets. A large national survey indicates that more than half of the American population doesn't eat a single piece of fruit, drink a glass of fruit juice, or munch even one vegetable on any given day of the year. Fewer than one in ten Americans eats the *minimum* recommended total of 5 servings of vegetables and fruits a day. For all those people, taking supplements seems a better course of action than doing nothing at all.

Megadoses: The Pros and Cons

Believing that more of something good must be better, many people take very large amounts of vitamins and minerals. They're cheap, after all, and available without a prescription. But just because a deficiency of a certain vitamin or mineral can make you sick, doesn't mean a carload of it will necessarily make you better than ever. Taking many times the RDA of any vitamin or mineral can give it the potency of a drug, and doctors rarely, if ever, recommend extremely high doses. Scientists are discovering that a moderate increase in certain vitamins can be beneficial for certain people. But they also know that large overdoses can definitely be dangerous. So, when taking supplements, it's wise to err on the side of caution, and check with your doctor before going too far.

Vitamin C. Nobel Laureate Linus Pauling was an early proponent of deliberately taking huge doses of a single vitamin to enhance health. In his book *Vitamin C and the Common Cold*, Dr. Pauling advocated doses as huge as 15 grams a day. (The RDA is 60 milligrams.) While some people continue to swear by the healthful effects of vitamin C megadoses, they can also have side effects, including nausea, abdominal cramps, diarrhea, and possibly kidney stones. Some laboratory tests, such as those for blood glucose, may provide inaccurate results for people who take more than 1,000 milligrams of vitamin C a day. Nevertheless, research into Dr. Pauling's hypothesis continues.

Niacin. Heart patients are often advised to take high doses of niacin (1,500 to 3,000 milligrams) to lower their cholesterol levels. Because niacin in large amounts can have uncomfortable side effects, such as a burning sensation in the skin or profuse perspiration, or dangerous ones, such as irregular heartbeats or liver damage, a doctor must monitor any such regimen closely.

Vitamin E. Some highly respected scientists support intake of relatively high doses of vitamin E (400 to 600 IU) by older people. They say the vitamin can protect against heart disease and help prevent macular degeneration, a serious eye problem that can lead to blindness. However, as with all vitamins and minerals, it's best to increase the amount you get in your diet before turning to a stripped-down supplement.

Dangers of Megadoses

But for the few vitamins or minerals that may be helpful in extra doses, there are many more that cause undesirable side effects.

Vitamin D. One of the more toxic of the vitamins, this substance can cause calcium to build up in the blood, creating a condition called hypercalcemia that can eventually damage the kidneys and cause soft tissues to harden, especially in the lungs, joints, stomach, and blood vessels.

Vitamin A. Adults who take more than 33,000 IU of vitamin A a day for several months (in the elderly, more than 5,000 to 10,000 IU; in infants and children, more than 14,000 IU) can end up with liver or bone damage, hair loss, and skin problems. The same is not thought to be true for large amounts of beta-carotene, which can turn the skin yellowish but is otherwise free of irreversible side effects. However, a few troubling and much-publicized studies have suggested that taking more than 5,000 IU of beta-carotene a day in supplements might be unwise until more proof of overall benefits is available.

Vitamin B$_6$. Taking 500 milligrams, or 250 times the RDA, of vitamin B$_6$ for any period of time can cause nerve damage; a tenth of that may cause other problems.

Iron. Large doses of iron can be toxic, even fatal. Each year, young children die after swallowing their parents' iron pills. The sweet coating formerly applied to make the pills more palatable has now been banned by law. Remember, too, that high doses of other supplements, such as vitamin C, can increase your absorption of iron.

Pills Versus Food:
Which Sources to Choose

Many nutritionists and major national health organizations insist that people can get all the nutrients they need from diet alone. "We do not advocate supplements," states Carolyn Clifford, Ph.D., chief of the Diet and Cancer Branch in the Division of Cancer Prevention and Control at the National Institutes of Health.

Others argue that while this may be true in theory, it's not reality for most Americans. The much-maligned American diet, while improving, remains overburdened with fat, salt, and sugar, and conspicuously lacking in vitamin-rich fruits and vegetables.

Ask a trusted doctor whether he or she regularly takes supplements, either multivitamins or a specific combination. The answer may very well be yes. Then ask whether he or she routinely recommends the same protocol to patients. Probably not. Whatever their private convictions, many doctors remain concerned that people will allow pills to take the place of a high-quality, low-fat diet.

The bottom line is this: The ideal course is to eat plenty of the fruits and vegetables that supply not only vitamins and minerals, but all the other phytochemicals we're learning to love. If you're not doing that, at least give yourself the more limited benefits of a well-balanced supplement (see the nearby box on "Tips for Choosing a Supplement").

Calculating Your Own Requirements

The Recommended Dietary Allowance (RDA) for vitamins and minerals as set by the federal government reflects the level of intake deemed *adequate* for most healthy people. Following the RDAs will prevent severe deficiency diseases, such as scurvy from lack of vitamin C and rickets from lack of vitamin D. However, there are certain situations in which more than the RDA may be called for. Many experts insist that the RDA can't cover everyday needs for everyone in this country at this time. (Supplements packaged after July 1995 must use an equivalent term, DV, for Daily Value, instead of RDA.)

Older People

People in their later years often eat inadequately, commonly missing out on important nutrients that a multivitamin/mineral would supply. For example, older people have less water in their bodies, so their level of water-soluble vitamins is lower, says James Scala, Ph.D., author of *Prescription for Longevity: Eating Right for a Long Life*. Because the absorption of nutrients declines accordingly, it may be wise for older people with less than optimal diets to increase the dose of certain vitamins and minerals as the years go

TIPS FOR CHOOSING A SUPPLEMENT

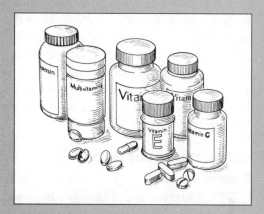

Shop wisely; some manufacturers make extraordinary claims for products that are ordinary or worse.

What to buy:

Because vitamin/mineral supplements are such a goldmine for hucksters, you're better off sticking with name brands from large, reputable companies. However, don't hesitate to comparison shop. Store brands offered by major chains such as Wal-Mart, K Mart, and Safeway are often identical to the national brands, and may be much cheaper. A 1994 survey by Consumer Reports showed price differences of up to fourfold for essentially the same products.

"USP," (for U. S. Pharmacopeia, an independent organization that sets standards for the purity and potency of drugs), on the label indicates that the contents will disintegrate (but not necessarily dissolve) promptly in your stomach. Some companies, including reputable ones, disapprove of USP testing methods.

If you have trouble digesting tablets, often the case for people over 60, consider capsules, available in health food stores. In whatever form, supplements should contain 100 percent of the RDA for at least the vitamins and minerals listed in the accompanying table. (Some people argue that because calcium can inhibit the body's absorption of iron, the two minerals shouldn't be contained in the same supplement.)

Be skeptical of high-priced special formulations. For instance, "stress-formula" vitamins were originally designed to help victims of extreme physical stress, such as burns or serious illnesses. Also watch the price of antioxidant formulas. It may be cheaper to take a standard multivitamin and buy beta-carotene, vitamin C, and vitamin E separately.

Be especially wary of unsolicited offers to sell you vitamins by phone. This is a fertile field for entrepreneurs of dubious reputability. Among the products and services sold through telemarketing, nearly one in five is a vitamin product.

Buying in bulk, such as during sales or from mailorder companies, may save money. But don't do it until you've tried one jar, even if it costs more that way. You may find that the product contains an additive (color or flavor) that disagrees with you.

Make sure that the expiration date doesn't extend beyond your ability to use up the contents. (If you can't read the label, reject the product.) As supplements age, their potency decreases, so keeping them around too long is no bargain. Furthermore, according to the Center for Science in the Public Interest, manufacturers can select expiration dates arbitrarily. A supplement that will expire in 9 months or less may have been on the shelf for years.

Chemical additives are never desirable, although they appear in many acceptable multivitamin products. A little starch may actually help the tablets disintegrate, while a tiny amount of sugar may make the pill taste less bitter.

Calcium. A multivitamin/mineral supplement may provide as little as 15 percent of the daily requirement. For more, choose a calcium supplement: 500 to 1,000 milligrams, usually in more than one tablet or capsule. Choose calcium citrate or calcium carbonate. Bone meal and dolomite (calcium magnesium carbonate) may contain lead or other heavy metals.

Iron. Because women have been told that they need more iron, especially during menstruation, you may jump at the chance to have more than 100 percent of the RDA—but don't. Only under the advice of your doctor should you have more than 18 milligrams a day. After menopause, when iron is no longer being lost with menstrual blood, it may be wise to take less than 100 percent of the RDA. Ask your doctor what is best for you.

Vitamin E. Many people take supplemental vitamin E because getting enough dietary vitamin E to yield the terrific effects that research has been tentatively uncovering—improving immunity and lowering the risk of heart disease, cataracts, and some cancers—would load your diet with fat and calories. Many experts advise buying the natural form, made from vegetable oil. (This is the only vitamin for which "natural" may possibly beat "synthetic.") Don't be deceived by the word "natural" on the label. Keep reading until you see d-alpha (not dl-alpha) tocopherol or tocopheryl. (Consumer Reports disagrees, claiming the distinction is unimportant.) The word "acetate" or "succinate" after that designation means the vitamin is more biologically active . . . fine, but not crucial. Typical daily supplement: 100 to 400 IU.

Vitamin C. The body can use or store only so much at a time and releases the rest, unused, in the urine. A typical daily supplement is 100 to 500 milligrams. If you take more, consider splitting up the dose—500 milligrams twice a day, for example—or buying the more expensive timed-release kind. Chewable vitamin C tablets can dissolve tooth enamel by increasing acid in the mouth. Swallow them. More than 4,000 milligrams a day can cause diarrhea and increase the risk of kidney stones or liver disease.

Take supplements with meals. Without a little fat (the equivalent of about a teaspoon of margarine), the body can't absorb beta-carotene and vitamins A, D, and E.

What Your Multivitamin/Mineral Should Contain

100% of RDA for Vitamins and Minerals Assigned RDAs

Vitamin A, preferably all as beta-carotene (5,000 IU)
Vitamin B$_6$ (2 milligrams)
Vitamin B$_{12}$ (6 micrograms)
Vitamin D (400 IU)
Folic acid[1] (0.4 milligrams)
Thiamin (1.5 milligrams)
Riboflavin (1.7 milligrams)
Pantothenic acid (10 milligrams)
Niacin (20 milligrams)
Copper[2] (2 milligrams)
Zinc[2] (15 milligrams)

100% or Less of RDA

Iron: Women after menopause and all men, 0 to 9 milligrams (0% to 50% of RDA) Women before menopause, especially those who bleed heavily and/or eat little or no meat, 18 milligrams (100% of RDA)

Magnesium: 100 to 400 milligrams (25% to 100% of RDA); but no more than 400 milligrams, to avoid diarrhea. This mineral is needed to prevent high blood pressure. However, if you have kidney disease you should check with your doctor before taking a supplement.

100% or More of RDA

Vitamin E: 100 to 400 IU (RDA is 30 IU)
Vitamin C: 1,000 to 3,000 milligrams (RDA is 60 milligrams)

Vitamins and Minerals Without RDAs

Chromium: 50 to 200 micrograms
Selenium: 50 to 200 micrograms

1. Older men and women should consider a product containing less than 50% of the RDA for folic acid. More than that could mask a severe deficiency of vitamin B12 leading to pernicious anemia, a dangerous blood disorder.

2. A product that contains zinc should also contain copper. Raising zinc levels without doing the same for copper can lead to a copper deficiency. Since copper is an oxidant, however, it should never be taken in amounts higher than the RDA.

on. According to Scala, you can consider taking as much as 800 IU a day of vitamin E, for example, go up to 3,000 milligrams of vitamin C, and take 25,000 IU of beta-carotene.

For other nutrients, the reverse is true. After about age 60, iron builds an "inventory" in the body for both men and women. Too much iron after that time can increase the risk of heart disease. For more on the dietary adjustments to consider in your later years, see Chapter 20.

Women's Special Needs

Women need more of certain nutrients at various points in their life. Three of the best examples are calcium to combat the bone loss that accompanies aging, iron to replace what is lost during menstruation, and a wide range of extra vitamins and minerals to ensure a healthy pregnancy.

Calcium. It takes a lot of calcium to prevent brittle bones (osteoporosis), which affects more than 25 million Americans, most of them women. Yet most American women get only about half the amount they need. By taking extra calcium, older women can help compensate for the bone loss that occurs with the departure of estrogen during menopause. However, the best time to build bone mass is much, much earlier. In fact, the buildup should start in childhood, since bone mass reaches 95 percent of its maximum density by age 18. After menopause, extra calcium is needed to protect the bone that remains, but it won't increase bone strength for the future.

While it's not yet certain, calcium may also help prevent colon cancer in men and

HOW MUCH CALCIUM DO YOU NEED?

Recommended daily calcium requirements were increased by experts at a National Institutes of Health conference in June 1994:

Group and Age	Daily Milligrams of Calcium
Infants	
Birth to 6 months	400
6 months to 1 year	600
Children	
1 to 5 years	800
6 to 10 years	800 to 1,200
Adolescents and Young Adults	
11 to 24 years	1,200 to 1,500
Men	
25 to 64 years	1,000
65 and over	1,500
Women	
25 years to menopause	1,000
Menopause to age 64	
Taking estrogens	1,000
Not taking estrogens	1,500
65 and over	1,500
Pregnant, breastfeeding	1,200 to 1,500

women alike. Researchers believe that when calcium encounters potentially cancer-causing fats in the bowel, the two materials combine, creating a harmless substance.

Calcium is found in many foods besides dairy products. Some examples are: figs, oatmeal, navy beans, and the all-purpose broccoli. Look for calcium-fortified foods, too. One cup of calcium-fortified orange juice contains the same amount of calcium as a cup of milk—about 300 milligrams.

If you take calcium supplements, the best way is to split them up over the day. If you're taking 1,000 milligrams a day, take one 500 milligram pill at breakfast and another at dinner, to keep calcium reserves building all night. Taking them separately also increases the total amount absorbed by the body and is less likely to cause constipation. Calcium carbonate is a little more likely than calcium citrate to cause constipation in some people, although most can digest either.

Don't take your calcium pill just before or after eating high-fiber wheat bran cereal, because the fiber can impede calcium absorption. If you take iron as well as calcium, don't take them together, since the calcium can inhibit the body's absorption of iron. Do, however, take vitamin D with your calcium—many calcium supplements contain both—because the body can't absorb calcium without it.

Any time your doctor prescribes a new medication, ask how it will interact with any vitamin and mineral supplements you take regularly. Taking calcium at the same time as tetracycline, for example, can prevent the antibiotic from working to its fullest capacity. If you have ever had kidney stones, you should ask your doctor whether it's safe to take calcium at all.

To figure out how much extra calcium you need, find the appropriate total daily dose in the nearby table "How Much Calcium Do You Need?". If you take a multivitamin, subtract the amount of calcium in the multi you take. Then subtract 300 milligrams for every serving of dairy products (yogurt, milk, cheese) you eat or calcium-fortified orange juice you drink on an average day. You may well find that you're already getting enough, or that a minor change in your diet will fully meet your needs.

Iron. The body needs iron to manufacture red blood cells, which contain hemoglobin, the protein that carries oxygen to other cells all over the body. Yet women lose iron each month in their menstrual blood, and ten percent actually have an iron deficiency every month. Don't take more iron supplements than multivitamins contain without your doctor's permission. To boost iron intake naturally, eat plenty of kidney beans, dried fruit, pumpkin seeds, and spinach. Liver contains iron, too, but should be eaten in moderation because it is high in cholesterol.

Since vitamin C increases iron absorption, swallow your iron pill with a glass of orange or grapefruit juice. Caffeine *decreases* iron absorption, though, so hold off on coffee, tea, cocoa, or cola.

Folic acid. One of the few absolute musts among a woman's vitamins is folic acid, also called folate or folacin. During pregnancy, folic acid is essential to the proper development of the baby. Without it, a baby may be born with severe birth defects of the brain and spinal cord. (See Chapter 16 "The Changes to Make When You're Pregnant"). According to the U.S. Department of Health and Human Services, the number of cases of neural tube defects in newborns would be halved if all women of reproductive age took 400 micrograms (0.4 milligrams) of folic acid a day. Don't wait until you know you're pregnant. Having folic acid in your body during the first few weeks of pregnancy, before you know you're pregnant, is crucial. Folic acid deficiency can also make women anemic, whether they're pregnant or not.

Zinc. Because the need for zinc increases during pregnancy, and many women don't get enough zinc anyway, doctors often recommend that pregnant women take a multivitamin containing the RDA of zinc. Healthy skin and the ability of wounds to heal require zinc as well.

Vitamin B$_6$. If you are pregnant, you will probably also need to take more B$_6$ since a developing baby can easily drain maternal stores of this vitamin.

Other Special Nutritional Needs

- People who are lactose intolerant—that is, unable to digest dairy products—may have to take calcium supplements.
- Very-low-calorie dieters may need extra vitamins and minerals, particularly iron, calcium, and vitamin B$_6$.
- Vegetarians may be deficient in iron and zinc, both of which are more easily absorbed from animal sources than from plants.
- Total vegetarians who eat no eggs or dairy products may have to take supplements of vitamin B$_{12}$, calcium, and vitamin D in order to get their RDA. Each is available from few sources other than animal and dairy products.
- Between October and March when daylight hours are shorter, it's almost impossible for anyone to get enough vitamin D except in the South or Southwest. Few home-bound invalids of any age get enough vitamin D from the sun year-round.
- Anyone who regularly takes anticoagulant drugs (blood thinners), including aspirin, should not take supplements of vitamin E. The combination of too much vitamin E and an anticoagulant can interfere with clotting. Talk to your doctor before mixing this or any vitamin or mineral supplement with medications.

- People who smoke, who are under great emotional or physical stress, or who have other health problems benefit greatly from extra boosts of antioxidants, especially vitamin C. "Ultra-athletes" who exercise extensively can become deficient in vitamin C as well, according to Dr. Kenneth H. Cooper, president and founder of the Cooper Aerobics Center in Dallas and the author of *Dr. Kenneth H. Cooper's Antioxidant Revolution.*
- Children, too, have special requirements. For details, turn to Chapter 18, "What's Right—and Wrong—for the Kids."

Proteins, Fats, and Carbohydrates

The major building blocks of everything we eat, the proteins, carbohydrates, and—yes—fats are all vital for health. Proteins are the raw material of every cell in our bodies. Carbohydrates are the body's main source of fuel. Fats serve as a high-capacity store house of energy, while supplying us with certain absolutely essential chemicals. If you somehow managed to completely eliminate any one of these three critical nutrients, you would die. The question around which much nutritional research revolves is not *whether* we need these nutrients, but rather in what proportions they do the most good.

PLANTS RICH IN PROTEIN

- Legumes (lentils, peas, dried beans, peanuts, soybeans)
- Seeds (sesame, sunflower)
- Nuts (cashews, almonds, walnuts, pecans)
- Whole grains (barley, bulgur, cornmeal, oats, rice, whole wheat)

What They Are

Proteins are composed of smaller units called amino acids. Our bodies can manufacture most of these acids, but nine are available only from the food we eat. Meat, poultry, fish, eggs, and dairy products such as milk and cheese are all concentrated sources of protein. It can be found in many plants, too; but you should know that in order to get all the necessary amino acids from plants, certain varieties must be eaten with others (rice served with beans, for example).

Infants, children, pregnant and breastfeeding women, and the elderly all need more protein than other people. Getting too little protein can lead to stunted growth, reduced immunity to disease, and lack of energy. When protein intake drops too low for too long, the body steals protein from muscle and other tissue.

In America, most people have the opposite problem. They eat almost twice as much as the recommended 50 grams a day (a piece of meat or chicken the size of the palm of a hand). Any excess protein you take in is immediately burned as energy or converted to fat. Because the body can't store proteins in their original form, they must be eaten every day.

Fats. The "fats" (lipids) that float through the bloodstream supply back-up energy for the body and help produce compounds that regulate blood pressure, blood clotting, and inflammation. Riding in the lipids are the fat-soluble vitamins A, D, E, and K, traveling through the body to perform their own crucial functions. It's fairly difficult to develop a fat deficiency: The equivalent of a tablespoon of olive oil a day is enough for all our needs.

Fat is a problem for most of us because every gram contains more than double the calories of the same amount of protein or carbohydrate. Since the average American diet gets more than 35 percent of its calories from fat—a little less than it used to, but still more than the 30 percent maximum that nutritionists recommend—calories are piling on. A recent Gallup poll indicated that a large majority of Americans are overweight, as walking down almost any street will tell you. Worse yet, in Western countries where a high proportion of daily calories comes from fat, (Americans eat eight times the needed daily amount) people have much higher rates of cancer of the breast, endometrium, prostate, colon, and pancreas than in countries where people eat modest amounts of fat (see Chapter 10, "What to Do About Fat"). This could be a coincidence, but experts haven't ruled out a possible link.

Carbohydrates. The body's main source of energy, carbohydrates come in two forms, simple and complex.

Simple carbohydrates (sugars) are found in many forms and under many names, including fructose, lactose, and sucrose. Natural sugars appear in fruit, milk, honey, and maple syrup. Refined sugars, such as table sugar, have been stripped of other nutrients, retaining little more than their calories. Often found in foods that are loaded with fat and calories, such as desserts, refined sugars contribute little to your health, but can add a lot to your weight.

Complex carbohydrates (starches), which must be split apart before they're absorbed, provide a more lasting source of energy than sugar. As an important dividend, the foods they're found in are loaded with vitamins and minerals. Complex carbohydrates are found in starchy vegetables (potatoes, corn, beans, peas), pasta, rice, some fruits, and whole grains, including whole-grain breads and cereals.

Seeking the Right Balance

Among the problems a low-fat, high-fiber diet can help fend off are heart disease, obesity, diabetes, and certain types of cancer. Remember that current recommendations make carbohydrates (especially complex carbohydrates) the centerpiece of good nutrition. Every day, we should all be eating 6 to 11 servings of grains (bread, cereal, rice, pasta), 3 to 5 servings of vegetables (raw, cooked, leafy, or juice), and 2 to 4 servings of fruit (raw, cooked, or juice).

Because what's officially counted as a "serving" may be much less than you'd put on your plate, servings can add up quickly. For example, one serving of bread is one slice; therefore, a sandwich contains two servings. One large baked potato counts as two or three servings of a vegetable. Half a cup of a cooked vegetable—not very much— is a serving. Since a medium banana provides one serving of fruit, a large one contains about a serving and a half. For the best foods to seek out, see the box on "Some Outstanding Sources of Carbohydrates."

Recent findings have debunked the notion that carbohydrates can be eaten in limitless amounts without adding much weight. In moderation, pasta remains a power food, especially if it's all or part whole wheat or made with vegetables such as spinach. But even a high-carbohydrate, low-fat diet will put on extra pounds if it's too high in calories. You should be particularly calorie-conscious if you're part of the 25 percent of

the U.S. population that overproduces insulin after eating sugar or starches.

Here's how everyone's daily intake of calories should break down after the age of two (infants' bodies use fat and cholesterol to build bones, muscles, and brains):

- 50 to 60 percent from carbohydrates,
- No more than 30 percent from fat (preferably much less) after age 2, and
- The rest from protein (10 to 20 percent).

SOME OUTSTANDING SOURCES OF CARBOHYDRATES

Fruits

Berries
Cantaloupes
Citrus fruits
Watermelons
Apricots

Vegetables

Cabbage
   (see also "The Potent Cruciferous Vegetables")
Carrots
Broccoli
Potatoes
Dried beans
Sweet potatoes
Spinach

Whole Grains and Whole-Grain Products

Oatmeal
Whole-wheat pasta
Bran
Bread

The Link with Cholesterol

The tendency of cholesterol to build up inside some people's arteries, thus leading to heart disease, is by now one of the best known facts in nutrition. Less well known is the fact that for the majority of the population, this doesn't happen enough to lead to problems. Nevertheless, since doctors can't tell whether or not cholesterol will affect you, the safest course is to keep your total blood cholesterol level below 200 milligrams per deciliter.

Cholesterol is most abundant in eggs and organ meats such as liver. However, eating animal fats also tends to raise cholesterol levels. That means keeping certain foods to a minimum and eating others in different forms. Instead of merely trimming the fat off red meat, for example, eat smaller portions less frequently. Switch to skim milk, which contains far less fat and cholesterol than any other kind. Downright fatty foods, such as richly marbled steaks and pizza dripping with grease, are best avoided altogether.

Fiber can help to remove excess cholesterol from the blood. Substituting olive oil for other types of fat also seems to help. Getting plenty of calcium, niacin, and vitamins C and E in foods and supplements reduces cholesterol levels as well.

The Better Side of Fat

Some of the elements in certain types of fat—the fatty acids—work together to promote health and growth. They come in "families" or series that vary according to where they're found.

Omega-3 fatty acids help build potent hormonelike substances. They're also vital for brain and eye development and may reduce the risk of heart attacks by preventing blood cells from sticking to the insides of blood vessels and building up as plaque. This family of fatty acids is derived from alpha-linolenic acid (ALA) and includes eicosapentaenoic acid (EPA), and docasahexaenoic acid (DHA). *What to eat:* Canola, flaxseed, and rapeseed oils, green plants, tree nuts (such as walnuts and almonds), and especially deep-water fish (salmon, tuna, mackerel, herring, shrimp), approximately 3 to 6 ounces two or three times a week. Fish oil supplements are not recommended.

Omega-6 fatty acids start with linoleic acid, from which gamma linoleic acid (GLA) and arachidonic acid (AA) are derived. A precursor to hormonlike chemicals known as prostaglandins, linoleic acid is called "essential" because it can't be synthesized from other nutrients in the body and must be obtained from food or supplements. It maintains the health of the skin and hair. *What to eat:* Corn, soybean, and other vegetable oils; foods that include those oils as an ingredient, ranging from bread to salad dressing; oils from seeds; beef, milk, and other products from animals that eat corn and grain.

Omega-9 fatty acids may help prevent breast cancer, according to recent studies. *What to eat:* Olive oil.

Fiber

Fiber (what used to be known as roughage) is the part of fruits, vegetables, whole grains, and bran that passes through the body without being digested. As it is carried through the digestive system and out of the body, fiber maintains health and lowers the risk of a number of diseases and conditions, probably including colorectal and perhaps other types of cancer. For sources of fiber, see the box "Not Just From Bran: Your Broad Choice of Fiber Sources."

Fiber is divided into two major types, soluble and insoluble. Fruits and vegetables contain a mixture of the two, although one usually predominates in any given food.

Soluble Fiber

This type of fiber is dissolved by water in the body. It's the sticky part of plants—like sap from trees. Soluble fiber is found in foods such as legumes (peas, peanuts, and lentils, for example), whole grains (barley, oats), some fruits (prunes, pears, apples), and many vegetables (broccoli, cabbages, carrots). Beans and oat bran are particularly good at clearing out the digestive system by softening bowel movements and stimulating the digestive tract to expel them. Oat bran can be bought in bulk and baked into bread and muffins or added to other foods, such as meat loaf or "veggie burgers."

Benefits of soluble fiber:

- It moderates the levels of glucose in the blood, important for everyone, and vital for diabetics.
- It tends to lower the levels of cholesterol in the blood, helping to prevent heart disease. Eating 2 ounces of oat bran or 3 ounces of oatmeal every day may lower blood levels of LDL ("bad") cholesterol by up to 5 percent.

Insoluble Fiber

This variety passes through the gastrointestinal tract in more or less its original form. Excellent sources include nuts, seeds, brown rice, unpeeled vegetables, whole-grain cereals (hot or cold) and baked goods, legumes, fruits, and especially wheat bran. A fine fiber-filled lunch: A bowl of pea soup with peanut butter spread on a high-fiber cracker.

Benefits of insoluble fiber:

- It makes bowel movements bulkier, helping to prevent constipation, hemorrhoids, and diverticulosis.
- It may lower the risk of colorectal cancer. Especially effective: raw wheat bran.

Both kinds of fiber make you feel full longer, controlling overeating and overweight.

How Much Fiber

American diets typically include only about half the fiber they should. Aim for at least 20 to 30 grams a day—a little less than an ounce. A high-fiber diet contains 25 grams of fiber for every 2,000 calories eaten. To obtain all the benefits that fiber has to offer, eat a

NOT JUST FROM BRAN: YOUR BROAD CHOICE OF FIBER SOURCES

You shouldn't have trouble adding fiber to your diet, considering that your options range from popcorn to prunes and from almonds to cabbage. The main reason many people associate fiber with bran is a series of successful advertising campaigns for breakfast cereals and bran muffins, which hit the media as soon as studies started suggesting that fiber could help prevent breast and colon cancers.

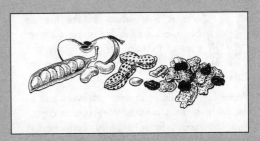

The table shows the amounts of dietary fiber in some fiber-rich foods. Dietary fiber is the total fiber content of the food. For instance, to get maximum fiber from oranges and apples eat the fruit whole; the juice alone has little fiber. Likewise, don't boil your vegetables into oblivion; this will allow vitamins and minerals to dissipate into the water and air. Wash, but don't peel, that baked potato.

Dietary Fiber,	in grams
Breads and Cereals	
Bran flakes, 3/4 cup	4.0
Raisin bran, 3/4 cup	4.0
Whole-wheat spaghetti, 1 cup	3.9
Wheat germ, plain, 1/4 cup	3.4
Bran muffin, 1 muffin	2.5
Oatmeal, cooked, 3/4 cup	1.6
Whole-wheat bread, 1 slice	1.4
Spaghetti, regular, 1 cup	1.1
Popcorn, air-popped, 1 cup	1.0
Rice, brown, 1/2 cup	1.0
White bread, 1 slice	0.4
Rice, white, 1/2 cup	0.2
Fruits	
Apple, 1 med.	3.5
Pear, 1/2 lg.	3.1
Strawberries, 1 cup	3.0
Prunes, dried, 3 prunes	3.0
Orange, 1 med.	2.6
Banana, 1 med.	2.4
Blueberries, 1/2 cup	2.0
Grapefruit, 1/2	1.6
Orange juice, 1/2 cup	0.5
Apple juice, 1/2 cup	0.4

Dietary Fiber,	in grams
Vegetables	
Peas, green, 1/2 cup	3.6
Corn, 1/2 cup	2.9
Potato, with skin, 1 med.	2.5
Brussels sprouts, 1/2 cup	2.3
Carrots, 1/2 cup	2.3
Broccoli, 1/2 cup	2.2
Sweet potato, 1/2 med.	1.7
Green beans, 1/2 cup	1.6
Bean sprouts (soy), 1/2 cup	1.5
Tomato, 1 med.	1.5
Kale, 1/2 cup	1.4
Cabbage, 1/2 cup	1.4
Summer squash, 1/2 cup	1.4
Spinach, raw, 1 cup	1.2
Celery, 1/2 cup	1.1
Lettuce, shredded, 1 cup	0.9
Onions, sliced, 1/2 cup	0.8
Legumes	
Kidney beans, 1/2 cup	7.3
Navy beans, 1/2 cup	6.0
Lima beans, 1/2 cup	4.5
Lentils, 1/2 cup	3.7
Nuts	
Peanuts, 10 nuts	1.4
Almonds, 10 nuts	1.1

Adapted from NIH Publication 87-2878, May 1987

WATER, THE FORGOTTEN FOOD

Water is everywhere in the human body, accounting for about 60 percent of its total weight. Totally deprived of water, we can survive for little more than days.

Water is the main component of every cell in the body. It plays a mandatory role in digestion, absorption, circulation, and elimination. It even helps the body regulate its temperature. Water keeps the mucous membranes of the nose, mouth, throat, lungs, and other areas moist. It washes food through the digestive system from beginning to end. It carries water-soluble vitamins and fiber around the bloodstream. It carries waste products away from the cells and out of the body.

We lose water constantly through perspiration, urine, sneezes, and even the tears that bathe our eyes and eyelids to keep them moist. No wonder the body's water has to be replenished all the time.

Drinking eight 8-ounce glasses of water every day (whether you feel thirsty or not), and more in hot weather, maintains the level your body needs. During exercise, take regular water breaks. Alcohol and beverages that contain caffeine increase urination, decreasing the amount of water in the body.

variety of foods that are rich in it. Avoid fiber supplements; you're much better off with the real thing, since you'll gain all the other health benefits that fiber-rich foods can offer.

Here's how whole grains make the difference. A slice of whole-wheat bread contains 1.4 grams of fiber, three and a half times more than a slice of white bread. Half a cup of brown rice contains a gram of fiber, five times more than the same amount of white rice. A cup of whole-wheat spaghetti contains 3.9 grams of fiber, more than three times as much as a cup of regular spaghetti. One easy way to get more fiber is to sprinkle three tablespoons of raw wheat bran on your food during the course of each day.

To prevent gas and diarrhea, increase the amount of fiber in your diet slowly. Drinking six to eight large (8-ounce) glasses of water every day will help the fiber move through your digestive system painlessly (see the box on "Water, the Forgotten Food"). □

CHAPTER 3

Health or Hype?
The Lowdown on
Natural Food

No preservatives, no pesticides, no additives, just pure whole food, the way nature intended. Sounds ideal, doesn't it? In practice, though, this "nutritional paradise" can be expensive and hard to find. Worse yet, in many cases it turns out that there's no strong evidence for the superiority of health foods over standard supermarket fare.

That doesn't mean that going natural for part or all of your diet isn't a valid choice. You might wish to purchase organic or health food products to spice up your dinner table or to make substituting grains for meat a bit more palatable. Some people buy organic products out of concern for the environment. Others simply prefer the taste of natural foods and grains such as quinoa or couscous. Whatever the reason for it, however, your choice of organic or all-natural food won't automatically make your diet healthier than it would be otherwise.

The fact is, you simply can't assume that everything sold at a health food store is better than what you can get at the supermarket, or that labels announcing a product is "natural" or "organic" mean that it's healthier. There are no federal definitions for those words and state regulations vary.

Both health food and conventional products have their pluses and minuses; which is best for you depends on your dietary goal. Do you want to reduce fat? Cut salt? Avoid artificial additives and pesticides? Eat less sugar and sweets? Read the small print on the label to see how each food stacks up. Health or natural foods may not be processed, for example, but could contain as much fat, sugar, or contaminants as their conventional counterparts.

Years ago, if you wanted to buy health food—a catch-all term for natural food, whole food, food grown organically, and food without additives, waxes, hormones, antibiotics or pesticides—you would usually have to shop in special health food stores or small, natural-food sections of certain supermarkets. In most regions of the country, that is no longer the case. Because of increased public interest in—and demand for—these foods, many more supermarkets are carrying them. Be cautious, however. It's often hard to distinguish them from more processed, additive-laden foods and they generally cost more. What you buy is always more important than where you buy it.

And what, exactly, should you buy? The key is to evaluate the caloric, fat, sugar, and salt content of each food, and to consider whether you are sensitive to any of its additives.

Supermarket Versus Health Food Store

If you sometimes shop at your local health food store, you are far from alone. The trade publication *Health Foods Business* estimates that in 1991 there were about 7,300 health food stores in the U.S. with total sales of $3.9 billion. Natural foods are becoming increasingly mainstream.

Many healthfood products moved to traditional stores when mainstream firms bought natural food companies, and today's health-conscious shopper can find most of his or her needs on ordinary supermarket shelves. As the big food conglomerates snap up more and more small natural food manufacturers, former "health foods" are becoming a major presence everywhere. That's how rice cakes and fruit-juice sweetened preserves, for example, became grocery-store regulars.

With less processed, additive-free, organic food now featured in most supermarkets,

ARE BROWN EGGS BETTER?

Some health food fans believe that brown eggs are healthier than white. Actually, shell color varies with species and breed of poultry, and has no effect on nutritional value.

natural food stores serve primarily as a source of variety. If your goal is to cut down on fat, sugar, and salt, you usually can find what you need in your local supermarket at a more reasonable price than elsewhere. But if you want wider selection of whole grain breads or harder-to-find products like bulgur or miso (fermented soy paste), a specialty store is still your best bet.

Natural food stores may also outshine supermarkets in terms of their willingness to obtain products for customers' special needs and their knowledge of unusual goods. But be wary of advice from health food store employees. While some clerks suggest that customers see their physician for serious medical problems, others are not so ethical. In 1989, volunteers of the Consumer Health Education Council in Houston surveyed 41 health food stores, asking about remedies for a fictitious HIV-infected brother. No less than 30 retailers reportedly claimed to carry products that would cure AIDS. Remember that employees may not be unbiased; always question what you hear.

"Natural" Best Bets

Remember, "natural" has no standard legal definition, and "natural" food is not necessarily healthy anyway. "Natural" foods may contain additives and be as high in sugar and fat as similar supermarket products. Natural frozen desserts, such as Ben & Jerry's Ice Cream, may be free of artificial ingredients but still be high in fat.

To be "natural" a food should be minimally processed and should contain no artificial additives or preservatives. By choosing such foods, you can avoid the extra fat, sodium, sugar, and additives generally used in processing. Some additives, such as sulfites, do pose hazards for some people. However, most do not; and aside from additives, no natural food has special health-promoting properties beyond its nutrients.

Which "Natural" Foods are Better than Processed?

Whole grain or enriched products are much more nutritious than refined versions and usually are no more expensive. For example, converted or refined white rice contains few of the nutrients present in brown rice. Precooked rice not only lacks many of its original nutrients, but is much more expensive in the bargain than unprocessed rice and much less nutritious. (See box on Grading the Grains.) The same is true of speciality breads. Enriched French or Italian breads cost up to three times more than whole grain bread with similar or better nutrition value.

In the cereal aisle, the situation is more complex. Many popular cereals have added nutrients and some offer 100% of the Recommended Daily Allowance—usually at a premium price. If your diet is adequate, however, this costly enrichment is unnecessary. On the other hand, some "natural" granola cereals, while free of unneeded enrichment, contain far more sugar and saturated fat than their processed counterparts. For example, 1/4 cup of Quaker 100% Natural

Granola cereal packs an average of 7 grams of sugar, 5 grams of fat, and 2 grams of fiber. One cup of General Mills Total or Wheaties beats Quaker on all counts, with 3 grams of sugar, 1 gram of fat, and 3 grams of fiber. However, there are some health food products that are both better and no more costly. Although Kellogg's Low-Fat Granola is lower in fat than most granolas, Health Valley Fat-Free Granola sells for about the same price, but has no fat at all. (See box on "The Best for Breakfast.")

Plant proteins such as grains, beans, nuts, and peas offer a low-fat, meatless way to get some needed protein. For instance, any of these trendy grain products can help you cut the fat in your diet while contributing to your protein requirements:

Amaranth: When cooked, amaranth has a slightly crunchy porridge texture with a corn flavor. Try it for breakfast topped with maple syrup. It looks like golden poppy seeds.

THE CURRENT WORD ON OAT BRAN. . .

If you have been wolfing down fiber-laden oat bran muffins every morning in hopes that your cholesterol will drop, maybe it's time to stop. In early 1990, researchers found that oat bran failed to lower cholesterol of young women. Among the foods studied:

- 1.25 cups cooked oat bran,
- 1.66 cups cooked oatmeal,
- 3.75 cups Cheerios,
- 10 slices of oatmeal bread,
- 4 granola bars.

By itself, all this oat bran reduces cholesterol by so small a percentage (five percent or less) that it is hardly worth the effort. Filling up on bran *will* cut your cholesterol level if it leaves no room for other, fattier foods. But it won't reverse the effects of a cholesterol-rich diet.

GRADING THE GRAINS

The Center For Science in the Public Interest (CSPI) calculated a "score" for each grain by adding up its percent of the U.S. Recommended Daily Allowance (RDA) for five nutrients plus fiber. There is no RDA for fiber, so CSPI used the new Daily Value (DV), of 25 grams.

For example, a five-ounce serving of quinoa has 9 percent of the DV for fiber (9 points), and 20 percent of the RDA for magnesium (20 points), 4 percent for vitamin B_6 (4 points), 8 percent for zinc (8 points), 14 percent for copper (14 points), and 18 percent for iron (18 points). That adds up to a score of 73.

Potatoes and pastas are included for comparison. Pastas are made from grains, and are quite healthy. The ten grains with the highest scores are CSPI's "Best Bites." Grains are ranked from highest to lowest score. Potatoes and pastas are not considered in awarding the "Best Bite" title.

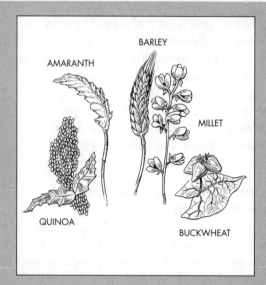

Grain (5 ounces, cooked)	Score	Fiber	Magnesium	B_6	Zinc	Copper	Iron
Potato, with skin	81	▲	●	▲	—	▲	▲
■ Quinoa[1]	73	●	▲	—	●	▲	▲
Macaroni or Spaghetti, whole wheat	69	▲	▲	●	●	▲	●
■ Amaranth[1]	66	▲	▲	—	●	▲	▲
■ Buckwheat groats[2]	64	▲	▲	●	●	▲	●
Spaghetti, spinach	61	na	▲	●	▲	▲	●
■ Bulgur	60	▲	▲	●	●	●	●

Barley: Individual grains look like smooth pearls. Barley is usually refined and is not sold as whole grain.

Bulgur: These tan-colored granules of cooked, dried, and crushed wheat have a nutty flavor. Bulgur keeps well when stored in a cool place inside a porous container; its food value is equal to that of whole wheat. Use it like rice: in broth, for example, or with black beans and corn.

Couscous: Sometimes called Middle Eastern pasta, these tiny yellow granules of finely cracked wheat have the texture of rice. Sales of this popular grain have more than doubled in recent years.

Grain (5 ounces, cooked)	Score	Fiber	Magnesium	B_6	Zinc	Copper	Iron
■ Barley, pearled²	59	▲	●	●	●	●	▲
■ Wild rice²	58	▲	▲	▲	▲	●	●
■ Millet	53	●	▲	●	●	▲	●
■ Brown rice	51	▲	▲	▲	●	●	—
■ Triticale¹	47	▲	▲	—	●	●	—
Spaghetti	42	▲	●	—	●	●	▲
■ Wheat berries¹	41	▲	●	—	●	●	●
Macaroni	39	●	●	—	●	●	▲
Kamut¹	37	na	▲	—	●	●	●
Oats, rolled	33	▲	●	—	●	—	●
Spelt¹	33	▲	▲	na	na	—	●
White rice, converted	26	—	—	—	—	●	●
Couscous	23	●	—	—	—	—	—
White rice, instant	18	—	—	—	—	●	●
Soba noodles	12	na	—	—	—	—	—
Corn grits	10	—	—	—	—	—	●

Key
■ "Best Bite"
▲ contains at least 10 percent of the RDA
● contains between 5 and 9 percent of the RDA
— contains less than 5 percent of the RDA
na not available.

Footnotes
¹ score is based on USDA estimates of all nutrients.
² fiber value is a USDA estimate.

Millet: Often used as a tasty base for meat or vegetarian chili, millet has rounded, ivory-colored beads.

Quinoa: A birdseed-shaped, mild-flavored grain, pale ivory to tan in color, quinoa can be used as a rice substitute. Before cooking, be sure to rinse it thoroughly under cold running water to remove its bitter coating.

Roasted buckwheat groats: These small brown pyramid-shaped bits are also known as kasha. They are used in cereal and many eastern European dishes.

When substituting grains for meat, be sure to include legumes such as beans or peas in your daily menu. Legumes and grains contribute different ratios of amino acids, the building blocks of protein, to provide the

THE BEAN BAG

All beans are nutritional powerhouses, but some are a bit more "powerhousey" than others. The Center for Science in the Public Interest came up with a score for each bean by adding its percent of the U.S. Recommended Daily Allowance (RDA) for seven nutrients plus fiber and potassium. There are no RDAs for fiber or potassium, so for fiber the CSPI used the new Daily Value (DV) of 25 grams. For potassium they used their "Nutrition Action RDA" (NARDA) of 3,500 milligrams.

For example: A cup of cooked lentils has 57 percent of the DV for fiber (57 points) and 19 percent of the NARDA for potassium (19 points). It also has 81 percent of the RDA for folic acid (81 points), 16 percent for magnesium (16 points), 33 percent for iron (33 points), 23 percent for copper (23 points), 15 percent for zinc (15 points), 25 percent for protein (25 points), and 16 percent for vitamin B-6 (16 points). That adds up to a score of 285.

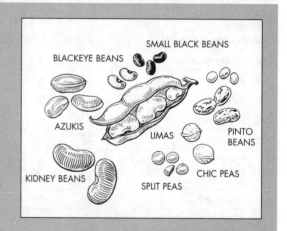

Small differences in score (25 points or less) are meaningless. Potassium and vitamin B-6 values are included in each score but don't appear on the chart. Numbers are for canned or cooked dried beans. Beans are ranked from highest to lowest score.

Bean (1 cup, cooked)	Score	Fiber	Folic Acid	Magnesium	Iron	Copper	Zinc	Protein
Soybeans†	300	●	▼	●	▲	●	▼	●
Pinto beans	287	▲	▲	●	●	▼	▼	▼
Chickpeas (garbanzos, ceci)	286	▲	▲	▼	●	●	▼	●
Lentils	285	▲	▲	▼	●	▼	▼	●
Cranberry beans*	278	▲	▲	▼	▼	▼	▼	●
Black-eyed peas (cowpeas)	273	●	▲	▼	●	▼	▼	▼

entire complement needed by the body. Legumes keep well in your pantry and can be prepared in a variety of ways. Many provide iron, zinc, and B vitamins. (See nearby box, "The Bean Bag".)

Tofu, a curd made from soy milk, is a bean-derived product that has provided low-cost protein to East Asians for 2000 years. A quarter-pound of tofu has 85 calories, 8 to 10 grams of protein, and 5 grams of fat, most of it the better unsaturated kind. The same amount of cooked chicken breast with skin has 223 calories and 8.8 grams of fat, (2.5 grams of which are saturated.) A quarter-pound of untrimmed, choice porterhouse steak delivers 346 calories and 25.1 grams of fat (10.1 grams saturated.) Because it's a plant product, tofu contains no cholesterol at all.

Bean (1 cup, cooked)	Score	Fiber	Folic Acid	Magnesium	Iron	Copper	Zinc	Protein
Pink beans*	269	●	▲	●	▼	▼	▼	●
Navy beans*	266	▲	▲	●	●	●	▼	▼
Black beans (turtle beans)	265	▲	▲	●	▼	▼	▼	●
Small white beans*	263	▲	▲	●	●	▼	▼	●
White beans	253	●	●	●	●	●	▼	●
Lima beans, baby	252	▲	▲	▼	▼	▼	▼	▼
Kidney beans, all types	243	●	▲	▼	●	▼	▼	▼
Adzuki beans*	238	●	▲	▼	▼	●	▼	▼
Great northern beans	228	▲	●	▼	▼	▼	▼	▼
Mung beans*	226	▲	▲	▼	▼	▼	▼	▼
Lima beans, large	224	▲	●	▼	▼	▼	▼	▼
Broadbeans (fava beans)*	197	●	●	▼	▼	▼	▼	▼
Peas, split (green)	192	▲	●	▼	▼	▼	▼	▼
Tofu, raw, (4 oz.)†	144	—	—	●	▲	▼	▼	●

Key
▲ contains at least 50 percent of the RDA
● contains between 25 and 49 percent of the RDA
▼ contains between 10 and 24 percent of the RDA
— contains less than 10 percent of the RDA

Footnotes
* Values for one or more nutrients are estimates.
† Soybeans are the only fatty bean. A cup has 15 grams of fat. A four-ounce serving of tofu, which is made from soybeans, can have anywhere from 2 to 7 grams of fat.

What About Herbs?

Most herbs are safe, but some are not. It's best to check with a health care professional before adding any to your diet. The warning also applies to herbal teas. Those made by major companies have a good safety record; avoid all others.

Certain herbal teas are reported to have caused serious liver disease. They contain pyrolizidine alkaloids, toxins that cause inflammation of the veins that drain blood away from the liver, a condition that can lead to scarring and obstruction. *Comfrey*-pepsin capsules, (a remedy for indigestion) and MU-16 (a tea containing comfrey) have been found to harbor the toxin. In one report, a woman who took comfrey-pepsin capsules and drank three cups of the MU-16 tea a day because she liked the taste, ended up with liver disease. Tests of the tea and capsules she consumed revealed that both contained pyrolizidine alkaloids.

Chaparral, promoted as an antioxidant, has been linked to two cases of acute hepatitis. *Germander, groundsel, skullcap, mistletoe,* and *senna,* have caused liver damage and death. Plants such as *woodruff* and *tonka beans* contain blood thinners. Patients taking anticoagulant medications, such as coumarin and warfarin, should avoid products containing these plants or their extracts. Teas prepared from *senna, buckthorn,* and *pokeroot* can cause severe diarrhea. *Mandrake, lobelia, burdock root, and jimsom weed* can lead to dry mouth, blurred vision, dilated pupils, and delirium. Some herbs are contaminated by dangerous plants. *Sassafras tea* has cancer causing properties and legal restrictions have been placed on the use of *safrole,* (a component of the oil of the sassafras tree bark) as a food additive. *Ginseng* can cause high blood pressure.

Is Kosher Healthier?

Most people associate the kosher label with purity, and the kosher food business is booming: Sales reached $30 billion in 1993. This growth has little to do with religious conviction, and everything to do with rigid standards.

Kosher meat has to pass inspection by a *bodek,* or Jewish food evaluator, who typically rejects more meat than does a federal official. A kosher label means that this inspection has been conducted. It also indicates that animals are slaughtered according to certain Old Testament directives and thoroughly drained of blood. Kosher and government inspectors look for different things: A bodek would not approve an animal with a blemish on the lung, whereas a government inspector likely would mandate that the lung alone be discarded. Lung scars have not been shown to pose significant health hazards, however, so this does not necessarily mean that buying kosher guarantees better protection from disease. Conversely, a government inspector checks an animal's glands for signs of infection that could pose public health problems, while bodeks are not trained to examine glands.

A kosher designation indicates nothing about nutritional value. Kosher hot dogs, for example, contain nitrites (sometimes associated with cancer) and lots of fat. Kosher meat may also have slightly more sodium, since salt is used to remove excess blood. Jewish inspectors examine products other than meat, but unlike government inspectors, they are not necessarily concerned with adherence to sanitation standards

Orthodox and conservative Jews, and even certain rabbis, disagree on the acceptability of certain kosher symbols. These are the most widely approved:

Star-K	OK
OU	KOF-K

If you see another symbol and buying kosher is important to you, check with a rabbi.

AN ORGANIC SAMPLER: WHAT PRICE "NATURAL"?

Brand Sold in Health Food Store	Brand Sold in Supermarket	Comments
Westbrae Natural 100% Organic Potato Chips	Lay's Potato Chips	The fat content of both chips are the same—56% of total calories. The oil used in the Westbrae chips is less saturated and the sodium content is appreciably less. But you're paying nearly twice as much for the natural, organic label.
Bearito's Organically Grown Tortilla Chips with Sea Salt	Tostito's Tortilla Chips	Nearly identical in price, fat and sodium contents. Corn, oil and salt are the only ingredients in both products. The difference: the health food store variety is made with organically grown corn and sea salt, neither of which offers any nutritional advantage.
Cascadian Farm Organic Grape Conserve	Polaner's All Fruit Grape Preserves	The ingredients may be the same—concord grapes, fruit concentrate and pectin—but the cost sure isn't. You pay a hefty premium for the organic grapes used in Cascadian Farm—$3.19 vs $1.89 for the same amount of jam, a 41% difference.
R.W. Knudsen Apple Juice	Redcheek Apple Juice	The health-food-store juice differs from its supermarket counterpart in two respects: it's made with organic apples and costs three times as much.
Santa Cruz Natural Apple Sauce	Grand Union Natural Apple Sauce	The ingredients are the same: apples and water. For organic apples, consumers pay four times more.
Cal's Organically Produced Blossom Honey	Golden Blossom Honey	Nutritionally, these products are the same, yet the health-food-store brand is more than twice as expensive as the supermarket variety.
Muir Glen Organic Tomato Paste	Hunt's All Natural Tomato Paste	Again, nutrition is not the issue, but cost certainly is. The health-food-store tomato paste costs a whopping five times that of Hunt's.
Jaclyn's Frozen Split Pea Soup	Tabatchnik's Split Pea Soup	Everything, down to the sea salt, is the same—but Jaclyn's costs 50 cents more per serving.
American Prairie Organic Oats	Grand Union Quick Oats	Once again, you're paying more for organic ingredients—two times more.
Earth's Best Organically Grown Baby Food Macaroni and Cheese Dinner	Gerber's Baby Food Macaroni and Cheese Dinner	Earth's Best provides more vitamin A, protein, calcium, iron and B vitamins than the Gerber's dinner. If you buy Earth's Best in a health food store, you'll pay about 2 1/2 times the supermarket price. Look for it on supermarket shelves and save about 30 cents a jar. When it comes to plain fruits and vegetables, Gerber's or Beech-Nut are nutritionally identical to, and cheaper than, Earth's Best.

Source: *Environmental Nutrition,* May 1993.

Is Organic Food Worth the Price?

Driven by fear of pesticides and additives, the organic food market has ballooned, doubling between 1987 and 1992, when sales reached $1.5 billion. Yet for most people, pesticides clearly pose little threat. Organic food still accounts for only a tiny share of the total U.S. grocery bill.

How real is the danger? For the U.S. Environmental Protection Agency (EPA), it's a major concern. Of the 350 pesticides allowed on food crops, the EPA considers 70 to be possibly or probably cancer-causing; and in 1987, the agency proclaimed pesticide residues third in terms of cancer risk among the 31 problems under its jurisdiction.

Many nutrition experts, on the other hand, say pesticide residues are insignificant in most people's overall diets. Pesticides exceed safe and acceptable levels in only a tenth of 1 percent of conventionally grown food. In up to 50 percent, there's no trace of common pesticides to be found. Simply washing produce and peeling fruit and vegetables removes most of what little remains. Avoiding imported products also cuts the chance of exposure.

Organic farming may further reduce the problem—but not by much. Shifting winds and water run-off can carry the chemicals from one field to another. As a result, some studies have found pesticide residues on organic and conventional foods to be similar. Meanwhile, organic fertilizers, while chemical-free, may carry disease-causing bacteria.

Certification.

The Organic Crop Improvement Association (OCIA) hires independent farm inspectors to certify that growing practices meet California standards—the strictest in the country. OCIA's seal has won worldwide respect. In addition, the U.S. Organic Foods Production Act of 1990 established a National Organic Standards Board to suggest guidelines. Processed foods containing at least 50 percent organically produced ingredients by weight (excluding water and salt) can use the word *organic* on the principal display panel—but only to describe the organically produced ingredients. Most experts believe that to be called organic, foods should not be waxed, artificially dyed, or sprayed with chemicals. Organic animal foods should come from animals raised without antibiotic or hormone treatment and prepared for market without the use of chemicals.

Avoid Imitations: When you do purchase organic products, you'll want to be certain you're getting your extra money's worth.

Additives: A Cause for Alarm?

Health food stores may be more likely than supermarkets to have packaged, quick-to-prepare products that are also additive-free. However, you need to read the fine print to be sure. You also have to remember that additives are not necessarily bad. Some, like vitamin fortifiers, enrich foods. Others prevent or slow spoilage; produce uniform color, texture, aroma, flavor and appearance; standardize thickening or stabilizing; preserve foods; and improve color or texture in the cooked product. A federal law prohibits use in food of any amount of a substance shown to increase the lifetime risk of cancer by as little as 1 in a million.

Some experts, such as Michael Jacobson, M.D., director of the Center for Science in the Public Interest in Washington, DC, argue

A CAUTION ABOUT ARTIFICIAL SWEETENERS AND CHILDREN...

For safety's sake, avoid giving saccharin-containing products to children under 2. Although studies of people who use saccharin have not uncovered any significant risk of cancer, the sweetener has been linked to cancer in laboratory animals. Young children may be more susceptible to such effects. Older children should also avoid artificial sweeteners. Mannitol and sorbitol can cause diarrhea. Table sugar, on the other hand, is as likely to calm children as to make them hyperactive, according to several studies.

that many additives have not been tested well enough to ensure safety. Some provide inexpensive ways of adding color and flavor when natural ingredients could do the job. Advocates of natural foods often argue that since many additives are unnecessary, and some may not even be safe, there's no reason to eat them. Most nutrition experts, however, stress that with a few exceptions, most additives make long-distance shipping and safe storage possible and pose little or no danger.

Here are some of the ingredients that manufacturers are routinely permitted to add to their food products.

Sweeteners: Products labeled "no sugar added" may still contain sweetening in the form of fruit juice or malt flavoring; diabetics, in particular, should note this fact. Remember, too, that baked goods can be sugar free, yet contain plenty of fat and calories.

For all practical purposes, there is no real difference between white sugar, brown sugar, honey, corn syrup, and concentrated apple or pear juices. Honey contains only trace amounts of B vitamins, iron, and calcium.

Blackstrap molasses is an excellent source of calcium and iron, but only if used in larger amounts than most people accept. Health food brands using sweeteners other than sugar and corn syrup provide little extra benefit, but typically cost a good deal more.

Salt: A "No Salt Added" label doesn't mean the food is not inherently salty. It may still contain plenty of sodium and therefore be inappropriate for someone on a low-salt diet. The term "low sodium" means the product has no more than 140 milligrams per serving, "reduced sodium" means at least 75 percent less sodium than a similar conventional food.

Oils: Many snack foods sold in health food stores contain heart-healthy nonhydrogenated oils while conventional snack foods often contain partially hydrogenated soybean, cottonseed, or canola oils. Even partial hydrogenation, which is used to solidify oils, can make fat more damaging to the heart.

MSG: Foods containing this additive need only be labeled if the MSG is 99 percent pure. Therefore, if you are sensitive to this substance, you may get a reaction from a food you think is safe. MSG, an ingredient in Chinese food and certain seasonings, can cause a throbbing headache, aching joints, nausea, dizziness, shortness of breath, numbness, weakness, and heart palpitations in certain people. Hydrolyzed vegetable protein usually contains up to 20 percent MSG. To minimize exposure to this additive, eat fresh foods rather than processed ones, read labels, and avoid all food that comes with a "flavor packet".

THE BEST FOR BREAKFAST

This chart lists nutrition numbers for one ounce of cereal. Remember, though, that surveys show that most people eat 3/4 ounces (about a cup) of light cereals—like Rice Krispies or Corn Flakes—and two or three ounces (1/2 to 2/3 cup) of dense cereals—like Grape-Nuts or granola. We have added, in parentheses following each name, how many cups of cereals equal one ounce. That way, you can figure out how much is in a serving of your cereal. For example, 1/3 cup of Kellogg's Bran Buds weighs an ounce. So if you typically eat about two-thirds of a cup, multiply the numbers in the chart by 2. "Best Bite" criteria: (1) predominantly whole grain, (2) at least 2.5 grams of fiber, (3) no more than two grams of fat, five grams of sugar, or 250 mg of sodium, and (4) free of BHA, BHT, and aspartame. Within each category, products are ranked from highest to lowest fiber.

Product	Fat (grams)	Fiber (grams)	Sugar (grams)
Whole Grain Cereal (50 to 120 calories)			
Kellogg's All-Bran w/Extra Fiber (1/2) a,b	0	14	0
General Mills Fiber One (1/2) a	1	13	0
Kellogg's Bran Buds (1/3) b	1	11	8
Kellogg's All-Bran (1/3)	1	9	5
Health Valley Raisin Bran Flakes (1/2)	0	6	na
■ Kellogg's Bran Flakes (2/3)	0	5	5
Kellogg's Fiberwise (2/3) b	1	5	5
Erewhon Right Start (1/3)*	0	5	na
Kölln Oat Bran Crunch (1/3)	1	5	na
Barbara's 100% Oat Bran (1/4)*	4	5	na
Nabisco Shredded Wheat'n Bran (2/3) b	1	4	0
Kellogg's Nutri-Grain Raisin Bran (3/4)	1	4	6
Kellogg's Cracklin' Oat Bran (1/2)	3	4	7
Post Fruit & Fibre Dates and Raisins (1/2) b	2	4	8
Kellogg's Fruitful Bran (1/2)	0	4	9
Kellogg's Raisin Bran (1/2)	1	4	9
Post Natural Raisin Bran (1/2)	1	4	9
Health Valley Oat Bran Flakes or O's (1/2)	0	4	na
■ Puffed Kashi (1-1/3)	0	3	0
Nabisco Shredded Wheat (1 biscuit) b	1	3	0
■ Kellogg's Nutri-Grain Wheat (2/3)	0	3	2
■ Weetabix (1-3/4 biscuits)	1	3	2
■ Post Grape-Nuts (1/4)	0	3	3
General Mills Total or Wheaties (1) b	1	3	3
Ralston Whole Grain Wheat Chex (2/3) b	1	3	3
Nabisco Fruit Wheats (1/2) b	0	3	5
Quaker Life (2/3) b	2	3	5
Kellogg's Frosted Mini Wheats (4 biscuits) b	0	3	6

Product	Fat (grams)	Fiber (grams)	Sugar (grams)
General Mills Raisin Nut Bran (1/2) b	3	3	8
Health Valley Real Oat Bran Raisin (1/4)	1	3	na
Grainfield's Oat Bran Flakes (3/4)	2	3	na
General Mills Cheerios (1-1/4)	2	2	1
General Mills Honey Nut Cheerios (3/4)	1	2	10
New Morning Oatios (1-1/4)*	2	2	na
Kellogg's Kenmei Rice Bran (3/4) b	1	1	4
General Mills Oatmeal Raisin Crisp (1/3) b	2	1	8
General Mills Wheaties Honey Gold (3/4) b	0	1	10
Granola and Muesli (90 to 130 calories)			
Arrowhead Mills Maple Nut Granola (1/4)	5	6	na
Familia 25% Bran (1/3)	2	5	6
Health Valley Healthy Crunch (1/4)*	1	4	na
■ Alpen (no salt/no sugar) (1/4)	2	3	5
Familia (1/3)	1	3	6
Kellogg's Müeslix Golden Crunch (1/3) b	2	3	6
Breadshop Fat Free Granola (1/3)	0	3	na
Health Valley Fat-Free Granola (1/4)*	0	3	na
Health Valley Real Oat Bran Crunch (1/4)	1	3	na
Rainforest Granola (1/3)	5	3	na
Quaker 100% Natural (1/4)*	5	2	7
Kellogg's Low-Fat Granola (1/3) b	2	2	8
Ralston Muesli (1/3)*,b	2	2	8
Refined Cereal (90 to 110 calories)			
Ralston Multi-Bran Chex (2/3) b	0	4	6
General Mills Basic 4 (1/2) b	2	2	6
Post Honey Bunches of Oats (2/3) b	2	2	6
Kellogg's Corn Flakes (1) b	0	1	2
Kellogg's Product 19 or Special K (1) b	0	1	3
Kellogg's Frosted Flakes (3/4) b	0	1	11
Kellogg's Rice Krispies (1) b	0	0	3
Kellogg's Nut & Honey Crunch (2/3) b	1	0	9

■ Best Bite b contains BHA or BHT
* average for the entire line na not available
a sweetened with aspartame

All information obtained from manufacturers.

Sulfites: These chemicals are used as preservatives in wines, dried fruits, and dried potato products, such as mashed potato flakes. About five percent of asthmatics have difficulty breathing within minutes of eating a food containing sulfites. The reaction can be fatal and requires immediate treatment at an emergency room. Sulfites occur naturally in almost all wines. Those bottled after mid-1987 must have a label stating that they contain sulfites if they have more than 10 parts per million of the additive. Organic wines are not necessarily sulfite-free, however most beers no longer contain sulfites. Although shrimp is sometimes treated with sulfites on fishing vessels, the chemical may not appear on the label. Avoid shrimp if you are allergic to sulfite. In 1985, the federal government banned addition of sulfites to most fresh fruits and vegetables. Fresh-cut potatoes and dried fruits are exceptions.

Antibiotics in meat: Antibiotics are given to animals to increase growth as well as to treat and prevent diseases. Regular exposure to low levels of antibiotics makes disease-causing organisms, such as salmonella, resistant, or less likely to respond, to those medications. Some of these antibiotic-resistant organisms can pass from animals to people. Farm and food workers are thought to be at risk, as is anyone who eats animal products. Researchers do not really know how often this happens. In 1988 the Institute of Medicine estimated that 15 percent of the 50,000 cases of salmonella infection in the U.S. each year result from organisms resistant to penicillin, tetracycline, and ampicillin, all of which are given to farm animals. However, the figure was based on incomplete data. An estimated 75 people die each year of salmonella resistant to those three antibiotics.

Some health advocates have warned of possible allergic reactions to antibiotic residues in meat. However, testing shows that most meat is antibiotic-free, and when a drug residue is found, the quantity is minute. Only two cases of allergic reactions to antibiotics in meat have been reported over the last two years.

BHA and BHT: There is considerable controversy about whether these preservatives are safe. Butylated hydroxyanisole (BHA) and butylated hydroxytoluene (BHT) are antioxidants that help keep oil in food from becoming rancid. Laboratory experiments with BHA have produced tumors in rats and hamsters. The cancer-causing potential of BHT is not so certain, with some studies showing an increased risk of cancer, and others finding a decrease. Some organizations such as the Center for Science in the Public Interest believe these additives should be gradually eliminated from the food supply. Government regulations require manufacturers to list both BHA and BHT on the labels of foods in which they appear.

Fat-free substitutes: Nutrition authorities view these as safe and, in themselves, an effective way of reducing fat intake. The problem comes when you eat a fat-free dessert, then "reward" yourself with an extra dish of real ice cream. You probably won't lose weight this way.

Tartrazine: this food coloring may cause a skin disease called atopic eczema in susceptible children.

Genetically Engineered Food: Any Real Risk?

In recent years, scientists' new-found ability to alter living organisms by tailoring their genes has been the source of much controversy and dread. The technique can be used to mass-produce exact replicas of natural substances like hormones, or even create new strains of existing plants and animals. Many experts view recombinant gene technology as a powerful new way of improving food safety, quality, and quantity. Opponents fear unintentional (or deliberate) creation of dangerous new organisms. Opposition to specific new products, however, focuses more on such issues as animal rights and the fate of small dairy farms than on any question of safety.

The Bovine Growth Hormone Scare

The Food and Drug Administration (FDA) made history in November 1993 when it approved rBST (recombinant bovine somatotropin), a genetically engineered growth hormone marketed by Monsanto, to boost milk production. That made rBST the first gene-tailored agricultural product to be approved for general use. The product duplicates BST, a cow's natural growth hormone. Injecting the hormone every 14 days increases a cow's ability to produce milk but does not affect milk quality.

There is no difference between natural and recombinant BST. Neither the biotech nor the natural version appears in milk and, in any event, the hormone is inactive in humans. The American Medical Association (AMA) and the American Dietetic Association (ADA) insist it poses no threat.

An FDA-authored paper reviewing 120 studies over 30 years attested to the hormone's safety. Milk from cows treated with rBST is identical to that from untreated cows and is equally safe. The FDA does not permit firms to say "free of BST" on their labeling,—although a label can read, "from cows not treated with BST"—and manufacturers need not identify products made with milk from rBST-treated animals.

A main argument against rBST is that it makes cows more susceptible to infection of the udder, thus increasing the need for antibiotic treatment and the chance of antibiotic residue in milk. The AMA says only insignificant amounts of antibiotics find their way into cows milk. However, humans drinking such milk theoretically could develop resistance to antibiotics. Monsanto, maker of rBST, claims that the increased risk of udder infection for the average dairy cow is one case every 10 years. Consumers Union, publisher of *Consumer Reports,* asserts that the rate is higher. One small Vermont study found seven times more cases of infected udders (mastitis) in rBST-treated cows. Those cows required treatment for six times as long as non-rBST-treated animals with the same infection. Some authorities recommend substituting other medications for antibiotics when udders develop infections.

The FDA checks all milk shipments for drug residue and pulls contaminated product from the market. States also check milk for antibiotics.

Government inspection is far from perfect, however. *The Wall Street Journal* found in its own 1991 study that 38 percent of the milk samples they tested had antibiotic residues. The Center for Science in the Public Interest in Washington, DC, found that 20 percent of samples it tested in the same year had residues of dangerous, sulfur-containing drugs. In response, the FDA has begun taking measures to improve its procedures.

Some rBST opponents feel that less chemically intensive agriculture is inherently better or that the hormone may reduce bovine fertility and suppress bovine immune systems, and thereby prove cruel to cows. Others fear that this expensive hormone could force small dairies out of business. Krogers supermarkets is one of the firms that does not use products from rBST-treated animals out of support for family farms.

Other Genetically Engineered Food Products

Calgene's Flavr Savr "MacGregor's" tomato, introduced in mid-1994, is slower to turn mushy than other tomatoes because genetic manipulation has neutralized the gene that causes softness. Two-thirds of cheese manufacturers in the U.S. use a genetically engineered enzyme called chymosin to coagulate milk. Chymosin mimics rennin, a natural animal enzyme formerly obtained by scraping the stomach lining of slaughtered calves. In the research pipeline are potatoes that absorb less fat when fried, squash that resists a damaging virus, and herbicide-resistant beans.

As of 1992, companies had to consult with the FDA before introducing genetically engineered foods if (1) there was a possible safety hazard or, (2) the alternative offering was dramatically different from, though as safe as, the existing product. For example, although the FDA does not require that all genetically engineered food be so labeled, any significant changes in nutritional content must be noted.

Irradiation: Safe or Not?

Irradiation exposes food to gamma, beta, or x rays from cobalt 60 or cesium in a closed room. This breaks chemical bonds in organisms such as insects and bacteria, thereby killing the pests so they cannot cause spoilage or food hazards.

Some people associate irradiation with nuclear power. However, cobalt 60 reportedly cannot explode. Food irradiation uses much lower energy levels and generates far less heat than does nuclear power. The World Health Organization and more than 30 countries have approved food irradiation to help ensure food safety. Other nations have banned the practice. The FDA permits its use on fruits, vegetables, grains, poultry, and spices.

Irradiated foods other than spices must display a special logo. The process can disinfect wheat, block sprouting in white potatoes, decontaminate herbs and spices, control trichinosis in pork and salmonella in poultry, slow ripening of fruits and vegetables, and kill insects in produce. However, because of widespread fear of irradiation in this country, few foods other than spices are treated this way here.

Is It Safe?

Researchers have been studying food irradiation for at least 40 years; it may be the most carefully examined food preservation process in use today. Because most radiation passes through food rather than remaining behind, a majority of scientists familiar with the procedure feel that it probably poses no danger and may have some benefit.

Irradiation has been used for years to sterilize medical equipment and consumer products. Half of all sterile medical supplies undergo irradiation as do cotton swabs, contact lenses, saline solutions, tampons, and teething rings. There is more controversy when it comes to food. Opponents argue that irradiation leaves nonradioactive byproducts. Experts disagree about whether these substances—which are also found in an estimated 90 percent of unradiated foods—can be hazardous to humans.

Some people object to radiation on principal. However, in some cases, irradiation may be safer than other decontamination processes. Nonirradiated spices, for example, are treated with ethylene oxide, a toxic, explosive, cancer-causing gas that poses dangers to workers, may pollute the air, and can leave a residue. This same substance was used to sterilize medical supplies until irradiation took its place.

How Does It Affect Food?

All commercial preservation methods destroy some nutrients. Irradiation reduces vitamin and mineral content by 10 to 15 percent, a figure that compares favorably with other techniques. For example, some nutrients are affected more by irradiation than by pasteurization; others react the opposite way. At the irradiation levels allowed by the FDA, there are no nutritional differences between irradiated food and products preserved by other means.

Irradiation can kill the dangerous salmonella bacteria found in as much as 60 percent of U.S. poultry. It also destroys the bacteria that causes trichinosis and kills *E. coli,* the organism that caused 500 cases of illness in people eating undercooked hamburger at fast-food establishments in the Northwestern U.S. in 1993. Some people claim that the amounts of radiation needed to kill all the salmonella in a heavily infested animal would reduce poultry quality to an unacceptable level. However, even a reduction in the amount of salmonella is better than no treatment at all, and makes proper refrigeration and cooking that much more likely to work.

While irradiation retards spoilage in some food, it makes others less marketable. For example, it speeds decay in produce with high water content, such as lettuce and peaches. Milk and other dairy foods give off unpleasant odors after irradiation. It may also alter the color of green vegetables. However, because allowable radiation levels are so low, changes in color, taste, and odor in foods coming to market are usually undetectable.

Smart Shopping: It's Not So Difficult

The good news is that the food you find in supermarkets is as healthy as the products available in most health food stores. There are legitimate reasons to spend more for organic, natural, and whole foods than for conventional products; but a major difference in nutritional value isn't one of them. To make healthier choices, check the fine print on labels. You may have to sort through a wealth of sometimes incomplete or misleading advertising claims, but you probably don't need to change your diet radically. □

CHAPTER 4

How to Pick a Nutritional Plan

When most people think about diet, they focus on weight loss—getting rid of those extra five or ten pounds they've been promising to shed. A booming industry caters to this fascination with weight and appearance, offering scores of books to help people shed weight, improve their sex lives, and look younger; promoting schemes to deliver a thinner you in a matter of weeks; and hawking diet plans based on "magic" foods, "power" foods, fast foods, convenience foods, even liquid foods.

At any given time, 20 million Americans are on a diet of some kind, and another 20 million are convinced they should be. Yet most of them fail to achieve their goals, dropping out because the programs they've chosen are too stringent, concentrate on foods they dislike, or conflict with their lifestyle. Even those who reach their objectives usually slip back, eventually returning to their original eating patterns.

This is not the way it has to be. A diet program needn't be a hardship, doesn't have to in clude foods you hate, and shouldn't be measured exclusively in terms of pounds lost. Instead, think in terms of your own health and enjoyment. If you simply follow what we know about nutrition today, you can protect your health, find an agreeable style of eating, and maintain a reasonable weight in the bargain.

Most experts, such as New York Times science and medical writer Jane Brody, believe that "unless you have a chronic illness like diabetes, or are genetically prone to heart disease, you need not become an extremist or an acetic, nor do you have to give up everything you love forever."

People adopt diets for two main reasons: 1) to improve their health and prevent serious medical problems or 2) to lose weight. In many cases, the same basic food plan—low fat, moderate protein, high complex carbohydrate—will accomplish both goals. In others, a more specialized program is necessary.

But before you start any new eating program, whether it be for weight loss or health, there are number of things you should consider. According to Stanley Gershoff, Ph.D., dean of the Tufts University School of Nutrition, you need to ask yourself:

■ **What is my motivation?** For example, if you believe losing weight will improve your love life or assure a job promotion, you are bound to fail. While a diet and fitness program can be a positive motivating factor, losing weight, in itself, does not guarantee your life will change.

■ **Why have I failed at other diets?** Perhaps it was not entirely your fault. You may have tried one of many fad diets that have been proven time and again to be ineffective. By examining your diet history, you may spot a trend. For example, extremely low calorie diets or organized diet plans may not work for you.

■ **Am I built like other members of my family?** Look at your close relatives. No matter how much you diet, you can no more change your genetically-given shape than you can change the color of your eyes.

■ **Do I have "special health considerations?"** Are you at risk for heart disease, high blood pressure, or diabetes? Do you have food allergies? Do you have high cholesterol, high blood sugar, or other medical conditions that might make certain diets harmful to you? Are your medications compatible with the program you're considering? If you do have a medical problem, ask your doctor to help you choose a program.

Eating Your Way to Good Health

Your diet can influence your risk of developing an imposing list of life-shortening diseases, including heart disease, cancer, stroke, diabetes, and high blood pressure, not to mention the less threatening but painful problems of tooth decay, bone fractures, and excess weight.

For example, almost everyone now knows that a diet rich in saturated fat plays a central role in the development of heart disease, America's number one killer. According to the American Heart Association, an ample body of scientific evidence shows that reducing dietary fat and cholesterol can lower the risk of heart and blood vessel disease in the general population.

Excess weight often goes hand in hand with high cholesterol. LDL, the so-called "bad" cholesterol, is known to promote atherosclerosis, the accumulation of plaque in the walls of the arteries that results in reduced blood flow and oxygen to the heart. Too much cholesterol in the blood invites this development. But, says Dr. Gershoff, for some people, slimming down to a healthy body weight will, by itself, completely correct elevated LDL concentrations.

Experts agree that any nutritional program aimed at preventing or improving heart disease should be based on a food plan that emphasizes low-fat, high-starch meals. It should also include sample menus and recipes; hints on how to eat at a restaurant, a dinner party, or a special occasion; plus information on such other risk factors as tobacco and alcohol. It should be neither so restrictive that it invites failure, nor so unstructured as to be confusing.

It should also include a medically approved exercise program. The Centers for

Disease Control and Prevention warn that the sedentary life-style of many Americans may be as great a risk factor for heart disease as high cholesterol or high blood pressure. On the other hand, aerobic exercise increases the strength of the heart, raises HDL (the "good" cholesterol), and alleviates stress on the heart.

Many other health problems respond favorably to this type of heart-healthy program. Certain types of cancer—including breast, colon, rectum, stomach, and esophagus—have been linked to the high-fat, low-fiber types of food that a heart-healthy diet restricts. Excess weight can also increase the risk of developing some cancers, so, as a heart-healthy diet brings down your weight, it reduces your cancer risk as well.

Some diseases, such as diabetes, require a more indivualized diet. A good diabetes diet, for example, groups foods according to their calories and their carbohydrate, protein, and fat content, and uses an "exchange" system to guide the dieter. With the help of a registered dietitian, these exchanges can be fine-tuned to accommodate your favorite foods while controlling blood sugar. Again, the emphasis is on weight control; a diet rich in starch and fiber, and low in fat; and regular aerobic exercise.

If you think you have allergies or food sensitivities, the first step is to get tested. Then you can work with your doctor or a dietician to eliminate the offending foods and develop a healthy eating plan.

Whatever your goal, be certain to discuss major changes in your diet with your doctor. He or she can tell you whether your medications could react unfavorably with certain foods, whether a particular diet can create problems with any medical condition you may have, and whether a program includes all the nutrients and calories you need.

Matching Nutrition to Your Principles

If religion or philosophy governs the type of food you eat, your choice of diet plans is automatically limited. Fortunately, there are a number of excellent programs to meet these special needs.

Vegetarian

Since 1970, there has been a 30 percent growth in vegetarianism in this country. Vegetarian restaurants, food stores, cookbooks, and nutritional programs are plentiful.

There are many degrees of vegetarianism. Lactovegetarians eat dairy foods but no animal protein including eggs. Ovolacto vegetarians eliminate animal foods from their diets, but do eat eggs and dairy products. Other vegetarians indulge in fish as well as dairy foods and eggs. Only vegans eat absolutely nothing from a creature that flies, walks, or swims.

If you are a vegetarian, you must choose a diet rich in the nutrients most Americans get from meat, poultry, fish, eggs, milk, and cheese. Your food plan should include vegetable protein from such sources as beans and soy products; starches from whole grains and a variety of fruits and vegetables; oils low in saturated fat; and nuts and seeds. You may also want to take vitamin and mineral supplements (especially vitamins B_2, B_{12}, and D, and iron, zinc, and calcium) to restore the essential elements that may be missing from your foods.

For vegetarians, most experts favor a diet program that permits you to combine foods for adequate nutrition. For example, during the course of each day nutritionists suggest you eat beans along with grains, or nuts and seeds; and eggs or dairy products along with any vegetable protein.

A good vegetarian diet program contains all the nutrients essential to good health and enough calories to support your ideal weight. It should include meal plans that allow you to choose among a variety of foods, and— ideally—recipes to help you cook them. It should also teach you how to plan your own menus.

Macrobiotic

Few nutritionists applaud a strict macrobiotic diet. It starts out as a balanced vegetarian diet, but can progress into a limited, extremely deficient intake of brown rice (or grain) only. Extreme macrobiotic diets can lead to scurvy, anemia, and dangerously low levels of blood sugar and protein. Some nutritionists call the diet "bizarre," and "repugnant."

Whole grains and vegetables are the key foods in a macrobiotic diet. They are supplemented by soups, soy products, beans, fruits, nuts, seeds, fish, and sea greens. Whole grain cereals make up 50 to 60 percent of the diet, fresh vegetables 20 to 30 percent, beans and sea greens five to 10 percent, and soup an

other five to 10 percent. Adherents are forbidden to eat artificial or chemically-processed products; refined sugars and grains; certain vegetables, fruits, and juices; red meat, poultry, eggs, and dairy products; saturated and refined fats and oils; caffeine, and carbonated beverages.

In its initial stages, a macrobiotic diet is not dangerous, although it may be deficient in certain essential nutrients. But if you choose this way of eating, nutritionists caution it's unwise to complete the transition to an almost complete reliance on grains. If, as its founder says, the diet's purpose is to "ensure survival of the human race and its further evolution on this planet," its prospects seem grim.

Kosher

It's easy to set a healthy kosher table, although it does require some tampering with traditional recipes.

Although Jewish dietary law requires separation of meat and dairy foods—they cannot be eaten at the same meals or on the same dishes—it's still easy to maintain a balanced diet. Approved meats come only from certain portions of animals that have split hooves, chew their cud, and have been killed according to a strict set of rules, but these restrictions still leave room for plenty of variety.

If you are an orthodox Jew, or if you eat only kosher, foods there is no reason your diet cannot meet the current standards for good health: you can still increase your fruits, grains, and vegetables and cut down on saturated fats. Jews from the Mediterranean countries typically eat that way, according to Bonnie Liebman, director of nutrition at the Center for Science in the Public Interest.

If you prefer traditional eastern European foods, even if only on holidays, you can still reduce their fat content. For example, use imitation sour cream and farmer cheese in blintzes and low- or no-fat cottage cheese in noodle pudding, defat homemade chicken soup, and make matzoh balls with egg substitute and fewer eggs.

While there are few specifically kosher diet cookbooks, you can modify recipes from a regular kosher cookbook or adapt recipes from others.

For those who prefer a formal weight control program with prepared meals, the 14-year-old Start Fresh program, based in Brooklyn, has developed a kosher diet low in fat, calories and sodium; moderate in protein; and high in complex carbohydrates. Participants can buy and prepare their own food or purchase the company's frozen breakfast, lunch, dinner, and snack foods.

Start Fresh also offers group, individual, and even telephone sessions that emphasize behavior modification. They cover topics such as how to shop for healthy food, how to feed the children when mother is on a diet; and staying on track before, during, and after special occasions. The plan also stresses exercise.

Losing Weight Without Losing Your Mind

The typical American man is now 20 to 30 pounds overweight, the typical woman, 15 to 30 pounds, and even children carry from 10 to 20 percent more weight than they should. Today's sedentary lifestyle is largely to blame. People gain weight when they take in more food than they can burn, and store the excess as fat. Our ancestors ate a great deal more than we do, but because they were physically active, they weighed less.

Simply maintaining a weight that falls within the normal range for your height and body type can increase your life expectancy by cutting your risk of high blood pressure, heart disease, diabetes, and other weight-related problems. But how do you choose a weight loss program once you—and your doctor—decide you need to lose weight? "A good diet is something you can stay on the rest of your life," says C. Wayne Callaway of George Washington University. "There's no advantage to short-term austerity programs. The more the weight fluctuates, the shorter your life expectancy." A sound program, should concentrate on behavior, not weight loss. "It should provide adequate food—not an excess—eaten in three daily meals, and include regular, moderate exercise you can live with."

For weight loss to be lasting, it must be based on permanent lifestyle changes that you can realistically stick to. A good nutritional program teaches you to set achievable short- and long-term goals; shows you how to recognize the reasons you overeat; and gives you enough information about foods, nutrients, and calories to make the right choices. It also maximizes your chance for success by providing practical methods to help you stick to your eating and exercise plan.

Quick weight loss diets do not work in the long run, most experts agree. A sensible program helps you shed from one-half to two pounds a week. Any more than that raises your risk of failure. Research has shown that the faster you lose, the more likely you are to regain the weight and the greater the danger to your health.

Today's best diet plans concentrate on lowering your intake of fat while raising your consumption of carbohydrates. Fat is usually limited to no more than 25 to 30 percent of total calories, and protein to 10 to 15 percent, with carbohydrates accounting for the remaining 55 to 60 percent. To lose weight safely, chose a program that recommends plenty of vegetables, fruits, and whole-grain products; and includes beans (legumes), as well as some nonfatty fish and poultry for protein and nonfat dairy products for calcium. Your meals should contain a minimum of foods high in saturated fats, such as cheeses, whole milk, beef, lamb, and pork.

That's a far cry from the high-protein, low-carbohydrate diet of the past, now believed to be a sure path to quick fatigue and poor performance.

The consensus is that calories do count, although extremely low-calorie diets can be unproductive. Your body type and lifestyle play a large part in determining your caloric requirements, but everyone has to burn 3,500 calories to lose a pound of stored fat. While some people can shed pounds on 1,500 calories, others may do better on 1,200 or 2,000. A tall 40-year-old man who has actively participated in sports from the age of 18 needs more calories while he is still active than he will as he grows older and more sedentary. A woman who never exercises may eat less than an athlete of the same age and build and still gain weight. Your physician, or a dietitian can help you determine how many calories you should eat to lose weight while still getting the nutrition you need.

Avoid diets that make you feel deprived. Chances are you will not be able to stick to them, and any weight you lose will quickly return. There is no reason to give up everything you love to shed pounds, and guilt is unproductive. Some approaches are:

- Splurge at a special occasion and give yourself an occasional treat. If you deny yourself completely, you will be more likely to binge. Eat some of your favorite foods, but take a smaller portion or a lower fat version.
- Choose a diet that gives suggestions on what to eat at a party or a restaurant.
- Learn how to compensate or trade-off. For example, if you eat a high fat food for breakfast, choose low fat foods for the rest of your meals.
- Make sure the program allows you to select from a variety of foods within each food group. A boring repetition can quickly lead to failure.

Be certain that your diet plan includes exercise. The best way to slim down and achieve fitness is with an easy program you can stick with and work into the rest of your daily activities; one that you can enjoy no matter how unfit you are to start with. The diet you choose should emphasize regular, moderate physical activity. Most experts agree that a good exercise program should include aerobic exercise to strengthen your cardiovascular system and muscle-building exercise as well. While losing weight, you need to exercise for more than 30 minutes three or

WARNING SIGNS OF FADS AND GIMMICKRY

"When it comes to diets . . . Americans are extraordinarily gullible," says Jane Brody. They will "swallow anything—dozens of eggs, hundreds of grapefruits, gallons of water, even wood pulp, vinegar, and seaweed—if it will keep them away, however temporarily, from the calorie-rich foods that have made them fat."

At best, fad diets are ineffective; at worst, they can seriously endanger your health. When choosing a program, watch out for the following danger signals:

■ **Excessively restrictive food choices.** Unless your diet is varied, you are likely to become bored and begin overeating. In addition, restricted programs often eliminate essential nutrients.

■ **Unrealistic promises.** "Lose 20 pounds in two weeks," shouts one plan. "You can eat everything you want (or often as you want) and still lose weight," claims another. There are no shortcuts when it comes to weight loss. While almost every diet works for a while, your initial weight loss is mostly water. You simply cannot lose fat quickly.

■ **Assertions that calories don't count.** If you consume more calories than you burn—whatever their source—you will gain weight.

■ **Nutritional imbalance.** Stay away from any diet that does not contain all of the carbohydrates, protein, fat, vitamins, and minerals you need to sustain health. Be wary when a program asserts that one element is a "no-no". Watch out especially for:

Low- or no-carbohydrate diets, such as the Dr. Robert C. Atkins' plan. Without carbohydrates, your body may begin burning protein, producing toxic waste products called ketones. In large amounts, these wastes can cause brain, liver, and kidney damage; nausea; fatigue; lethargy; and, over time, heart problems. When protein must be used for energy, it cannot build and replace tissues as it should. These diets are also too high in saturated fat and too low in fiber and essential vitamins and minerals.

Crash diets. The 'crash' in crash diets comes afterward, when we start gobbling food to meet the demands of our depleted bodies.

Unsupervised all-liquid diets, especially liquid protein.

Fasting. The pounds will come off quickly, but without essential nutrients, you will lose muscle as well as fat. Although a day or two probably will not hurt, you also run the risk developing a serious, even life-threatening disease or psychological condition if the fast persists too long.

■ **Ineffective, or dangerous gimmicks.** Over the past few years, several popular plans have sung the praises of special foods, supplements, and medications whose "magic" properties practically guarantee weight loss. Remember that shedding pounds involves sensible, healthy eating, and lifelong behavior modification, not a "miracle" potion that, at best, does not work, and at worst, could endanger your health. Be especially alert to claims made for:

—Appetite suppressants
—Hormones (including thyroid and human chorionic gonadotrophin [HCG])
—Diuretics
—Laxatives
—Fiber Pills
—Vinegar
—Certain types of fruit, especially when the dieter eats nothing else for days (or weeks) at a time
—Any diet that relies on only one food or class of foods (for instance, rice, grain, or water)

■ **Tie-ins with a specific manufacturer.** There's no reason to eat one company's product if another has equivalent food value.

four times a week. Once you've reached your goal, 20 to 30 minutes will do.

Maintaining your target weight is important. Yo-yo-ing up and down is unhealthy. Any good nutritional program should also help you determine why and where you overeat, so you can develop lifetime strategies to help eliminate the problem and *keep off* those unwanted pounds. Remember, though, not to be discouraged if a few pounds return. If you've taken off more than your body can handle, it will inevitably seek its natural weight.

Picking a Diet That Suits Your Personality
Good nutrition and diet programs stress self-sufficiency. Even if you choose a "structured weight control program" initially, it is likely that the more comfortable you become with selecting your own nutrition and fitness plan, the less obsessed you will become with food and the less likely you will be to binge.

Even so, dieters have different needs. Some require individual counseling and encouragement, others are more comfortable in groups; a few can diet on their own. A plan with plenty of flexibility and choice is perfect for one person, a rigid food plan is ideal for another. If your program fails to match your personality, you are less likely to achieve your goal.

Your diet plan also should be individualized to fit your special needs. In weight loss and maintainance, "one-size-fits-all" usually does not work. If you are a vegetarian or a diabetic, or if your religion places restrictions on your foods, ask a counselor to customize the standard diet for you.

Be wary of organizations that require purchase of their prepared foods unless you have neither the time nor the talent to cook your own meals. Though convenient, the products can be expensive. Some even include un-

healthy ingredients, like excess salt or sugar. A reputable company gives you the option of shopping for and preparing your own food.

If you need the support and encouragement of a group of like-minded dieters, pick an organization like Weight Watchers. If you would rather work one-on-one with a counselor, turn to Diet Center, Jenny Craig, or a similar program. For more on the leading organizations, turn to Chapter 6, "Best Strategies for Losing Extra Pounds."

To Choose Or Not To Choose
If you have trouble making choices when it comes to food, your program should include preplanned menus complete with portion sizes and recipes. Duke University Medical Center provides meal plans, shopping lists, and recipes for the entire four weeks of its maintenance program.

If you like to cook, or if you are adventurous, you'll want more flexibility. The Tufts University School of Nutrition, for example, offers sample menus, but does not insist you eat specific foods at specific meals. It does, however provide helpful information on subjects such as ways to balance your diet, methods of reducing the fat in your food, the nutrients in fresh vegetables and fruits, and the sodium and fat content of various cheeses.

Liquid Diets
If you are severely overweight and at risk for serious health problems, your doctor may recommend a medically supervised liquid diet regimen. Optifast, Medifast, HMR, and other similar products, unlike the liquid pro-

teins that caused deaths in 1970s, include both high-quality protein and necessary amounts of vitamins and minerals. More than 300,000 people, including television talk show host Oprah Winfrey, have chosen this type of weight-loss program.

Like any dieting plan, a liquid protein regimen is not for everyone. You must be at least 50 pounds overweight or 30 percent above your ideal weight range on the Metropolitan Life Insurance Company charts. If your physician puts you on a strict liquid protein diet, you will need to be under the supervision of a clinic or hospital. Although you need not be an in-patient, you may require frequent—even daily monitoring. Five times a day for 12 weeks you will drink a beverage consisting of protein/nutrient powder mixed with water—and eat or drink nothing else. After the initial period, solid, healthy foods will be reintroduced. While you are dieting, you will also be taught to modify your eating behavior so that you will not regain weight when you return to normal meals.

The good news is: four out of five people who complete this kind of program lose an average of 40 pounds.

The bad news is: one-half of those who start the plan drop out, and most of those who make it through eventually regain the weight they lose, just as Oprah did. According to Tufts nutritionist Stanley Gershoff, if you lose weight this fast you are three times more likely to regain it than if you go more slowly. A second drawback is that while some dieters lose fat, others lose lean muscle tissue. A third problem is the cost: This kind of diet program is expensive. However, some health insurance plans will pick up the charges.

A second type of liquid diet is less expensive, does not require supervision, and, when used for a short period of time (e.g., 10 days) or to replace one meal a day, is not considered to be dangerous. Products such as Slimfast and Sweet Success are available in supermarkets and pharmacies at reasonable prices. However, if you consume only liquid, you are not learning how to cope with real food in the real world.

Hallmarks Of a Sound and Sensible Plan

A good nutrition plan not only helps you lose excess pounds, but also teaches you how to set your own goals and take lifetime responsibility for your weight and your health. Your program should contain the following features:

■ **Easy-to-follow instructions.** If the instructions are too complex, you will never stick to the plan. Your diet should fit easily into your life, not take it over.

■ **A healthy, balanced diet.** Nowadays the emphasis is on complex carbohydrates; fat is a "no-no". While we all should cut down or eliminate *saturated* fats, we do need some fat or oil in our diet—up to a recommended limit of 30 percent. We must also consume vegetable or animal protein and essential vitamins and minerals. Your diet should not eliminate any of these elements.

■ **Sufficient calories.** Different people require different numbers of calories to lose weight. The calorie count of your diet depends on your build, your level of activity, your lifestyle, and the number of pounds you need to shed. While you should not consume more calories than you can burn, you must have enough to maintain your health. Remember: extremely low-calorie diets never work in the long run, and can be dangerous.

■ **A variety of foods.** If you stick to one food or group of foods (fruits, for example) to the exclusion of others, your boredom may lead you to binge or to quit the diet completely. It may also be unhealthy.

■ **Readily-available foods.** Unless you enjoy browsing in specialty gourmet shops, choose a diet that lets you shop in your neighborhood supermarket. You do not need persimmons and jicama to lose weight.

■ **Meal plans and recipes.** It is helpful to know how to combine foods and when to eat them. And recipes are wonderful when you are learning how to cook a new, healthy way.

■ **An exercise plan.** Aerobic and muscle-building exercise are an important part of any weight-loss program. A good diet book or counselor should include exercise in the program, helping you plan a regular program of activity for the rest of your life. (see Chapter 8 for more on exercise.)

■ **Behavior modification.** You are bound to gain back the weight you have lost unless you understand why you overeat and learn how to change your habits permanently.

The array of diet books available to you—if you choose the do-it-yourself approach—is truly staggering. The brief "Buyer's Guide" that follows will give you an overview of today's leading titles. The books have been rated by their overall soundness by the Board of Consultants of *The PDR Family Guide to Nutrition and Health*.

BUYER'S GUIDE TO DIET BOOKS

Key to the ratings

■ ■ ■   Highly recommended
■ ■   Recommended
■   Not recommended

Rating	Name of Book	Author/Publisher	Description

Improving Your Health

Arthritis

Rating	Name of Book	Author/Publisher	Description
■	Freedom from Arthritis	Philip J. Welsh, Tree of Life Publications	May be a healthy diet, but there is no conclusive evidence that diet cures or relieves arthritis.
■	The Arthritis Relief Diet	James Scala, Plume	A balanced diet, but no single approach will work for everyone.

Cancer

Rating	Name of Book	Author/Publisher	Description
■	Cancer And Nutrition	Charles B. Simone, Avery Publishing Group Inc	Ten-point plan including diet tips to prevent development of cancer.
■	The Cancer Prevention Diet	Michio Kushi, St. Martin's Press	Macrobiotic diet to stave off cancer; inadequate nutrient intake; risky.
■ ■	The Cancer Recovery Eating Plan	Daniel W. Nixon, Random House	What to eat after diagnosis; eating plans for different types of cancer; recipes.

Diabetes

Rating	Name of Book	Author/Publisher	Description
■ ■	The Diabetic's Food Exchange Handbook	Clara G. Schneider, Running Press	Good information on food exchanges, calorie counts, and sodium values for nearly 4,000 popular foods.
■ ■ ■	The American Diabetes Association and The American Dietetic Association Family Cookbook	American Diabetes Association, American Dietetic Association, Simon & Schuster	Good information, menus, and recipes; easy to use.

Rating	Name of Book	Author/Publisher	Description
Heart Disease			
■ ■	Controlling Cholesterol	Kenneth H. Cooper, Bantam	Everything you ever wanted to know on the subject.
■ ■ ■	Dr. Dean Ornish's Program for Reversing Heart Disease	Dean Ornish, Ballantine	Diet, exercise, and lifestyle changes, plus a very low fat and cholesterol, high fiber and carbohydrate diet. Good for motivated people.
■ ■	Eater's Choice— A Food Lover's Guide to Lower Cholesterol	Ron Goor, Houghton Mifflin	Basic information, shopping tips,recipes; well-balanced nutri tion; easy to follow.
■ ■ ■	The Living Heart Diet	Michael DeBakey, et. al., Raven Press	Sound advice, diet, and food guides for heart health.
Intestinal Problems			
■	Breaking the Vicious Cycle— Intestinal Health Through Diet	Elaine Gottschall, Kirkton Press	High carbohydrate diet that claims to alleviate Crohn's disease, ulcerative colitis, diverticulitis, celliac disease, cystic fibrosis, and chronic diarrhea. However, dietary requirements for these diseases are varied.
Allergy			
■ ■ ■	Food Allergy: A Primer for People	S. Allan Bock, Vantage Books	Explains the differences between allergies and intolerances. Discusses proper testing. Scientifically-based information.
■	No More Allergies	Gary Null, Villard Books	The author's theories on allergies; includes diet, menu plans, and recipes. Not scientifically substantiated.
■ ■	Understanding Allergy, Sensitivity, and Immunity	Janice Vickerstaff Joneja, Rutgers University Press	Includes section on menu planning
AIDS			
■ ■	Surviving with AIDS: A Comprehensive Program of Nutritional Co-Therapy	C. Wayne Callaway, Catherine Whitney, Little Brown	Clinically tested low-fat, high-calorie program to help stop rapid wasting. Practical advice.

Rating	Name of Book	Author/Publisher	Description
Miscellaneous			
■ ■	The Food Pharmacy Guide to Good Eating	Jean Carper, Bantam	Foods for colon, lung and other health problems, with emphasis on fruits, vegetables, and low-fat foods; includes recipes.
■	The Healing Power of Foods	Michael T. Murray, Prima Publishing	Vegetables that supposedly heal, plus foods for specific diseases. Not scientifically substantiated.
■	The Save Your Life Diet	David Reuben, Random House	This 1975 high-fiber diet promises protection from disease. Questionable claims. Fiber must be part of balanced diet.
Promises, Promises			
■	Eat Smart, Think Smart	Robert Haas, Harper Collins	Special foods and supplements to increase intelligence, lose weight, forestall aging, and improve sleep.Not scientifically substantiated.
■	Power Foods	Liz Applegate, Rodale Press	"High Performance" drinks, "power eating" strategies. Not scientifically substantiated.

Weight Loss and Fitness

Rating	Name of Book	Author/Publisher	Description
■ ■ ■	Eating on the Run	Evelyn Tribole, Leisure Press	Smart eating plan loaded with ideas for busy people.
■ ■ ■	Outsmarting the Female Fat Cell	Debra Waterhouse, Hyperion	Weight control for women; entertaining.
■ ■ ■	Jane Brody's Nutrition Book	Jane Brody, Bantam	A good general guide to weight control and better health; sensible advice; easy to understand.
■	Dr. Lendon Smith's Low Stress Diet	Lendon Smith, McGraw-Hill Book Company	"Recognizing and managing stresses that create the cravings, addictions, binges, and unhealthy eating patterns that make you overweight." Not scientifically substantiated.

Rating	Name of Book	Author/Publisher	Description
■	Fit for Life	Harvey Diamond, Warner Books	Claims "it's not what you eat, but when and how." Emphasizes fresh foods, especially vegetables, eliminates dairy products. Contains misinformation. May lead to nutrient deficiencies.
■ ■	Jenny Craig's What Have You Got to Lose	Jenny Craig, Villard Books	Program advocated by this national organization. Good basic information (although sometimes not accurate). Expensive and time-consuming.
■	Lean Bodies	Cliff Sheats, The Summit Group	Lose body fat by increasing calories—25% protein, 65% carbohydrate, 10% fiber and essential fatty acids. Protein intake too high. Fat intake too low.
■ ■	One Meal at a Time	Martin Katahn, Warner Books	By the author of the T-Factor diet. Counts fat grams. Meal plans and recipes for dieters of all ages. Good concept, but eating too many calories still makes a difference.
■	The Beverly Hills Diet	Judy Mazel, Macmillan	Fad fruit diet. Not scientifically substantiated.
■	The Carbohydrate Addict's Diet	Rachel F. Heller, Richard F. Heller, Signet	High-fiber, low-fat, low-carbohydrate diet. Certain "complementary" foods must be combined at specific meals. Meal plans and recipes. Gives misinformation. Not scientifically substantiated.
■	The Carbohydrate Craver's Diet	Judith J. Wurtman, Houghton Mifflin Company	Low-calorie, high-carbohydrate diet with sweet or starchy snacks at daily "peak craving time." Not dangerous, but no scientific substantiation.
■	The Diet Center Program	Sybil Ferguson, Little Brown	Low-fat diet and lifestyle changes recommended by this national program. Too low in fat. No evidence that it works in the long term.

Rating	Name of Book	Author/Publisher	Description
■	The Doctor's Quick Weight Loss Diet	Irwin M. Stillman, Prentice-Hall	This 1968 best-seller emphasizes protein, eliminates carbohydrates. But eliminating an entire food group is unhealthy, and weight loss is too rapid.
■ ■ ■	The Duke University Medical Center Book of Diet and Fitness	Michael Hamilton, et. al., Fawcett Columbine	Excellent all-around plan for taking weight off sensibly and keeping it off through balanced diet and exercise.
■	The Hilton Head Diets (separate books for metabolism, people over 35, children and teens)	Warner	Rigid week-by-week meal plans for people with different amounts of weight to lose. May be too restrictive.
■	The McDougall Program for Maximum Weight Loss	John A. McDougall, Dutton	Low-fat, high-carbohydrate weight-loss diet promises to lower blood pressure and cholesterol, reduce risk of heart disease and cancer, eliminate most food allergies. Claims not scientifically substantiated.
■ ■	The Mediterranean Diet Cookbook	Nancy H. Jenkins, Bantam Books	Emphasis on fruits and vegetables, grains, legumes, breads, and fish, with small amounts of lean meat. Large amount of olive oil raises fat level too high. Diet may not include enough calcium.
■	The Pritikin Program for Diet and Exercise	Nathan Pritikin, Grosset & Dunlap	Promises you will feel and look younger. Emphasizes exercise. But it's too low in fat (less than 10%), calcium, iron, and vitamin B_{12}, and weight loss is too rapid (13.3 pounds in four weeks).
■	The Salad and Salmon Diet	Ronald Hoffman, The Hoffman Center, New York. (Available only by mail from Hoffman Center)	Low-saturated-fat diet with plenty of vegetables, few fruits and dairy products, and no refined foods. No portion sizes, meal plans, or recipes. Too restrictive.
■	The T-Factor Diet	Martin Katahn, W.W. Norton & Company	Claims protein and carbohydrate calories don't matter; fat does. But too many calories still produce fat, no matter what the source.

Rating	Name of Book	Author/Publisher	Description
■	The Two Day Diet	Glenn Cooper, Random House	Special "fat-burning, appetite depressing" food combinations two days at a time, anything you want the other two. Impossible to stick with over the long term. A fad diet.
■ ■	Thin for Life	Anne M. Fletcher, Chapters Publishing Ltd.	Low-fat diet, plus information on lifestyle changes and exercises.

Vegetarian and Macrobiotic Diets

Rating	Name of Book	Author/Publisher	Description
■ ■ ■	Diet for a Small Planet	Frances M. Lappé, Ballantine Books	Nutritional bible for vegetarians, complete with recipes. Information on "complimentary proteins" may be out-of-date.
■	Making the Transition to a Macrobiotic Diet	Carolyn Heindendry, Avery Publishing Group Inc.	A fairly basic vegetarian diet that could be dangerous if you make the transition to an all-rice or all-grain regimen. Theories not scientifically substantiated.
■	Macrobiotic Diet	Michio and Aveline Kushi, Japan Publications, Inc	Starts out as a basically healthy vegetarian diet, but progresses to dangerously restrictive all-rice or all-grain regimen.

Pocket "Counters"

Rating	Name of Book	Author/Publisher	Description
■ ■	The Cholesterol Counter	Annette B. Natow, Jo-Ann Heslin, Pocket Books	For "heart-healthy" dieters.
■ ■	The Dieter's Calorie Counter	Corinne T. Netzer, Dell	10,000 listings.
■ ■	The Fast Food Nutrition Counter	Annette B. Natow, Jo-Ann Heslin, Pocket Books	Handy when eating out.
■ ■	The Fiber Counter	Corinne T. Netzer, Dell	Covers brand name and generic foods.
■ ■	The Low Fat Supermarket Shopper's Guide and The Low Fat Fast Food Guide	Jamie Pope-Cordle, Martin Katahn, W.W. Norton & Company	Lists foods by brand names.
■ ■ ■	T-Factor Fat Counter	Jamie Pope-Cordle, Martin Katahn, W.W. Norton & Company	Counts fat, cholesterol, calories, fiber, and sodium.

Keeping Your Weight in Check

CHAPTER 5

How Much Weight Is Too Much: Setting a Healthy Goal

In the U.S., food is abundant, diverse, delicious, ... and very often, high in calories. The result of this embarrassment of riches is an alarming rise in the number of fat Americans. Overweight is a particular problem for those under the age of 50, especially women and minorities. Yet younger fat people stand to benefit even more from weight reduction than do the middle-aged and elderly.

The American Phenomenon of Overweight

The average weight of Americans age 25 to 30 rose a substantial 10 pounds from 1985 to 1992, to 173 pounds for men and 148 pounds for women. It is estimated that approximately 34 million Americans—30 percent of the population—are overweight. Nine percent are severely obese.

Obesity and overweight are not the same thing, though the experts don't agree as to what, precisely, obesity is. In general, the term "obesity" is applied when an individual is from 20 to 30 percent over the average weight for his or her age, sex, and height.

The economic cost of battling these excess pounds is substantial: over $40 billion in healthcare costs and at least $30 billion a year in efforts to lose or control weight. The costs in terms of human suffering cannot be so easily quantified.

The Health Consequences

Overweight encourages high blood pressure, high cholesterol, heart disease, diabetes, and a variety of other diseases.

For example, high blood pressure is almost six times more common among overweight people age 20 to 44 and twice as common in those 45 to 74. Overweight people are also three times more likely to develop diabetes. In fact, the Nurses Health Study, one of the largest disease-risk studies ever undertaken, showed that women who

FIGURING YOUR BMI

The Body Mass Index (BMI) incorporates both your height and weight to assess your weight-related level of risk for heart disease, diabetes, and high blood pressure.

To find your BMI, multiply your weight in pounds by 700, divide by your height in inches, then divide by your height again. For example, if you're 5 feet, 10 inches and weigh 185 pounds, the math would go like this:

- 185 pounds x 700 = 129,500
- 129,500 ÷ 70 inches = 1,850
- 1,850 ÷ 70 inches = 26.4

Indications of Risk:

- BMI of 25 or less: very low to low risk
- BMI between 25 and 30: low to moderate risk
- BMI of 30 or more: moderate to very high risk

gain 15 excess pounds increase their risk of diabetes by 50 percent.

For men, the consequences of being overweight can be even more pronounced. A recently completed 27-year study of more than 19,000 middle-aged men found that those at their ideal weights lived significantly longer than those just 2 to 6 percent above what's considered ideal. That's not a lot of excess baggage. For a medium-framed man who's 5 feet, 10 inches tall, 6 percent of an ideal weight of 158 pounds is only nine-and-a-half pounds.

The heavier the men in the study, the shorter their life expectancy. Those who were 20 percent overweight had a risk of death from heart disease that was two-and-a-half times that of men whose weight was ideal.

Cancer and More

Obesity has also been linked with gallstones, back pain, sleep apnea (a condition characterized by brief periods when breathing stops during sleep), heartburn, stroke, gout, varicose veins, and even some types of cancer, including colon and prostate cancer in men, and uterine, endometrial, and breast cancer in women.

When researchers looked at 735 women who were treated for stage II and III breast cancers, they found that among women who were more than 20 percent over their ideal weights the risk of recurrence was a third higher than among their slimmer counterparts. As a result, many researchers regard obesity as an independent indicator of a poor prognosis for breast cancer, even when the best medical treatments are administered.

What seems clear is that the biochemical disruptions caused by being overweight are more complex and more prevalent than we thought. In just the last year or two, medical researchers have discovered links between excess weight and an astonishing variety of health problems, ranging from osteoarthritis of the hands and knees to birth defects. All of these discoveries underscore the wisdom and benefits of weight control.

Osteoarthritis. It makes sense that there's a link between osteoarthritis of the knees and being overweight: carrying an extra 50 pounds of baggage can wreak havoc on the knee joints. But recent research from the University of Michigan found that people who were 20 percent or more overweight were also three times more likely than slimmer people to have osteoarthritis of the hands, and that their arthritis was more severe.

Carpal-Tunnel Syndrome. Excess weight may also be a major contributing factor to a nerve conduction problem in the hand, commonly known as carpal-tunnel syndrome, or CTS. The Portland Hand Surgery and Rehabilitation Center found that overweight was the strongest single predictor of CTS—twice as influential as age. Surprisingly, the kind of work people did had virtually no bearing on whether or not they developed the problem.

Immune Deficiencies. An intriguing study from Japan suggests that obesity may also be a threat to the body's immune system. Indeed, when obese people were put on strict diets, losing an average of 50 pounds each,

activity of the T lymphocytes—the body's defender cells—nearly doubled.

Birth Defects. Preliminary research also indicates that women who are extremely—not just moderately—obese have about twice the risk of giving birth to babies with very serious defects, including spina bifida, when protective bone fails to close around the spinal cord.

Social, Economic, and Psychological Stress. A certain degree of social contempt is probably the most damaging psychological consequence of overweight. People with weight problems have traditionally been regarded as sloppy, lazy, and lacking will power or self-control. They suffer discrimination at school

THE WAGES OF FAT

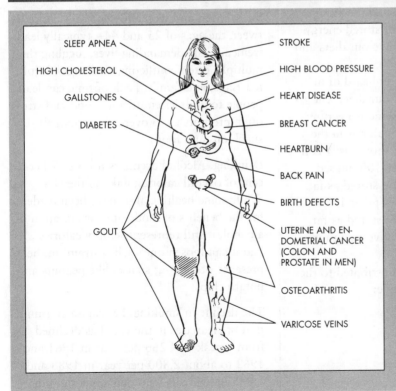

SLEEP APNEA
HIGH CHOLESTEROL
GALLSTONES
DIABETES
GOUT

STROKE
HIGH BLOOD PRESSURE
HEART DISEASE
BREAST CANCER
HEARTBURN
BACK PAIN
BIRTH DEFECTS
UTERINE AND ENDOMETRIAL CANCER (COLON AND PROSTATE IN MEN)
OSTEOARTHRITIS
VARICOSE VEINS

Excess weight is not responsible for everything that ails you, but it definitely is associated with some of America's most dangerous disorders, including high blood pressure, heart disease, diabetes, and recurrent breast cancer. If you are overweight, your chances of developing high blood pressure are at least double what they would otherwise be, and your chances of becoming diabetic are triple. Among men tipping the scales at 20 percent above the norm, the rate of heart disease is two-and-a-half times the rate among men whose weight meets the ideal.

and in the workplace. Indeed, public mockery of fat people is one of the last remaining socially-sanctioned forms of prejudice. Repeatedly fruitless efforts to control their weight and years of subtle put-downs and overt criticism can tear away at the self-esteem of overweight men and women.

How It Happens

Why is overweight so prevalent in America? The answer is simple: Many of us are taking in more fuel than our bodies need.

Evolution perfected the fat storage mechanisms of the human body. For millennia, periodic food shortages—as a result of drought, or catastrophe—were a way of life for our ancestors. Those people most likely to survive were those who during good times could convert extra food into body fat that served as insurance against the famine. At approximately 3,500 calories per pound, fat is an extremely efficient repository of stored energy.

But life has changed, as have our diets and activity levels.

Today, periodic famine is unheard of in the industrialized world, yet our diets tend to be richer than ever. Indeed, Americans now consume 34 percent of their calories in the form of dietary fat, the food most easily converted to body fat. (For every 100 unused calories taken in as fat, 97 are stored as fat. For every 100 unused calories taken in as carbohydrates, only 77 are stored as fat; the rest fuel the process of converting those carbohydrates to fat.)

Other factors that have contributed to the epidemic of overweight include:

Highly processed foods. While there are exceptions to the rule, the healthiest foods tend to be subject to the least processing by food manufacturers. Whole grain cereal is more nutritious—and lower in calories—than fatty, sugary granola. A fresh peach is nutritionally preferable to a slice of peach cobbler. Many of us, unfortunately, have developed the habit of eating foods laced with excessive amounts of fat, sugar, and sodium.

Lack of exercise. While our caloric intake has increased, our caloric expenditures have declined. We Americans are leading far more sedentary lives than our parents and grandparents did. We have countless labor saving devices at home and at work; and our leisure time is more likely to be spent in front of a computer or a television than on a softball field or a bike, or even just walking.

Stress. Men and women—especially those between the ages of 25 and 44—typically lead tremendously demanding lives, juggling the multiple, often conflicting challenges of job, marriage, and family. Lack of time can lead people to grab less nutritious food and stress often prompts us to overeat or routinely snack on junk food.

Drinking. Alcohol accounts for 5 to 7 percent of overall caloric intake in the U.S. While some health claims have been made for the benefits of moderate consumption of alcohol, it still represents empty calories . . . and it can loosen one's self-restraint in the presence of high-fat snacks like peanuts and potato chips.

The decline in smoking. Per-capita consumption of cigarettes in the U.S. has declined from a peak of 4,266 per year in 1961 and 1962 to about 2,800 per year in 1988 and 1989. Individuals who quit smoking often experience a 4- to 6-pound weight gain. It is important to remember, however, that smoking is far more dangerous than is a relatively small gain in weight.

Sex Matters

It's sad but true: Women gain weight more easily than men do; and women have to work harder to get it off. It's all a matter of biochemistry.

A fat cell is designed to store calories (lipogenesis) when you don't need them and release fat (lipolysis) when you do. The enzymes that help store fat are called lipogenic enzymes; the ones that help release fat are lipolytic enzymes.

Women tend to have more lipogenic enzymes for fat storage; and the more you can store, the bigger the fat cell. Men have more lipolytic enzymes for fat release and, therefore, smaller fat cells.

Testosterone, the male sex hormone, activates the lipolytic enzymes for speedy release of fat. Estrogen, the female sex hormone, activates and multiplies the lipogenic enzymes. (This explains the extra deposits of fat that women experience during puberty and pregnancy, and when they are taking oral contraceptives or getting estrogen-replacement therapy.) Estrogen not only stimulates the storage of fat, but also directs where most of it will be stored, concentrating it in the hips, buttocks, and thighs.

Having evolved as protection against periods of famine, these fat-storage mechanisms are governed by the needs of each gender. A man's body generally contains enough fat to protect itself for a few months. A woman's

WHEN DIETING RUNS AMOK

For far too many Americans, the feast/famine cycle of our earliest ancestors has resurfaced as the binge/diet cycle of today. Approximately eight million Americans suffer from such eating disorders as anorexia (a refusal to eat due to an obsessive fear of fatness) and bulimia (binge eating followed by purging through vomiting or laxatives). Women seem to be particularly vulnerable to an abnormal preoccupation with food and a distorted body image.

Thirty years of deifying slimness in the media have led to this sad state of affairs. The fact is that five or ten excess pounds doesn't make you obese, and thin does not equal fit or healthy.

While about a third of U.S. women are actually overweight, as many as 77 percent believe that they are too fat and 40 percent are on a diet at any given time. For many, it's completely unnecessary.

body, on the other hand, stores nine months' worth of fat—enough to protect her and her unborn child for the length of a full-term pregnancy.

Throughout their lives, women have more body fat than men. Even the bodies of young girls contain a higher percentage of fat than young boys' bodies do. And at certain milestones in the female lifecycle—puberty, pregnancy, and menopause—women tend to put on more fat. That means that the older a woman gets, the more likely she is to stray from society's ideal of female beauty.

To make matters worse, the thigh, hip, and buttock fat that estrogen helps deposit is metabolized more slowly than fat elsewhere, making those particular pounds especially difficult to reduce.

Overweight or Over-Fat?

Don't trust only your scale or your mirror; they tell just half the story. It is body fat, rather than weight, that maybe the best indicator of whether or not you need to trim down.

Fat comprises about 15 to 18 percent of the total body weight of a healthy, physically fit man. For a woman, the ratio is slightly higher: from 20 to 25 percent. Remember: you can be overweight without being over-fat and over-fat without being overweight.

For example, a 6-foot-tall, 275-pound linebacker may be overweight according to formal height-weight tables. But, as a professional athlete, his body-fat content may be as low as 10 percent, making him fit, not fat. Conversely, a man whose weight falls within the "normal" range, but who gets little exercise and whose body fat measures 18 percent, could be classified as over-fat.

There are a number of techniques for calculating body fat. Most are based on pinching and measuring subcutaneous fat (the fat below the skin). However the most accurate method involves being weighed in a water tank, since the measurement takes into account the fat that may be marbled through your muscles. Fat—like cream—floats; lean muscle mass and bone, which are heavier than fat or water, sink. The fatter you are, the less you will weigh submerged in water.

This is one of the reasons why a tape measure can be a better tool than a scale for measuring the success of a weight loss program. Since muscle weighs more than fat, your weight may seem to stabilize or even increase as you build muscle mass. Don't be discouraged. If you're wearing smaller-sized clothes or you've lost inches from your hips, waist, or neck, you are actually leaner and healthier than when you started.

Apple vs. Pear

At least as important as total weight is where the fat tends to settle on your body. While fat in the hip, thigh, and buttocks is mainly stored just under the skin, fat in the midsection is stored deeper in the body.

It has now been well-established that having an "apple shape," in which fat collects around the midsection, is more dangerous than having a "pear shape," in which excess fat gravitates to the hips and thighs.

Experts theorize that abdominal fat releases more fatty acids, leading to a rise in blood cholesterol and triglyceride levels. While this can be a serious health problem in and of itself, it also may interfere with the action of insulin in the body, thus increasing the risk of diabetes. Some researchers also believe that "apple shape" obesity may increase the availability and activity of estrogen, leading to an elevated risk of breast cancer. The good news is that, to some degree, you can modify your shape, whether apple or pear, through exercise and diet modification.

It's Not Just A Matter of Will Power

Most of us realize that our dissatisfaction with our bodies is the result of our society's love affair with the ultra-slim ideal of beauty personified by underfed "waif" models. We have also bought the myth that our bodies are infinitely adjustable.

Obesity researchers are discovering, however, that our capacity to change our weights is actually quite limited. In addition to our gender, we can partly blame our genes. Even before discovery of the "fat gene" in mice, researchers had decided that genetic factors can be twice as important as lifestyle in determining adult weight.

Although for many centuries obesity was considered simply a result of gluttony, it is now well established that there is a genetic propensity for it in some individuals, families, and larger social groups with a shared heritage. For example, studies have shown that twins with a genetic tendency toward fatness are likely to grow up fat, even if adopted separately by thin families.

Researchers have also found that one person's basal metabolism (the rate at which he

APPLE OR PEAR

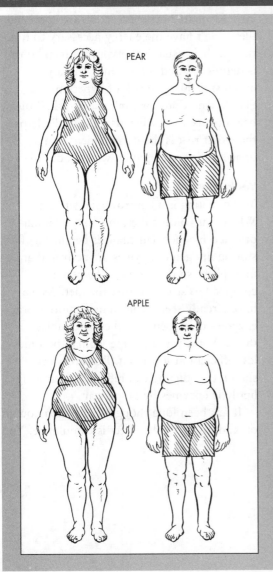

PEAR

APPLE

People with apple-shaped figures (heavy around the abdomen) have a higher risk for cardiovascular disease than do pear-shaped people (heavy around the hips and thighs).

To find your waist-to-hip ratio:

1. Use a tape measure to find the circumference of your waist at its narrowest point when your stomach is relaxed.

Waist:_____ inches

2. Measure the circumference of your hips at their widest (where your buttocks protrude the most).

Hips:_____ inches

3. Divide your waist measurement by your hip measurement.

Waist ÷ hip = _____ Waist-to-hip ratio

The higher the ratio, the more apple–shaped; and the greater the risk of disease. Women should have a ratio of 0.8 or less. For men, a waist-to-hip ratio of less than 0.95 to 1.0 is recommended or she expends energy) can differ from another's by as much as 400 to 500 calories a day. There can also be differences in the ways individuals store or burn off extra calories. One person may need to consume 4,000 calories each day to gain weight, while another may see an increase on just 1,000 calories a day.

And, in particular ethnic groups—for example, the Pima Indians of Arizona—there is an extraordinarily high prevalence of obesity. Genetically equipped to retain fat in times of famine, they respond to today's ready availability of food and reduced activity with an especially quick and substantial weight gain.

The influence of genes is far from clear-cut. To confuse matters, ethnic, religious, and class factors all seem to play a role in obesity. For instance, researchers don't know whether it's a cause, an effect, or a coincidence, but it's a fact that excess weight tends to accompany low social status. Ironically, people who live below the poverty line are more likely to be fat than those at the top of the economic pyramid.

Diets Alone Don't Do It

Regardless of your background or genetic make-up, it *is* possible to keep your weight in check. Radical and repeated dieting, however, is not the answer—even though physicians routinely recommend dieting for heavy patients. Extreme dieting poses dangers associated with continual food restriction, and statistics show that 80 to 90 percent of all dieters regain the weight they lose.

Prescription and over-the-counter medications rarely work either. Although they may help take off pounds temporarily, there is little evidence that they can help maintain long-term weight loss.

Very Low Calorie Diets

Physician-supervised commercial semi-starvation diet plans, which offer participants just 400 to 600 calories daily for a period of months, are supposed to help the dieter's body shed excess fat rather than muscle. But there have been many reports of adverse side effects, including at least 67 deaths.

Very low-calorie diets, particularly those that concentrate on one or two foods, often lack adequate nutrients. People on restricted diets don't have the energy necessary to function at their usual activity levels; metabolism is depressed; and see-sawing weight gains and losses raise the risk of hypertension. People who don't or can't stick to their diets begin to see themselves as failures. Perhaps the worst risk is the development of a dangerous preoccupation with food.

Yo-Yo Dieting

Yo-yo dieting is a controversial subject. When you go on a diet, the body's famine-oriented biochemical changes begin. The fat-storing lipogenic enzymes are activated and multiplied, so that you will be better equipped to store fat after the diet. As we have already seen, women have more storage enzymes than men, and dieting doubles them. Worse yet, a dieting woman becomes less efficient at losing fat. Research has shown that dieting can reduce fat-releasing lipolytic enzymes by 50 percent.

It has been long thought that when you go on and off diets, the effect is cumulative. You supposedly manufacture even more storage enzymes and fewer releasing enzymes after every diet cycle, so that each time you go on a diet, you will lose the weight more slowly and gain it back more quickly. However, the National Institutes of Health have been unable to find any evidence that yo-yo dieting actually does make weight loss more difficult the next time around. Nevertheless, it's still a good idea to avoid it.

Easier than Dieting: a Matter of Eating Right

So, if dieting isn't the answer, what is? It's how you eat—not just what you eat—and how you live.

Keep a food diary. For four days, including one weekend, write down the foods you eat, how much, where, when, and under what circumstances (for example, watching TV at night, when you're angry, when you are cleaning up the kitchen). This can help you see whether you have an eating pattern that is blocking your efforts to control your weight. (Are you confusing anger, anxiety, or boredom with hunger?)

Stop dieting. Diets are restrictive, boring, and punitive. Eating healthy, however, is a satisfying lifetime proposition. Increase your consumption of nutrient-rich foods like vegetables, fruits, and whole grains, while cutting back on "empty" calories and fatty fare. (But keep your favorite foods on the menu—at least once in a while—so you won't feel deprived.)

Eat slowly. Smell, taste, and savor your food. If you eat too fast, you'll be stuffed before you feel full.

Burn the fat. Exercise is critical for healthy weight loss. It doesn't have to be vigorous exercise: a brisk walk or other form of aerobic exercise for 30 minutes every other day is enough to raise your metabolism and condition your cells to release and burn fat. Building muscle mass helps, too. It increases the number of mitochondria, the fat-burners in your muscle cells. Strength-building exercise for 30 to 60 minutes 4 days or more per week increases muscle mass and doubles the efficiency of the mitochondria in your muscle cells.

Be a daytime eater. While metabolism is highest during your first 12 waking hours, the typical American eats about 70 percent of the day's calorie allotment after 5:00 p.m.,

STARTING YOUR CHILDREN OFF RIGHT

In the last trimester before birth, the baby begins to accumulate fat cells. For the first six months of infancy, the number of fat cells continues to increase, then slows through childhood. The total number of fat cells accumulated (generally 30 to 40 billion in the average adult) depends on genetic and lifestyle factors, especially nutritional ones.

Although some researchers believe that obesity in childhood predisposes a person to obesity for life, not all fat babies grow into fat adults.

Obviously, it's better—and easier—to prevent gain than it is to try to take off excess pounds after they have accumulated. For the best ways of keeping your child's weight in line, see Chapter 18, "What's Right—and Wrong—for the Kids."

WHAT'S THE RIGHT WEIGHT RANGE FOR YOU?

Standardized height-weight tables should be merely a starting point for an understanding of your natural weight. The best weight for many people is simply the lowest they have been able to maintain for a year as an adult without a struggle.

Body shape is another factor you should consider when calculating your ideal weight. Fat concentrated on the hips, thighs, and buttocks (the classic "pear shape") is less dangerous than fat you carry on your abdomen (the "apple shape"). So, individuals with slender arms, legs and hips, who are thick around the middle, should probably dip below the standard for their height to reduce their risk of developing fat-related illnesses like cardiovascular disease and diabetes.

Most obesity experts prefer the Metropolitan Life Insurance Company Weight table for determining recommended weight ranges for optimum health. Remember that less can be more here. In a study of Harvard alumni, researchers found the lowest mortality among individuals who weighed, on average, 20 percent less than the U.S. average for men of comparable age and height.

1. DECIDE ON YOUR FRAME

Bend your forearm upward at a 90° angle. Keep your fingers straight and turn the inside of your wrist toward your body. Place the thumb and index finger of your other hand on the two prominent bones on either side of your elbow. Measure the space between your fingers on a ruler. Compare with the figures below listing elbow measurements for *medium-framed* men and women. If your measurement is lower than those listed below it indicates a small frame. Higher measurements indicate a large frame.

Men		Women	
Height (in 1" heels)	**Elbow Breadth**	**Height (in 1" heels)**	**Elbow Breadth**
5'2"-5'3"	2 1/2"-2 7/8"	4'10"-4'11"	2 1/4"-2 1/2"
5'4"-5'7"	2 5/8"-2 7/8"	5'0"-5'3"	2 1/4"-2 1/2"
5'8"-5'11"	2 3/4"-3"	5'4"-5'7"	2 3/8"-2 5/8"
6'0-6'3"	2 3/4"-3 1/8"	5'8"-5'11"	2 3/8"-2 5/8"
6'4"	2 7/8"-3 1/4"	6'0"	2 1/2"-2 3/4"

when metabolism is lowest. If you wake at 7:00 a.m. and your body needs 1500 calories a day, it will burn about 75 percent of those calories (or 1,125 calories) from 7:00 a.m. to 7:00 p.m., and only about 25 percent (or 375 calories) after 7:00 p.m. Any additional calories after 7:00 p.m. will stay around to haunt you.

Shrink and multiply your meals. Eat five or six meals a day instead of three, but eat only the amount of food that you would ordinarily have eaten at three meals distributed evenly over the course of the day.

Look for support. Not all of us can go it alone. Turn to friends, family, and the local chapters of organizations like Overeaters Anonymous or Weight Watchers to provide the encouragement you may need when your commitment to a healthy lifestyle falters.

2. FIND YOUR PLACE IN THE TABLE

The following weights at ages 25-59, based on lowest mortality, are given in pounds according to frame (in indoor clothing weighing 5 lbs. for men and 3 lbs. for women; shoes with 1" heels).

Men Height Ft In	Small Frame	Medium Frame	Large Frame	Women Height Ft In	Small Frame	Medium Frame	Large Frame
5 2	128-134	131-141	138-150	4 10	102-111	109-121	118-131
5 3	130-136	133-143	140-153	4 11	103-113	111-123	120-134
5 4	132-138	135-145	142-156	5 0	104-115	113-126	122-137
5 5	134-140	137-148	144-160	5 1	106-118	115-129	125-140
5 6	136-142	139-151	146-164	5 2	108-121	118-132	128-143
5 7	138-145	142-154	149-168	5 3	111-124	121-135	131-147
5 8	140-148	145-157	152-172	5 4	114-127	124-138	134-151
5 9	142-151	148-160	155-176	5 5	117-130	127-141	137-155
5 10	144-154	151-163	158-180	5 6	120-133	130-144	140-159
5 11	146-157	154-166	161-184	5 7	123-136	133-147	143-163
6 0	149-160	157-170	164-188	5 8	126-139	136-150	146-167
6 1	152-164	160-174	168-192	5 9	129-142	139-153	149-170
6 2	155-168	164-178	172-197	5 10	132-145	142-156	152-173
6 3	158-172	167-182	176-202	5 11	135-148	145-159	155-176
6 4	162-176	171-187	181-207	6 0	138-151	148-162	158-179

Source: Courtesy of Metropolitan Life Insurance Company *Statistical Bulletin*.

Take it easy. Trying to lose too much too fast by following a diet that is too stringent just won't work. Target a slow, but steady weight loss not to exceed one-half to 2 pounds a week. (Aim for a loss of more than 1 percent of your body weight per week.) An exercise-induced burn of 300 calories a day plus a daily calorie reduction of only 200 calories is often enough to lose a pound a week.

Be flexible. Don't set rigid targets; and don't let your menu dominate your life. Listen to your hunger, and stop when it subsides.

Whatever else you do, be sure to get up and move around. A recent study at the University of Washington among overweight, but otherwise healthy men over age 65 found that trimming off five pounds by walking, jogging, or bike riding raised "good" cholesterol—high-density lipoproteins (HDLs)—even more than did losing 20 pounds by cutting calories alone.

So What Weight Is Right For You?

Recent research suggests that if you repeatedly have trouble reaching—and maintaining—your ideal weight, you may be better off surrendering that elusive goal altogether and focusing instead on what your body really wants to weigh: your natural weight.

Natural weight is the weight your body goes to and maintains when you're eating reasonably and not drastically cutting calories, exercising vigorously, or otherwise trying to shed pounds. It will never be a fixed number, but, rather, a range of 5 to 8 pounds (since weight normally varies slightly with changes in general health, activity, hormone levels, and the time of day).

Of course, that doesn't mean that any weight is healthy. If your weight is 20 percent or more over the top of the ideal range for your height and frame (see the nearby table), you should consider trimming down to stay healthy.

Gauging Your Natural Weight

To determine your current natural weight range, consider the following factors.

Your personal weight history. Try to remember the lowest weight range you have successfully maintained as an adult, without dieting, for a period of a year or more. That is your baseline natural weight range.

Your family. Make a mental picture of your parents, grandparents, aunts, and uncles when they were about the age you are now. Because genetics is a powerful variable in terms of size and shape, family resemblance can help define your natural weight. (Remember, however, that even if you come from a long line of very heavy people, if your weight seems dangerously high, it's wise to check with your doctor about the need to shed some pounds.)

Your exercise habits. Think back to that period when you maintained your lowest-ever weight. If you exercised regularly then and don't do it now, you may need to add several pounds to your baseline weight range—or start exercising again.

Your age. As the years pass, metabolism slows and weight tends to creep upward. There is a great deal of controversy about whether or not you can afford to put on a few extra pounds as you get older without risking your health. Nevertheless, while not all of us gain weight with age, few can expect to have as sleek a profile at 40 as at 25. Your target—all things being equal—should be to keep your weight no higher than the current height-weight recommendations.

Then What?

Once you have determined your natural weight range, what do you do with the information? If your weight is excessive for your height, you should try to lose weight gradually by adopting a low-fat, moderate-calorie, healthful diet and boosting your exercise level. Remember that crash diets and furious bouts of exercise don't work; moderation and consistency do.

If your natural weight and shape check out healthy, however, your only real task may be to abandon the image of that impossibly svelte ideal and begin the process of becoming comfortable with the body you have. □

CHAPTER 6

Best Strategies for Losing Extra Pounds

Yes, you *can* reach and maintain a healthy weight. Despite the discouraging news of failures in many diet programs and America's growing problem with obesity, researchers are finally beginning to pin down just which strategies work—and which fail—to help long-term weight control.

Let's start with the bad news. "You are what you weigh" is one of the more pervasive—and destructive—messages of contemporary American culture. But ironically, our preoccupation with the numbers on the scale and our excessive admiration for the slender figure seem to be leading to an increase in obesity. In 1980, 25.4 percent of the U.S. population was overweight; by 1991, the figure had jumped to 31.1 percent—a trend that includes all races, ages, and genders, according to a 1994 report by the National Center of Health Statistics. Overall, a third of Americans are overweight, with adults weighing an average of 8 pounds more than they did a decade ago.

Though many have difficulty managing their weight, it's not for lack of trying. An es-

timated 50 million Americans will go on diets this year, seeking advice from books, TV diet gurus, support groups, and clinical programs. Women's magazines report that 95 percent of their female readership is on a diet. Desperate dieters have turned the weight-loss business into a booming industry, with annual revenues of $30 to $50 billion. However, while some will succeed in shedding those extra pounds, some studies show that perhaps as few as 5 percent manage to keep them off. The report from the National Center of Health Statistics also warns that "weight reduction through calorie-restricted dieting ...ultimately [is] not very effective."

Hold on! Does this mean diets don't work? Of course not. "Diets do work. It's the maintenance programs that don't work," says Dr. Arthur Frank, Medical Director of the George Washington University Obesity Management Program. "Most people who do get involved with a weight-loss program stay with it. Most people who stay with it

TIP-OFFS OF RIP-OFFS

When it comes to weight-loss schemes, the Food and Drug Administration warns you to be particularly skeptical of claims containing words and phrases like:

- easy
- effortless
- guaranteed
- miraculous
- magical
- breakthrough

- new discovery
- mysterious
- exotic
- secret
- exclusive
- ancient

do, in fact, lose weight. The problem is that most people still have a difficult problem maintaining weight at the new lower level." The notion that diets don't work is a roundabout way of saying that there are no magic ways to keep pounds off permanently; obesity is a chronic condition that requires lifelong attention.

In addition, the studies showing that most people regain the weight they lose may not apply to most of us. These studies have been done in clinical programs on people with the most severe weight problems. "Most people who are successful in losing weight do so on their own," says Dr. Xavier Pi-Sunyer, Director of the Division of Endocrinology and Nutrition at St. Luke's-Roosevelt Hospital, New York, and Professor of Medicine at Columbia University. "They are seldom included in studies. We also have very little data about how people do one-on-one with a physician, dietitian, or nutritionist." So do-it-yourself dieters may have more reason to be optimistic about their chances for success.

Instead of a quick fix, self-starters tend to be motivated to change their overall eating patterns, with better long-term results. Still, the secret lies in finding the nutritional strategy that works best for you. "Adults and children with weight problems need tools for making better decisions about how to lose weight," says Judith Stern, ScD, RD, Professor in the Departments of Nutrition and Internal Medicine at the University of California, Davis. A healthy skepticism is a good place to start. Beware of claims of weight-loss miracles: "Lose weight while you sleep;" "Eat all you want and get thin;" "This secret method will work where others fail." If a diet claim seems too good to be true, it probably is.

The sections that follow are designed to help you sort through and discard the diet claims that are confusing, costly, misleading, even hazardous to your health. They will help you choose a weight-loss plan that is suited to your individual needs. The next chapter focuses on effective techniques for maintaining a healthy weight, once you achieve it.

It's Not All Heredity

An understanding of the basic causes of overweight can help you analyze your own strengths and weaknesses and choose a diet plan that will maximize your chances of success. To some extent, obesity is hereditary; but scientists now believe that heredity accounts for only a third of the problem, with the remaining two thirds stemming from cultural factors.

Though every culture in the world has overweight individuals, the problem is most pervasive in America. "The United States is one of the richest countries in the world, giving us a bounty of food at relatively little cost," says Dr. Frank, co-author of the 1995 National Academy of Sciences dieting guidelines. "In addition, we have perfected snack food. The difference in snack-food consumption between this country and western Europe is enormous. For example, Americans eat more than twice as many calories in snack foods than do the French." Overall, our rich and diverse food supply tends to be high in fat, sugar, and calories.

In addition, over the years Americans have come to expect larger portions. "A 'normal' meal to us looks massive to foreigners," says Dr. Pi-Sunyer. "We'll scarf down a 12-ounce slab of beef without thinking; while most of the world would be happy with 4 ounces. We think nothing of a three-scoop ice cream cone, yet elsewhere one small scoop of sherbet is considered a luxury." Adds Judith Stern, "You can super-size anything for 35 cents in most convenience stores or fast food places." In the land of 64-ounce shakes, things certainly have raged out of control.

Inactivity is also a culprit. Most Americans lead sedentary lifestyles, relying on cars rather than walking, watching sports instead of playing them, plowing through paperwork rather than fields. The upshot? "We eat more and exercise less; we take in more calories and expend fewer. We're like a car with too much gasoline," says Dr. Pi-Sunyer.

The Genetic Thermostat
Some people will never be able to achieve the American ideal of super-slimness, no matter how healthfully they eat or how regularly they exercise. It's just not in the genetic cards. Studies have shown conclusively that an individual's body size and shape is genetically coded as surely as the color of the eyes. The body's normal weight range varies considerably among individuals and is overwhelmingly determined by heredity. The weight to which your body naturally inclines is like a preselected temperature on a thermostat. Your genetic make-up guides your body towards its natural weight through both hunger cues and metabolism. "Obesity is not simply the lack of self-control," says Dr. Pi-Sunyer.

Although the genetic mechanisms underlying obesity are still largely unknown, our understanding is rapidly increasing. Scientists have recently discovered a gene which, when mutated, is associated with great obesity in mice. "These animals cannot get to a normal body composition," says Dr. Dale R. Romsos, Professor of Nutrition, Department of Food Science and Human Nutrition, Michigan State University, who was involved in the groundbreaking research. "If you restrict the mice's food intake, you make them smaller, but they are still obese. They do lose body weight, but in tissue, not in fat." The gene is similar to one in humans. "It may be a contributing factor in a subset of obese humans, but it is very unlikely to be the problem in a person who is 10 or 15 pounds overweight," says Dr. Romsos.

This discovery is only the beginning of unravelling the genetics of weight control. "Human obesity springs from numerous genes, and it is likely that a combination of as many as 20 or more may be involved," says Dr. Pi-Sunyer. Nor does a genetic predisposition automatically yield obesity. In certain environments, people with a genetic inclination towards obesity might never be overweight. But combined with the cultural factors in the U.S. where food is plentiful, diets are high in fat, and people tend to be sedentary, a genetic tendency towards obesity can blossom to its full potential.

In the Eyes of the Beholder

Being severely overweight carries with it a social stigma unlike any other health condition. A person with asthma or diabetes is not "blamed" for his or her condition. But Americans regard obesity "as a disease of willful misconduct," explains Dr. Frank. "This view holds that you are fat because you are not a good person, you have misbehaved." As a result, dieters tend to punish themselves when the results they seek are not achieved; they feel like they're "cheating" when they go off their regimen. Worse yet, our worship of the svelte has produced an alarming increase in eating disorders. Efforts to acquire the "ideal" body are leading more and more people, especially women, to diet at the cost of their health.

To combat this social stigma, the idea of fat—or size—acceptance has gained a growing following. Groups such as Largesse and the National Association to Advance Fat Acceptance promote "size esteem" and work to dispel the "myth" that overweight people are less disciplined than others. Instead of thinking thin, they say, "think health." Adopt the philosophy of Dr. John P. Foreyt of Baylor University: "Not everyone can be skinny, but everyone can be healthier."

There is wisdom in this for us all. Before embarking on a weight-loss program, it really is important to try to separate social pressures from valid medical reasons for improving nutrition. This involves answering three questions: 1) Should I be worrying about my weight at all? 2) If so, what are the motivations leading me to overeat? 3) What type of weight-loss program will offer me the best chance of success?

Should You Even Be Worried?

Two thirds of the American population is not overweight at all. So before plunging into a diet, we should all carefully analyze our motives and our need to lose weight.

The medical definitions of weight problems are based on deviations from standard height/weight charts:

- "Overweight:" 10 to 20 percent higher than normal
- "Obesity:" 20 percent or more above normal weight
- "Morbid obesity:" 50 to 100 percent over normal weight, more than 100 pounds over ideal weight, or sufficiently overweight to have severe problems with health or normal functioning.

However, many experts today discard the notion that there is such thing as an "ideal" weight, a predetermined number to which everyone of a certain age and height should aspire. The concept of "healthy" weight—which varies from person to person depending on genetic background, health condition, and age—is beginning to win acceptance.

Standard weight tables can be off by as much as 20 to 30 pounds for any given person, notes Dr. Covert Bailey in *The New Fit or Fat*. The height/weight table may say 120 pounds is ideal for a person of your age and height. But if you currently weigh 160, your

SCALE SAVVY

There's a natural tendency for dieters to weigh themselves often, perhaps several times a day. But, be prepared: your weight goes up and down throughout the day depending on your activity level and food and fluid intake. Even your day-to-day weight will fluctuate, due to varying degrees of fluid retention. Women tend to gain "water weight" during their menstrual periods, and both men and women tend to retain extra fluids after eating sodium-rich foods. Instead of torturing yourself with these meaningless changes, it is probably best to weigh yourself less often, perhaps once a week in the beginning, and once a month thereafter. Another approach is to average your daily weights to obtain one weekly figure. Or, plot your weight on a graph each day, and look for a gradual downward slope, ignoring the occasional sharp peaks and dips.

For the most accurate readings:

- Stand on the scale at the same time of day. In the morning, before breakfast, is best.
- Wear approximately the same amount of clothing—or none.
- Always use the same scale.
- Concentrate on trends in your weight pattern rather than specific numbers.

family history, activity level, and lifestyle may make 140 or 145 a more reasonable goal. In addition, your weight is only a very rough indicator of the amount of fat your body contains, and most physicians believe the percentage of your weight that comes from fat tissue is far more important than your total body weight (which includes not only fat but also muscles, bones, and bodily fluids). Height/weight tables could indicate that a lean, but very muscular person is "overweight," while a person whose weight is within the "normal" range might actually be carrying around more fatty tissue than is healthy.

Some of the best indicators of whether you need to change your eating patterns have nothing to do with numbers. Some people have abandoned the scales entirely, preferring to rely on signs such as these:

- How do you feel? Energetic and vibrant, or drained and wiped out? Are you able to walk up a few flights of stairs without panting? Can you accomplish the daily tasks you need to?
- Do you have health problems such as back pain, diabetes, or high blood pressure that would improve with weight loss?
- Can you "pinch an inch" of fat at your waist or behind your arm?
- What is your overall muscle tone? Are you flabby?
- How well do last year's clothes fit?
- Has your doctor actually said you should lose some weight?

If you've been overweight since childhood or adolescence, you may not even know what a "healthy" weight for you would be. The point at which excess pounds become a significant danger to your health is signaled by your Body Mass Index (BMI) and your waist-to-hip ratio, both of which tell whether you're heavy enough to be at increased risk of heart disease. For detailed advice on gauging your "personal best" weight level, see Chapter 5, "Setting a Healthy Goal."

Why Do You *Really* Eat?

If you've decided you do need to lose weight, due to your own assessment or that of your doctor, it's helpful to begin by examining your current eating patterns. Human beings don't eat simply because they are hungry. "People eat because of stress, fatigue, and distraction," says Dr. Frank. "People eat for social, cultural, and religious reasons. They eat at festivals and because it's their birthday. They eat because their friends or family are eating." Evidently, there are powerful psychological forces governing the way we eat. These enormously confounding motivations are the reason it's so difficult for people to control their eating behavior. It's not simply a matter of willpower.

This doesn't mean that emotional eating is always a bad thing. Real adults in the real world have high-stress days, and occasional overeating can bring well-deserved comfort and pleasure. What's important is to identify this behavior when it occurs. This will help you sort out emotional cues from actual hunger signals, and help you pinpoint the reasons you eat when you are not hungry.

What type of eater you are can affect what type of eating modification you should make. Consider the following types, described by an article in the August 1994 *Harvard Health Letter:*

■ **Restrained eaters:** These people eat less than the recommended minimum calorie counts, but still think they weigh too much. They may need objective evaluation by an outside source. It might be that their body image needs revising more than their diet.

■ **Moderate eaters:** People in this group don't consciously restrict the kinds or quantities of foods they eat, but naturally limit their calorie intake. They might need to im-

prove their nutrition, but not necessarily in order to lose weight.

■ **Binge eaters:** Some people severely restrict the amount and types of food they eat, then periodically binge out of anxiety, stress, or boredom. They may need to incorporate the connection between food and emotions into their diet plans by making sure they derive enough pleasure and emotional satisfaction from their every-day meals. If carried to extremes, this pattern can lead to yo-yo dieting and even bulimia.

■ **Unrestrained eaters:** This group tends to consume large amounts of high-calorie, high-fat foods in one sitting, and may feel uncomfortably full later on. They may be out of touch with the body's signals that they have had enough to eat. Consulting a professional nutritional counselor may be helpful.

Strategies for Successful Weight Loss

Wherever you fall on the eating spectrum, you need to choose an eating plan—whether it's a commercial plan like Weight Watchers or one you devise yourself—that suits your needs and cravings. Do you need the control of weighing and measuring every bite you eat, or do you need the freedom to eat whatever quantities of low-fat, nutritious foods satisfy your hunger? Do you feel most in control when you eat 3 square meals a day, or when you "graze" on 5 or 6 small meals throughout the day? Have long-standing eating habits suddenly started adding on pounds that a fresh approach could take off? Do you need to ease into a new eating plan gradu-

TO LOSE WEIGHT:

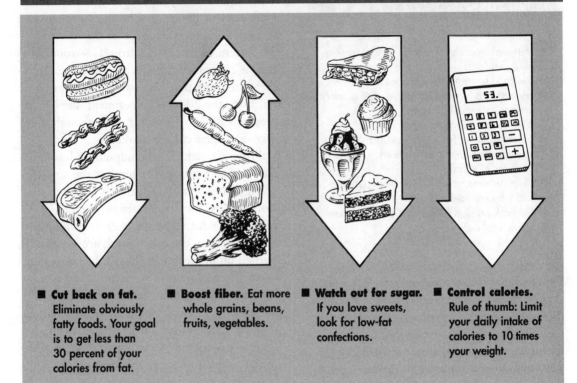

- **Cut back on fat.** Eliminate obviously fatty foods. Your goal is to get less than 30 percent of your calories from fat.

- **Boost fiber.** Eat more whole grains, beans, fruits, vegetables.

- **Watch out for sugar.** If you love sweets, look for low-fat confections.

- **Control calories.** Rule of thumb: Limit your daily intake of calories to 10 times your weight.

ally, adapting to new low-fat, high-fiber foods week by week, or would you be more motivated by a single clean sweep of all the junk in your diet? Doing what works for you may not be the same thing that worked for your best friend or your spouse.

When it comes to improving your eating patterns, any change is better than none at all. The "Shape Up America!" campaign launched in 1994 by former Surgeon General C. Everett Koop promotes the benefits of even modest weight loss. "Eat sensibly. Exercise regularly. Drop a few pounds. Shape up," Koop advises. Remember, a little will go a long way for your long-term health and your self-image.

The "D" Word

The word "diet" is often interpreted as "a temporary regimen that leads to permanent weight loss," rather than its original meaning of "how one eats." The effectiveness of "a temporary regimen" to lose weight has been questioned by certain weight-control specialists. Some research seems to show that yo-yo dieting, the common cycle of repeatedly losing and regaining weight, may be as bad for you as weighing too much in the first place.

FAT-REDUCING STRATEGIES FOR WEIGHT LOSS

- Increase amounts of whole grains, vegetables, and fruits
- Switch to low-fat milk and cheese
- Try reduced or non-fat mayonnaise, margarine, and salad dressing
- Trim fat and skin from meats
- Switch to lower-fat meats and fish (such as skinless chicken, water-packed tuna, and lean cuts of meat)
- Limit the amount of full-fat butter, cheeses, and fatty red meat
- Cut back on high-fat pastries and ice cream
- Try non-fat desserts

Other studies find it poses no risk (other than that of incessant frustration). A growing anti-diet movement urges people to throw away their calorie counters and concentrate on modifying their eating patterns. Meanwhile, the diet industry continues to thrive.

The difference between the pro-diet and anti-diet factions is, however, largely a matter of semantics. The fact is, if you want to lose weight, you're going to have to become conscious of and carefully control, what you eat for a period of time, and monitor what you eat thereafter. Whether you consider this a diet or not really doesn't matter.

Focus on Dietary Fat

In determining the success of a weight-loss program, fat consumption may be more important than the number of calories eaten. Researchers found that the percentage of fat in the diet was the single strongest predictor of weight gain among 294 adults monitored for 3 years by Memphis State University investigators. By contrast, total calorie consumption had only a weak relationship to weight gain for women, and none at all for men. In another approach, researchers at the University of Illinois at Chicago switched 18 women volunteers from a diet that derived 37 percent of its calories from fat—roughly the fat content of the average American's diet—to a diet that was only 20 percent fat. Over the 20-week experiment, the women lost 4 to 5 pounds, even though they *increased* their caloric intake.

From a weight-loss standpoint, a low-fat diet is ideal because it minimizes the amount of fat readily available for your body to store. Excess dietary fat can be pumped directly into your fatty tissue. Proteins and carbohydrates, on the other hand, are usually burned up immediately. They'll be converted to fat when present in sufficient quantities, but that requires extra (calorie-burning) work in the process. Researchers are finding that, for certain overweight people, eating excessive amounts of carbohydrates can add to the problem. For the majority of us, however, carbohydrates remain distinctly preferable to fat.

But how low is low? The American Heart Association, the National Academy of Science, the American Cancer Society, and many other groups recommend that we get a maximum of 30 percent of our calories from fat, (with no more than 10 percent of total calories from saturated fats). Another body of nutrition experts, including Nathan Pritikin and Dr. Dean Ornish, suggest that even lower levels of fat (10 to 20 percent of total calories) are much better than 30%, and can actually reverse existing heart disease.

If you decide to aim for the low end of this range, it might be advisable to consult your doctor. And totally eliminating fat is not only impractical, but extremely unwise. Our bodies do require a small amount of fat for lubrication, essential fatty acids, and fat-soluble vitamins. The necessary amount is all too easy to come by, however; so limiting all pure fats, (butter, margarine, and cooking oils) and high-fat foods, (full-fat dairy products, fatty red meats, pastries, and nuts) should be a key part of your weight-loss strategy. This doesn't mean that you should always avoid high-fat foods—only that you should balance them with lower-fat foods such as grains, vegetables, and fruits.

The new "Nutrition Facts" labels make it easier to determine exactly how much fat is in the food you are eating. They indicate how many grams of fat one serving contains. Each gram contributes about 9 calories toward the total number of calories per serv-

ing—more than twice as many calories as protein or carbohydrates. To determine what percentage of the calories in a food comes from fat (if it's not already listed on the label), multiply the weight of the fat (in grams) by 9, then divide by the total number of calories in a serving. Or, for a simpler rule of thumb, just aim for a total daily intake of no more than 30 to 50 grams. Most people can lose weight at this level.

What about foods that are not labeled with nutrition information? Fruits, vegetables, berries, grains, legumes (peas and beans), and egg whites generally have little fat. (Avocados, olives, nuts, soybeans, and seeds are exceptions.)

Boost Your Fiber
Fiber has many benefits, but one stands out when you're losing weight: it fills out the stomach and intestinal cavity, producing a feeling of fullness. Fiber is found chiefly in nonprocessed foods such as whole grains, beans, peas, fruits, and vegetables. Fiber

BEST BETS FOR FIBER

	Size of Serving	Fiber Content
Bran cereal	1 cup	6 to 21 grams
Beans (baked)	1/2 cup	10 grams
Blackberries	3/4 cup	7 grams
Baked potato	1 large (8 ounces)	6 grams
Winter squash, cooked	1 cup	6 grams
Cranberries	1 cup	5 grams
Split peas, cooked	1/2 cup	5 grams
Artichoke, cooked	1	4 grams
Kiwi fruit	1 medium (4 ounces)	4 grams
Orange	1 small (6 ounces)	4 grams

may be added to processed foods in the form of bran, which is the outer coating from a grain such as wheat or oats.

The typical American diet is high in processed foods, most of which contain little or no fiber. Most people get only around 10 to 12 grams of fiber per day, while 25 to 30 grams are needed to get real health benefits. If your current diet is low in fiber, it's important to increase your intake gradually over a period of weeks or months (a sudden jump can cause bloating, cramping, and gas). Try having a small serving of a high-fiber, low-fat cereal with your breakfast; as your system becomes used to the higher fiber levels, start substituting whole-grain breads, cereals, and pastas for refined (white flour, low fiber) varieties. Increase your consumption of fresh fruits and vegetables, and eat edible peels and skins, (apples, potatoes) instead of trimming them.

Calories Still Count

Your body needs a certain number of calories per day to maintain bodily functions—referred to as your Basal Metabolic Rate (BMR). You can estimate your BMR by multiplying your current weight (in pounds) by 10 for women, 11 for men. For example, a woman who weighs 120 pounds would require about 1,200 calories per day just to maintain her bodily functions. You'll also need some percentage of calories above your BMR to provide energy for your daily activities; the percentage will vary widely based on your metabolism and activity level. A moderately fit and active person might need 30 to 50 percent more calories than her BMR to maintain her current weight. Example: a 120-pound woman would need approximately 1,680 calories per day [1,200 + (1,200 x 40%) = 1,680]. A person who is

very fit and exercises frequently might burn as much as 100 to 200 percent more than his or her BMR.

If your goal is to lose weight, you'll need to take in fewer calories than you use up, or burn off extra calories through exercise, or both. If you choose to decrease calories, aim for the amount needed daily to maintain your target weight, not current weight. Most experts recommend that women take in a minimum of 1,200 calories and men a minimum of 1,600 per day. Lower calorie levels are unlikely to supply all the essential nutrients you need, and may slow down your metabolism, making weight loss even more difficult. For gradual weight loss, some professionals recommend a daily calorie target of 10 times your weight. At this level, they say, you can expect to lose half a pound per week.

Good (And Bad) News About Sugar

The "empty calories" of sugar have gained a bad reputation. Yet sugar by itself isn't a problem. It's the high levels of fat in sugary foods such as ice cream and pastries that really put on the pounds. In terms of weight loss or maintenance, sugar becomes objectionable only when you fail to keep your intake down to moderate levels. Sugar is a carbohydrate, thus it is normally burned by the body immediately, and is converted to fat only if it's present in quantities too large to be used at once.

Nevertheless, some people find that even moderate amounts of sugar stimulate cravings for yet more sweets, often of the high-fat variety. If you are one of these

BEFORE JOINING A COMMERCIAL PROGRAM, ASK THE FOLLOWING:

- What are the health risks?
- Are there data that prove the program actually works?
- Do customers keep the weight off after they leave the program?
- Does the plan have a maintenance program?
- What kind of professional supervision is provided?
- Is the importance of moderate exercise for weight loss and weight control emphasized?
- Does the weight-loss strategy emphasize a gradual loss? (1 percent of body weight per week is healthy; 3 or 4 pounds or more per week is potentially dangerous.)
- Concentrate on trends in your weight pattern rather than specific numbers.

people, you may find it helpful to eliminate processed sugars from your diet, relying instead on the natural sweetness of fruits, vegetables, and grains. Artificial sweeteners can be an effective aid if you have occasional cravings for sweets, but probably won't work for those of us with an active sweet tooth. The taste of artificial sweeteners can trigger sugar cravings about as easily as the real thing can.

Choosing a Diet

Once you've decided it's time to shed some extra pounds, the big question is How? The basic principles—less fat, fewer calories, more fiber—are enshrined in hundreds of dieting schemes, all of them clamoring for your attention. At any given time, there are over 300 diet books in print. In 1991, about 8,500 commercial diet centers were in operation across the country (many owned by about a half-dozen national companies). Each year, approximately 8 million Americans enroll in some kind of structured weight-loss program. All these choices can be grouped into four categories:

- Do-it-yourself efforts that involve "going solo," or using diet books and support groups as aids
- Nonclinical programs that employ counselors to teach weight loss and nutrition
- Clinical programs, where licensed doctors may offer drugs or surgery
- One-on-one consultation with a registered dietitian

The choices can be overwhelming because the weight-loss industry is largely unregulated. We may soon see some improvement, however. New 1995 guidelines on safe and effective dieting have been developed by The Institute of Medicine, an arm of the National Academy of Sciences. "The current system is chaos," says Dr. Frank, co-author of the guidelines. "None of these programs gives any information." To give dieters a basis for choosing the right program, the guidelines call on weight-loss programs to issue comprehensive data about patients' long-term weight loss, improvements in obesity-related diseases, and improved health practices.

The guidelines recommend that you:

- Pick a program that incorporates your individual needs
- Ask a trusted health care professional if the program is sound and appropriate
- Carefully assess your health before and during weight loss

- Remember that programs promising results without dieting and exercise won't work
- Make sure the company requires breast-feeding women, children, and patients with any chronic disease to undertake weight loss only under medical supervision
- Check that sufficient exercise is part of the program.

Matching the Diet with Your Needs

Choosing a diet depends a lot on your personal needs. "At the extremes, the decision is easy," says Dr. Frank. "If you weigh 350 pounds and you are recovering from your second heart attack, it's dangerous for you to go to Weight Watchers. If you are 15 pounds overweight, 23 years old, and in good health, it doesn't make sense for you to go into a clinical program." However, most people fall between such extremes. The program you choose, counsels Dr. Frank, depends on your personal view, and how much time, money, and effort you're willing to put in.

"There is no one best way to lose weight," says Dr. Pi-Sunyer. "People are individuals and they do it different ways." To determine which type of diet—self-created, a commercial program, or a book—suits your personality, ask yourself the following questions:

Does the diet fit my lifestyle? Any diet should include foods you like, eaten when and where you prefer. Personal input in meal-planning gives most people a sense of self-control and motivation. Some people, however, would rather be relieved of decisions and purchase food directly from a program.

Will I be eating the same foods as my family? Eating unfamiliar or tiny servings of food while your family dines on its regular fare can be hard to keep up. Such a stringent or limited diet can make you feel deprived, resentful, and rebellious.

Is a variety of foods from all food groups included, with no total exclusions? Even fats and sugars should be allowed in moderation. When you cut back on certain types of foods too far, it can be difficult to meet your nutritional needs.

Can you afford the weight-loss plan you've chosen? Take into account the cost of membership, weekly fees, food, supplements, maintenance, and counseling. Check if the costs are covered under health insurance. Beware of programs that require large sums of money up front. A pay-as-you-go system is safer.

Do I need someone to talk to about my goals? Professional counseling can help you learn how to control your eating habits and provide structured support. However, if you're self-motivated, just talking to your spouse or a close friend may give you the support you need.

Do I need group support and encouragement? Many studies show that people who diet with the help of support groups are more likely to control their weight successfully. A support group doesn't have to be a commercial program; it could be a community-based group or just a group of friends.

Do I need to learn how to prepare low-calorie, low-fat meals? If you don't understand food labels, food preparation methods, or nutrition, seeking help is advisable.

Are the recommended foods easily found at any regular grocery store? For some, going to specialty or health food stores is bound to prove tiresome after a while.

Do I have time to put a program together by myself?

Tips for Do-It-Yourselfers

If you're the go-it-alone type, keep these tactics in mind. You'll need to make up for the support that comes automatically with enrollment in a program.

Find a good time to start. "I'm going on a diet tomorrow," is a sentence that often heralds failure because it's sparked by a momentary impulse (or guilt after a triple-decker ice cream cone) rather than a well-thought-out plan. Weight loss is tough, and you should give it the same careful consideration you would give to changing your career or buying a house. Think it through. Create a plan that really suits your lifestyle. Find a starting date during a relatively quiet time in your life, not while you're also moving to another state or dealing with a crisis at work.

Create a diet "campaign." Some people prefer to start with an exercise program, and add nutritional changes later on. For others, the reverse strategy works best. And for "all or nothing" types, starting both programs on a particular day can increase motivation.

Choose a good book for companionship. Some people prefer a diet plan book, while others do best with a low-fat, low-calorie cookbook. For a guide to the leading diet books, see Chapter 4. Turn to Chapter 36 for the experts' advice on cookbooks.

Check with your doctor if you have any medical problems. You need to make sure that the eating and exercise strategies you've chosen are suitable and safe.

Decide whether you need a "quick start." Quick-start programs, in which you change your eating habits drastically for a few weeks, are likely to deliver the most dramatic changes on the scale. For example, The Bloomingdale's Diet starts off with 3 days of vegetable-only menus. This helps you break with your former eating patterns and gives you a chance to appreciate the appealing flavors to be found in very low-calorie foods. Other food groups are then reintroduced one by one. This kind of food plan requires a good deal of concentration during the initial phase and may not be suitable if you're pressed for time. For many people, however, this approach serves as a great motivator. After you've lost those first exciting five pounds, you can modulate the plan into one you can continue life long.

Consider "gradualism." This strategy works best for people who don't have too much weight to lose, and those who can accept the idea of slow—but steady and permanent—change. One approach is to modify one daily meal at a time. For example, during the first week, you can concentrate on low-fat low-calorie dinners, assembling menus and creating tasty meals. In the second week, you can turn to lunch, and so on. Or, you can tackle one food group at a time. A switch to low-fat dairy products is a good start. The second week, pay attention to lower fat meats and fish, and to learning how to create one or two vegetarian dinners a week. (Be careful, though: Some vegetarian recipes are amazingly high in fat.)

COMPARING THE TOP FOUR PLANS

Weight Watchers

Plan: "Personal Choice," an exchange-type plan, allows a certain number of servings daily from each "selection" group (breads, fruits, vegetables, proteins, dairy, and fats). Makes allowances for a certain number of "optional" (free) calories per week to do with as you please. A "Fat and Fiber" plan was added in December 1994. It encourages members to eat low-fat meals (15 to 35 grams daily; men and youths can go up to 45 grams a day) and get plenty of fiber (20 grams or more daily).

Cost: There is an initial membership fee ($15 to $20), plus a fee for each meeting attended ($9 to $12). Members who attain their "goal weights" become lifetime members, and can attend meetings for free as long as they maintain their new weights. WW markets several types of processed foods not necessarily low in calories but designed to fit easily into the program. Use of WW foods is completely optional.

Rate of Loss: The number of selections you're allowed per group per day depends on how fast you wish to lose weight; the program recommends a maximum loss of 1 1/2 to 2 pounds per week. You set your own goal weight based on a Weight Watchers height/weight chart. If you lose more than this, you'll be instructed to slow down the rate of loss. This practice, unique among the programs, fits with current medical thinking about the hazards of too-rapid weight loss.

Meetings: Weekly meetings, which feature a "weigh in" for each member (confidential) and various activities such as motivational videos, discussions, and distribution of program materials and recipes.

Counseling: Each counselor employed by Weight Watchers is a former client who has achieved and maintained his or her goal weight on the program. Gaining the weight back is grounds for dismissal.

Exercise: Encourages moderate exercise in combination with the diet plan.

Jenny Craig

Plan: Requires dieters to buy and consume only company-brand foods (except for a few items such as fresh dairy products and produce). Prepackaged meals are said to help dieters learn "portion control" while freeing them from the necessity of weighing, measuring, and preparing food.

Cost: One-time registration fee: $79. Jenny Craig foods cost about $60 to $70 every week. (The cost drops slightly as you approach your goal weight and start eating some regular food). Supplemental vitamins: $2.25 per week. Weight maintenance: $99 for one year. Additional home lifestyle counseling tapes: $75.

Rate of Loss: The average weekly loss is 1 to 2 pounds for women; 2 to 3 pounds for men. Goal weight determined by a height/weight chart.

Meetings: Group class in behavior modification, which teach participants how to make healthy food choices once they've been weaned off the Jenny Craig foods.

Counseling: Uses one-on-one counseling for clients.

Exercise: Exercise is encouraged.

Nutri-System

Plan: Requires dieters to buy and consume only company-brand foods (except for a few items such as fresh dairy products and produce).

Don't forget fluids. Drinking the equivalent of eight glasses of water a day is recommended for everyone, but especially for those trying to lose weight. The fluids fill you up, prevent the shakiness and fatigue of dehydration, and give you something to put in your mouth when you're trying to forget about eating.

Eat slowly and savor your food. Give your internal "portion control" monitor a chance to get through to you. Some foods, such as

Cost: Basic enrollment fee: $79, including all meetings, counseling, and materials. Food: about $69 per week (7 days) until you are halfway to your goal weight; then $49 per week (5 days).

Rate of Loss: Average loss of 1 1/2 to 2 pounds per week.

Meetings: Weekly 30-minute group meetings teach basic food exchanges and portion control; continuing until weight loss is achieved.

Counseling Weekly 10-minute meetings with counselors, who are usually trained employees rather than registered dietitians.

Exercise: Encourages exercise.

Diet Center

Plan: Offers varying amounts of protein, vegetables, fruits, dairy, and grains; low in sugars and fat. Participants must take Diet Center food supplements. The food plan provides a range of 1,000 to 2,175 calories per day for men and women. Maintenance program lasts for one year.

Cost: Depends on the amount of weight to be lost. Enrollment fee: $52 to $79; Reducing phase: $37 to $53 per week; "Sta-b-lite" phase: $37 to $53 per week; weight maintenance: $110. DC offers a line of frozen main dishes, along with other products, but these purchases are not mandatory.

Rate of Loss: Estimated to be 2 pounds per week.

Meetings: No group meetings.

Counseling: Daily weigh-ins with a diet counselor (flexible).

Exercise: Encourages exercise by setting and monitoring exercise goals.

vegetables prepared without added fat, can be eaten in large quantities to satisfy hunger and prolong the pleasure of a meal. Pastas, potatoes, bread, and rice are filling foods that round out a meal, but should not be eaten with abandon. Other foods, such as cheeses, meat, and sweets, give extra zing to meals and, in very small portions, can be part of a weight-loss plan.

Keep track of your progress. The scale helps some people and tyrannizes others. If you find that the number on the scale affects your self-esteem for the day, find another way to measure progress. Try on a once too-tight skirt or pair of jeans each morning. Or keep a food diary of what you eat each day. Tracking progress is important. It's a reminder that you've started a change, and rewards you with a hint of the final results.

Don't punish yourself. If you "fall off the wagon" and indulge (or even overindulge) in something you think you shouldn't have eaten, it's not a disaster. An episode of un-controlled eating does not mean that you or your diet failed. Learning to climb back on the wagon is a key to long-term success.

Survive the "plateaus." While the first pounds often come off quickly, many dieters hit plateaus where their weight remains steady for weeks even though their fat and calorie counts are low. Getting through these periods requires a bit of faith and "stick-to-it" spirit. Your metabolism is making noble efforts to keep up your fat levels, in the mistaken belief that starvation is near. But weight loss will start again once this plateau is passed.

Get the right support. You may need to ad-vise your spouse and friends on how to help you. They shouldn't appoint themselves your "diet cop"—this will only bring out the rebel

CUSTOMER SATISFACTION WITH THE LEADING DIET PROGRAMS

Consumer Reports asked readers to tell about the problems they encountered with different weight-loss programs.

Did the program have higher costs than you were led to believe?

Extra more likely:
Jenny Craig (47%), Nutri-System (47%).
Extra less likely:
Weight Watchers (7%), HMR (17%).

Was there strong pressure to buy the program's products?

More pressure:
Jenny Craig (55%), Nutri-System (55%).
Less pressure: Weight Watchers (5%).

Was there strong pressure to join or stay in the program?

More pressure:
Nutri-System (34%), Jenny Craig (31%).
Less pressure:
Medifast (11%), Weight Watchers (12%).

Was the dieting method artificial and difficult to incorporate into daily life?

More artificial: Medifast (40%), Optifast (37%), Nutri-System (31%).
Less artificial: Weight Watchers (6%).

Were you always hungry?

More hunger: Medifast (22%).
Less hunger: Weight Watchers (10%).

in most people. But neither do they need to tempt you unnecessarily by insisting you taste their dessert or order something "more exciting" in restaurants.

Reward yourself. Small treats and large pleasures will help you celebrate everything from sticking with your plan on Day One to reaching your target weight, along with whatever small markers you create in between. Some people find going into a store and trying on clothes they could never wear before is a great reward—even when they're not ready to buy. Others give themselves free time— an hour to sit in the sun and dream; an afternoon at the movies; a walk in the park at sundown—for whatever they truly enjoy.

Checking Out the Enrollment Programs

Cost, comfort, and common sense are the basics to look for when shopping for a commercial program. These plans generally attract women who have a moderate weight problem and men who are moderately to seriously overweight. All the top four commercial weight-loss programs—Diet Center, Jenny Craig, Nutri-System, and Weight Watchers—include a low-calorie diet of about 1,000 to 1,500 calories a day and some kind of supportive counseling.

None of the top four emerges as better at helping individuals to lose weight and keep it off, according to a 1994 Consumer Reports survey of 95,000 readers who had attempted to lose weight in the past 3 years. Overall, however, Weight Watchers tended to be the clear favorite among those polled. It costs less than the others, emphasizes healthful dietary habits, encourages relatively slow weight loss, and generally appears to provide the most satisfying support. In contrast, Nutri-System and Jenny Craig cost more and

FEELING DUPED?

To file complaints about weight-loss products or programs, write any of the following:

- **Federal Trade Commission**
  Correspondence Branch
  Washington, D.C. 20580

- **Food and Drug Administration**
  Consumer Affairs and Information
  5600 Fishers Lane, HFC-110
  Rockville, MD 20857

- **Your State Attorney General**
  Office of Consumer Protection
  Your State Capital

are more likely to use high-pressure sales tactics. But, as Deralee Scanlon, RD points out in *Diets That Work:* "The monetary aspect does not in itself lessen the potential effectiveness of a program—in fact, some people take these programs more seriously precisely because of the financial investment."

Clinical Programs (Liquid fasts)

These are the most drastic weight-loss programs, designed for people with a serious problem. No one should go on a liquid-fast program without a compelling medical reason to do so. Liquid fasts are generally appropriate only for people with a BMI in the 30s, or people with BMIs in the high 20s who have a serious weight-related risk factor, such as severe high blood pressure or diabetes. For long-term maintenance of healthier weight, the programs are no better than any other. They are available only through hospitals or doctors' offices and require regular physical checkups and blood tests. Three popular liquid-fast programs include: Health Management Resources (HMR), Medifast, and Optifast. Medical complications may include such "adjustments" as dizziness, sensitivity to cold, slower heart rate, brittle nails, rashes, fatigue, diarrhea or constipation, muscle cramps, and bad breath. They generally cost between $2,000 and $3,000.

Liquid diets a la Oprah Winfrey, who lost 67 pounds on the Optifast program and gained it all back, show that short-term solutions are meaningless without long term change. These days, Oprah has replaced diet shakes with a personal chef, focusing on intensive exercise and nutritional changes she can follow for life, rather than just a goal weight. "Changing the way you think about food is the first step toward achieving and maintaining a desirable weight," Oprah writes in the best-seller *In the Kitchen with Rosie* (which contains delicious low-fat, low-sugar, low-salt recipes you can cook yourself, even if you can't afford a private cook).

Potentially Dangerous Diet Strategies

In the diet industry, anything goes. "Appetite suppressing eyeglasses" boast colored lenses that are said to project an image on the retina that dampens the desire to eat. "Magic weight-loss earrings" are custom-fitted to the purchaser to stimulate, it is claimed, the acupuncture points controlling hunger. (Neither has been proven effective.) Much of the diet advice you encounter may be misleading, and some of it can be downright dangerous. Beware of the following weight loss wonders.

Diet Pills. Over-the-counter "diet aids" really do work—but only for a while. They contain phenylpropanolamine, a stimulant chemically similar to amphetamine that stimulates your central nervous system and decreases your appetite, and/or mild diuretics which cause you to eliminate fluids more quickly than normal. These pills can temporarily cause your weight to drop, but they won't eliminate body fat. As soon as you stop taking them, your weight is likely to bounce back to its previous level. Side effects can include dizziness, nausea, and increased urination. The pills can be dangerous for people with heart problems, thyroid disease, and high blood pressure. "Pills are not the answer," says Dr. Pi-Sunyer. "The answer is diet and exercise. There is effort involved in weight loss."

Very Low-Calorie Diets. Studies show that people who lose weight slowly over a reasonable amount of time are more likely to keep the weight off. A weight-loss diet of at least 1,200 calories a day works best for most people. Consuming less than this can deprive you of essential nutrients. New studies suggest that diets very low in fat may actually endanger your health. Diets very low in calories (less than 1,000 calories a day) can also be harmful and should be attempted only under the care of a doctor. If you lose more than 1 or 2 pounds per week, you're almost certainly losing muscle, not just fat tissue. Make sure the diet you choose allows you enough food to keep you from feeling overly hungry.

Fasting. As with very low-calorie diets, when you fast, you lose muscle before fat. After a day or two of fasting, many people succumb to a high-calorie binge. Long-term fasting is hazardous, since it weakens your immune system and places a strain on vital organs.

Skin Patches. These "diet patches," which supposedly contain an appetite suppressant, have not been proven safe or effective. The Food and Drug Administration has seized millions of these products from promoters.

Diuretics. The weight you lose is only water weight. The loss is temporary and doesn't include any fat. Diuretics can promote dangerous dehydration and cardiac problems.

Electrical muscle stimulators. These devices, which have legitimate medical uses in physical therapy, have no place in weight loss or body toning. You just can't zap off the fat. When used incorrectly, the devices can cause electrical shocks and burns. □

CHAPTER 7

How To Keep
the Lost Pounds Off

"The challenge of losing weight is very different from the challenge of maintaining the loss," notes James Hill, PhD, associate professor of Physiological Psychology at the University of Colorado in Denver. "Most Americans trying to lose weight think, 'okay, I'll subject myself to this program for 12 weeks. I can put up with anything for that long.' But they don't give a lot of thought to the changes in behaviors that will help them maintain the loss."

Until recently, this way of thinking was aided and abetted by the diet industry, which also devoted more attention to weight loss than to maintenance. A section on maintenance is tacked on to most diet books and programs mostly as a "post script" that basically says "keep it up." The traditional assumption was that the nuts and bolts of an intense weight loss program—counting fat grams and calories or weighing portions— could easily become a permanent part of life. But the reality is that weight maintenance involves switching from a restricted reducing diet to a more flexible set of eating patterns that will keep you at your desired weight. By their nature, those new habits are harder to set down as a simple set of rules.

A wake-up call to focus on weight maintenance was sounded in 1994, when dieting guidelines published by the National Academy of Sciences revealed that the average dieter regains two-thirds of lost weight within one year and almost all within five years. The report noted that although different weight-loss programs use different diets and strategies, none have been able to overcome this basic pattern. "My impression is that the success people have in maintaining their weight loss appears to be entirely unrelated to how they lost the weight," says Dr. Arthur Frank, medical director of the George Washington University Obesity Management Program. "Most weight loss diets do work in the short term. The problem is, we have not yet evolved good techniques for maintenance."

Happily, this is beginning to change, and there are now a lot of clues as to how and why some people succeed at "keeping it off," while others seem to return to their old weights just as soon as they've purchased a smaller-sized wardrobe. This chapter looks first at the success stories—the characteristics and approaches of people who manage to control their weight long-term. It then explores how to cope with the psychological implications of having a healthier, slimmer body; and, how to develop weight maintenance techniques that fit your own personality and lifestyle.

Principles of Success

What can we learn from the few people who DO succeed at long-term weight control? A number of researchers have begun to answer this question through innovative efforts such as the National Registry of Successful Weight Losers. This program keeps track of several hundred people from around the country who have succeeded at long-term weight maintenance. Other research has compared groups of dieters who regain their weight to those who are able to maintain their new, lower weight for several years or more.

Perhaps the most significant finding is that even the most successful long-term weight losers admit that staying on track is a major challenge. When asked how difficult it was for them to maintain their weight, their answers ranged from "moderately hard" to "very hard." Even people who have never

had to lose weight often report that they have to work hard to avoid gaining.

Accepting the fact that weight maintenance is a difficult task may be an important first step towards success. The triumph of losing weight makes it easy to develop illusions of invulnerability—"I'll never backslide; I'm going to stick to this diet for the rest of my life." Recognizing that the task is hard, and that some degree of failure is inevitable, will prepare you to cope with the obstacles ahead. You can set aside the notion that now that you've lost weight, your problems are solved and you can go back to being spontaneous, forgetful, and unconscious about what you eat. People who do acknowledge the difficulty of weight maintenance seem to be able to rise to the challenge and formulate realistic goals that they can take pleasure in meeting.

Overcoming the Body's Inertia

"There seems to be a powerful but elusive signal that makes people return to their original weight," endocrinologist F. Xavier Pi-Sunyer, director of the Obesity Research Center at St. Luke's-Roosevelt Hospital Center in New York told the New York Times. "We now know that it is unrealistic to expect a very heavy person to be thin."

Indeed, recent research at Rockefeller University has revealed a "self-adjusting" mechanism at work in the body's metabolism. When you lose weight, your metabolism slows down, burning fewer calories than before, and making calorie control all the more imperative. We don't know whether this compensatory change is permanent, but it's definitely a problem in the months immediately following a diet.

For many people, therefore, maintaining modest weight loss is a more appropriate goal than struggling to remake themselves completely. Very heavy people can often substantially improve hypertension, cholesterol, and blood sugar levels, and sometimes even decrease their risk of cardiovascular disease, by losing just 10 percent of their body weight, said Dr. Pi-Sunyer. If they can keep this weight off for a year, they can then try for another 10 percent, he suggests.

Studies comparing weight maintainers to regainers have yielded some interesting insights that may help you devise a weight maintenance program to suit your needs and abilities.

Weight History

The ease of maintaining dietary changes that produce weight loss seems to be related to individual weight history. In a worksite study at a large Midwestern university campus between 1987 and 1990, the dieters involved had been overweight since they were anywhere from 5 to 60 years old. But researchers found that the problem had begun earlier among those who regained weight— on average, at age 26, compared to age 33 for those who succeeded in maintaining their weight loss. Only one of the weight maintainers—but seven of the regainers—reported being overweight as a child.

If you have a long history of being overweight, you should recognize that maintenance may be especially challenging. You may need to seek long-term medical and/or social support to help you create and stay with a maintenance program. A 1993 study from the *Annals of Internal Medicine* found that physician advice and encouragement helped individuals both lose weight and maintain the loss.

Weight Cycling

A history of dieting and regaining weight may also make it more difficult to finally become a maintainer. In one study, subjects averaged six cycles of losing and regaining weight within the past 5 years. Dieters who had been through fewer weight "yo-yos" had an easier time maintaining weight than those who had lost and regained many times. Though some reports now insist that past weight cycling does *not* make future maintenance more difficult, a tendency to yo-yo is, if nothing else, a signal that you really need to make weight maintenance a serious, long-term priority. Trying to lose weight may actually be a mistake during periods in life when more urgent needs, such as coping with a personal, family, or career crisis, demand your attention. A strong effort to lose and then maintain your weight when other conditions in your life are more settled, may allow for greater success. This is bound to be better than the frustration of many half-hearted attempts at inopportune moments.

Education

Dieters who keep their weight off tend to have more years of education than those who regain weight, according to a 1994 study in the *Journal of the American Dietetic Association*—(a mean of 14.2 years of education for regainers, compared to 15.8 years among maintainers).

This finding seems to reinforce the notion that learned skills are the key to weight maintenance. It doesn't mean that if you have less education, you are bound to fail, but you may need to mount a deliberate effort to learn necessary maintenance skills. If "book learning" is not your style, you can try videos or an audio tape behavior modification program.

Food Awareness

Successful maintainers report that they use a variety of approaches, including reducing calorie and fat content of their food, and increasing activity. Most often, maintainers alter their lifestyles and food choices but don't completely deny themselves favorite foods. Unlike regainers, maintainers are always aware of their food consumption and quickly respond to weight gain with changes in habits. Relapsers, on the other hand, tend to rely on diet foods or formulas, attend weight-control groups—and continually feel deprived.

Taking a positive approach to weight maintenance means making sure that your eating plan is both pleasurable and fun. And keeping track of your results allows you to nip an incipient gain in the bud.

Activity Levels

The amount of leisure time devoted to physical activity is among the key differences between weight maintainers and regainers found in every study thus far. The differences are dramatic. A large study at Kaiser Permanente Health Care group in Freemont, California found that 90 percent of maintainers—but only 34 percent of relapsers—exercised regularly. Interestingly, most maintainers (90 percent) chose walking as their exercise. The fact that they liked this form of exercise helped them stay with it. Exercise helps weight maintenance by burning excess calories, squelching appetite, and increasing lean muscle tissue, which in turn increases your metabolism.

The message here goes beyond the obvious (and important) recommendation to make exercise or some kind of physical activity an integral part of your life. It's also a warning that you can be especially vulnerable to weight gain during periods when you cannot exercise. Bad weather, minor illnesses or injuries, and a stretch of intense busyness or personal crises, can all interfere with your exercise schedule. While it may not be possible to overcome these barriers immediately, watching what you eat during these times can help you maintain your weight until you're able to exercise again.

Skills and Support

Research shows that people who maintain weight loss generally get more help from others and attack problems more easily than those who do not. "Maintainers had a better social support network; most had three or more people they could turn to," according to a study published in the *American Journal of Clinical Nutrition*, by Judith S. Stern, Sc., professor of Nutrition and Internal Medicine at University of California, Davis. "Maintainers also had better problem-solving skills. When faced with a relapse, regainers more often used escape-avoidance—'I'll deal with this problem tomorrow'—while maintainers knuckled down and tried to analyze and solve the problem."

It may be helpful, therefore, to view stabilizing your weight loss as a difficult set of puzzles to solve. As soon as you get one puzzle figured out—for example, devising a shopping schedule to keep fresh fruits and vegetables in the house—another one crops up. Holiday dinners, business luncheons, travel, a sprained knee that keeps you from exercising, a new office mate who brings in your favorite butter cookies, your mate giving up and gaining 10 pounds, a personal crisis . . . . The list is endless. But you can develop skills for solving each dilemma and find help in this effort by seeking out support from smart and sympathetic friends. "Continued contact with formal weight loss programs is a predictor of maintenance success," notes Stern.

Personalization

One of the most interesting research findings is that weight maintainers choose from a wide variety of strategies, personalizing their weight loss programs to reflect their own needs, tastes, and lifestyles. In the Kaiser study, both those who maintained and those who relapsed used many of the same strategies to lose weight, but those who maintained their weight loss adapted these strategies in ways that were specific to their own lifestyle. Maintainers were more likely than relapsers to devise a personal eating plan and to make attempts to avoid feelings of deprivation when changing their eating patterns.

The Psychology of Weight Maintenance

A weight loss diet is comparable to a sprint to the finish line: exciting, fast-paced, goal-oriented, and all-consuming. But maintenance is more like a long distance run: it requires pacing, picking yourself up after a fall, and nurturing your own motivation and enthusiasm.

Along with the nuts and bolts of staying nutritionally aware and active, maintenance also involves a subtle process of adjusting to and accepting your new, thinner self. Some people regain weight because they can't get comfortable in their slimmer bodies. Significant weight loss often requires people to adjust to changes in their relationships, and to manage the excitement and pressures

that their trim new look can provoke.

In our weight-obsessed society, the successful pound loser is apt to receive a lot of attention. While lapping up compliments might seem like an easy task, you may also face jealousy and subtle put-downs. Unexpected reactions may make you feel insecure and even overwhelmed at first. The repercussions of changing any long standing pattern of self destructive behavior, such as overeating, can throw you and your self esteem into a psychological tailspin.

Dealing With Jealousy

"When people notice you slimming down it can be threatening at first," says Helen Singer Kaplan, MD, PhD, director of the human sexuality program at New York Hospital-Cornell Medical Center. The king-size reactions you're likely to get from friends and family can be disconcerting, ranging from "Wow, you look great;" to such backhanded compliments as "you should have done this ten years ago;" to the outright hostility of "I hate you—I wish I could lose 20 pounds." There may also be frequent demands to know your "secret" and "how you did it," which can lead you into long, dull conversations about dieting.

A good way to deal with these reactions is to be prepared. Try role playing with family or a trusted friend, or just with yourself, in the mirror. Think of what people are likely to say and prepare your replies in advance. Often a casual "thank you" and a swift change of subject is best. One woman decided to answer the "how did you do it?" question with "the usual way, less eating and

MAKING FRIENDS WITH YOUR SLIMMER SELF

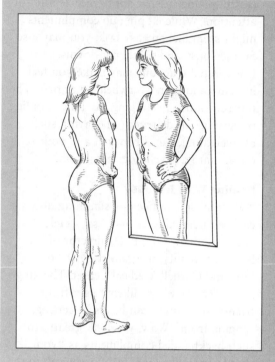

Incredibly, many weight losers have trouble accepting as "real" the body they've worked so hard to create. After years of living with excess pounds, their new physique doesn't quite seem natural—as though it belongs to someone else.

If you find yourself succumbing to this feeling, you must take steps to get over it. The idea that somehow you really should be heavier can easily become a self-fulfilling prophecy.

Make a deliberate effort to get used to your new appearance as quickly as possible. Study yourself on a daily basis. Get new clothes that fit your body to its best advantage. Spend more time on grooming and beauty care. This all may seem rather self-absorbed, but it's a necessary psychological step towards your goal of maintaining a healthy weight long-term.

more exercise." Also, find comfortable responses to jealous reactions from a spouse or friends. Explaining that keeping the weight off isn't easy is one way to counteract the implication that some special ability is allowing you to succeed easily where others have failed. Directly asking for the other person's support ("It would help me stick to my plan if you didn't insist that I try your dessert,") may also help temper envious responses.

Dealing with Sex
Increased attention from the opposite sex, including flirtation from co-workers and glances and comments from strangers, may be an unexpected (or desired) result of weight loss. If this occurs, it's a good idea to examine how you feel about it. While the attention may be flattering, it can also be disconcerting and inappropriate. For some people, the loss of weight means a loss of protective covering that must be replaced with new ways of handling people. Don't fall into the trap of regaining weight to retreat to more comfortable and familiar social relationships. Learn to politely but firmly discourage unwanted attention. If sexual harassment becomes a genuine danger and you can't seem to cope, don't hesitate to seek counsel from an appropriate therapist.

Accepting Your New Self

Along with dealing with others in a new way, you may have to talk with yourself about the "new you." The weight comes off your body first, but you need to give your mind time to get used to it. Most people find they need to accept both who they are now, and who they were when they were heavier—rather than demonize their old self as "fat" or "disgusting." Some feel an odd sense of disloyalty to their former, heavier self when they enjoy their new shape. They may also face a sense of unreality, or image anxiety, and need to remind themselves that "I'm still the same person, though others may not see it that way."

You can help yourself accept your new appearance with a number of simple steps. One is to look at yourself naked in the mirror every day—to get used to the way your body has changed and acknowledge it as your own. Try to avoid being critical about what you see and instead view yourself as kindly as you would a good friend. It helps to remember that "you are what you think you are," and to feed yourself positive thoughts.

Learning to claim and enjoy your new body is a good way to hold on to it. Some people "show off" in the privacy of their own home, wearing attractive, form-fitting clothing or lingerie around the house to get used to seeing a positive reflection. Body-nurturing, grooming, and beauty rituals also promote a healthy body image. Try some simple acts of kindness to yourself, such as soaking in an aromatic bath, applying body lotion, and taking special care of your hair, nails, and skin.

While laying claim to your new body, cultivate a positive self-image, as well. The following exercises can help you reinforce self-esteem:

- Make a list of your personal assets—personality traits and behaviors that you believe make you a valuable person. Ask trusted friends to help you add to this list. Then consult it frequently to encourage positive self-thoughts.
- Add a creative project or endeavor to your leisure time pursuits—something you really like to do or a new activity you've been interested in trying. Think of this as a well-deserved gift to yourself.
- Do something to streamline and simplify your life, and to reduce everyday annoyances. This can be as simple as cleaning out closets or programming your phone for automatic dialing, or as complex as putting your financial records in a computer so you can save time when you pay bills each month.
- Take time to relax. Set aside some time each day to regroup and appreciate yourself and your life. Turn off the radio and the television. Experiment with deep breathing, muscle relaxation, or just sitting still and counting your blessings.
- Explore activities that increase body awareness and strength: Take a dance class; try yoga or meditation.

Weight Maintenance Skills

Once you've lost the weight and have come to accept your new appearance, you have to develop new skills to hold onto your hard won gains. While there is no simple formula for keeping weight off, there are skills you can develop that will help you maintain your desired weight and make maintaining it more automatic.

KEYS TO CONTINUED MOTIVATION

- Make a specific decision to maintain weight loss, separate from the decision to lose weight.
- Commit yourself to following through on your decision.
- Continue to define small nutritional goals for each day.
- Practice positive thinking by concentrating on your goal, not your limitations.
- Visualize success. Success is the knowledge of what to do and commitment to do it.
- Be as patient and kind to yourself as you are to your good friends.
- Chart your progress and reward your efforts.

The "C" Word

Long-term weight management requires a conscious commitment—one just as strong, or stronger than the one you made in deciding to lose weight. Permanent commitments can seem daunting; "for the rest of my life," has a tone of finality that may evoke a rebellious spirit—"how do I know, at this point, what I want to do for the rest of my life?"

So with maintenance, as with any large project, it's a good idea to break the task down into smaller, do-able segments. Many people find it easier to make a commitment to maintain their current weight for one year. Your maintenance pledge can be made on a memorable day—New Year's, Valentine's Day, your birthday—and be up for reconsideration and renewal 12 months later (after a suitable celebration of your first year's success).

The commitment should be specific—something like: "I will continue to go to exercise class 3 times a week. I will continue to use vegetables for my snacks. I will continue to restructure the way I think and act about food so that I can maintain a healthy weight.

I know this is a major challenge and that I may occasionally slip up, but I can do this. It's my responsibility and although I may ask others for help, I understand this is something no one can do for me."

Once the commitment is made, keep visualizing your success. Imagine yourself a year from today, still able to get into your current sized jeans. Imagine yourself relaxed and happy, eating foods you like that are also good for you.

Create New Habits

Habits are an economical use of our mental energy. Most of us develop a set morning routine, for example, so that we don't waste time when we wake up wondering whether or not to brush our teeth today. Years ago you decided to brush your teeth every morning and now you just do it without thinking.

In the same way, weight maintenance becomes a much easier proposition once you've established good nutritional habits. Simplification and preparation are the key to getting new habits in place. For example, if you don't habitually eat breakfast but have decided to do so to boost your morning energy and prevent overeating at lunch, start with a simple approach. Dr. Stern suggests eating the same breakfast every day until the habit is firmly embedded. Prepare by keeping the things you want for breakfast always on hand.

In times of stress, notes Dr. Stern, your old poor eating habits and non-nutritional lifestyle may prove stronger than newly learned habits. To avoid falling back into old habits, you need to trigger your new habits on a daily basis. For example, put a note on the mirror reminding yourself to eat break-fast, and set out dishes and some ingredients the night before.

Simplifying your approach to food makes it easier to form new habits. Choose a nutritional plan that feels comfortable and do-able. If possible, reduce your plan to a simple-to-remember formula. For example, plan to eat a fruit or vegetable with each meal or snack, or set a fixed number of por-tions from each food group to eat every day. Keep your plan in your wallet and look at it before you buy your lunch. And remember to drink plenty of fluids. Dehydration causes you to feel weak, tired, and light-headed. These symptoms also mimic hunger and may lead you to snack when all you really needed was water or juice. Drinking eight glasses of water a day will also help you feel more energetic and fit.

Connect with Hunger

People who have never had a weight problem tend to eat when their body says "I'm hungry." But hunger signals may be a

mystery to those of us who have been through various deprivation diets. Judith Matz, co-director of the Chicago Center for Overcoming Overeating, suggests it's possible to relearn to identify and respond to hunger signals and to eat when they occur. "With practice you can reconnect your eating with internal cues," she says. Doing so helps you distinguish between a bodily urge for nour-ishment and the desire for emotional comfort from food." This doesn't mean you should never reach for food out of emotional hunger, but that you should know it when you do. Sometimes you may choose to satisfy an emotional hunger with food, but other times you may decide to fill it with a phone call to a good friend or another more direct satisfaction of your emotional needs.

If you often feel hungry between meals, consider adjusting your food choices. Some foods have "staying power," notes Sybil Ferguson of The Diet Center Program. They stay longer in your system, helping you feel more satisfied and energetic. Many foods low in calories, such as prepackaged conve-nience diet foods, are also low in "staying power" because they're digested quickly. Natural foods with lots of fiber, such as oatmeal, vegetables, and fruits—are helpful for maintenance because they take longer to chew and to digest, and they create a full feeling in your stomach.

Skipping meals, either because of time crunches or out of guilt from previous overeating, interferes with the steady state of satisfaction that makes maintenance easier.

HEALTHY, FILLING SNACKS

- Celery (3 stalks), 10 calories
- Broccoli, raw (3 stalks), 25 calories
- Carrot, raw, 30 calories
- Peach, raw, 40 calories
- Graham cracker (one whole), 50 calories
- Orange juice (1/2 cup), 55 calories
- Cantaloupe (half), 60 calories
- Bread, whole wheat (1 slice), 65 calories
- Apple, 80 calories
- Cottage cheese, 1 percent fat (1/2 cup), 80 calories
- Milk, low-fat (1 cup) 125 calories
- Potato, baked (plain), 140 calories
- Yogurt, low-fat (8 ounces), 100-250 calories
- Hard pretzel, (1, 1 ounce), 110 calories

When the body has been deprived of food for many hours, your blood sugar level drops, leading to cravings for immediate energy boosts. Eating a balanced selection of foods on a consistent schedule helps stabilize your blood sugar level and hunger sensations, so you can continue to make intelligent decisions about eating.

Avoid Deprivation

A sense of deprivation ("oh, I wish I could eat that," "you're lucky, you can eat anything," "I used to be able to finish a whole cake at one sitting") is a prime enemy of long-term weight maintenance. Tyrannical diet programs do work well for short-term weight loss, but over the long haul, we all need to eat for pleasure as well as nourishment. Meals are among the most pleasurable social events in life, and it pays to learn to take pleasure in the foods that are good for you.

Keep a list of foods or dishes you particularly like that also fit in with weight maintenance. One man's list includes: pancakes with fresh strawberries, grilled mushrooms, mussels marinara, linguine with tomato sauce, crusty Italian bread, and sorbet. When he finds himself missing his old bacon, eggs, and steak diet, he treats himself to all of his favorite nutritious foods in the same day. It keeps his spirits up without expanding his waistline.

Whenever you feel hungry, there's always something you can eat that will be satisfying without threatening your weight stability. Try keeping the refrigerator stocked with fresh fruits and vegetables—especially when you'll be spending a lot of time at home for a few days. Treat yourself to exotic and out of season fruits and vegetables when they look inviting in the market. You're probably spending a lot less than you used to on meat and sweets, so this is not such an extravagance. Nibble on red peppers, fresh young carrots, and cucumbers dipped in a low-fat sauce (no-fat salad dressing makes a quickie dip).

Monitor Your Weight

Some people use the scale. Others keep a food journal. Still others check in with a certain skirt or pair of pants. But most successful weight maintainers use some kind of daily weight check-up. If they find they've put on a pound or three, they quickly try to ease themselves back on track. This may involve relaxation efforts, visualizing more nutritional eating, or being extra careful for a few days. But once a 5-pound gain has occurred— you should consider it a "weight emergency" and construct a relapse recovery plan.

Return from Relapse

"Everyone should expect to have slips from their weight maintenance program," says Professor James Hill. "The trick is not to let it go on too long. After you've gone off a routine for several days, its easy to slip into complete relapse. The most important thing is to recover as soon as possible."

The first step in recovery is to identify the problem(s). List all possible reasons to finish the sentence, "I've started gaining weight again because ...." Your list may include: "I've been unable to exercise," "I've been too busy to grocery shop and cook," "I have the winter blahs," "I've been under a lot of stress," "I got tired of eating sensible foods."

Then adopt an optimistic stance about your ability to bounce back from hard times. Assume responsibility for your actions and beliefs—this puts you firmly in control of your future. Come up with some solutions for each of the stresses that undercut your program. For example, a new low-fat cookbook or cooking class can help you combat food boredom. If grocery shopping is the sore point, perhaps you can enlist a family member to help out.

When you've patched together a recovery plan to meet your needs, gather strength for the new change by tapping into your support network. Everyone needs at least one person to talk to about weight maintenance—someone who is positive and reinforces your decisions. If you were part of a formal weight loss program, check in with the support group whenever you need to recover from a lapse.

Relapses can be a bit humiliating. After all, you may have spent 18 months carefully keeping yourself in nutritional balance, and now, in what seems like a short time, you've gained 10 pounds. But focusing on your own strengths, remembering previous accomplishments, and setting realistic goals for the future can soon have you back on the maintenance track.

Feed Your Emotional Needs

The trick to avoiding relapses—and coping with those that occur— is to remember that you're a capable, lovable human being who can accomplish your goals. Nurturing your own self esteem can help you cope with the stress and burn-out that so often leads to overeating. When you feel tired, bored, quick to anger, withdrawn, rigid and ineffective, you're most apt to abandon your nutritional program. It helps to remember the positive side of your weight loss experience: feelings of being in control, reaching goals, making peace with your appetite, taking care of yourself. It's easy to believe in yourself when things are going well. It's when the going gets tough that you need to reinforce your self-confidence.

Making positive life changes that improve your body and mind are a good way to foster self esteem. Consider taking a stimulating class or workshop, or try a new exercise program, such as fencing, basketball, or power walking. Developing a relaxation ritual, which may involve breathing exercises, chanting, or muscle tension and relaxation, is another excellent technique for caring for yourself.

The Maintenance Mantra

Why do you want to maintain your weight loss? What's the most important factor for you? The reasons vary from person to person. For some, lowering blood pressure or a high cholesterol level is most important. For others, cosmetic concerns loom largest. Naming your motivation proudly and loudly, at least to yourself, can help you stay on track.

"Usually people go out and lose as much weight as they can, then see how much they can keep off," notes Professor Hill. "Maybe we should do the reverse. First, make the right nutritional changes, then, based on our ability to stick with them, accept the resulting weight." □

CHAPTER 8

Exercise: The Other Half of Weight Control

Let's face it: Dieting is difficult, and permanently upgrading your eating habits takes determination too. When making these changes, you need all the help you can get—and luckily there's one inexpensive, medically approved strategy that will not only boost the effectiveness of your diet, but also keep the pounds from coming back. For good measure, it will give you a better-looking body, and a healthier, happier life.

The strategy is simple: Eat less. Exercise more.

Why Dieting Isn't Enough

If you still secretly believe, as so many people do, that you can slim your body and keep it slim forever with one crash diet, you're headed for disappointment. At first, your efforts may be successful. But if you diet without exercising, you're at risk of becoming a fat person in a temporarily thin body. Remember that 95 percent of all dieters will eventually regain the weight they've lost if they don't make permanent changes in their eating habits—and don't increase their level of physical activity during (and after) a diet.

In addition to boosting the results of your diet and keeping extra pounds off afterwards, exercise offers you these valuable health bonuses:

- Lower blood pressure
- Reduced risk of heart disease
- Increased endurance, strength, energy, and productivity
- Reduced stress
- Improved body tone and enhanced attractiveness
- Reduced risk of osteoporosis
- Protection against adult-onset diabetes
- Help with smoking cessation

And there's more. Exercise not only increases your body's metabolic rate and helps you burn calories faster, it also stabilizes your body's insulin and blood sugar levels, and can decrease your appetite. Regular exercise also fights the effects of aging and can even extend life. A study conducted by the

TEST YOUR EXERCISE IQ

The National Heart, Lung, and Blood Institute developed this quick quiz for checking your exercise savvy.

True or False:

1. Exercise increases your energy.
2. Some exercises are better for you than others.
3. A good exercise regime takes several hours each week.
4. We need less exercise as we age.
5. The more athletic you are, the easier it is to exercise.

Answers:

1. True: Exercise energizes the body by increasing metabolism. Biochemical reactions induced by exercise also help relieve stress and fight fatigue.

2. True: Choose sustained exercise, such as brisk walking, swimming, running, and cycling. Activities like isometrics and yoga can tone muscles or increase flexibility. But to burn calories, increase metabolism, and provide cardiovascular benefits, include aerobic and muscle-building activities in your exercise plan.

3. False: You'll get results with a program lasting 20 to 40 minutes, performed at least three times a week.

4. False: You need to maintain physical activity throughout your lifetime. A 70 year-old can exercise less rigorously than a 30 year-old, but both should exercise regularly for 20 to 40 minutes, at least three times a week.

5. False: Anyone can exercise, no matter how athletic. In fact, research indicates that those who benefit most from exercise are those who start at the lowest fitness levels.

National Institutes of Health indicated that men and women aged 86 to 96 tripled the muscle strength of their legs when they worked out with weights. This is especially good news for older seniors, who may be able to avoid life-threatening hip fractures and other disabling injuries if they embark on well-supervised exercise regimes. Other studies have shown that weight-bearing exercise can help reduce the risk of osteoporosis, the "brittle bone" condition that afflicts many women in their postmenopausal years.

How Muscle Building Helps

If you think that muscle-building exercise (weight training) is only for the bulging biceps crowd, think again: Muscle-building exercise is one of our strongest allies in the war against fat.

Here's why: Both fat and muscle tissue burn calories just to maintain themselves. A pound of fat burns two calories a day—but a pound of muscle burns 30 to 50 calories a day. The more muscle tissue you have, the more calories you burn each day—even if your day's most strenuous exercise is channel surfing.

On the average, muscle mass shrinks by 10 to 12 percent between the ages of 30 and 65. Middle age tends to be a time in life when people slow down and become less active, which itself depletes muscle tissue. And when muscle tissue shrinks, a vicious circle begins: Your ability to burn calories plummets—and your fat deposits grow.

Trying to reverse this process with a crash diet alone may just make matters worse: Crash diets can rob the body of muscle as well as fat. In a quick 30 pound weight loss, for example, 4.5 pounds of muscle could vanish—and that lost muscle means that your body will burn calories much more slowly than it did before. The obvious solution: You need to build—or at least maintain—muscle while you're losing weight.

For shedding pounds and keeping them off, for maintaining your health and extending your life, for improving your looks and boosting your outlook—for all these things, exercise needs to be a regular part of your life.

Beginning an Exercise Program: When to See Your Doctor

If you're under 35 and in good general health, you can probably begin most exercise programs without permission from your doctor—as long as you start out slowly, warm up and cool down as recommended, and build up to peak levels over a period of time.

But if you're over 35, seriously overweight, habitually inactive, or a smoker, it's wise to consult a physician before you begin. (Seek your doctor's approval, too, if you're planning to work out with weights for the first time.)

No matter what your age, the President's Council on Physical Fitness and Sports recommends that you see your doctor before beginning an exercise program if you have any of the following:

- High blood pressure
- Heart trouble
- Diabetes
- A family history of strokes or heart attacks
- Frequent dizzy spells

MAKE EXERCISE AN ALL-DAY EVENT

Here are ten good ways to get more exercise out of your daily routine

1. Hop off the bus a stop early and walk to your destination.
2. Get off the elevator a floor below yours and take the stairs.
3. Don't drive from store to store when shopping—park far away and walk.
4. Don't call pals in other offices at work—walk over to see them.
5. Walk to work—or walk at least part of the way.
6. Don't order in lunch—walk out for it.
7. Never sit when you can stand, or ride when you can walk.
8. Reserve part of your lunch time for walking and/or stretching.
9. Do your own house and yard work.
10. After a while, get off the bus or elevator two stops sooner; speed up your walking.

- Extreme breathlessness upon minor exertion
- Arthritis or other bone problems
- Severe muscular, ligament or tendon problems
- Any known or suspected diseases or conditions, including back problems

If you have any of these conditions, your doctor may recommend an exercise stress test. It's a simple, painless procedure that takes about 30 minutes to complete. As you use a treadmill or stationary bike, your heart rate, blood pressure, and other readings will be monitored. Based on your test results, your doctor will help you design a safe and effective exercise program for your individual level of fitness.

EXERCISE THOSE CALORIES AWAY

Many dieters know that a 4-ounce serving of ice cream contains about 300 calories. But how many people know they can work off those calories by: dancing energetically for a half hour, cycling for three-quarters of an hour, or gardening strenuously for an hour and quarter?

According to Dr. James Rippe, you can exercise your way to weight loss. In his book, *The Exercise Exchange Program,* he suggests you burn 200 to 300 calories a day doing something energetic. Choose an activity, using the guide below. (Figures are based on men weighing 154 pounds and women weighing 128 pounds.)

Make sure your activity is fun and fits your personal level of fitness, and do it for the recommended amount of time:

Activity	Minutes to Burn 100 Calories	
	Women	Men
Rock 'n' Roll Dancing	10	9
Boxing	10	8
Running (12 minute mile/5 mph)	11	9
Aerobic exercise (high impact)	13	11
Hiking (no backpack)	14	12
Shoveling snow	15	1
Tennis (Singles)	15	12
Aerobic exercise (low impact)	17	14
Cycling at 9.4 mph	17	14
Climbing stairs	17	14
Tennis (Doubles)	21	17
Walking at 4 mph	21	17
Weeding the garden	24	20
Swimming (20 yards per minute)	26	21
Grocery shopping	28	25
Mopping floors	28	25
Walking at 3 mph	30	25
Raking leaves	32	26
Bowling	34	29

Consider this: For people in good health, the risks of inactivity are potentially far more dangerous than those associated with vigorous exercise.

Once you begin your program, you'll notice sustained results within eight to twelve weeks. You'll find you have plenty of energy to perform your daily routines—with energy in reserve to meet peak demands. You'll have the vigor for leisure time pursuits, whether you enjoy hiking through a museum or up a rocky hillside. You'll gain endurance and be able to walk, jog, run, or swim farther than you could before you became fit. Your muscles will be strengthened and your body will become more limber and flexible.

As you approach your "personal best" level of fitness, your body fat will decrease; your muscle mass will increase. You'll have a leaner, more attractive body, and you'll experience a generous boost in your self-esteem.

What's the Right Exercise Program for You?

You've made the decision to incorporate exercise into your life. Now you face a dizzying array of options from which to choose. What kind of exercise is best? How can you find the time to exercise? Should you exercise with or without supervision?

Think about your lifestyle. If the exercise program you're considering doesn't fit into it, it will be hard to stick with that program over time. Consistency and regularity guarantee the success of your weight loss/fitness exercise program, so choose a program that can become as much a part of your daily routine as brushing your teeth.

Think of your new exercise plan as a package of components that you can vary according to your needs, your moods, and your individual level of fitness. If you seek maximum weight loss and health benefits, two of these components, aerobics and muscle-building exercise, are essential. You can combine both in some kinds of exercise (like fitness walking and jogging), vary your exercises, and add other options for variety.

Aerobics

The most important component of your exercise program should be aerobic ("in the presence of oxygen") exercise. An aerobically fit body uses oxygen efficiently during exercise; over time, aerobic exercise conditions and strengthens the body's heart and respiratory systems so that it can function well during sustained physical activity. Your weekly program should include at least three 20 minute sessions of continuous, rhythmic aerobic exercise using the large muscle groups.

Aerobics provides exercise for your heart muscle, which, like other muscles, needs a

DETERMINING YOUR "THR"

Subtract your age from 220, then multiply that result by .65 and .85 to get the lower and upper limits of your Target Heart Rate range. The THR range of a 40 year-old, for example, is 180 (that's 220 minus 40) times .65 and .85, or 117 to 153 (heartbeats per minute). Take your pulse by counting the number of heartbeats for 10 seconds; multiply by six to find your heartbeats per minute.

regular workout in order to maintain its strength. For your heart to receive maximum benefits from aerobic exercise, it must be worked at (or near) the upper end of a "target heart rate" (THR) range, where it is being effectively but safely stressed. For the way to calculate your THR, see the nearby box.

Start by working toward the low end of your range; build slowly over time to the higher end. If you've consulted a doctor before beginning your exercise program, be sure to follow his or her advice with regard to your THR.

How Long Should Your Aerobic Workout Be? You should build up to a session that includes at least 20 minutes of exercise at your THR. Begin with 5 to 10 minutes of low-intensity warm-up stretches; the high-intensity middle portion of your routine should last at least 10 minutes at the beginning of your program; work comfortably up to 30 minutes or more over a few weeks. Follow with a 5 to 10 minute cool-down.

EXERCISES, BENEFITS AND CALORIES BURNED

Key: ■—Especially Good ●—Good

Exercise	Aerobic Conditioning	Flexibility	Endurance	Builds Muscle	Relieves Stress	Good for Beginners	Cal per hr.*	Expense Factor
Dancing (rock)	■	■	■		■		290-575	free
Boxing	■	■	■		■		400-600	can be expensive
Badminton	●	●				●	230-515	moderate
Basketball	■	■	■	■			170-515	inexpensive
Bicycling								
Outdoors	■		■	Leg	●	■	170-800	one-time equipment investment
Stationary	■		■	Leg		■	85-800	one-time equipment investment
Bowling						■	115-170	moderate
Canoeing	depends on speed	■	●	Upper body	■	■	170-460	can be expensive
Gardening					■		115-400	free
Golfing no golf cart							115-400	can be expensive
Handball, Racquet ball and Squash	■	■	■	■	■		345-690	moderate to expensive
Rowing	■		■	■	■	■	170-800	can be expensive

How to Warm Up. Five or 10 minutes of warm-up stretches will help you avoid muscle stiffness, soreness, and even injuries. Stretching also enhances your body's flexibility, a key component of overall fitness. Finally, stretching adequately before your principal exercise prepares you mentally for the activity at hand.

When performing general warm-up stretches, hold each stretch for at least 30 seconds; do not bounce. When you feel a definite, but not painful, pulling sensation, you will know that you are stretching adequately. Make sure to stretch the muscles you'll be exercising; runners, for example,

Exercise	Aerobic Conditioning	Flexibility	Endurance	Builds Muscle	Relieves Stress	Good for Beginners	Cal per hr.*	Expense Factor
Running								
5 mph (12 min mi)	■	■	■	■	■	■	460	cost of good shoes
7 mph (9 min mi)	■	■	■	■	■		690	cost of good shoes
Skating (Ice/Roller)	■	■	■	■	■	■	230-460	can be expensive
Skiing								
Cross Country	■	■	■	■	■	■	290-800	can be expensive
Downhill	■	■	■	■	■	■	170-460	can be expensive
Soccer	depends on game						290-600	varies
Stair Climbing	■	■	■	leg		■	230-460	free
Swimming	■	■	■	■	■	■	230-690	varies
Tennis	■	■	■	■	■		230-515	can be expensive
Walking								
2 mph (30 min mi)	■				■	■	115	cost of shoes
4 mph (15 min mi)	■	■	■	leg	■	■	260	cost of shoes

Note: Calories burned are estimated for a 120 to 130 pound person; a person weighing 170 to 180 pounds burns calories about 40 percent faster. Low end estimates are for minimum efforts; high end estimates are for maximum efforts. To gain aerobic benefits for any activity, work within your Target Heart Rate (THR) (see box) and do the activity continuously for at least 20 minutes. To burn fat, continue for more than 20 minutes.

should concentrate on leg and lower back muscles; rowers should stretch arm and upper body muscles.

The Cool Down. After a workout, let your heart rate return to normal while you do a low-intensity exercise, such as slow walking. Do cool-down stretches—which can be the same as your warm-up stretches—to keep blood from pooling in your legs, to prevent dizziness after a strenuous workout, and to help prevent muscle soreness. Spend at least 5 minutes cooling-down.

Muscle-Building Exercise
Exercising with weights or resistance-type exercise machines such as Nautilus is essential for dieters (and everyone else), for these

A CIRCUIT TRAINING PROGRAM FOR GYM OR HOME

This circuit workout was developed by Petra Kolber, a fitness expert from the Molly Fox Fitness Club in New York City. It is designed to condition every major muscle group within a short period of time, no matter what your level of fitness.

Before you begin to circuit train:
■ Check with your doctor if you've never worked with weights before.
■ Remember to breathe during each exercise.
■ Keep stomach muscles tight, back straight, shoulders relaxed, and chest lifted.
■ Repeat each exercise 15 to 20 times.
■ Take 10 to 15 second breaks between each set of the various exercises.

1. Triceps Extension: Stand with right foot in front of left, right knee slightly bent and right hand resting on thigh for support. With weight in left hand, bring arm back to about shoulder level. Return to original position; switch arms.

Beginners: No weight or 2–3 lb weights
Intermediate: 3 lb weights
Advanced: 5–8 lb weights
At the gym: Use the Triceps Extensor

2. Standing Squat: Stand with feet apart, toes out at a 45 degree angle, making sure your weight is placed on your heels. Lower body to just above knee level with knees over toes and feet flat on floor. Squeeze buttocks briefly; return to original position.

Beginners: No weights (keep hands on thigh)
Intermediate: 5–8 lb weights resting on thighs
Advanced: 5–8 lb weights resting on shoulders
At the gym: Use the Leg Press Machine

3. Standing Inner Thigh: Place your weight on the left leg, knee slightly bent. Extend the right leg forward. Leading with the right heel, squeeze the inner thigh and draw right leg across the front of the left leg as far as you can. Hold for two seconds and return to original position; switch legs.

Beginners: No weights; legs only
Intermediate: Use a medium resistance exercise band
Advanced: Use a high resistance exercise band
At the gym: Use the Adductor Machine

4. Biceps Curl: Stand with feet hip distance apart, knees relaxed, weights lightly held in hands, arms at sides with palms facing front, elbows at waist. Bend elbows, slowly bringing hands to shoulders. Hold for three seconds; return arms to original position.

Beginners: 2–3 lb weights
Intermediate: 3–5
Advanced: 5–8 lb weights
At the gym: Biceps curl

5. Calf Raise: Standing with feet hip-distance apart and toes facing forward, raise up on toes, lifting heels from floor. Lower heels to original position.

Beginners: No weights
Intermediate: 3–5 lb weights resting on shoulders
Advanced: 5–8 lb weights resting on shoulders
At the gym: Seated or Standing Calf Raise

exercises build calorie-burning muscle. In one study, a group of people followed the same diet and exercised for 30 minutes three times a week. Half performed aerobics exclusively; the other half cycled for 15 minutes and worked on Nautilus machines for 15 minutes. After eight weeks, the aerobics-only group lost 3 pounds of fat and a half pound of muscle. But the group that combined aerobics and strength training lost 10 pounds of fat—and *gained* 2 pounds of muscle.

6. Shoulder Press: Stand with feet hip-distance apart and knees slightly bent. With weights in hands at shoulder height and palms facing forward, slowly extend arms (do not lock elbows) overhead; slowly lower arms to original position.

Beginners: No weights
Intermediate: 3 - 5 lb weights
Advanced: 5 - 8 lb weights
At the gym: Shoulder press

---

7. Push-Ups: Kneel on all fours, making sure your weight is placed just above the knees, and crossing legs and arms slightly wider than shoulder width apart. Flex elbows and slowly lower body until chest touches the floor. Using arms and chest muscles, return to original position without locking elbows.

Beginners: Do a "standing push-up" against a wall
Intermediate: Do this version
Advanced: Classic, straight-leg push-up with weight on toes, not knees
At the gym: Chest or bench press

---

8. Abdominal Crunch: Lie on floor with knees bent and lower back pressed into floor, hands behind head, elbows out to sides. Gently lift shoulders off floor while tightening abdominal muscles; lower to original position.

Beginners: No weights
Intermediate: 5 lb weights resting on chest
Advanced: Bring legs, crossed at ankles, toward ceiling; as you lift shoulders, tighten abdominal muscles.
At the gym: Use the Abdominal Machine

The American College of Sports Medicine, which once recommended aerobics alone for fitness, has now added muscle-building exercise (strength training) to its guidelines. They suggest two weekly sessions, 8 to 12 repetitions each, of 8 to 10 different exercises. Lifting free weights, working out on Nautilus machines, and doing exercises like sit-ups and push-ups are good. Make sure you learn how to use any equipment properly so you can get the maximum benefit and minimize your risk of injury. As with aerobics sessions, make sure your strength training sessions include an adequate warm-up and cool-down period.

Circuit Training

Circuit training combines the heart and respiratory benefits of aerobics with the muscle building and toning benefits of strength training. It differs from strength training in two ways: it uses lighter weights and more repetitions; and, unlike strength training or exercise machine work-outs, where several sets of repetitions of each exercise are performed before moving on, in circuit training you move quickly from one exercise to another in sequence. Depending on your level of fitness, you repeat the circuit one or more times.

Studies show that circuit training burns more calories than strength training, and is a real energy booster. An added benefit: Those who enjoy this fast-paced work out say it helps beat boredom.

Circuit training can be done in a gym or health club, where staffers can design a program tailored to your needs (see the section on "What to Look for in a Gym or Health Club"), or in your own home (follow the program in the nearby box).

Whether you circuit-train in the gym or at home, you're likely to gain muscular strength and cardiovascular endurance in two or three weeks; after five to eight weeks, you should begin to see an improvement in muscle tone.

The Big Four: Biking, Running, Swimming, Walking

Fitness experts call these the "Big Four," since when it comes to aiding weight loss, aerobic conditioning, fitness, and general well-being, these activities are among the best. In addition, each is easy to learn, adaptable, relatively inexpensive, and can be done alone or with others. If you're lucky enough to enjoy doing these exercises, they can also make up most of your fitness program. Bad weather's no deterrent, either; today stationary cycles and treadmills take exercise indoors.

Walking. According to Casey Meyers, an expert on walking and author of two books on the subject, this most natural and basic of human activities has been recognized as a serious form of exercise only since the mid-1980's. In his book, *Walking* (Random House, 1992) he argues that, mile-for-mile, once you shift to a run you are *using less energy (burning fewer calories) and less oxygen than if you had increased your speed while still walking*. This fact, he claims, dispels the myth tale that running is superior to walking for weight loss and aerobic fitness.

When it comes to weight loss, whether you run a mile or walk it briskly (15 minute per mile), you'll burn the same number of calories.

There are four levels of intensity for fitness-walking.

- *Low (Strolling):* 18 to 30 minutes per mile. Start with strolling when you begin walking for fitness, especially if you're seriously overweight or haven't been getting exercise.
- *Moderate (Brisk Walking):* 14 to 17 minutes per mile. Most fit walkers can handle a 15-minute-per-mile pace in comfort.

- *High (Aerobic Walking):* 10.0 to 13.5 minutes a mile. At this intensity, walking and running overlap; at this pace, a slow run or jog begins. You are walking aerobically only when you reach your THR.
- *Very High (Race Walking):* Less than 10.0 minutes a mile. This is considered a track and field event and has been part of the Olympics since 1908; it is a competitive sport and not a daily exercise.

As with any other form of exercise, studies show that you'll reap the most rewards from walking if you walk three times a week for at least 20–30 minutes each time, reaching your THR. Your goal, over time, should be to walk three miles every time, no matter what your pace. However, the faster your pace, the more aerobic benefits you'll realize and the faster you'll burn calories.

Running/Jogging. Running or jogging is arguably the most popular form of aerobic exercise in America today. Millions of runners now take to city streets, country lanes, and parks everywhere as part of their regular exercise routine.

Is there a difference between running and jogging? According to running expert Bob Glover, the only difference is the spelling. He calls everyone a runner, no matter how fast or slow their pace.

Who can run? Almost anyone in good health, with no history of chronic illness. As with any other form of exercise, however, if you're over 35, smoke, or have any of the medical conditions listed earlier, check with your doctor before you begin.

Getting off to a running start is simple. All you need is the right footwear. Good running shoes must fit perfectly, and be light, flexible, and durable. Look for these qualities:

- Thick, layered sole from heel to toe
- Resilient heel wedge and reinforced heel cup
- Molded Achilles tendon pad
- Flexible midsole
- Padded tongue
- Studded rubber sole

Before you run, do 10 minutes of stretching and warm-up exercises. Once you're running, begin slowly, and aim to run a mile or so in 15 to 20 minutes, three to five times a week. Alternate running with brisk walking, especially when you first start your running program; work up to your THR over time.

When you can run a mile comfortably, you can increase your distance gradually—but not by more than 10 percent a week.

Running is not without risks. Injuries are common to runners—it is estimated that nearly 60 percent will suffer at least one injury serious enough to temporarily prevent training. Many injuries are caused by easily avoided conditions such as ill-fitting shoes; rocks, bumps, holes and other unfavorable road or track conditions; running farther or faster than your fitness level allows; and bad running technique. You are more likely to sustain injury if you run competitively.

Heat-related conditions such as dehydration, heat stroke, heat exhaustion and heat cramps can be very serious. They are also easily avoidable. Wear light clothing; do not run on very hot and humid days; and drink plenty of fluids during longer runs. On hot days, drink about eight ounces 15 minutes before you run, and every two miles during the run. Always include 10 minutes of cool-down exercises after your run.

IF YOU DECIDE TO JOG...

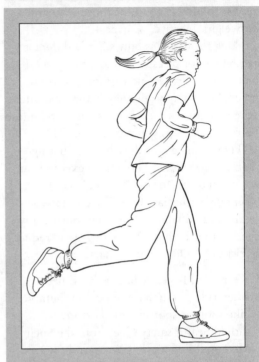

For safety's sake, keep these key points in mind.

- Begin slowly, allow yourself 15 to 20 minutes to run a mile.
- Increase distance gradually—no more than 10 percent a week.
- Drink plenty of fluids when running in hot weather.
- On really hot days, don't run at all.

Biking. Nearly 100 million Americans are bikers. People ride for transportation, fun, fitness, and competition. But no matter what the reason, biking is a great aerobic conditioner and muscle-toner. It also promotes flexibility, especially of the hip and knee joints. Since it's a non-weight-bearing exercise, biking is good for those who are overweight, inactive, or over 40.

Biking for fitness is only slightly different than biking for pleasure. Follow the general guidelines for an aerobic workout; warm up and cool down appropriately before and after biking; and bike steadily for about 20 minutes at a rate that keeps you within your THR.

There is one major drawback to biking—it can be hazardous. Though no exercise can ever claim to be "perfectly safe," according to running enthusiast Bob Glover, more people are injured when biking than during any other aerobic activity. You can greatly reduce the risks by following these safety tips:

- Wear a hard-shell helmet at all times when riding. Purchase one at a reputable bike shop or sporting goods store; it should bear a safety label from the Snell Memorial Foundation™. Learn how to adjust the helmet for a snug, safe fit.
- Remember: Bikes are vehicles. Ride *with* the traffic. Obey all traffic signals and signs. Signal your intentions to those around you.
- Make sure you are visible—the brighter, the better. Apply reflective tape to your bike, including the spokes.
- Anticipate! Watch ahead for turning cars, jaywalkers, car doors that may fly open in front of you, and dogs.
- Wear a whistle around your neck or equip your bike with a loud horn, buzzer, or other noise-making device.
- *Never* listen to music through headphones while biking.

Swimming. A water workout is great aerobic exercise. And because water packs 12 times the resistance of air, it's ideal for toning mus-

cles while burning fat. In water, your weight shrinks to just 10 percent of what you weigh on land. This eliminates stress on ligaments and joints, and lessens the risk of fractures, sprains, and strains. This is particularly important for the elderly or pregnant. Water-based exercises are ideal for those with arthritis, as well as for obese and sedentary people. Exercising in a swimming pool can also be a real physical and psychological stress beater.

At a hefty 600 calories a mile, swimming expends more energy than almost any other form of exercise. Experts advise using the crawl or backstroke when swimming for fitness. Be careful that water temperature is not too cold or warm—the ideal is 82 to 86 degrees; avoid eating heavily before your swim.

Water exercise also offers a wide range of workout possibilities. Special exercises have been developed for use in the water. For example, try the "water jog," which is nothing more than jogging in water while pumping the arms. You should begin slowly, aim for a 10 minute jog, and build up over time to 20 to 30 minutes sessions. For a more challenging workout, jog in water that's chest-deep.

Aquatic equipment like boots, wings, barbells and other devices are also available for water exercises, as are flotation devices that allow non-swimmers to do water workouts.

If you swim or exercise frequently in a pool and find yourself irritated by chlorine, you can purchase eye goggles; nose clips and water-tight ear plugs are a good idea, too.

For Fun, For Variety, Try . . .

Many less traditional and some previously out-of-style forms of exercise are in vogue now. Football players study dance to improve their footwork and coordination; women are entering the boxing ring; and children and adults are taking up all forms of martial arts. Different forms of exercise can add variety and interest to your routine. You can probably find classes for most of them at your local gym, health club, adult education center, or Y.

Calisthenics, the "granddad" of modern exercise regimes, are the exercises you remember from gym class: jumping jacks, squat thrusts, toe-touches, push-ups, and sit-ups. Performed correctly, they are excellent calorie-burners, can provide aerobic conditioning, and can tone and strengthen muscles.

Use calisthenics as a warm-up to your regular routine, for a break, or even as your entire routine with an aerobics component. As with any exercise program, be sure to include a warm-up and cool-down period, and to work at your personal level of fitness, building up gradually over time.

Yoga. Whether you think of it as a way of life or as a way of exercising, yoga can reduce stress and enhance your mental well-being. On the physical side, certain yoga exercises are good for increasing flexibility and strengthening muscles. In addition to classes, and private instruction, there are a variety of books and videotapes for everyone from beginners to advanced practitioners.

Plyometrics. Remember the medicine ball? It's making a comeback as a fun addition to your regular aerobic workout. Plyometrics, the stretching and sudden contraction of

DO'S AND DON'TS FOR AVOIDING EXERCISE INJURIES

Do warm-up exercises for 5 to 10 minutes before you start.

Do cool-down exercises for 5 to 10 minutes at the end of sessions.

Do exercise regularly and consistently at least 20 minutes three times a week.

Do stop at once if you experience unusual discomfort.

Don't exercise at a pace that's too fast for you.

Don't over do it. If you can't speak while exercising, slow down.

Don't double distance or duration overnight; increase gradually.

Don't give up . . . just slow down! It may take 8 to 12 weeks to condition a body that's been sedentary for its entire adult life. Be patient with yourself.

muscles as when catching a heavy ball, can build muscle strength and increase power. For more information on these exercises, including a routine for wheelchair athletes, read *Plyometric Exercises* by sports physiologist Dr. Donal Chu (Bittersweet Publishing Company, Livermore, CA).

For a change of pace in your aerobics workout, substitute a medicine ball for hand weights. Make sure to start out with a small, lightweight ball, about 18 inches in diameter, weighing from two to nine pounds. The weight you select should depend on your personal level of fitness; the lower the level, the lighter the ball. Medicine balls are generally available at fitness retailers.

Dancing. Ballroom dancing. Line dancing. Square dancing. Disco dancing. When done continuously and energetically for a half-hour or more, dancing is a great form of aerobic exercise—and a fun way to meet people.

The martial arts, including karate, t'ai chi ch'uan, kung-fu, judo and aikido, vary in their efficacy as total exercise programs, but all may aid your ability to fight stress and remain calm under duress. Some, like karate, are ancient forms of self-defense; others, like t'ai chi ch'uan, are considered "soft martial arts" rather than training for protection.

These disciplines are taught in martial arts schools and many community centers. Before you sign up with a martial arts school, check its credentials and get references to make sure they have an appropriate program for you.

Boxing. You don't have to be a fighter to consider boxing as a fitness activity. In gyms across the country, women, as well as men, are discovering that boxing is an excellent aerobic workout that conditions upper body and leg muscles. If the notion of sparring with a partner seems too aggressive, try a punching bag to absorb your energy. Check the yellow pages under "boxing instruction," or call health clubs to find a program in your area.

When to Stop

How much exercise is too much? It all depends on you and your personal level of fitness. But, fit or not, knowing when to stop is vital in order to avoid injury.

While you should feel sweaty and *slightly* breathless in the middle of your aerobic workout, and be able to hear your heart pounding in your chest, you should not become dizzy or nauseous, or feel sharp pain. If you do, stop and take a rest; see your doctor before resuming exercise if symptoms continue. But if you experience:

- Pressure or discomfort in your chest
- Faintness
- Shortness of breath
- Bursts of very rapid, slow, or irregular heartbeat
- Excessive fatigue
- Severe joint or muscle pain

STOP exercising at once, and consult your doctor before going back to your program.

The Family that Exercises Together Stays Healthy Together

Fitness experts tell us that we are raising a generation of unfit children.

Television, computers, video games, and other sedentary pastimes seem to be making our children more indoor-oriented than ever before. Sadly, safety concerns in many neighborhoods have also limited our ability to allow children outside for unsupervised play.

We need to make exercise as important a part of our children's routine as their schoolwork, regular medical care, and proper nutrition. Begin introducing energetic activity in infancy—even if it's watching you work out—so that your children develop healthy exercise habits that last. Make exercise a fun family affair, and you'll help your children remain fit and active throughout their childhood, and beyond.

Here are some tips for making exercise part of your family's life:

- Set up a room for active play. Remove anything breakable, carpet the floor, and equip the room with active toys only: Blocks, balls, riding toys, etc. A great addition: an old mattress kids can jump around on. Banish from this room TVs and video games.
- Check out kids' sports programs in your area, and sign your children up as soon as they're ready. For example, AYSO (American Youth Soccer Organization), welcomes children aged 5 and up and emphasizes the fun of the game rather than on winning.
- Take your child with you when you exercise. If you bike or jog, put your baby in a special seat or stroller (remember baby's bike helmet!) See if your gym has baby exercise classes—or check programs like "Gymboree," "Mommy and Me," or others that encourage parent-child fitness activities.
- Take family vacations at activity-centered resorts—or plan family camping and hiking trips or biking excursions.
- Some kids shy away from sports or competition. Build self-esteem by interesting them in individual activities—ballet, tap dancing, swimming, or horseback riding. Get private or group instruction if you can; join your child if he or she is willing.
- Encourage your child to walk. If possible, walk instead of driving with your children; take walks for fun. Explore your neighborhood on foot.

Fitness For Sale

If you're the kind of person who needs a maximum of motivation to get on the exercise track, going it alone in your living room probably isn't the right choice for you. Your commitment to a regular exercise program may get a needed boost if you join a gym or health club, book yourself a package of exercise classes, or hire a personal trainer.

What to Look for in a Gym or Health Club
Health clubs range from the Spartan to the luxurious, from no-frills-basic-gyms to carpeted comfort domes where everything is provided for you but the sweat. Choosing a facility is a matter of personal taste, style, and budget. Here are some tips to help ease your choice:

- The closer a club is to your home or office, the more frequently you're likely to use it. Experts agree: You'll exercise more regularly at a club with a convenient location.
- Tour clubs at high-traffic time, like right after work and during lunch hours or at the time you are most likely to use the facility. Is there a wait for frequently-used stationary bikes? The aerobic benefits of circuit-training won't be yours if you're standing in line to use the equipment.
- Is the crowd dressed for success? If your gym wear is torn sweats, you might not feel at home. Also, consider whether you want a single sex or coed gym.
- If you're not going to swim, take classes or get spa-treatments, then you don't need a club that offers these extras. Instead, get the most for your money by selecting a simpler facility. Similarly, if you're not going to use much of the high-tech equipment, opt for a place that offers classes and the basic fitness equipment.
- See if the club is affiliated with the Association of Quality Clubs, whose members follow a uniform code of conduct, or the Association of Physical Fitness Centers; most members are clubs run by Bally that follow set guidelines.

QUICK HEALTH CLUB CHECKLIST

- Is the club well-maintained, clean, and well-lit?
- Is the range of equipment adequate for your needs?
- Is the equipment easily accessible and comfortably placed?
- Are there instructions posted on each machine?
- Are any of the machines broken or out of service?
- Are time limits for popular equipment posted and enforced?
- Are you comfortable with the pace, the clientele, and instructors?
- Are staffers friendly and well-informed?
- Do you get a full tour and demonstration?
- Does the club offer a couple of trial sessions?

- Be sure instructors are certified by such organizations as:

ACE	American Council on Exercise
ACSM	American Council of Sports Medicine
AFAA	Aerobic and Fitness Association of America
AFB	Association for Fitness in Business
CIAR	Cooper Institute of Aerobic Research
IDEA	International Dance Exercise Association
NSCA	National Strength and Conditioning Association

- All instructors should be certified to perform CPR; swimming teachers should have a Water Safety Instruction Certificate.
- Get all promises in writing. If equipment is to be added, or the pool is being enlarged, have it written into the contract. Have the contract include other services you may want, such as child-care. Try for a month-to-month deal; if that's not possible, make sure that there is a termination-clause so that you can cancel your membership if you move, change jobs or become otherwise unable to use the facilities. At a minimum, clubs should have a "freeze" policy if you are unable to workout due to illness or injury.
- Check with the Better Business Bureau to make sure the club has a satisfactory "business performance record."

Fitness Classes

A recent magazine round-up revealed that fitness classes are becoming more interesting—and exotic—than ever before. Classes like "YogaRobics," "Bench Defense," and "Yokibics" are cropping up, indicating that when it comes to exercise, east is meeting west. The idea is that the more interesting the class, the more likely you are to stick with it.

Another addition to the exercise scene is the "Step Reebok Cross-Training Circuit Work-Out," which is making its way into health clubs across the country.

For information on interesting fitness classes, check health clubs, Y's, and your yellow pages.

Personal Trainers

For the ultimate personal fitness regime, there's the personal trainer. A good one will design a work-out program specifically for your needs, and will put you through your paces on a regular basis.

You can choose to work out with your trainer at home or in a gym—usually, your trainer will be affiliated with one. In Washington, DC and other cities around the country, the latest fad is the trainer with a well-equipped exercise van that comes to your home or office.

Some trainers are also nutritionists, and will help you with diets and eating programs. Some will go so far as ridding your refrigerator of fat and sugar-laden taboos.

To find a trainer, check with Y's and health clubs. Make sure a trainer is certified by one or more of the organizations listed above. Ask him or her for a list of client references, then call to check up. You can expect to pay $25 an hour and up for the services of a qualified personal trainer.

A Gym of One's Own—A Guide to At-Home Exercise Equipment

Never have there been so many options in at-home exercise equipment—or so much high technology. In exercise bikes—the best-selling category—choices range from simple to sublime. At the low end are stationary bikes, with little more than pedals and handlebars, that start at about $200.

On the deluxe side, there's a Virtual Reality Bike with a video screen and even a fan to simulate the wind in your hair. It retails for around $8,000.

When purchasing any piece of exercise equipment, make sure to get adequate instruction from your salesperson, especially if you're unfamiliar with exercise techniques.

Try any piece of home exercise equipment thoroughly before you buy, either at a friend's, a gym, or in the store. Give it at least a twenty minute test to make sure you'll be comfortable. (If that makes the retailer uncomfortable—shop elsewhere.) Read the manual before you use your new machine, and keep it handy for reference.

Cross-Country Ski Exercisers give a complete upper and lower body workout. Used correctly, they place less stress on the joints than other aerobic exercisers but they do require coordination.

Look for: Adjustable hip rest for balance; tension on poles or pulleys, and height of poles or length of pulley cords should be easily adjustable. Poles or cords should allow as full a range of forward-to-back motion as possible.

Rowing Machines are second only to ski machines for a well-rounded aerobic work-out. There are two main types, those with pistons and those with flywheels; the latter is closer to a real on-the-water workout in a shell.

Look for: A heavy duty steel frame; a pulley or pair of oars that moves smoothly through the full range of motion; a seat that glides easily on wheels or ball bearings; a "stop" at the back of the seat track; and an easy-to-reach resistance setting. Tall or heavy-set people may find that units low to the ground are difficult to use comfortably.

Treadmills are most effective when they push you to maintain a pace, so motorized versions are the best choice. Treadmills with adjustable incline features add to your workout's efficiency by providing uphill exercise. Some treadmills offer a choice of laps, random, or pre-set courses, allowing you to vary your workout.

Look for: Front and side rails that help you keep your balance; make sure side rails allow arms to swing. Speed and incline controls should let you make adjustments while you're moving on the machine. Gauges for time, distance, and pace are essential and a speedometer is good for serious workouts. The emergency on/off switch should be clearly marked and easy to reach.

Stationary Bikes. Usually, the heavier the machine, the better the quality. Make sure the model you choose is easy to pedal and has an easy-to-reach and read resistance adjustment knob.

Look for: Seat height and angle that are adjustable in the stem; and handlebar height that is adjustable in the neck; foot straps to let you use muscles as you push up as well as pull down on the pedal. Gauges should include a resistance monitor and speedometer.

Home Gyms. According to *Consumer Reports* (November 1993), "The attempt to produce a multi-purpose device at a price suited to the consumer market too often resulted in design compromises that could drive you from the gym bench to the sofa." The magazine recommended joining a health club or taking aerobic exercise classes as an alternative to buying poorly-designed multi-purpose home gym equipment.

Exercise Videos—Workouts with the Stars

These days, you can exercise in your living room with everyone from Cher to Debbie Reynolds—but how do you know who'll provide the best—and safest—workout?

Is it a good idea to select a video just because you like the celebrity? The answer, according to experts, is maybe. Peg Jordan, RN, is editor of *American Fitness,* the magazine of the Aerobics and Fitness Associations of America (AFAA). She believes that few celebrities know much about exercise, but that at least some (Cher, for example), have qualified trainers designing and conducting the exercises.

Here are hints for selecting safe, enjoyable exercise videos:

- Check the credentials of the instructor or consultant. He or she should be certified by one or more of the organizations listed previously. Look for degrees in kinesiology or exercise science.
- Choose exercise that's suitable for your level of fitness.
- Rent and try, then buy.
- Look for a complete routine, with adequate warm-up and cool-down exercises. Programs should progress from beginning to more challenging levels. The instructor should regularly remind you to maintain proper form.
- Make sure you'll enjoy hearing the instructor—and the music—over and over again.
- Find out whether you will need equipment and whether your exercise area will be large enough to accommodate the workout you've selected.

Exercise Books: A Buyer's Guide

Exercise/fitness books have their own large section in well-stocked book stores. Today, it seems as if almost every body part has a manual devoted to reducing or increasing its size. Unless you're a real fitness fanatic and near-expert yourself, you'll probably want an exercise and fitness book that's general in its scope, rather than one that limits its concentration.

If you're choosing one book for general reference, check the author's credentials. Books by doctors or highly-trained exercise specialists are likely to be more informed and comprehensive than those by celebrities or media personalities.

Consider these books . . .

■ *Health & Fitness Excellence,* by Robert H. Cooper, Ph.D. This clear, well-written book offers a comprehensive, aerobics program with a good mix of exercises, as well as solid dietary information. Illustrated exercises are easy-to-follow.

■ *Fitness and Your Health,* by David C. Nieman, Dr. P.H., FACSM (Bull Publishing, 1993). This book contains interesting quizzes that test your fitness level and knowledge. It helps you decide whether you should seek medical advice, and explains which fitness programs are best suited for you. Includes easy how-to advice about switching to a healthier lifestyle.

■ *The Exercise Exchange Program,* by James M. Rippe, MD. and Patricia Amend (Simon & Schuster, 1992). A highly versatile, easy-to-follow program combining solid nutritional advice and exercise information. Comprehensive programs that include all the significant exercise formats (aerobic, strength training, flexibility) are clearly presented.

■ *Walking,* by Casey Meyers (Random House, 1992). A top motivational book that makes you want to get outside and walk. The author discusses all aspects of walking for fitness and provides concise guides to walking-for-fitness programs for all age groups.

■ *The Family Fitness Handbook,* by Bob Glover and Jack Shepard (Viking Penguin, 1989). Glover, the man who propelled running from a solitary pleasure to a national pastime, takes on American family fitness in this readable, information-packed volume. Programs for running, swimming, biking, walking, and aerobics are covered and there are chapters on kids' sports, nutrition, stress, and fitness for physically and mentally challenged children.

But not these:

■ *Kathy Smith's WalkFit™ for a Better Body* by Kathy Smith (Warner Books, 1994). This book by video exercise star Kathy Smith takes a sound, though cursory, look at exercise advice, nutritional information, and walking programs. Casey Meyers' *Walking* is far more interesting and motivational.

■ *Technique,* by Tony Little with Paula Dranov (Time Warner, 1994). The book opens with praise from the many celebrities whose bodies Little has helped shape; clearly, he is a superior and enthusiastic personal trainer. But the exercise photos of the authors are poor and the directions are difficult to follow.

■ *Stop the Insanity,* by Susan Powter (Simon & Schuster, 1993). Self-made media star Powter has a great personal story to tell about losing lots of weight, but her book is filled with questionable information that could prove dangerous for some readers. For example, she dismisses as unnecessary physical exams for most women considering first-time exercise programs, and pooh-poohs drinking eight glasses of water a day— advice most fitness experts deem essential.

■ *Callanetics,* by Callan Pinckney (Avon Books, 1994). A runaway best-seller, *Callanetics* is a body-sculpting program that boasts proven results. The exercises appear to be sound, but the instructions are hard to follow and the accompanying photos are poor. The author recommends a one hour-plus program that is probably too long for most readers to follow. □

CHAPTER 9

Going Too Far: Anorexia, Bulimia, Bingeing

Nearly everyone has seen the images: an impossibly thin young girl, obsessively toying with food but never eating it, the details of her skeleton clearly visible through her dry flesh; or the young woman with bulimia, compulsively stuffing herself with thousands of junk-food calories, then vomiting back everything she has eaten and doing it all over again, sometimes many times a day.

Rooted in deep psychological, cultural, and physical dysfunctions, an eating disorder is one of the most stubborn problems a person can face. In recent years, these mysterious illnesses have received a torrent of media attention—as the subject of television movies and talk shows, and as grist for the tabloids. One celebrity after another (usually female) has revealed her personal battle with these disorders. Some, like Princess Diana and actress Jane Fonda are bulimics. Others, such as TV actress Tracy Gold, are anorexic. Perhaps the most dramatic and horrifying stories are those of anorexic women who have starved themselves to death: rock and

roll star Karen Carpenter, only 32 when she died in 1983; or more recently, gymnast Christy Henrich, 22, who weighed just 43 pounds at the time of her death, which was attributed to multiple organ failure.

Anorexia nervosa and bulimia nervosa have long been classified as psychiatric illnesses. A third eating disorder, binge-eating syndrome, has just been added to the basic psychiatric guidelines. Together, they can be viewed as variations on a theme of extreme eating and behavior—from not eating at all (anorexia), to binging-and-purging (bulimia), to eating nearly all the time (binge-eating syndrome). It takes a combination of medical, psychological, and nutritional therapy to overcome any of these disorders. Treatment usually involves the patient's family as well, especially in the case of anorexics, who are frequently adolescent girls.

Eating disorders can be found around the world, but they are most common in industrialized western nations where food is abundant. In the United States, there are many strong cultural influences at work that most experts agree contribute to the development of eating disorders. Women in particular are the target of a constant barrage of subtle and not-so-subtle "thinner-is-better" messages, and by most counts, they account for about 90 percent of those with eating disorders.

Estimates of the number of people with eating disorders vary, in part because the disorders are often characterized by secretive behavior and can remain undetected until serious health problems develop. Some studies estimate that one percent of adolescent and young adult women in this country have an eating disorder, with concentrations in some subgroups such as college students and athletes. The National Association of Anorexia Nervosa and Associated Disorders (ANAD), an educational and self-help organization, estimates that seven million women and one million men in this country have eating disorders.

Eating disorders usually begin early in life. The period between 14 and 18 years old is the riskiest; and by age 20, fully 86 percent of people with eating disorders have already experienced symptoms, according to ANAD. These symptoms, which vary by disorder, can continue for years, or even decades. And it is important to remember that individuals with problems serious enough to be diagnosed as eating disorders represent only a fraction of those people who have fasted or binged or purged at some point in their lives. Serious problems may begin as diets that go out of control, or as an obsession with food that grows out of a seemingly healthy interest in good nutrition.

In the past two decades there has been a growing interest in eating disorders in the medical and psychiatric communities. Many programs now exist to treat them, and family physicians and other health professionals are becoming increasingly sophisticated in recognizing symptoms. Nutritional education at an early age, especially for young athletes and others who are considered high-risk, can sometimes prevent eating disorders from developing or from going out of control.

Anorexia, bulimia, and binge-eating have much in common. All are centered on food, and all involve extreme control or lack of control in eating behavior. They can overlap or alternate in the same person, with anorexics sometimes developing binge/purge behavior and bulimics going through periods of fasting. Despite these similarities each is a distinct disorder with its own symptoms, patterns, and treatment.

Anorexia Nervosa

Anorexics don't eat; but that doesn't mean they lack an appetite. Indeed, anorexics often display an obsessive interest in food. A typical anorexic will read about food, shop for, cook, and constantly think about food, in fact, will do everything with food except eat it.

According to the American Psychiatric Association, from one-half to one percent of women between ages 15 and 30 suffer from anorexia. The number of cases appears to have increased in recent decades, although it is not clear whether this is due to an actual increase or better reporting.

Anorexics have usually been described as high-achieving, perfectionist, and compliant white adolescents from comfortable or affluent families. The stereotype has its limits, however. Increasingly, cases are being reported among African Americans and Hispanics. Those studying the spread of anorexia and other eating disorders have found that while age and gender are closely related to development of eating disorders, ethnic background and economic status are not.

Hallmarks of Anorexia

According to current diagnostic guidelines, you are anorexic if you:

- Refuse to maintain a minimally normal body weight. This is estimated at 85 percent of what is considered normal weight for your height.
- Have an intense fear of gaining weight or getting fat.
- Have a distorted perception of what your body actually looks like. If you are an anorexic, you will look in the mirror at what may be an emaciated image and honestly believe that you are overweight and need to lose weight.
- Stop having your menstrual periods. Depriving the body of nutrition interferes with the hormonal cycles that regulate menstruation, bringing it to a halt. (If you are male, this obviously does not apply, although hormonal abnormalities are also seen in male anorexics.)

Anorexia typically begins to develop between ages 12 to 14, or later in adolescence, at about age 17. Some cases have appeared before puberty and some as late as the early 30s. The cause is unknown, although a variety of cultural and psychological factors are probably involved. Eating disorders seem to run in families, and a girl has a 10 to 20

WARNING SIGNS OF ANOREXIA

Anorexia nervosa does not develop overnight, and early treatment can head off severe illness and even save lives. Some warning signs are clear; others more subtle.

- Unnatural or obsessive preoccupation with food, dieting, and weight
- Distorted body image and intense fear of gaining weight
- Denial of hunger
- Avoidance of social situations with food
- Poor eating habits and decreasing daily intake of food
- Cessation of menstrual periods
- Lack of energy, weakness, fatigue, and depression
- Abdominal cramps and other aches and pains
- Excessive exercising
- Decreased coordination
- Inability to concentrate
- Indecisiveness

times greater risk of developing anorexia if she has a sibling with the disease.

Many anorexics come from close-knit families that allow their members little room for individuality. Rebellion against this restrictive environment often takes the form of refusing to eat.

There are two types of anorexia. With the restricting type, you lose weight primarily through dieting, fasting, and excessive exercise. The binge-eating/purging type is more complicated because it can be confused with

RAVAGES OF ANOREXIA

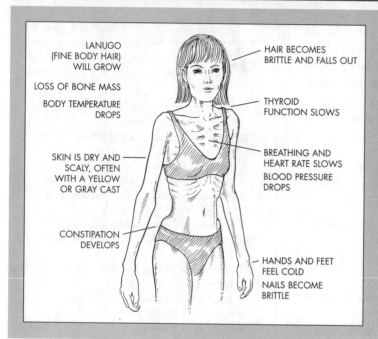

LANUGO
(FINE BODY HAIR)
WILL GROW

LOSS OF BONE MASS

BODY TEMPERATURE
DROPS

SKIN IS DRY AND
SCALY, OFTEN
WITH A YELLOW
OR GRAY CAST

CONSTIPATION
DEVELOPS

HAIR BECOMES
BRITTLE AND FALLS OUT

THYROID
FUNCTION SLOWS

BREATHING AND
HEART RATE SLOWS
BLOOD PRESSURE
DROPS

HANDS AND FEET
FEEL COLD

NAILS BECOME
BRITTLE

Fatal in up to 10 percent of cases, anorexia can cause irreversible damage in those who survive. The severe malnutrition that accompanies the disorder can bring on osteoporosis, the brittle-bone disease underlying many of the fractures suffered by the elderly. Dry, scaly, yellowish skin and noticeable hair loss are other unpleasant signs of this insidious disorder that, ironically, begins with the pursuit of perfection.

bulimia. This type of anorexic may binge-eat, then purge by vomiting and misusing laxatives, diuretics, or enemas, or even purge regularly after eating only small amounts of food.

What Happens To Your Mind and Body
Many anorexics describe the beginning of their disorder as a reaction to a comment such as "you really need to lose some weight." They begin to diet and enjoy the positive feedback that comes with weight loss and the sense of control that they feel over their bodies. But then they somehow lose perspective on what a healthy or attractive body image really is, and want only to

continue losing weight. While they feel they are controlling their diet, the diet ends up controlling them.

"I controlled everything through my food," said Tracy Gold, a young TV actress whose battle against anorexia was well-publicized in gossip columns and fan magazines. She described this control as turning into a tremendous fear of food that became nearly impossible for her to overcome. "To me it was like an evil force inside of me," she said. "You want to live; you want to get better; but you literally don't know how."

Christy Henrich, the 22-year-old gymnast who died in July 1994 weighing 43 pounds, used similar words to describe what her life had become. "My life is a horrifying nightmare," she said when she went public with her illness a year before her death. "It feels like there's a beast inside of me, like a monster. It feels evil."

Psychologically, in addition to these feelings of fear and evil, anorexics often suffer from other psychological problems, such as obsessive-compulsive behavior, social isolation, anxiety, a revulsion toward fat and self-indulgence, and compulsive and excessive exercising. Often, a hidden depression lies at the core. Like people suffering from involuntary malnutrition, anorexics may also exhibit any of the following additional symptoms:

- Insomnia
- Lack of concentration
- Indecisiveness
- Preoccupation with food
- Mood swings
- Irritability
- Fatigue and lethargy

In the most extreme cases, mental functioning becomes severely impaired.

A number of medical conditions characterize anorexia, some stemming from what are believed to be underlying psychological issues. For example, teen age anorexics are often described as fearful of growing up and attempting to thwart their emerging sexuality. By fasting these girls not only keep their breasts and hips from developing, but also block the process of menstruation.

Emaciation is a second, more obvious condition that develops, but more important is the body's protective response to the effects of starvation. Vital organ function begins to decline, as if shifting into a lower gear of operation. Breathing and heart rates decline. Blood pressure drops. Thyroid function slows. Body temperature goes down.

Most anorexics cannot tolerate cool temperatures and always feel cold, particularly in their hands and feet.

They may develop constipation due to water imbalance. Deprived of protein, their nails and hair may become brittle and their hair may fall out. Vitamin deficiencies will eventually cause their skin to become dry and scaly, often with a yellow or gray cast to it. As anorexia progresses, a type of fine body hair called lanugo will grow. This downy covering is probably an attempt by the body to compensate for the loss of muscle and fat tissue.

The breakdown that anorexia causes in hormone production also often results in osteoporosis, the loss of bone mass that leads to brittle bones. It is comparable to the condition that develops in postmenopausal women whose bodies have almost stopped producing estrogen. Some long-term studies have found that once osteoporosis develops in older women, it cannot be reversed.

The course and progression of anorexia varies considerably, depending on when the condition is detected, what supports are in place, and how it is treated. Up to ten percent of those with anorexia nervosa eventually die of the disease. Most others go on to lead healthy and productive lives.

Treatment for Anorexia: What to Expect

There are two important points about treating anorexia. First, denial is one of the most consistent features of the disorder, and most anorexics resist treatment. It is usually up to a family member or close friend to recognize the problem and get the patient into treatment.

Second, continued treatment and monitoring is crucial because anorexia can be a chronic and recurring condition. This means that one successful course of treatment does not necessarily cure the disease and that even "cured" patients may suffer setbacks. In fact, some studies have found that as many as half of anorexics who have been hospitalized for treatment will relapse after what has been considered a successful course of treatment. So, for most patients, treatment will be a long-term process.

Most patients undergo a combination of psychological and medical treatment. In many cases, this means hospitalization to begin dealing with the physical effects of starvation. Hospitalization is usually advised if you weigh less than 70 percent of your recommended body weight, have rapidly progressing weight loss, and have symptoms such as irregular heartbeat, dizziness or fainting, and low potassium levels. Anorexia is probably the only psychiatric illness for which the most effective initial treatment is often a long stay in the hospital.

The first step is called "refeeding," which can be done on an in- or outpatient basis, depending on the severity of your condition and whether or not you're ready to cooperate. Some patients have to be force-fed through nasogastric or intravenous tubes; there are even cases in which courts have ordered such treatment in order to keep the victim alive.

While refeeding goes on, you'll begin to receive behavioral therapy, psychotherapy, and nutritional counseling. You'll be encouraged to develop your eating plans, which will start with small amounts of food that you can feel safe with, gradually increasing the number of calories you consume and broadening your selection of foods. Your doctor will keep a close watch to avoid potential physical problems that can develop with refeeding such as abdominal bloating, consti-

pation, and swelling. If a slow and gradual approach is taken, these can usually be avoided or lessened.

Therapy is typically a lengthy process. A variety of different approaches are used, alone or in combination. These include cognitive behavioral therapy and individual or group psychotherapy. Recently, as doctors began to realize the role the family plays in development of the disorder, family therapy has become increasingly common. Self-help groups such as Overeaters Anonymous are also a major source of therapy. Nutritional counseling remains an absolutely crucial part of treatment.

A number of different medications have been used for anorexia. Some have helped, although no single medication stands out. Anti-anxiety drugs may work in some cases, while antidepressants are frequently prescribed if you have symptoms of depression.

The prognosis for anorexia varies, depending on the severity of the disease and your ability to cooperate with treatment. If you are able to acknowledge the severity of the problem, get help, and successfully re-build your self-esteem, you have every right to be confident of recovery.

Bulimia Nervosa

Though still uncommon, bulimia is not as rare as anorexia. Doctors estimate that it occurs in as many as five percent of adolescent and young adult women. Only 10 to 15 percent of bulimics are male. Of the three eating disorders, it is the one most easily kept hidden, since many bulimics maintain a normal body weight, even while they engage in the extreme and destructive binging and purging that characterizes the disease. As a result, the actual number of bulimics may be twice as high.

In the last decade, the secrecy cloaking bulimia has been brushed aside as celebrity confessions and widespread media reports about the disorder have multiplied. Many colleges now have programs through their student health centers to deal specifically with bulimia, since it is so widespread on campuses. Some studies claim that 10 to 20 percent of female college students have practiced bulimic behavior at some time in their lives. Like anorexia, bulimia is also associated with certain athletic and artistic pursuits, such as running, gymnastics, competitive swimming, and dancing.

Bulimics may consume astounding quantities of food in the binge phase of their cycle.

WARNING SIGNS OF BULIMIA

Although some of the warning signs bulimia are similar to those of anorexia, most are associated with purging. Bulimic behavior can accelerate quickly. To stave off potentially serious physical consequences, early recognition is a must.

- Avoidance of social eating situations
- Disappearance after meals; long visits to the bathroom after eating
- Secretive eating
- Denial of hunger
- Hidden stashes of food, particularly high calorie food such as candy, chips, etc.
- Intake of potassium pills
- Use of laxatives, diet pills diuretics, emetics
- Bloodshot eyes (from vomiting)
- Abrasions on the back of the hand (from inducing vomiting)
- Compulsive exercising
- Swollen salivary glands

A typical binge lasts about two hours. The following description from "My Name is Caroline" (Doubleday, 1988), a book by recovering bulimic Caroline Miller, vividly illustrates what was a characteristic binge for the author, and many other bulimics:

...I give my order for a double-thick vanilla frappe.... Colorful jimmies, peanuts, chocolate chips, coconut and other ice cream accouterments beckoned. I wanted to ask the woman to toss some jimmies and chocolate chips into my shake, but I knew that normal people didn't do that kind of thing....[At] my next destination, David's Cookies,...I quickly picked out two pounds of cookies. I crammed a few cookies in my mouth while I paid....Baskin Robbins was next....I ordered a mixture of pralines 'n cream and jamoca almond fudge....With the cookies in my pocket I was going to make a huge crunchy mess and finish it all myself.

Ms. Miller then describes her purge, a graphic, unpleasant, but accurate portrayal of what a bulimic goes through:

I jammed two fingers down my throat and felt the familiar bile rising. Harder and harder I thrust, gouging the back of my throat in the process....All of a sudden the food came up in gushes, splattering all over the toilet seat, the floor and my clothes. Disgusted yet elated at my success, I kept probing, trying to make sure I was getting everything up....

THE HIGH COST OF BULIMIA

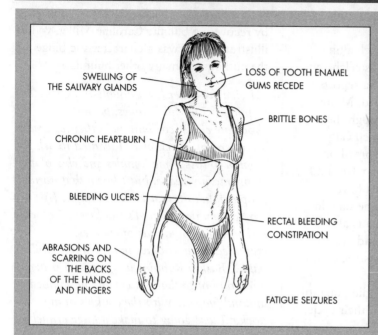

SWELLING OF THE SALIVARY GLANDS

LOSS OF TOOTH ENAMEL GUMS RECEDE

BRITTLE BONES

CHRONIC HEART-BURN

BLEEDING ULCERS

RECTAL BLEEDING CONSTIPATION

ABRASIONS AND SCARRING ON THE BACKS OF THE HANDS AND FINGERS

FATIGUE SEIZURES

Although it's not as lethal as anorexia, bulimia can cause severe and permanent disfigurement. As stomach acids erode the gums and etch the teeth, a bulimic's smile may become ragged. In the end, all teeth may need extraction. Constant trauma to the digestive system can lead to ulcers, hemorrhage, and rectal bleeding. As in anorexia, irreversible osteoporosis may result.

What Qualifies as a True Bulimia

To be diagnosed as a bulimic, you must meet the following diagnostic criteria:

- You engage in recurrent episodes of binge-eating. This is defined as consuming larger than normal amounts of food within a two-hour period, and feeling a lack of control over eating during the episode.
- You repeatedly compensate for the binge-eating with purging behavior to prevent weight gain. Purging behavior can include self-induced vomiting; misuse of laxatives, diuretics, enemas, over-the-counter diet pills, or other medications; fasting; or excessive exercise.
- You binge and purge at least twice a week for three months.
- Your self-evaluation is unreasonably influenced by body shape and weight.

It is important to remember that while these precise standards must be met for a medical diagnosis, you may be one of many people who does not meet the strict criteria but is still moderately to severely impaired by bulimic behavior.

What Happens to Your Mind and Body

Bulimia, too, has its psychological and physical components, including its own set of personality characteristics. Researchers have suggested that many bulimics suffer low self-esteem, intolerance of frustration, and an inability to appropriately recognize and express their feelings. Some have even theorized that childhood sexual abuse may be a factor in later development of bulimia, but this link has never been proved, and is certainly not the case for all bulimics.

Like anorexics, bulimics are likely to be preoccupied with food, at the expense of other, healthier pursuits. Their obsessiveness and secretiveness is comparable to the behavior of many substance abusers. In fact, bulimia has been linked to substance abuse, and other impulsive actions such as overspending, shoplifting, and promiscuity. The hidden nature of a bulimic's bingeing and purging activities can lead to social isolation, although many bulimics manage to function appropriately and keep their behavior secret.

Depression has also been associated with bulimia, and some studies have found that more than half of all bulimics have experienced clinical depression. However, it is unclear whether depression causes the eating disorder, or vice versa.

Some research has also found irregularities in the brain chemistry of bulimics, particularly in the release and processing of the chemicals that regulate the feeling of being full. While most people eat only when hungry, bulimics respond to the mere presence of food.

Bulimia can remain hidden for years, while the bulimic persists in her unhealthy eating habits. Eventually, however, physical signs of the disease are likely to become difficult to conceal. Extreme purging can cause dehydration and imbalances in the body's level of potassium, sodium, and other chemicals, which in turn can lead to fatigue, seizures, irregular heartbeat, and brittle bones.

Vomiting, the most commonly used method of purging, can also lead to tell-tale signs—and even serious injury:

- It can damage the stomach and the esophagus, sometimes resulting in bleeding, ulcers, loss of the gag reflex, and chronic heartburn.
- Stomach acids can have very damaging effects on the mouth. They cause gums to recede and tooth enamel to erode, leading to ragged teeth. Tooth enamel is not replaceable, and some bulimics finally need to have all their teeth extracted.
- Repeated vomiting also causes salivary glands to swell, resulting in a chipmunk-like appearance.
- Many bulimics have abrasions and scarring on the back of the hands, caused when they stick their fingers down their throats to induce vomiting.

Overusing laxatives results in a different set of problems. Constipation and bloating are common, and laxative abuse may also lead to bowel abnormalities and rectal bleeding.

Getting Treatment for Bulimia

Bulimics are usually more willing than anorexics to admit their problem and accept help. The disorder is generally considered less complicated to treat than anorexia, and bulimics rarely need hospitalization. Exceptions are cases of extreme chemical imbalances, serious gastro-intestinal complications, or severe depression.

Cognitive behavioral therapy that helps you re-evaluate unrealistic expectations and demands on yourself is usually regarded as most effective in treating bulimia. One technique is to keep a diary of food consumption and eating behavior. For example, your therapist may have you write down everything you eat over a certain time period—a chore that can very effectively interrupt a pattern of binging.

Cognitive therapy also helps you recognize what triggers your binge/purge behavior and helps you come up with other ways to deal with those triggers. It also helps you deal with the unrealistic messages about body image that permeate our culture. Therapy should be combined with nutritional counseling, to help you learn how to plan regular, balanced meals.

Group therapy can also work well, particularly for those in college. Family therapy is often helpful if you live at home.

Antidepressant medication can be very beneficial if you are one of the many bulimics who suffer from a depressive disorder. A variety of these drugs have been used with bulimics and doctors are currently excited about fluoxetine (Prozac), which acts on the system that regulates serotonin, the brain chemical that controls feelings of being full.

Regular dental care is also an important part of treatment for bulimics.

Like anorexics, bulimics are prone to relapse. The episodes can be caused by stressful life events, anything from final exams to career change to divorce. Some kind of continuing therapy or access to a support or self-help group can often prevent relapse, or make it easier to quickly move through the relapse back to healthy eating patterns.

Binge-Eating Disorder

Now regarded as a psychiatric problem unto itself, binge-eating disorder is, essentially, bulimia without the purging. Binge-eaters do not force themselves to vomit, take laxatives, or otherwise rid themselves of their food, and hence, are almost always extremely overweight. They are also referred to as compulsive overeaters.

Some degree of binge-eating takes place in a substantial percentage of people in weight-control programs—anywhere from 15 to 50 percent, according to various studies. General surveys have found that as many as four percent of Americans may engage in binge-eating, often after completing a weight-control program or attaining weight goals.

When Does Binge-Eating Become a Disorder?

Because binge-eating disorder has only recently been recognized as a true illness, it has not been studied to the same extent as anorexia and bulimia. The official diagnostic criteria are still viewed as general guidelines, and shouldn't be considered definitive.

Binge-eaters eat large amounts of food, sometimes when they are not even hungry. They usually eat alone, feeling embarrassed about the amount they consume. After a binge, they often have feelings of self-disgust, guilt, or depression.

For those with a true disorder, the episodes occur, on average, at least twice a week for six months. Like bulimics, people with binge-eating disorder are likely to eat very quickly, continuing even after they feel uncomfortably full. While binging, compulsive overeaters feel they are unable to stop.

What Happens to Your Mind and Body

Studies have found that people with binge-eating disorder are more prone to major depression, anxiety disorder, and other psychiatric conditions. They are also more likely to have a family history of substance abuse. However, doctors are not sure whether binge-eating causes the psychiatric problems or vice versa—or even if there is any relation at all.

Binge eaters often suffer from frustration and low self-esteem, and may connect other difficulties, for example, problems with relationships or employment, to their eating habits. The secretive nature of their disorder may cause social isolation, as it does for bulimics.

The most common physical consequence of binge eating is weight gain, and often obesity. Along with this comes increased risk of a number of diseases associated with being overweight: high blood pressure, clogged blood vessels, heart attack, stroke, diabetes, and sometimes bone and joint problems.

Treating Binge Eating

For a binge eater, food is an addiction—in some ways harder to treat than an addiction to drugs or alcohol. If you have a substance abuse problem you can learn to completely avoid drugs or alcohol. But it's impossible to totally give up food. Moreover, certain foods that are likely to cause eating problems— such as sweets or high-fat foods like potato chips—are often part of everyday social activities. If you are a binge-eater, it can be very difficult indeed to successfully negotiate these potential pitfalls. Learning what triggers a binge and substituting a healthier reaction when you encounter a trigger can be a major help.

Like other eating disorders, binge-eating can be treated with behavioral therapy and psychotherapy. However, support and self-help groups are especially important. Overeaters Anonymous, for instance, is a 12-step program that is often helpful for those with binge-eating disorder. Remember, though, that the habits that mark this disor-der have often developed over a long period of time, making them difficult to fix. Therapy is often a long-term process, punctuated with relapses. Still, just as with alcohol or drugs, it *is* possible to control this most insidious of all addictions. □

Section Three

Food and Your Heart

CHAPTER 10

What to Do About Fat

It's the buzzword of the Nineties. Today, just about everyone has heard that fat and cholesterol are bad for you. Fat, we're told, makes you overweight, and may be linked to some types of cancer. Too much cholesterol can lead to a heart attack.

Yet we all know very old folks who have cholesterol-laden eggs for breakfast each day. And now we hear reports about "good" cholesterol and "better" kinds of fat. Things are not as simple as they seemed.

There's good and bad news in this. On one hand, we now have to worry about the *kind* of fat we eat. On the other, we don't have to eliminate every scrap of it from our diets.

How Fat Fits In

First of all, it's important to differentiate between the fat we wear and the fat we eat. In addition to the muscles, bones, and other organs that make up *lean* body mass, humans have body fat distributed throughout the tissues, beneath the skin, and floating free within the bloodstream. Fat accounts for about 15 to 18 percent of the total weight of a healthy, physically fit man.

For a woman, the proportion is slightly higher: about 20 to 25 percent.

Everyone needs a reasonable amount of body fat. It provides you with the essential fatty acids (linoleic and linolenic acids) needed for normal reproduction and growth. It is also essential in the production of several hormone-like compounds, such as prostaglandins, that help regulate blood pressure and other vital bodily functions. Fat maintains healthy skin and hair, cushions the bones and vital organs, protects the body from extremes of temperature, and carries essential nutrients (notably vitamins A, D, E, and K) throughout your system. Its main function, however, is to serve as fuel for the muscles. Fat alone provides about 65 percent of the energy your muscles require.

Our bodies manufacture this fat from a wide variety of substances, including protein, carbohydrates... and other fats. Any

FAT FORMULA #1:
YOUR FAT ALLOWANCE

You should get no more than 30 percent of your calories from fat. But what exactly does that mean in terms of your own daily diet? Here's a simple way to tell.

Multiply your daily calorie intake by .30 (the percentage of your calories that should come from fat) and then divide the resulting total by 9 (because there are 9 calories in every gram of fat).

$$\left(\frac{\text{daily calorie allowance x .30}}{9}\right) = \begin{array}{l}\text{total fat}\\\text{allowance}\\\text{in grams}\end{array}$$

If you eat 1,800 calories a day, you would multiply 1,800 by .30 for a total of 540, then divide 540 by 9. The new total is 60, so your total daily fat allowance is 60 grams.

If you don't want to be bothered with an exact calculation, the table below will give you a fair approximation of your allowance. But remember: however you get the figure, it's still a *ceiling*. Just because you have a budget of a certain number of fat grams per day, doesn't mean you have to spend it. The less fat you eat, the better off you are.

Total Daily Calories	Fat Allowance (in Grams)
1500	50
1600	53
1700	57
1800	60
1900	63
2000	67
2100	70
2200	73
2300	77
2400	80
2500	83
2600	87

portion of our diet not immediately needed as fuel gets converted into body fat. Since the fat in our food is the easiest part to convert, a high-fat diet is more likely to leave us with the excess pounds that we dread. That, however, is only one of the problems with too much fat.

How Much Fat Can We Handle?

All fat is a treasure trove of calories. At 9 calories, one gram of fat has more than twice the calories of a gram of protein or carbohydrate. What does this mean in terms of your daily diet? A cheeseburger contains about 30 grams of fat. For that same 30 grams, you could eat 80 cups of broccoli, or 30 cups of pasta, or 45 pears, or 30 cups of kidney beans.

Many experts feel that we should get no more than 30 percent of our daily calories from fat. This works out to 73 grams of fat in a 2,200-calorie diet. Nevertheless, the average American diet is still over 35 percent calories from fat. Just eating the recommended number of servings from each of the major food groups (milk, vegetable, meat, fruit, and bread) automatically gives you up to half your daily allowance of fat—even if you pick low-fat foods and add no fat or oil during preparation. Indeed, a single tablespoon of corn oil is enough to meet your entire daily physiological requirement for fat. In contrast, the average American actually consumes eight times that amount—the equivalent of a full stick of butter every day.

Total intake is only part of the story, however. There are many *types* of fat; and not all fats are created equal.

Saturated Versus Unsaturated

Most of the fats we eat are triglycerides—three fatty acids attached to a glycerol molecule. These fatty acids vary in the extent to which they are saturated with hydrogen atoms. Fats containing mostly saturated fatty acids are called "saturated;" those with fatty acids that are mostly polyunsaturated or monounsaturated are labeled "unsaturated." In general, the more saturated the fat, the more likely it is to be solid at room temperature—and the more dangerous it is for your health.

Saturated Fats

Because these fats tend to raise your cholesterol level, they represent the biggest threat to your heart. Often solid at room temperature, they congregate in well-marbled meats and whole-milk dairy products. Some veg-

VEGETABLE OILS: THE BEST AND THE WORST

The lower the level of saturated fat and the higher the level of unsaturated fat (including both mono- and polyunsaturates), the better the oil. It is important to note that coconut and palm kernel oils—two of the so-called "tropical oils"—are even higher in saturated fat than butter (included here for purposes of comparison only). Canola, almond, safflower, and sunflower are among the oils lowest in saturated fats (and, therefore, highest in unsaturated fats). Olive, almond, and canola oils are the highest in monounsaturated fats, believed by experts to lower the level of cholesterol in the blood without producing a reduction in levels of HDL, the "good" cholesterol.

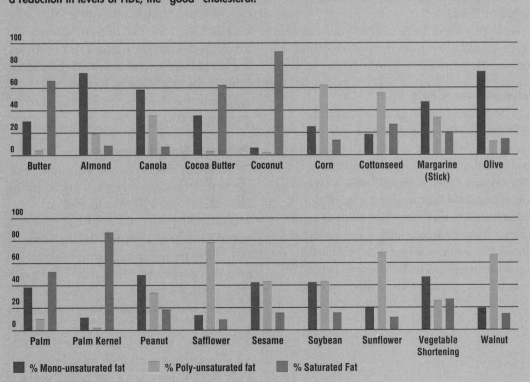

etable fats—including palm, palm kernel, and coconut oils—are also saturated.

Butter, whole milk, cheese, ice cream, egg yolks, and fatty cuts of beef, pork, and lamb are all particularly high in these potentially dangerous fats. Because these are among most Americans' favorite foods, we tend to consume two to three times as much saturated fat as we should (a recommended 7 to 10 percent of total calories).

Monounsaturated Fats

Many experts believe that if you substitute monounsaturated fat (olive, peanut, canola, avocado, and certain fish oils) for the saturated fat in your diet, you can lower your blood cholesterol levels and thereby reduce your risk of heart disease. In Mediterranean countries, where olive oil is a major part of the diet, people do in fact have fewer heart problems.

Between 10 and 13 percent of your caloric intake should come from monounsaturated fats.

Polyunsaturated Fats

Fats from such sources as corn, soybean, safflower, sunflower, and sesame seed oils— and certain fish—help to lower blood cholesterol and should make up 10 percent of your calories. The "omega-3" oils, a type of polyunsaturated fat found in tuna, salmon, mackerel, and other fatty fish, seem to act as a blood thinner, decreasing the risk of lethal blood clots and possibly staving off hardening of the arteries. The best way to get omega-3 oils is to eat two to three servings of fish per week. Fish oil capsules should be taken only with your doctor's approval.

Even though polyunsaturated oils appear to be better for you, don't make the mistake of *adding* fat to your diet. In general, the less fat you eat, the better off you are. Instead, switch from the more harmful saturated fats to the more benign unsaturated varieties.

Hydrogenated Fats

Many food manufacturers solidify unsaturated liquid fats through a process called hydrogenation. This technique is used to create margarine or shortening for use in deep-fat frying or as an ingredient in baked goods and candy. However, hydrogenation turns an unsaturated fat into a polyunsaturated fat containing trans-fatty acids. Some studies indicate that because they increase blood levels of the "bad," artery-clogging type of cholesterol, trans-fatty acids may increase your risk of heart disease. The extent of this danger remains to be proven, but if you want to cut down on trans-fatty acids in the meantime, substitute oils and tub margarine for the stick variety and cut back on fried foods.

Fat and Heart Disease

Heart disease is, unfortunately, as American as baseball and apple pie. It is the nation's chief killer, accounting for 940,000 deaths a year—one out of every two. Five million people in the U.S. suffer from angina pectoris—severe, recurring pain caused by partial blockage of the coronary arteries. And the economic costs of heart disease are staggering: more than $108 billion in 1991 alone.

Over their lifetime, men in the U.S. face a 42 percent chance of developing heart disease. But it's not just a male health problem.

THE CORONARY ARTERIES: WHERE THE WORST PROBLEMS ARISE

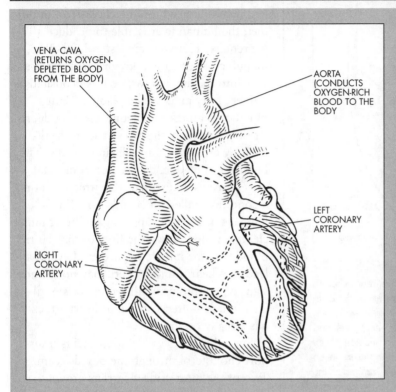

VENA CAVA
(RETURNS OXYGEN-
DEPLETED BLOOD
FROM THE BODY)

AORTA
(CONDUCTS
OXYGEN-RICH
BLOOD TO THE
BODY

LEFT
CORONARY
ARTERY

RIGHT
CORONARY
ARTERY

All arteries are essential; they supply the body's organs with the oxygen-rich blood they need to survive. But the coronary arteries are especially crucial, for they feed the heart muscle itself. Without a constant flow of blood from the coronary arteries, this muscle will weaken and die.

When fatty build-up inside a coronary artery restricts the flow of blood, the heart warns of diminished supply with the severe chest pains known as angina. If a blood clot completely blocks the already constricted artery, the result is a heart attack— a "myocardial infarction" in which the patch of heart muscle served by the artery dies from lack of blood.

In fact, the risk of cardiovascular disease among postmenopausal women exceeds that of men. A quarter of a million women over the age of 60 die of heart attacks every year—six times the toll from breast cancer.

Many factors contribute to the risk of developing heart disease. High blood pressure, diabetes, and too much cholesterol in the blood all can play a role. Lifestyle factors such as cigarette smoking, obesity, and physical inactivity can add to the danger. Indeed, the majority of heart attacks occur in people whose total blood cholesterol levels are between 180 and 240 and who have other risk factors—for example, smoking, a sedentary lifestyle, or a family history of heart disease.

None of these risk factors—or even a combination of them—*guarantee* that you'll develop a heart problem. A majority of people with high cholesterol, for instance, never die of heart disease. However, since the experts have no way of predicting whether or not you'll be among the lucky ones, the only wise course is to keep the odds in your favor. This means attacking all the risk factors you can, and, on the dietary front, working to reduce your cholesterol levels.

DANGEROUS PLAQUE

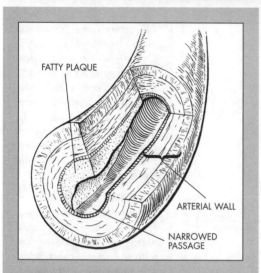

FATTY PLAQUE

ARTERIAL WALL

NARROWED PASSAGE

Excess cholesterol becomes a threat when it begins forming deposits at points inside the arterial walls. Mixed with debris from the wall itself, the resulting build-up narrows the vessel and stiffens the wall, leading to the condition called atherosclerosis. If the constriction occurs in an artery serving the brain, there's danger of the total blockage called a stroke. If a coronary artery becomes clogged, the result is a heart attack.

For every one percent decrease in cholesterol, according to many experts, your chance of having a heart attack declines by *two percent.*

The Truth About Cholesterol

Cholesterol is not intrinsically bad. This waxy, fat-like substance is, in fact, a necessary part of your body chemistry. It is found in all animals and in all animal products (such as meats, eggs, milk, and cheese). There is no cholesterol in any plant product—fruits, grains, legumes (dried peas and beans), vegetables—or the oils made from them.

There's no need for any cholesterol in our diet; the human liver is able to produce all we require. Excessive cholesterol, whether manufactured by the body or eaten, finds its way into the arteries, where it is deposited as a thick, fatty gunk called plaque. White blood cells attack the plaque, creating debris. At the same time, the artery tries to heal itself by growing more cells in its walls. The build-up of plaque, debris, and additional cells narrows and stiffens the artery, creating a condition called *atherosclerosis.* If this happens in a vessel supplying the heart muscle, it can slow down the flow of oxygen-rich blood that the muscle requires and eventually lead to a heart attack. There may not be any signs or symptoms of atherosclerosis until it's too late—after a stroke or heart attack has already occurred.

Special carriers called lipoproteins transport cholesterol through the bloodstream. Two of the most critical carriers are *low-density lipoproteins* (LDL) and *high-density lipoproteins* (HDL). The more abundant form is LDL, commonly referred to as "bad cholesterol." High levels of LDL are associated with an increased risk of heart disease. High levels of HDL—the "good cholesterol"—seem to prevent the disease (while low levels seem to encourage it). So the lower your total and LDL cholesterol levels and the higher your HDL level, the better off you are.

According to the National Cholesterol Education Program you should aim for:

- a total blood cholesterol level less than 200 milligrams per deciliter (one tenth of a liter) of blood;
- an LDL level less than 130 milligrams per deciliter; and
- an HDL level greater than 35 milligrams per deciliter.

A man with a total blood cholesterol level of 240 is twice as likely to have a heart attack as one with a level of 200, all other factors being equal. A level of 300 carries five times the risk of a level of 200. Conversely, a 25 percent drop in blood cholesterol levels can cut the risk of a heart attack in half.

Total blood cholesterol tells only part of the story, however. The *type* of cholesterol makes a big difference, too. While LDLs contribute to artery-blocking deposits of plaque, the HDLs seem to vacuum excess cholesterol from the bloodstream. So a high level of LDLs—more than 130 milligrams per deciliter—is not good. Neither is a low level of HDLs—below 35 milligrams per deciliter. A good measure of risk, therefore, is the ratio of total cholesterol to HDLs. You can figure your ratio by dividing your total cholesterol level by your HDL level. A ratio of 2.5 or lower is good; a ratio of 4 warrants further discussion with your doctor.

UNDERSTANDING BLOOD CHOLESTEROL READINGS

Doctors now recommend that you should have your blood cholesterol levels checked regularly, beginning at age 20. Since heredity and lifestyle factors are critical variables, your doctor is in the best position to interpret the results and suggest a course of action. (The most common therapy for high cholesterol includes a low-fat diet, regular exercise, losing weight, giving up smoking, and—for some people—medication.) The classifications shown here will be part of the physician's evaluation. Remember that LDL cholesterol is "bad" and should be low, while HDL cholesterol is "good" and should be high. If your LDL level is too high, chances are that your triglycerides will be high as well.

Total Blood Cholesterol	Classification
Less than 200 milligrams/deciliter	Desirable
200-239 milligrams/deciliter	Borderline High
240 milligrams/deciliter and over	High

LDL Cholesterol	Classification
Less than 130 milligrams/deciliter	Desirable
130-159 milligrams/deciliter	Borderline high
160 milligrams/deciliter or higher	High

HDL Cholesterol	Classification
40-50 milligrams/deciliter (for men)	Desirable
50-60 milligrams/deciliter (for women)	Desirable
Less than 35 milligrams/deciliter	Low

Triglyceride Levels	Classification
Less than 200 milligrams/deciliter	Normal
200-400 milligrams/deciliter	Borderline high
400-1,000 milligrams/deciliter	High
More than 1,000 milligrams/deciliter	Very high

A low triglyceride (blood fat) level may also be important to the health of your heart. While there is no direct link between high triglyceride levels and atherosclerosis, excessive triglycerides often accompany higher total cholesterol and LDL levels and lower HDL levels. Ideally, your triglyceride levels should be less than 200 milligrams per deciliter. The same dietary and lifestyle changes that reduce total cholesterol and LDL levels should have a positive impact on triglycerides as well.

Lowering Your Cholesterol

When you attack your cholesterol, cutting it out of your diet is only part of the answer. Don't forget that saturated fat can also raise blood cholesterol, and in fact is by far the worst offender. Keeping it under 10 percent of your total calories is a crucial first step.

Nevertheless, with dietary cholesterol too, a good rule of thumb is "less is best." Try to limit your cholesterol intake to no more than 300 milligrams per day. A three-ounce serving of broiled liver, for example, contains 331 milligrams of cholesterol; an equivalent portion of beef has 76. The cholesterol count for packaged foods appears on the label under **Nutrition Facts.**

For most people, relatively minor changes in the diet, (eliminating butter and rich desserts, for example) can lower cholesterol by 10 to 15 percent. Keeping your quota of meat to about 6 ounces per day can also work wonders, since it cuts down your intake of both cholesterol and saturated fat. And regular exercise—the only proven way of raising your "good" HDL levels—is yet another essential weapon in the war against high cholesterol. The results can be rewarding. An 8 to 20 percent reduction in blood

DIETARY CHOLESTEROL COUNTS

Too much cholesterol in your food can leave you with too much in your blood; and for many people, that can mean an increased risk of heart disease. According to the American Heart Association, the average American woman consumes about 320 milligrams of cholesterol a day; the average man, 450 milligrams. People's tolerance of cholesterol varies, but as a general rule of thumb, your dietary intake should be no more than 300 milligrams daily. How much is that? The chart below will give you an idea. (For additional counts, see the table at the end of the book.)

Food	Milligrams of Cholesterol
American cheese (1 ounce)	27
Avocado (8 ounces)	0
Bacon (3 slices)	15
Beef liver, pan-fried (3 ounces)	551
Beef sirloin (4 oz.)	101
Bologna (1 ounce)	15
Brazil nuts (6)	0
Butter (1 tablespoon)	31
Chicken, breast meat (4 ounces)	79
Chicken, thigh meat (4 ounces)	108
Chocolate cake, frosted (2 ounces)	20
Danish (1)	56
Duck (4 ounces, no skin)	101
Egg yolk (1)	213
Egg white (1)	0
Halibut (3 1/2 ounces)	30
Ice cream, premium (1/2 cup)	44
Lobster (4 ounces)	82
Milk, skim (8 ounces)	4
Milk, whole (8 ounces)	35
Pumpkin pie (2 ounces)	39

cholesterol levels means a 20 to 40 percent reduction in heart attacks.

When cholesterol levels do not respond to diet and exercise, your doctor may prescribe a medication. Most cholesterol-reducing drugs act by preventing the body from manufacturing cholesterol, reducing absorption of dietary cholesterol, or combining with cholesterol and removing it from the body. The most common cholesterol-lowering drugs are niacin, lovastatin (Mevacor), cholestryamine (Questran), gemfibrozil (Lopid), probulcol (Lorelco), colestipol (Cholestid), and fluvastatin (Lescol), the newest member of the "statin" family. For people with heart disease, these drugs are proven life savers. However, they can be expensive and may occasionally cause side effects, so your doctor is likely to prescribe one for you only if you already have heart disease or are threatened by some of the other risk factors that can lead to it.

Kids and Cholesterol

According to the American Health Foundation, one in four children in the U.S. has a high cholesterol level—not surprising given American eating habits. Depending on age, a child in the U.S. gets between 10 and 15 percent of his or her daily calories from snacks and fast foods, traditionally high in fats and cholesterol. While you don't have to eliminate all these treats from your child's diet, most cardiologists agree that limiting fat intake—*from age two on*—will help reduce the risk of heart disease later in life. All high-risk children, such as those with a parent or grandparent who develops any cardiovascu-

HEALTH BOOSTERS

The following foods are richest sources of the omega-3 fatty acids that help to reduce the risk of heart disease by lowering blood pressure and reducing the likelihood of blood clots. Experts recommend two to three servings of omega-3 fish every week.

Bluefish	Sable
Herring	Salmon
Mackerel	Sardines
Pompano	Tuna
Rainbow trout	Whitefish

lar disease (including high cholesterol) before the age of 55, should have a cholesterol test—if only to establish a basis for later comparison.

Limit fat to 30 percent of your child's total daily allotment of calories, with less than 10 percent of those calories coming from saturated fat. Keep cholesterol consumption to no more than 100 milligrams for every 1,000 calories consumed.

Beware of starting the program too early, however. Dietary fat and cholesterol are critical for normal brain development in infants and toddlers, so wait till the child is two to start him or her on the path to a lifetime of healthy, low-fat eating. (For more on the healthiest way to feed very young children, see Chapter 17, "Giving Your Baby an Ideal Diet.")

Fat, Cancer, and More

The link between fat intake and certain types of cancer is controversial. Nevertheless, there's no denying that breast cancer occurs more frequently in countries where women have high average intakes of both total fat and saturated fat.

(American women, for instance, are six times more likely to develop breast cancer than Japanese women, whose eat far less fat.) Some studies indicate that a high-fat diet also increases the risk of cancer of the colon and possibly even of the ovary, uterus, endometrium, and prostate. One theory suggests that

FAT FORMULA #2: THE FOOD FAT PERCENTAGE

Supermarket shelves, and freezer cases overflow with "lite" and "low-fat" goods. Many manufacturers tout the fat content of their products (for example, "only 5 grams of fat per serving"). But calorie for calorie, some foods will use up your daily allowance of fat much faster than others. To find out whether a product is out of balance, you need to check the share of its calories delivered by fat. Look on the food label for **Nutrition Facts**, and find the amount of calories from fat. Divide that number by the number of total calories, then multiply by 100 to get the fat percentage.

$$\left(\frac{\text{calories from fat}}{\text{total calories}}\right) \times 100 = \frac{\text{percent of calories}}{\text{from fat}}$$

For example, one serving of ready-to-eat roasted chicken thigh, without skin, totals 160 calories, 90 of which come from fat. Ninety fat calories divided by 160 total calories equals .5625, which, when multiplied by 100, equals 56.25 percent. In other words, more than half of the calories from that single serving of chicken are coming from fat calories.

Since the American Heart Association recommends that only 30 percent of your daily caloric intake come from fat, the rest of your meal will have to be very shy of fat calories if you hope to keep them within recommended bounds. Remember, it's perfectly acceptable to eat foods that are over 30 percent fat—as long as you're willing to counterbalance them with items below the 30 percent target.

as dietary fat intake increases, so do sex hormone levels, which may cause cancer in the reproductive organs. We do know that diets high in fat increase the amount of cholesterol and bile acids in the colon. The bacteria that live in the lower digestive tract may then convert these substances into cancer-causing by-products. (For more about foods that may cause cancer, see Chapter 13.)

Other serious health problems associated with a high intake of fat include diabetes and high blood pressure.

Fat is not only a high-calorie food that threatens your waistline, it's also a demonstrated health risk. Remember the number 30: no more than 30 percent of your daily caloric intake should come from fat.

Keeping Your Fat Intake at Safe Levels

Cutting the amount of fat in your diet not only improves your odds of continued good health, it also makes it easier to lose weight. Remember that while the body readily burns carbohydrate and protein calories, it stores fat calories as body fat. Moreover, the body uses more energy burning carbohydrate and protein calories than fat calories.

Whether you are interested in reducing your fat intake to look and feel better— or because it could be a matter of life and death—the following tips may make the process a little easier.

■ Read labels carefully to determine both the type and amount of fat in processed foods, and check the calorie figures, too. The Food Fat Percentage Formula (see box near-

HEART-FRIENDLY CHOICES

Reducing your fat intake is not as hard as it seems. It's really just a matter of making a series of relatively easy substitutions. None is any real hardship, yet together they will have a major impact on your diet. Following is a list of commonly available lower-fat substitutes you and your family can learn to love. Fat content is based on average single-portion servings. Fat counts of these and many other foods can be found in the tables at the end of the book.

Eat	Instead of	For a fat saving of...
bagel	apple muffin	8 grams
slice of angelfood cake	glazed doughnut	14 grams
hot-air popped popcorn	microwave butter popcorn	8 grams
pretzels	potato chips	9 grams
water-packed tuna	oil-packed tuna	6 grams
cocoa powder	baking chocolate	13 grams
roasted chestnuts	dry-roasted peanuts	13 grams
sorbet	premium ice cream	25 grams
lean roasted ham	salami	8 grams
Manhattan clam chowder	New England clam chowder	13 grams
baked potato	fast-food french fries	11 grams
salmon	T-bone steak	22 grams
spaghetti marinara	fettuccini alfredo	90 grams
baked taco chips	fried taco chips	5 grams
a shredded wheat cereal	granola	5 grams
two slices raisin bread	one croissant	10 grams
chicken (white, no skin)	chicken (dark, with skin)	20 grams
trimmed pork loin	pork spareribs	18 grams
jam	butter	11 grams
skim milk	whole milk	8 grams
peach	peach pie	16 grams

by) can be especially helpful here. For example, if you think that 2 percent milk is low in fat, you're wrong. That "2 percent" refers to fat content by weight. In terms of *calories* from fat, it registers a hearty 33 percent— a bit *more* than the 30 percent balance you should strike in your diet as a whole.

■ **Eat less saturated fat.** In practical terms, that means eating less meat, cheese, eggs, and whole dairy products. Replace fat-laced meat with leaner cuts, or with skinless chicken, turkey, and fish. Instead of whole eggs, use egg whites. And dip your bread in olive oil instead of slathering it with butter or margarine.

■ **Go meatless occasionally.** Prepare legumes (dried peas and beans), pasta, and rice dishes for your main course, using low-fat or non-fat dairy products. Don't think automatically of cheese or nuts as a healthy meat-substitute. Like ice cream, many cheeses have a fat calorie ratio of 60 to 70 percent, while nuts may derive as much as 85 percent of their calories from fat.

■ **When you do eat meat, eat less and eat leaner.** The American Heart Association recommends eating no more than 6 ounces of cooked lean meat, poultry, fish, or seafood per day. (A 4-ounce portion is the size of a deck of cards.) Choose cuts with a minimum of visible fat. "Select" grade meats tend to be lower in fat than "Choice" or "Prime." Wild meats such as venison, buffalo, and rabbit tend to have even less fat. Avoid domestic duck and goose, which are very high in fat, in favor of turkey and chicken. And choose white meat over dark, which can be as much as six times higher in fat. Be sure to trim all visible fat from meat and remove the skin from poultry before eating.

■ **Eat more unprocessed whole grains, fruits, vegetables, and beans.** These filling foods not only serve as stand-ins for richer meat and dairy products, but also deliver powerful arterial plaque fighters: carotene, vitamins C and E, selenium, and soluble fiber. The exceptions to the rule are coconut, olives,

KEY FACTS

- There are 9 calories in a gram of fat.
- The ceiling for fat in an average 2,200-calorie diet is 73 grams a day.
- Saturated fat (mainly from animals) is worse that unsaturated fat (mainly from plants)
- The ceiling for cholesterol is 300 milligrams a day.
- High blood levels of LDL cholesterol can be dangerous.
- High levels of HDL cholesterol are desirable. Exercise can raise your HDL levels.

and avocado, which are high in fat. If you want to indulge occasionally, eat small portions of avocado and olives—they are high in monounsaturates—but try to avoid coconut, which is high in saturated fats.

■ **Beware of "hidden" fat.** A handful of peanuts, granola cereal, egg-laden breads and pastas, nondairy creamers, even some fast food "diet" meals can be astonishingly high in fat. A fish filet sandwich at McDonald's, for example, has almost 26 grams of fat and 45 milligrams of cholesterol, more than the same restaurant's cheeseburger. A large bucket of unbuttered movie theater popcorn that has been popped in coconut oil has the equivalent of three days' allotment of heart-clogging saturated fat.

■ **Watch the portions.** A 3-and-a-half-ounce helping of meat or fish is sufficient for one serving. In general take a serving that is about the size of the palm of your hand or a deck of cards.

■ **Try to steam, bake, or broil foods instead of sautéing them.** If you do want to sauté, use a nonstick skillet and substitute broth for fat. Don't even think about deep-fat frying.

■ **Avoid undermining healthy foods by dressing them in butter, margarine, mayonnaise, or other high-fat sauces.** One tablespoon of Caesar salad dressing, with 8 grams of fat, can raise the fat ratio of half a cup of Romaine lettuce to 88 percent. Experiment with spices to add palate-pleasing flavor. Reduced broth or puréed vegetables make a healthful low-fat alternative to conventional—and risky—cream- or butter-based sauces.

■ **Use skim or low-fat products instead of the full-fat varieties.** Choose skim or 1 percent milk instead of whole milk, a frozen fruit juice bar or low-fat frozen yogurt over ice cream, a slice of angelfood cake over a brownie. Don't, however, assume that "low-fat" is the same as "low-calorie." Because fat is what helps you feel full, it's easy to overindulge in lower-fat foods. If you are taking in more calories than you can burn up, those calories will be stored as fat, even if they come from carbohydrates and proteins.

■ **Don't assume that vegetarian or "health" foods are low in fat.** Check the labels. A half cup of granola has a fat calorie ratio of 50 percent . . . that's a higher percentage of fat than a Snickers bar (45 percent).

■ **Graze all day—on low-calorie munchies.** Snack frequently, but stick with modest portions of low-fat foods: rice wafers, dry cereals (but not high fat granolas!), whole grain breads, fruits and vegetables, nonfat or low-fat cottage cheese.

■ *Remember: you are what you eat.* □

CHAPTER 11

Heart-Healthy Ways to Perk Up Your Diet

"Whenever people talk about what's healthy for your heart, they tell you what you shouldn't be eating," sighed a middle-aged woman with a family history of heart disease. "I wish someone would tell me what I should eat."

It's true that eating for a healthy heart has usually been presented in terms of what to avoid. However, as research turns more towards uncovering the positive benefits of various foods, it's becoming clear that *increasing* your intake of certain items can make a genuine contribution to your cardio-vascular health. These foods include not only the vegetables and fruits frequently touted for a variety of nutritional purposes, but also less obvious choices such as garlic, vegetable oil, and even wine.

The fact is, a heart-healthy diet doesn't have to be boring. For most of us, it does mean cutting back on the animal fat and cholesterol that can lead to clogged arteries (see Chapter 10). But it can also mean adding an exciting array of delicious new recipes to your weekly menu—with fish, vegetables, and seasonings that you might otherwise have missed. The secret is in knowing what to add; and on that score, the experts now have plenty to tell us.

Some Clues from the Mediterranean

In the 1950s, scientists began studying the diet and health of almost 13,000 men in seven countries: Greece, Italy, Finland, Japan, the Netherlands, Yugoslavia, and the United States. The result of their 15-year investigation was the Seven Countries Study. One of the most notable findings of this study was the remarkably low rate of heart disease among people living on the island of Crete in the Mediterranean Sea off the coast of Greece. Only 4 percent of the deaths of middle-aged men in Crete were from heart

HEART-HEALTHY FOODS TO FOCUS ON

Add more of these foods to your everyday diet for a healthier heart—and extra variety, too.

Beans	Green leafy vegetables
Bran	Orange vegetables
Citrus fruits	Oatmeal
Garlic	Potatoes

Fish:

Anchovies	Salmon
Bluefish	Sardines
Herring	Tuna
Mackerel	Whitefish

disease, compared to 46 percent of the deaths of their counterparts in the United States.

These statistics sent scientists hunting for explanations. One of the factors scrutinized most closely was what the men were eating, and what the scientists found was a diet very different from that of most Americans. It featured large amounts of vegetables, fruits, grains, and fish. Olive oil was used extensively in food preparation and as an accompaniment to some foods; garlic was often used for seasoning; wine was frequently drunk with meals; meat rarely appeared.

The benefits of this diet probably come from a combination of factors. Omega-3 fatty acids found in some fish help prevent blood clots that can lead to heart attacks and strokes. Many studies have linked moderate wine drinking to increased levels of HDL, the cleansing "good" form of cholesterol that helps keep arteries clear. Fruits and grains are rich in vitamins called antioxidants that have been found to discourage clogged arteries and may have an anticlotting effect as well. Olive oil is one of several unsaturated fats that lower LDL, the "bad" cholesterol

that leaves fatty deposits on the walls of arteries. Garlic has been shown to lower triglyceride (fatty acid) and total cholesterol levels, while leaving "good" HDL levels undisturbed.

With all these elements as the foundation of a diet, the healthy hearts of the people of Crete no longer seem such a mystery. Other things may also be involved, such as exercise and lifestyle, but subsequent studies testing this type of diet against others continue to show the same indisputable cardiovascular benefits.

You don't have to adopt the cuisine of Crete to realize these benefits, either. Since we now know exactly which nutrients are responsible, you can choose among a variety of ways to add or increase them in your diet. Here's a closer look at the items to focus on.

Antioxidants: A New Twist on Some Old Vitamins

Oxidation can be very harmful, as we know from reactions that occur outside our bodies. For example, when metal is exposed to oxygen the result is rust; when butter oxidizes it becomes rancid.

Oxidation also happens within the human body. The compounds that cause oxidation are called free radicals. These unstable molecules scavenge the body, combining with molecules from healthy cells. Oxygen is the most common of the free radicals. While these compounds do perform a number of useful functions, a surplus can damage cells. Some of the harm caused by free radicals is thought to lead to heart disease and cancer.

(The relation of antioxidants to cancer is covered in Chapter 14.)

A number of factors such as cigarette smoke, excessive consumption of alcohol, polluted air, and radiation can promote excessive formation of free radicals. The body counters this process by producing antioxidants. These compounds combine with free radicals to keep the oxidation process in check.

Scientists have theorized that the antioxidants we eat serve the same role as internally manufactured antioxidants—they, too, may inactivate free radicals. Three of the best dietary sources of antioxidants are vitamin C; vitamin E; and beta-carotene, a form of vitamin A found in plants. Each of these acts in a different way and seems to have its own protective role to play. While opinion is not unanimous, many experts are coming to believe that daily intake of these vitamins should be increased considerably to take full advantage of their antioxidant properties. However, there is no general agreement on what the best amount should be.

Other antioxidants may also play a role in cardiovascular health. Selenium is an essential mineral that works as an antioxidant. Glutathione, which is found in plant and animal tissue, is thought to be one of the key players in the antioxidant protection process.

Flavinoids—natural components of all plants—are being studied for their antioxidant properties. Some researchers have theorized that they may be as effective as vitamins C and E in stabilizing free radicals. There are thousands of different flavinoids, and one research project has narrowed its examination to five that seem to have an antioxidant effect. A good source of flavinoids is kale, which also has high levels of vitamin C and beta-carotene. In a study of more than 800 elderly men in the Netherlands, higher flavinoid intake corresponded with lower rates of heart disease. Major sources of flavinoids in their diets were tea, onions, and apples.

Vitamins and Minerals That Help Your Heart

Along with their antioxidant properties, Vitamins C and E and beta-carotene have been associated with a wide range of other protective characteristics. Other vitamins and minerals, such as the B vitamins and potassium, also appear to help maintain a healthy heart. All of these nutrients are readily available in heart-healthy amounts from a wide array of common foods.

Vitamin C

Nearly 50 years of research have linked vitamin C to positive health benefits. Much attention has been given to the role of vitamin C in staving off colds and other infections. However, some studies now suggest cardiovascular benefits as well: Researchers have found that heart disease patients tend to be deficient in vitamin C, while patients taking vitamin C supplements are less likely to develop clogged arteries.

Vitamin C is also important for the production of collagen, the fiber that reinforces blood vessel walls and other parts of the body. If the body perceives a shortage of vitamin C, it compensates by producing a form of LDL to repair blood vessels that have been weakened by the vitamin shortage. This can lead to high LDL counts, which we know are linked to clogging of the arteries.

Vitamin C is considered a first line of antioxidant defense. Vitamin C molecules, which are water soluble, scavenge free radicals before they can enter cells and begin their damage.

Vitamin C can be found in a variety of foods, particularly citrus fruits, green vegetables such as broccoli and kale, and potatoes. A diet that includes the minimum daily recommendation of five servings of fruits and vegetables probably includes enough vitamin C to realize its benefits to the heart.

Vitamin E

Several studies of people taking large doses of vitamin E have linked it with reduced rates of heart disease. Harvard Medical School's Nurses Health Study, which tracked 87,000 women for up to eight years, found that women who took vitamin E supplements for over two years had 41 percent fewer heart attacks than women who did not. Another study of 39,000 men found that those who took at least 100 International Units (IUs) a day of vitamin E (more than three times the current RDA of 30 IUs) for at least two years, had 37 percent fewer heart attacks and bypass surgery procedures than men who got vitamin E only from their diets.

Vitamin E is fat-soluble. It is carried in LDL, and does most of its work within the cell. It has been shown to have a potent antioxidant effect, and has been linked to reduced plaque build-up in coronary arteries. It has also demonstrated its ability to reduce the stickiness of blood platelets, which may help prevent blood clots from forming. However, some scientists caution that finding a reduced

rate of heart disease among people who take large doses of vitamin E doesn't prove the vitamin is the cause. Before changing our diets, they say, we need more research.

If you want to increase your vitamin E intake right now, good dietary sources include vegetable oils, nuts, wheat germ, egg yolks, margarine, tuna fish, oatmeal, and a few vegetables such as asparagus and turnip greens. However, most vegetables are not a major source of vitamin E. In fact, it is very difficult to get from food alone the 100-plus IUs of vitamin E thought to be beneficial for the heart. This is particularly true in a low-fat, low-cholesterol diet, which is not likely to include large amounts of eggs and seed oils (such as sunflower or sesame-seed), the best sources for vitamin E. Vitamin supplements can provide the difference, and are increasingly recommended for their cardiovascular benefits. There have, however, been some negative effects associated with supplemental doses of vitamin E (for example, acceleration of an hereditary eye disease called retinitis pigmentosa was seen in one study, and increased rates of stroke and lung cancer were seen in another). So if you're thinking about adding a vitamin E supplement to your diet, it would be wise to talk to your doctor first about risks, benefits, and your optimal dosage.

Beta-carotene

Beta-carotene is a substance found in plants that is converted to vitamin A by the liver. An increasing number of studies are showing that beta-carotene provides benefits of its own, aside from its role as vitamin A. Scientists are investigating its effects not only on heart disease but also on cancer, cataracts, and various aspects of aging. Studies have found reduced rates of heart disease in groups with high dietary beta-carotene intake and in groups taking beta-carotene supplements. For example, a six-year study of 300 male physicians showed that those taking beta-carotene supplements had 50 percent fewer strokes, heart attacks, cardiac deaths, and angioplasties, compared with those taking dummy pills instead.

Beta-carotene—which is a form of an orange pigment called carotenoid—is found in large amounts in orange vegetables and fruits, such as carrots, sweet potatoes, butternut squash, pumpkin, cantaloupe, and papaya. It is also present in dark green, leafy vegetables like kale, spinach, collard greens, and leaf lettuces. If you include generous portions of these vegetables in your diet, you are probably getting the amount of beta-carotene that you need to help keep your heart healthy.

B Vitamins

Several recent studies have found that increased levels of heart disease are associated with high blood levels of a chemical called homocysteine. One study of 15,000 men over a 13-year period found that those with the highest levels of homocysteine were three times more likely to get heart attacks than those with lower levels.

The B vitamins, particularly B_6, B_{12}, and folate (also called folic acid), act on this chemical to keep it from accumulating in the blood. Unfortunately, nutritional surveys show that Americans typically have diets low in B_6 and folate; and many people have difficulty absorbing B_{12}, especially as they get older.

The richest sources of B vitamins are liver and kidney. However, these are not recom mended in a low-fat, low-cholesterol diet. B vitamins are also found in a number of fruits, vegetables, and grains. Folate—which is also important in the diet of women of child-bearing age because it helps prevent congenital defects such as spina bifida—is in dark green leafy vegetables, citrus fruits and juices, dried beans, nuts, oatmeal, wheat germ, and brewer's yeast. Some cereals are fortified with folate (usually listed in the ingredients as folic acid.)

Vitamin supplements are another way to get adequate amounts of B vitamins in your diet. In particular taking B_{12} in pill form may be a way to get around any absorption problems that you may have.

Potassium

Potassium-rich foods have been found to help your heart and cardiovascular system by lowering blood pressure. This can be an important factor in reducing the risk of strokes, and is discussed in detail in the next chapter.

Good dietary sources of potassium include bananas, beans, potatoes, grapefruit, peppers, squash, grapes, and apples. Most high-potassium foods have the added benefit of being high in fiber and low in sodium and fat.

The Virtues of Garlic

Healing, strengthening, and preventive powers have been attributed to garlic through the ages. Garlic, ancient historians reported, was an important food in the diet of the Egyptian pyramid builders. Greek athletes ate garlic before their competitions. French priests chewed garlic to ward off the bubonic plague, and European soldiers of later generations ate it and rubbed it into their wounds to prevent battlefield infections. And, of course, the most enduring lore about the effectiveness of garlic concerns its ability to protect against vampires.

Studies on vampires are still pretty inconclusive, but garlic has convincingly proved its worth in a number of areas where scientific study can yield measurable results. In laboratory testing, it has destroyed a wide range of organisms that cause human disease: bacteria, viruses, fungi, parasites, and protozoa. It has even been effective in destroying bacteria that have become resistant to antibiotics. In Europe and Asia, garlic supplements have become best-selling over-the-counter drugs.

As garlic has drawn increasing scientific attention, researchers have observed a number of benefits to the cardiovascular system. The chemicals in garlic seem to work in at least three ways to protect against heart disease: by lowering total cholesterol and raising HDL; by lowering blood pressure; and by making platelets less sticky, which can help prevent blood clots from forming. Both laboratory and human tests have shown positive results from garlic in a variety of forms: raw, cooked, concentrated in supplements, and in powders and oils. Onions, have been found to have similar beneficial effects.

A compound known as allicin is suspected to be the source of garlic's benefits. However, it is only one of several active ingredients in garlic (and onion) and knowledge about the way these ingredients actually work on the cardiovascular system is still preliminary. Studies on garlic have not yet been large or long enough for researchers to make definitive recommendations about the amounts to include in your diet or what form is most beneficial. Allicin, which is released by cutting or crushing a clove of garlic, is destroyed by heat, suggesting that raw garlic may have more potent effects than cooked garlic.

The situation becomes more confusing when you look at the many forms of garlic supplements that are currently on the market. These garlic pills, powders, and capsules are not regulated; not always labeled for potency; and not standard in composition. The amount of allicin and other ingredients released by garlic powder tablets, for example, has been found to vary nearly 20-fold among different products. The chemical composition of fresh garlic also varies, depending on growing conditions and variety.

Garlic and garlic supplements probably pose little risk for most people and can be a health-promoting addition to your diet. However, because of garlic's apparent blood-thinning properties, if you regularly take aspirin or another anticoagulant drug, you should consult your doctor before adding large amounts of garlic to your diet.

Garlic is a very pungent herb, and the side effect that people complain about most is bad breath. You may be able to avoid this with synthesized forms of garlic in pills or capsules, but reactions to these are not always predictable, since individual body chemistries react in different ways to the chemicals responsible for bad breath. In addition, these chemicals travel through the bloodstream after garlic is ingested, even if you take it in concentrated pill form, so this side effect is very difficult to avoid. (Even garlic rubbed on the skin is likely to eventually show up on your breath.) As you might expect, work is underway to develop a smell-free or less odoriferous form of garlic.

BLOOD CLOTS: THE GREATEST DANGER TO YOUR HEART

A build-up of cholesterol inside the arteries sets the stage for trouble; but it's usually a blood clot that finishes off the job. If a clot develops or lodges inside an already fat-clogged coronary artery, the situation is especially grave. These arteries supply the heart muscle itself with oxygen rich blood. Denied this life-giving source of energy, the patch of heart muscle served by the artery quickly weakens and dies (note pale area in diagram).

Such a blockage is called a myocardial infarction. Clot-busting drugs such as Activase and Streptase are now used to reestablish blood flow to the heart muscle. But the best treatment is prevention, including a low-fat diet, blood-thinners like the omega-3 fish oils, and, if necessary, cholesterol-lowering drugs and blood thinners, like aspirin.

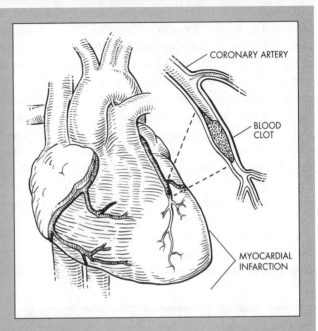

CORONARY ARTERY

BLOOD CLOT

MYOCARDIAL INFARCTION

Foods That Fight Clots

One way in which heart-healthy foods can improve cardiovascular health is their blood-thinning effect, which can help prevent the formation of blood clots. Clotting is a crucial function of blood, necessary for healing cuts and scrapes. It is caused by tiny blood cells called platelets that stick together to begin building a clot. But when platelets become too sticky, clots may form within the bloodstream, preventing the flow of blood to the heart or brain, and leading to heart attacks and strokes.

Many people take aspirin regularly for its blood-thinning properties, and there are some foods that may offer similar benefits. Both garlic and some of the antioxidant vitamins are thought to have some ability to make platelets less sticky.

There are other foods that have also been shown to have blood-thinning effects. In generations past, a popular tonic thought to cure many ills was cod-liver oil. It turns out that grandmother's home remedy may actually have had a scientific basis. Research over the past 20 years has shown that omega-3 fatty acids—which are abundant in fish oils and fatty fish—may have important blood-thinning properties and work in other beneficial ways on the heart. These acids are thought to be one of the significant health-promoting elements of a Mediterranean-style diet.

Omega-3s are a type of polyunsaturated fat found in large quantities in fatty fish like salmon, mackerel, sardines, herring, anchovies, whitefish, and bluefish. Other fish and shellfish also have fair amounts of omega-3s. Scientists became interested in these fish oils in the early 1970s when Danish scientists found that the Eskimos of Greenland had very low rates of heart disease despite their high-fat, high-cholesterol diets. When some of the subsequent research results proved contradictory, interest in fish oil waned. However, recent studies have done much to restore its reputation.

Other sources of omega-3 have also been identified. Linolenic acid is a fatty acid, found in some plants, that the body can convert to the omega-3 chemicals. This acid is in linseed oil, walnuts and walnut oil, soybeans, spinach, and mustard greens. It is also found in rapeseed, which is used to make canola oil, an increasingly popular cooking ingredient.

While the exact mechanisms of omega-3 fatty acids are not yet completely understood, they are thought to displace another, less beneficial type of fatty acid called omega-6 for control of certain biochemical reactions in the body. Besides working as a blood-thinner, the omega-3s have been shown to reduce blood pressure, total cholesterol and LDL levels, and fatty acid (triglyceride) counts.

Tests have shown that while taking fish oil supplements provides some of the cardiovas-

HOW FIBER HELPS THE HEART

Fiber, which passes through the *digestive* system, seems an unlikely candidate for helping the *cardiovascular* system. But, by removing the excess cholesterol from the body—and hence the blood it does indeed help the heart. The key steps are shown here.

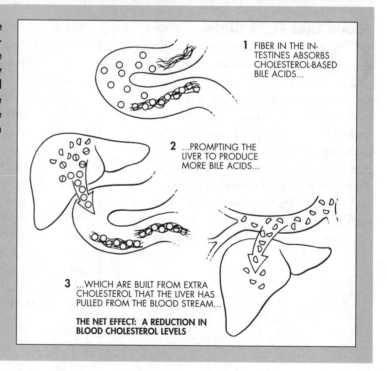

1 FIBER IN THE INTESTINES ABSORBS CHOLESTEROL-BASED BILE ACIDS...

2 ...PROMPTING THE LIVER TO PRODUCE MORE BILE ACIDS...

3 ...WHICH ARE BUILT FROM EXTRA CHOLESTEROL THAT THE LIVER HAS PULLED FROM THE BLOOD STREAM...

THE NET EFFECT: A REDUCTION IN BLOOD CHOLESTEROL LEVELS

cular benefits available from fish itself, eating the real thing seems to supply a broader range of protection. Two or three servings of fish or shellfish a week is probably sufficient to supply beneficial amounts of omega-3 fatty acids. In fact, there are some indications that ingesting too much can be detrimental. Studies have found depressed immune functions and an increased risk of some types of stroke in people who eat fish more than once a day.

Most experts also advise against taking fish oil capsules, unless they are prescribed by your doctor. The capsules supply such concentrated forms of omega-3s that overdosing is possible. This can lead to excessive bleeding, undesirable interactions with other drugs, and other health problems. Diabetics, particularly, should consult with their doctors about the role of fish oil in their diet, because some studies have shown fewer benefits for them than for non-diabetics.

Through the years, there have been searches for other naturally-occurring food products that might bestow the blood-thinning benefits of fish oil. After all, aspirin, the most commonly used anticoagulant, comes from the bark of the willow tree. A form of Chinese mushroom called "tree ears" has been tested and found to have significant blood-thinning effects. However, since these are fairly rare in the U.S. not much further study has been done on them.

How Fiber Figures In

We've heard a lot about how important fiber is in our diets, particularly to prevent constipation and encourage regularity, and as protection against colon cancer. In recent years, fiber has also been promoted as a way of lowering cholesterol, thus helping prevent heart disease. A rush of excited publicity a few years ago about oat bran as a cholesterol-lowerer led to a flood of oat bran products on the supermarket shelves. The hype has settled and oat bran is now seen as just one of a number of fiber-rich foods that can promote heart health.

Scientists theorize that bran, dried beans and other legumes, psyllium (a grain which is used to make some cereals), barley, and other foods high in soluble fibers (fibers that dissolve in water) all lower cholesterol by trapping bile acids in the digestive system. The liver manufactures bile acids from cholesterol. When fiber pulls these acids out of the digestive system, the liver draws cholesterol from the bloodstream to manufacture replacement acids.

Some fibers are more soluble than others, and more effective in lowering cholesterol. How much you can lower your cholesterol by including fiber in your diet also depends on how much fiber you eat. One study found that on average, you have to eat one cup of cooked oat bran or more than two cups of cooked beans a day to get a 5 to 10 percent drop in cholesterol. Eating natural fiber—rather than fiber supplements of the refined fiber found in many breakfast cereals—is the best way to get the health advantages of fiber in your diet.

How (A Little) Wine Can Help

The cardiovascular benefits of alcoholic beverages is a subject that immediately opens the doors to controversy. As we know, alcohol can be a dangerously addictive substance that is associated with a host of medical and social maladies. Alcoholism remains a serious and pervasive public health problem, and the suggestion that alcohol may be good for your health is bound to meet with resistance and skepticism.

However, years of research showing the same pattern of results cannot be ignored. The fact is that study after study has linked light or moderate drinking with reduced amounts of heart disease: Moderate drinkers have been found to have less heart disease than both heavy drinkers and non-drinkers. The phenomenon has been called "the French paradox," from a study published in 1992 that found 40 percent lower rates of coronary heart disease among moderate wine drinkers, despite all the fat in French cuisine.

There are two important points to emphasize about these findings:

- Moderation is key. There is no evidence that increased alcohol intake leads to increased benefits. Levels that have been found beneficial are one to two drinks a day. (A standard drink is defined as 12 ounces of beer, 4 ounces of wine, or 1.5 ounces of 80-proof spirits.) Drinking in excess of these amounts may lead to serious health problems—including heart disease.
- There are some people who should never drink, including recovering alcoholics and pregnant women.

There are at least two theories about the mechanism by which alcohol reduces the risk of heart disease. Some scientists have suggested that alcohol raises artery-cleansing HDL levels; others have observed that it has an anticoagulant effect on platelets. It may be that a combination of both mechanisms contributes to the effect.

The alcohol that was consumed in the "French paradox" was primarily red wine, but other studies have found similar protective results from white wine, beer, and distilled spirits. It has been suggested that drinking with meals, with the balancing caloric intake of food—as is the custom with wine—is healthier than drinking cocktails or beer without a meal. Another theory about the benefits of wine concerns resveratrol, a substance in grapes that may have protective cardiovascular effects. Other compounds called phenolics are also part of the nonalcoholic content of wine and may have antioxidant effects. So it is possible that some of the positive effects of drinking could come from nonalcoholic grape juice as well.

Whether to drink or not, and how much, is an individual decision. No one should view scientific findings about possible benefits of drinking as a license for irresponsible behavior, or even permission to begin a habit that could potentially be destructive. These findings are just one small part of a much larger picture. You need to weigh risks and benefits of all your options in a comparative way.

A New Medley for the Health of Your Heart

It is almost surely a combination of several factors, each contributing in its own way, that will lead to maximum health for your heart. The key to building a heart-healthy diet is to creatively combine as many of the different elements described here as you find you are comfortable with.

Clearly, frequent and substantial servings of fresh fruits, vegetables, beans, and grains are a critical element of a heart-healthy diet. And while the focus of this chapter has been on what is good for you, not what is bad, it is equally important to minimize high-fat and high-cholesterol foods in your diet.

Since meat is a major source of saturated fat and cholesterol, some people advocate vegetarianism as an obvious path to heart health. However, most nutritionists agree that small and well-spaced amounts of meat and dairy products are an efficient way to supply a number of necessary nutrients without any significant increase in your risk of heart disease. If you center most of your meals around large servings of meat, you should probably re-think your menu planning, but there's no need to eliminate meat altogether.

It is also important to remember that none of the foods suggested here are panaceas that will single-handedly solve all of your cardio-vascular problems. Nor are they antidotes for bad habits. Don't think, for example, that if you drink wine with dinner, it will off-set the harm done by cigarette smoking, or that eating lots of garlic means you can eat all the red meat and ice cream that you want. Instead, take what we know about heart-healthy eating as an opportunity to expand the variety in your diet, working all the best foods into a menu plan that's not only good, but good for you. □

CHAPTER 12

The Dietary Approach to High Blood Pressure

The most familiar diet advice for people with high blood pressure is to cut down on salt. That "common knowledge," however, is currently a hot scientific controversy. Though reducing salt intake does make a difference for some people, for many others it has no practical effect. Ask any two doctors what to do about salt, and you're likely to get two different answers.

Given this confusion among even the experts, a "correct" decision is almost impossible to make. A wise one, however, remains a possibility—once you know the issues. Here's what we can currently say with certainty, and what remains to be resolved.

There's no question that a heart-healthy diet—low in saturated fat and other fats—can cut your overall risk of cardiovascular disease by reducing artery-clogging levels of blood cholesterol and helping you maintain an appropriate weight. It's also possible that an increased intake of certain nutrients—

and, possibly, a decrease in salt—may help keep blood pressure down.

Fortunately, there are two points about high blood pressure that the experts do agree on:

- Bringing high blood pressure under control saves lives.
- Effective control of high blood pressure does *not* mean you have to eat a bland, highly restricted diet or start a perpetual round of visits to the doctor.

High Blood Pressure: Take It Seriously

About 50 million Americans, or about one in four adults, have high blood pressure, also called hypertension. It has been called "the silent killer," because it usually causes no symptoms until you are struck by one of its dangerous complications, including heart attack, stroke, heart failure, and kidney problems. Many Americans don't know they have high blood pressure until the damage to their cardiovascular system has already been done. That's why it's so important to have your blood pressure checked

HOW PRESSURE BUILDS

As the arteries conduct oxygen-rich blood deeper and deeper into the tissues, their circumference steadily shrinks, ultimately ending at the arterioles. These tiny vessels, which feed blood into the network of capillaries supplying the individual cells, play a crucial role in maintaining your blood pressure. When their muscular walls tighten, there's less room inside and blood pressure rises. If the muscles relax, the available space increases and blood pressure falls.

Some high blood pressure medications (the so-called ACE inhibitors) work by relaxing the walls of the arterioles. Others (diuretics) take the opposite approach, reducing the volume of blood the constricted arterioles must contend with. Diuretics do this by prompting the kidneys to wring salt and water from the bloodstream. If you are taking this type of medication, extra salt in your diet will counteract its effect.

regularly, and to work with your doctor to lower it if it becomes too high.

Even mildly elevated blood pressure, left untreated, raises the risk of complications—especially if, like many people with mild hypertension, you have other cardiovascular risk factors such as high blood cholesterol, diabetes, or excess weight. Treatment to lower high blood pressure, usually with medication, has saved thousands of people from disability and death. Diet and other so-called "lifestyle measures" can play an important role, helping to control blood pressure with less medication or, in some instances, with no medication at all.

Blood Pressure Basics

Most cases of high blood pressure have no known cause. But it's well known how blood pressure works, and why too high a pressure is risky.

Blood pressure is the force that the bloodstream exerts against the walls of the arteries as they carry blood from the heart to the rest of the body. (Blood returns to the heart through the veins.) At the end of each artery, tiny blood vessels called arterioles circulate blood to all the body's tissues. The pressure inside these vessels varies as they open up (dilate) or clamp down (constrict)—in much the same way that water pressure inside a garden hose will go up or down depending on whether the nozzle is shut or open wide. Your blood pressure fluctuates in time with a number of factors, including emotional stress, bodily position, and time of day.

The body regulates blood pressure through a complicated system that involves the heart, kidneys, and many different substances in the bloodstream, including hormones and minerals such as sodium, potassium, magnesium, and calcium. For adults, normal blood pressure ranges from about 110/80 to as high as 140/90, measured in millimeters of mercury (mm/Hg), the standard unit on a blood pressure measuring device. The higher number is the *systolic* pressure, measured as the heart contracts; the second and lower number is the *diastolic* pressure, measured as the heart rests between beats.

Here is what hypertension experts recommend to physicians: Unless a patient's blood pressure is very high, don't make a diagnosis of hypertension until the reading has been elevated on three separate occasions. That's because blood pressure can vary significantly from day to day. Treatment is usually recommended if blood pressure *persists* at 140/90 or above after several check-ups.

Diet, Drugs, Or Both?

If you are diagnosed as having mild high blood pressure (140/90 to about 160/100), your doctor may suggest that you make certain lifestyle changes before starting medication, including eating less salt, getting more exercise, losing weight if you are overweight, and quitting cigarettes if you smoke. Such measures alone lower blood pressure to a safe level in about one out of four cases. Eventually, most people with high blood pressure will still need medication to control their condition, but in the meantime these non-drug methods will cut the risk of heart disease just as effectively.

In theory, doctors should recommend about 6 months of lifestyle modification before prescribing medication to a patient with mild to moderately high blood pressure. After all, medication costs money, can cause side effects, and may need to be taken for life. Yet in practice, many physicians prescribe blood pressure-lowering drugs right away. Why? Because they believe that patients are more likely to stick with a regimen of pills than with "harder" changes such as diet, weight loss, and exercise. That is true for some people, but it may not be true for you. If your doctor recommends high blood pressure medication before you have tried these measures—and you feel willing and able to carry them out—let your doctor know.

The Great Salt Debate

"You've got high blood pressure? Uh-oh, no pretzels or potato chips for you!" Most Americans feel at least a twinge of guilt when they reach for the salt shaker. After all, everyone has heard that too much sodium (as in sodium chloride, or table salt) is a culprit in high blood pressure, and that cutting down on salt can keep pressure down.

There's just one problem: Nutrition scientists aren't so sure any more. Some researchers argue passionately that salt really is the villain. According to this camp, slashing the sodium from our current high-salt diets would practically wipe out high blood pressure, America's most common chronic disease, in a single generation. Other scientists contend, just as ardently, that while research has shown some intriguing connections between sodium and blood pressure, there is nowhere near enough cause-and-effect evidence to justify a widespread salt shakeout, even for people with high blood pressure.

So what's a pretzel lover to do?

At this point, moderation is still the best course. A moderate cutback on salt can be accomplished quite easily, and still leave your diet full of flavor. This kind of modest sodium restriction can't hurt and may help if you have high blood pressure or are at risk of developing it. Whether or not a stricter reduction in sodium intake is necessary, or even wise, is another matter.

What We Know About Salt

Researchers know that sodium and blood pressure are interrelated; they just can't agree on the implications.

Small amounts of sodium are essential to maintaining the body's fluid balance. But no one on a typical American diet needs to worry about that. The body requires only about 500 milligrams a day to function; and a prudent daily maximum has been estimated at 2,400 to 3,000 milligrams. Americans, however, consume an average of 4,000 to 6,000 milligrams a day, and sometimes more! Normally functioning kidneys handle the excess by flushing out sodium and water, thus keeping a lid on blood volume (the space blood takes up in the vessels) and the resulting blood pressure.

Clearly, too much salt can raise blood pressure too high, at least in some people, based on the following evidence:

■ Before the introduction of blood pressure-lowering drugs in the 1950s, dangerously high blood pressure was routinely treated with an extremely strict low-salt diet or a demanding weight-loss diet such as the so-called "Rice Diet."

■ Studies of laboratory animals have shown that those fed sodium-rich diets tend to have higher blood pressure and more strokes and related problems than animals on lower-salt diets.

■ Populations with a high sodium intake (usually, in more developed countries where foods are highly processed and preserved) have more cases of high blood pressure per capita than the populations of countries with low-salt diets, where people live mainly on fresh, unprocessed foods.

So, the less salt, the better, right? Not necessarily. In a frustrating twist, scientists have failed to make a clear-cut connection between salt intake and blood pressure *in specific individuals*. Almost all Americans consume excess salt, but not all of us develop high blood pressure; and among those who do get hypertension, not all have a particularly salty diet. Some people with high blood pressure who switch to a low-salt diet see no effect on blood pressure, and a few even experience a rise in pressure. Thus, your uncle, the junk food lover, may live to a ripe old age with low blood pressure—while your aunt, the health food maven who wouldn't touch a grain of salt, just might wind up with high blood pressure anyway.

It's clear that some people are more sensitive to the effects of sodium on blood pressure than others are. These "salt-sensitive" individuals may retain more sodium in their bodies, leading to fluid buildup and, finally, to high blood pressure. Part of the puzzle may lie in genetics. African-Americans and people with a family history of hypertension are both more likely to be salt-sensitive, and are also at higher-than-average risk of hypertension. People over age 40 may also be more susceptible to the pressure-raising power of salt, possibly because the kidneys become less efficient at excreting salt as we get older.

One obvious solution would be to test everyone for sensitivity to sodium, and then recommend low-sodium diets only to those who would benefit. However, scientists have been unable to develop a simple and practical test for sodium sensitivity, in part because high blood pressure is affected by so many factors besides diet. Lacking this convenient shortcut, the only way to test yourself for sodium sensitivity is to cut back on sodium for several months, and see whether your blood pressure responds.

What's Right For You?

Can you lower high blood pressure—or keep it from ever rising too high—just by restricting sodium?

That depends on several variables: personal salt sensitivity, how much your blood pressure is elevated, and how successfully you can really restrict sodium, which is present even in many of the salty-tasting commercially prepared foods. Many people find they can cut their salt intake approximately in half without too much difficulty, just by making simple and gradual substitutions in everyday food choices.

On average, this step reduces blood pressure by 3 to 4 points. However, results vary widely from one individual to the next. If you turn out to be salt-sensitive and your pressure is only a little too high, moderately restricting your sodium intake may do the job. But for many people, lowering blood pressure enough to make a difference may require dietary changes big enough to be burdensome, especially if you often dine out or depend heavily on packaged and convenience foods.

Special Salt Warning

For some people, there's no question that salt restriction is worthwhile. For instance, a cutback is definitely in order for people taking blood pressure-lowering medications called diuretics ("water pills"), such as hydrochlorothiazide (HydroDiuril), furosemide (Lasix) or amiloride (Moduretic). These drugs work mainly by helping the kidneys to flush out salt and water, which in turn helps reduce the amount of blood pushing against arterial walls; and a high-salt diet can counteract their effects. Other medical problems may also call for serious sodium restriction: They include heart failure, kidney (renal) disease, and other conditions that can cause fluid retention and swelling of the hands and feet.

EAT THESE HIGH-SODIUM FOODS SPARINGLY WHEN CUTTING BACK

- Anchovies
- Bacon
- Barbecue sauce
- Bologna
- Buttermilk
- Cereal, dry*
- Cheese*
- Chips, potato and corn*
- Crackers*
- Cured meats
- Frankfurters
- Ketchup
- Meat, canned or frozen in sauce
- Mustard
- Nuts, salted*
- Olives, green
- Pastrami
- Pepperoni
- Pickles
- Pizza
- Salami
- Sausage
- Seeds, salted*
- Soup, canned*
- Soy sauce*
- Worcestershire sauce

* Low- or no-salt versions available

Adapted from: Starke RD and Winston M.
American Heart Association Low-Salt Cookbook.
New York: Times Books, 1990.

Cutting Back On Salt Without Losing Flavor

If you decide to try a moderate cutback in sodium, you'll find that it's one of the easiest health-boosting changes to make—*if* you do it with small, gradual adjustments. Scientists who research the human senses believe that a taste for salt, unlike a sweet tooth or a craving for fat, may not be inborn. So after "weaning" yourself from salty food, your tastes may actually change, making foods you once enjoyed seem unpleasantly salty.

A typical sodium-restricted diet calls for no more than 2,000 to 3,000 milligrams per day. There's no need to be rigid or obsessive about numbers, however; if you pack away pizza and salted peanuts at a party, you can compensate by choosing low-salt foods the next day.

The first steps to a lower-sodium diet are to eat smaller portions of high-salt foods, choose alternatives to them when possible, and go easy on adding salt in cooking and at the table. Experiment with lemon juice, vinegar, wine, pepper, herbs, spices, onions, and garlic to add zest to your cooking. (For suggestions, see Chapter 35, "Herbs and Spices: Your Allies for Healthier Meals.")

Shop more carefully, choosing fresh foods instead of processed ones whenever possible. The lion's share of sodium in the U.S. food supply is not added at the table or stove; more than one-third is added by food manufacturers, often to foods such as breakfast cereal and bread that may not seem salty. Thanks to public concern over salt, many traditionally high-sodium products such as crackers, canned soups, and tomato sauce are now available in lower-sodium versions. Some may taste unacceptably bland compared to the original, but others may surprise you.

One Step At A Time

Remember, the key to success is not to make big changes all at once. Try making one adjustment or substitution a week. Here are some suggestions:

- When choosing packaged foods, read labels and keep an eye on sodium content. (See box, "How Low is 'Low'?")
- Ease up on the salt shaker—taste food before you salt it. Later, leave the salt shaker off the table.
- Add little or no salt in cooking water for pasta, rice, and cereals.

EASY TRADE-OFFS

It's wise to keep sodium intake to no more than about 2,000 to 3,000 milligrams a day. Simple substitutions can make a big difference. For instance:

Choose:	Sodium (milligrams)	Instead of:	Sodium (milligrams)
Lemon juice (1 tbsp.)	0	Soy sauce	1,320
Fresh cucumber (1 medium)	14	Dill pickle	1,900
Salt-free bouillon (1 cube)	31	Regular bouillon	960
Fresh peach	0	Canned fruit (1/2 cup)	10
Fresh green beans (1 cup)	5	Canned green beans	925
Orange juice (1/2 cup)	1	Tomato juice	320
Fresh ground beef (3 oz.)	57	Beef frankfurter	425
Frosted Mini-Wheats (1 oz.)	0	Rice Krispies (1 oz.)	290
Popcorn, plain, air- popped (3 cups)	0	Potato chips (1 oz.)	133
Orange drink (16 oz.)	20	McDonald's Chocolate Milkshake	240
McDonald's hamburger	500	McDonald's Big Mac	950

Adapted from: Moser M and Becker B. *Week by Week to a Strong Heart*. Emmaus, Pa.: Rodale, 1992.

- If there are some foods, such as hard-boiled eggs or French fries, that you simply must eat with added salt, choose them less often and enjoy them, salted, when you do.
- Instead of canned vegetables, choose fresh or plain frozen ones (without added sauce).
- Choose fresh meat, poultry, and fish over canned and processed versions: for example, lean roast beef instead of a meat sandwich-spread or bologna.
- Use smaller amounts of high-sodium condiments like ketchup, mustard, and soy sauce.
- Use regular convenience foods in moderation and choose low-sodium versions whenever available. Items to be careful with include frozen entrées, canned soups, bottled salad dressings, and most dry instant mixes.
- Reform your snacking: Choose low-salt crackers, plain pretzels, unsalted peanuts, fresh fruits and vegetable sticks, and plain air-popped popcorn more often than potato or tortilla chips, salted pretzels, or salted nuts.
- If you eat out frequently, ask for sauce on the side or request that dishes be prepared without added salt.
- At salad bars, go easy on salty additions such as dressing and bacon bits.

HOW LOW IS 'LOW'?

Here is how the Food and Drug Administration defines various terms and nutrition claims used on food labels:

Sodium

- *Sodium-free:* less than 5 milligrams per serving
- *Very low sodium:* 35 milligrams or less per serving
- *Low-sodium:* 140 milligrams or less per serving
- *Light in sodium:* at least 50 percent less sodium per serving than the average amount for the same food with no sodium reduction
- *Lightly salted:* at least 50 percent less sodium per serving than the regular item
- *Reduced or less sodium:* at least 25 percent less per serving than the regular item

Salt (Sodium chloride)

- *Salt-free:* sodium-free (see above definition)
- *Unsalted, without added salt, no salt added:* a.) no salt added during processing, and b.) the food it resembles and for which it substitutes is normally processed with salt

Potassium

- *High-potassium:* 700 milligrams or more per serving
- *Good source of potassium:* 350 milligrams to 665 milligrams per serving
- *More or added potassium:* at least 350 milligrams more per serving than the regular item

Calcium

- *High-calcium:* 200 milligrams or more per serving
- *Good source of calcium:* 100 milligrams to 190 milligrams per serving
- *More or added calcium:* at least 100 milligrams more per serving than the regular item

Table salt is about 40 percent sodium by weight. Other common sodium-containing compounds include monosodium glutamate, the flavor enhancer; sodium bicarbonate, or baking soda, used in antacids; and various preservatives such as sodium citrate. It may be that salt, and not other sodium compounds, is the culprit in high blood pressure, but scientists aren't sure. If you're serious about sodium restriction, it wouldn't hurt to watch intake of these other sources of sodium as well.

How Low Should You Go?

If moderate sodium restriction doesn't seem to lower blood pressure, would a stricter cutback work?

You can't count on it, say hypertension experts. It is certainly advisable to keep sodium intake reasonably low whether or not it actually brings down your blood pressure: Don't chuck it all and go back to pickling everything. But many physicians who specialize in hypertension are reluctant to urge further salt restrictions on their patients, including those with high blood pressure. Here's why:

- Blood pressure can usually be controlled without the inconvenience of a highly restricted diet if you follow your doctor's recommendations regarding medication and lifestyle changes, such as weight loss.
- Many people find an extremely low-salt diet too difficult to follow for the long term, since it requires avoiding most convenience and fast foods.

- Cutting out salt often means avoiding many highly nutritious foods such as meat, dairy products, canned beans, and grain foods including bread and muffins. The less variety in your diet, the greater your chance of nutritional shortfall. The net result may be a poorer diet if you don't plan food choices with extreme care.
- Very low salt intake may be unwise for some people, including pregnant women, athletes, laborers, or others involved in heavy physical exertion, especially in warm climates where fluid losses due to perspiration are high.

The bottom line: Ask your doctor before putting yourself on a super-low-sodium diet.

Replacing The Salt Shaker

So far, neither nature nor the food industry has come up with a perfect salt substitute for people who like to pour it on. Before you use a commercial salt substitute, read the label carefully. Some seasoning blends contain sodium as well as other ingredients. "Light"

GOOD SOURCES OF POTASSIUM

Ample potassium in the diet may help keep blood pressure from rising too high. For adults, the recommended daily intake of potassium is about 3,500 milligrams per day. People with certain medical conditions or those who take certain medications may need more, but ask your doctor before taking supplements. Among the best sources of potassium are the following foods:

400 milligrams or more	200-399 milligrams
Banana, 1 medium	Apple juice, 1 cup
Cantaloupe, 1 cup, cubed	Beef, lean, cooked, 3 ounce
Honeydew melon, 1 cup, cubed	Beets, cooked, 1/2 cup
Milk, skim, 1 cup	Blackberries, 1 cup
Nectarine, 1 large	Brussels sprouts, fresh, 1/2 cup
Orange juice, 1 cup	Carrot, raw, 1 large
Potato, 1 medium	Celery, 3 (five-inch) stalks
Prunes, 10 medium	Cherries, raw, 15
Prune juice, 3/4 cup	Chicken, cooked, 3 ounce
Red beans, cooked, 1/2 cup	Flounder, cooked, 3 ounce
Tomato juice, salt-free, 1 cup	Grapefruit, 1/2
	Grapefruit juice, 1 cup
	Lentils, cooked, 1/2 cup
	Lima beans, green, 1/2 cup
	Orange, 1 medium
	Pork, fresh, lean, cooked, 3 ounce
	Salmon, unsalted, canned, 3 ounce
	Spinach, cooked, 1/2 cup
	Strawberries, sliced, 1 cup
	Tomatoes, unsalted, canned, 1/2 cup
	Tuna, water-packed, unsalted,
	1/2 cup Turkey, unprocessed, 3 ounce
	Watermelon, 2 cups, cubed

Adapted from: Starke RD and Winston M.
American Heart Association Low-Salt Cookbook.
New York: Times Books, 1990.

salt products may contain sodium diluted with fillers such as maltodextrin, a corn byproduct. Others contain only herbs, spices, or derivatives from vegetables, including seaweed. Some substitutes contain modest amounts of minerals that may be beneficial, such as calcium and magnesium (see below).

One ingredient to handle with care is potassium chloride, the chief component in some salt substitutes. It may leave a bitter or metallic taste, and should not be added to food during cooking. More importantly, potassium-containing substitutes can actually be dangerous if used along with:

■ Potassium-retaining diuretics, including triamterene (Dyrenium, Dyazide) and amiloride (Midamor, Moduretic), which help the body conserve this mineral
■ Potassium supplements such as Micro-K, sometimes recommended for people taking diuretics that deplete potassium
■ ACE inhibitors such as benazepril (Lotensin) and captopril (Capoten), which can also cause blood potassium levels to rise

The combination of any of these drugs with a potassium-based salt substitute could cause a harmful excess in your body. Potassium is vital to body functioning, and many people may not get enough of it. Too much of the mineral, however, can cause problems such as heart rhythm irregularities. If you are taking any sort of medication, check with your doctor before you start using any salt substitute that contains more than just herbal seasonings.

Other Changes To Consider

Who says there's never any good news from the nutrition police? According to recent research, it's quite possible that eating more crisp salads, fresh juicy fruits, low-fat yogurt, and tasty whole grains may help lower blood pressure, perhaps even more effectively than giving up salt. Certain nutrients found in these foods, along with dietary fiber, just might play a key part in keeping high blood pressure at bay.

In particular, various studies have shown that people with a higher dietary intake of magnesium, potassium, and fiber had significantly lower blood pressures than those with lower intakes. Calcium, too, may play a protective role. The final word isn't in yet, but since foods high in these substances are also among the building blocks of a healthy, low-fat diet, it's worth taking a closer look at their potential benefits on blood pressure.

Potassium

Some scientists now believe that a shortage of this mineral, and not just an excess of sodium, may be an overlooked culprit in the high rates of hypertension that plague Western cultures. Higher potassium intake may also protect against stroke, independent of its effect on blood pressure. Other researchers suggest that it may be the *ratio* of sodium to potassium, rather than just levels of sodium or potassium alone, that regulates blood pressure, making lower sodium and higher potassium intake a good two-pronged strategy.

The recommended daily intake of potassium for an average adult is about 3,500 milligrams per day. Rich food sources of potassium include vegetables, fruits, meats, fish, and poultry. For most people, the safest and most enjoyable route is to include

STUCK ON SALT? OTHER WAYS TO HELP LOWER BLOOD PRESSURE

Sodium reduction won't bring down high blood pressure for everyone, and it's not the top priority anyway. The following measures are just as important, or more so, in reducing elevated blood pressure:

■ **Quit smoking.** Cigarette smoking and high blood pressure both increase the chance of heart disease and stroke. Together, they're a double threat. A long-term smoking habit doesn't cause high blood pressure, but it increases the risk of heart and blood vessel disease so much that quitting is a must for those with hypertension.

■ **Lose those extra pounds.** According to some high blood pressure experts, weight loss is the most single most effective method of reducing blood pressure without drugs. Staying trim may also prevent blood pressure from rising too high in the first place.

■ **Get regular, moderate exercise.** A gentle workout of 20 minutes or so at least 3 times a week makes the heart work more efficiently, lifts the spirits, and helps banish stress. It may also help achieve a modest reduction in blood pressure. Athletics aren't needed; a brisk walk is safer and just as effective.

■ **Get a handle on stress.** Being tense doesn't cause hypertension; some laid-back people get it, too. But chronic stress may worsen the condition by raising levels of the body's "fight or flight" hormones. Stress-beaters like exercise, meditation, hobbies, volunteer work, and recreation turn down the pressure cooker of a stressful life, and may help lower blood pressure, too.

■ **Take medications as directed.** For most people with high blood pressure, the cornerstone of therapy is medication. If you are prescribed drugs to lower blood pressure, take them faithfully as directed, even if you're feeling fine. If you experience side effects, don't just quit taking medication; discuss the problem with your doctor, who can probably clear up the problem by adjusting dosage or changing drugs.

potassium-rich foods such as bananas, orange juice, beans, and potatoes in their daily diet. The official recommendation of at least five servings of fruits and vegetables daily will go a long way toward meeting this goal. (See the nearby box for good sources of potassium.)

Don't, however, try to boost potassium intake by using supplements or potassium-containing salt substitutes unless your doctor specifically recommends it. Extra potassium is not a proven "treatment" for high blood pressure, although it may be prescribed for some people taking medications, such as diuretics, that cause excess potassium loss. Certainly, if your doctor prescribes a diuretic, you should ask whether you will need extra potassium.

Calcium And Magnesium

These two minerals play a closely linked role in blood vessel constriction, and may also help govern blood pressure. The first hint of this came from studies showing lower rates of cardiovascular disease in communities with hard water, which is exceptionally high in minerals. Studies in laboratory rats also suggest that adequate levels of dietary calcium and magnesium protect against high blood pressure.

The results in human testing have been less conclusive, and no major health organization yet recommends magnesium or calcium supplementation as a preventive or treatment for high blood pressure. But many Americans get *less* than the recommended daily level of both minerals, so at the very least you should make sure you're getting enough.

The official recommended daily intake of calcium is 800 milligrams for adults over 24 years old and 1,200 milligrams for adolescents; and many experts advise several hundred milligrams more than that, especially for pregnant, nursing, and post-menopausal women. To reach that goal, eat plenty of low-fat dairy products and other calcium-rich foods such as broccoli, and salmon. Women, who may reap the added benefit of preventing osteoporosis (thinning of the bones), should also ask their doctors whether calcium supplements are advisable.

Up to three-quarters of the U.S. population gets less than the recommended amount of magnesium (400 milligrams a day). Those most likely to be deficient in magnesium include the elderly, diabetics, moderate or heavy drinkers, and people taking diuretics. Doctors use magnesium to treat heart rhythm abnormalities and it *may* even help prevent clogging of the arteries. High-magnesium foods include oats, bran, nuts, and legumes (beans and peas). Other good sources are fruits, vegetables, and fish. As for supplements, again—ask your doctor before taking them. They often cause diarrhea; and in any case, a varied diet offers benefits you can't get from a pill.

Fiber

Although many scientists still doubt its validity, some research has suggested a link between increased fiber intake and reduced blood pressure. Given the well-known preventive benefits of fiber-rich foods for many other conditions, from heart disease to colon cancer, this is just one more reason to include fruits, vegetables, and whole grains in your daily diet.

Can Cutting Down On Coffee Help?

Coffee has long been suspected of a host of harmful effects on the heart and other organs, and has been the object of extensive study. However, any evidence of potential harm is conflicting and not very strong. Some researchers have noted that blood pressure may rise in heavy coffee drinkers (more than about 5 cups a day), but more modest intake seems to make no difference. If you have hard-to-control high blood pressure and drink a great deal of coffee or other caffeinated beverages (including tea and some soft drinks), it may be worth cutting down or making at least a partial switch to decaffeinated brews. Some caffeine is also present in chocolate and cocoa products, and in many non-prescription medicines.

Can Cutting Down On Alcohol Help?

Heavy drinking and high blood pressure go hand in hand. It's well proven that more than 2 ounces of hard liquor daily is associated with higher pressure, and more than 3 ounces with actual hypertension. Heavy drinking also boosts your risk of stroke and liver problems and, of course, carries with it the risk of addiction.

If you drink regularly, just cutting alcohol intake down or out can have a noticeable impact on too-high blood pressure. The usual recommendation is to limit daily alcohol intake to no more than 1 drink for women, 2 for men. (A drink equals an ounce and a half of liquor, 1 average glass of wine, or a standard can of beer.)

Is it better still to be a teetotaler? There's no scientific evidence that the alcohol intake described above causes harm to most people. In fact, some studies suggest that modest alcohol intake may actually protect the heart, possibly by raising levels of HDL, or "good" cholesterol.

But when it comes to drinking, the risks are much better proven than the benefits. Alcohol is a source of nutritionally empty calories—a concern for people with high blood pressure who are watching their weight. Certain blood pressure and heart medications should not be mixed with alcohol. And some people should *never* drink: pregnant women and anyone with a personal or family history of alcoholism or any signs of liver disease. □

Cancer: Foods That Could Cause It—or Fend It Off

CHAPTER 13

Cut Back on These Foods to Cut Your Cancer Risk

Can you fend off cancer simply by adjusting your diet? The answer is Yes . . . in a way. Upgrading your diet does not guarantee that you'll always remain cancer-free, but it can yield a dramatic improvement in the odds.

In the past 30 years the National Cancer Institute has devoted an increasing share of its research dollars to the relationship between nutrition and cancer. By the mid 1960s, research had already suggested that diet has a major role in the development of many cancers and that reducing or excluding certain foods from the diet might play a significant part in cancer prevention. By the late 1970s, scientists were able to put a number to the risk. They estimated that diet contributed to cancer deaths in as many as 40 percent of the cases among men and 60 percent of the cases in women. A 1982 study

followed up with a comparable estimate: 35 percent of cancer deaths were said to be related to certain elements of the diet. Since then, we've learned more and more about specific culprits in cancer, even though scientists have yet to find any sure-fire means of prevention.

What's holding us back? Part of the problem lies in the tools available to researchers. For instance, many major studies rely on surveys of the eating habits of large population groups, drawing conclusions by comparing their dietary patterns and health outcomes to those of other groups. If women in countries with high-fat diets (such as the United States) have higher incidences of breast cancer than women in countries where less fat is consumed (for example, Japan), it can then be theorized that a high-fat diet may be one of the causes of breast cancer. If further studies show that when Japanese women move to the United States and adopt a higher-fat diet their incidence of breast cancer goes up, that hypothesis is strengthened.

This, however, is far from proof of a cause/effect relationship, nor do such studies pinpoint the specific compounds within certain foods that may cause cancer. For more definitive proof, researchers analyze the effects of certain foods on animals; but this too falls far short of certainty. What happens to rats or mice in the laboratory is not always the same thing that happens to humans in their normal environment.

The only way to be reasonably certain of the effects of diet on health is to stage a large, scientifically controlled study that carefully monitors the diets of human subjects and notes the diseases they develop over a period of years. Although these studies are very expensive and results may take decades, they are still being performed. For example, the National Cancer Institute is sponsoring several long-term prevention trials at participating medical centers around the country.

As the growing body of research about diet and cancer indicates, this is an extremely complex subject. "People are always looking for the magic bullet, some simple answer for what causes cancer or what can prevent it," says Carolyn K. Clifford, Ph.D., chief of the Diet and Cancer Branch of the National Cancer Institute. "But the fact is, there is no simple answer. Overall dietary patterns— and not just one single food—are what must be examined. There is enough evidence available to permit formulation of some dietary guidelines related to cancer, but we keep learning more."

A brief overview of how the disease develops can help in understanding the relationship between nutrition and cancer. There are three major stages in cancer development:

- **Initiation,** in which a cancer-causing agent first damages a cell's genetic material.
- **Promotion,** when cells in which initiation has occurred are exposed to chemicals that speed up cell division. Such chemicals cannot initiate cancer themselves: generally long-term exposure to these promoters is necessary for cancer to develop. Nutritional factors are thought to have their greatest impact on cancer in this stage.
- **Progression** is the final stage of cancer development when cells become fully malignant and acquire the ability to metastasize, or spread, to other parts of the body.

A number of foods have now been implicated in the development of cancer. They include both naturally occurring substances and artificial additives. Cooking and food preservation methods may also influence the development of cancer. And cancer-causing agents found in pesticides or even in packaging sometimes get into our bodies through the food we eat.

Not all research ends in a guilty verdict, however. Several foods initially denounced as cancer-causing have later been cleared of all charges. We'll take a look at these substances as well, and see where they stand today.

Your Best Bet: Cut Dietary Fat

There is more research on fat and its relationship to cancer than on any other component of the American diet. While the results are far from conclusive and shed little light on the reason, there is no question that groups with a high fat intake also have a higher cancer rate. As the findings about American and Japanese breast cancer rates indicate, population studies have shown a strong correlation between fat and cancer—especially in the breast, colon,

HOW FOREIGN CHEMICALS HELP CANCER TAKE HOLD

Chemical agents—both natural and artificial—can be found on the scene at each phase in the hidden growth of cancer.

1. Initiation. Cancer begins when the DNA governing a cell's growth and division is sabotaged by a foreign invader, such as a virus, a toxic chemical, or radiation. Note that irradiation to preserve food does *not* leave any cancer-causing radiation behind.

2. Promotion. When already damaged cells are bathed in a cancer promoting chemical for an extended period of time, they eventually break loose into uncontrolled proliferation. It's at this stage that regular consumption of harmful dietary chemicals plays its biggest role. The culprit can be a natural ingredient, an additive, or a chemical created during cooking.

3. Progression. Growth can continue unnoticed for years. But it is only when the abnormal cells gain the ability to colonize distant parts of the body that the cancer becomes truly—and almost inevitably—lethal.

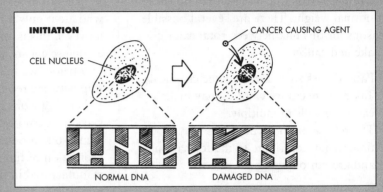

INITIATION

CELL NUCLEUS

CANCER CAUSING AGENT

NORMAL DNA   DAMAGED DNA

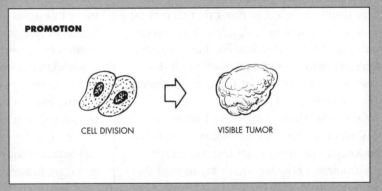

PROMOTION

CELL DIVISION   VISIBLE TUMOR

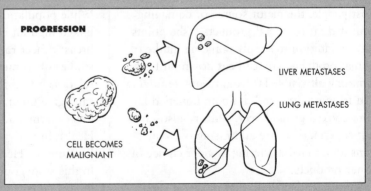

PROGRESSION

LIVER METASTASES

LUNG METASTASES

CELL BECOMES MALIGNANT

prostate, rectum, and lining of the uterus. One study even found higher rates of skin cancer among people who eat an appreciable amount of fat. Most research suggests that it's *total* fat intake, rather than a specific type of fat (such as saturated, monounsaturated, or polyunsaturated) that shows a link with cancer.

It should not be surprising, therefore, that excess weight itself is a risk factor for cancer.

Research has found that heavy people have a greater risk both of developing cancer and of dying from the disease than do those of normal weight. There are several possible reasons for this link between total caloric intake and cancer:

- Fatty tissues store carcinogenic chemicals.
- Taking in excessive calories may make it easier for cells to multiply.
- The release of hormones from fatty tissues may contribute to the formation and growth of malignant tumors.

Despite all the suspicious statistics, however, there is still no definitive proof that dietary fat encourages cancer. Indeed, a few studies seem to disprove the connection. Further research is necessary before we can be certain that decreasing the amount of fat you eat can protect you from this dread disease.

Of course, there are plenty of other reasons to cut back on fat—most notably its tendency to promote heart disease. So it's important to know where the fat in your diet is coming from, says the NCI's Clifford. "For most people, the major source of damaging saturated fat is animal products," she points out. In addition to simply reducing intake of animal products, you can cut down on fat by trimming all visible fat from meats, removing skin from poultry, and draining liquefied fat from cooked ground beef. Clifford also notes that supermarkets are addressing our concerns about fat by offering a wider choice of leaner products.

Some scientists think that red meat carries special risks of cancer, particularly colon cancer. Red meat certainly has higher levels of fat than poultry or fish, and Harvard University's study of 88,000 nurses found that women who ate red meat daily were more than twice as likely to develop colon cancer as those who ate it only a few times a week. Again, however, this is an area of disagreement among scientists, and more research is necessary before we fully understand the relationship between red meat and cancer.

Fat may work in a number of different ways to promote cancer. In the colon, for example, bile production may play a role in the promotion of tumor growth. Bile is a fluid manufactured in the liver to aid in the digestion of fats; the more fat you consume, the more bile acids your liver produces, and an excess of bile acids may encourage cancerous tumors to grow. Saturated fat in particular is associated with colon (and rectal) cancer.

Fat consumption may also stimulate the production of estrogen, and high levels of estrogen promote the growth of breast tumors. Decreasing the amount of fat in the diet has been shown to lead to reduced levels of estrogen. However, there the evidence of a fat/breast cancer relationship stops short. While population and animal studies have linked high fat consumption to increased breast cancer rates, some large controlled studies of women have failed to bear out the relationship. If there is one fact that scientists can agree upon at this point, it is that larger, longer term studies are needed. The Women's Health Initiative, begun by the National Institutes of Health in 1994, is one attempt. In this study, one group of participants is limiting their fat intake to less than 20 percent of their total calories.

While the average American now gets nearly 40 percent of his or her calories from fat, many experts say fat intake should be limited to 30 percent—and some scientists believe even that figure is too high. In testimony before Congress in 1993, Dr. Peter Greenwald, director of the National Cancer Institute's Division of Cancer Prevention and Control, said that 30 percent is "a practical target," but "data could be used to justify an even greater reduction."

Alcohol: Another Leading Suspect

Your health can be affected not only by what you eat, but also by what you drink. Although it's now thought that moderate amounts of alcohol may have a *beneficial* effect on your heart, the same is not true for alcohol and cancer. Most studies in the latter area suggest a higher risk of cancer among those who drink. According to the National Cancer Institute, alcohol is associated with an estimated three percent of cancers in the United States. A wide range of laboratory and population studies show that it can influence all three phases of cancer: initiation, promotion, and progression.

Again, however, these findings are far from definitive. While the pattern of alcohol consumption and increased cancer rates continues to be confirmed by population studies, ethanol—pure grain alcohol—does not appear to cause cancer in laboratory animals. However, the alcohol you drink is metabolized in your body to a substance called acetaldehyde, which has been found to have carcinogenic effects in laboratory studies.

High alcohol consumption has been linked most often to cancer of the liver, breast, rectum, mouth, esophagus, pharynx, larynx, digestive tract, bladder, and lungs. In addition many studies have observed a "synergistic" effect between alcohol consumption and cigarette smoking; that is, cigarettes and

A CANCER-CAUSING FUNGUS

For world travelers, here's something else to worry about. Aflatoxin is a naturally occurring mold that grows on grains and legumes—most commonly, on peanut plants. Aflatoxins are carcinogenic, and are particularly associated with liver cancer. They are thought to interact with the hepatitis B virus, making the pair a leading cause of liver cancer.

For Americans, liver cancer is not considered a major problem. It is far more prevalent in Asia and Africa, where high rates of liver cancer in some areas coincide with exposure to aflatoxins. In this country, aflatoxins are closely monitored by the Food and Drug Administration and need not concern us. But beware when traveling abroad, especially if you have been exposed to hepatitis B.

alcohol, working together, have a greater likelihood of causing cancer than either does alone. This is especially true of cancers of the mouth and throat; as many as three-quarters of oral cancers in the U.S. are attributed to the alcohol/tobacco combination. According to one theory, alcohol increases the body's absorption of the carcinogens in tobacco.

Researchers disagree on the ways in which alcohol works as a cancer-promoting agent. Many studies have shown that alcohol depresses your immune system, and thus may impair your body's ability to recognize and eliminate cancerous cells. Alcohol also seems to decrease levels of vitamins A and E, two important antioxidant vitamins that are thought to have a role in preventing cancer. (For more information, see Chapter 14.)

It is also possible that other ingredients in alcoholic beverages could be implicated in the alcohol/cancer association. For example, the cancer-causing substances called nitrosamines are found in some alcoholic drinks, particularly beer. Indeed, according to one theory, rather than actually being a cancer-causing substance itself, alcohol instead works with other substances (such as tobacco) to promote the growth of malignancies.

Some of the most confusing data come from breast cancer research. Many studies have shown an association between alcohol consumption and breast cancer, but the link has not always been strong, and scientists have not always ruled out other possible explanations. However, some of this research has turned up surprising results. The Nurses' Health Study, for example, found that women who drank only moderately (one or two drinks a day) had a 50 percent higher rate of breast cancer than those who did not drink at all (although the risks of the two groups equalized somewhat after their four- and eight-year follow-up evaluations).

In another study, women who drank about one ounce of pure alcohol (the amount in two average drinks) daily for three months were found to have higher levels of the suspected cancer-promoting hormone estrogen than did non-drinkers.

Most of the more than 50 extensive human studies conducted in the past 35 years, have found an association between alcohol and cancers of the colon and rectum. Beer-drinking seems to put both men and women at higher risk than consuming other types of alcoholic beverages. Alcohol is thought to promote colon and rectal cancers in several ways: by suppressing the immune system, changing bile metabolism, and dosing the area with cancer-causing nitrosamines.

Excessive drinking can bring on liver disease, and alcohol seems to play a role in the promotion of liver cancer. One study found that heavy drinkers have more than four times greater likelihood of developing liver cancer than those who drink lightly or not at all.

Why Cured Meat Is Sometimes a Problem

Nitrosamines are substances that occur naturally in some foods. They form during the metabolism of nitrites and nitrates—two closely related compounds made of nitrogen and oxygen and used to cure and preserve meats. The bad news is that nitrosamines have been found to be potent carcinogens. But there is also good news about nitrosamines: In the two decades since these carcinogenic substances were first found in food, the amount of nitrites and nitrates in the American food supply has decreased significantly.

In the early 1970s scientists identified nitrosamines—already known to be carcinogenic—in a variety of foods, including cooked bacon and sausage, cured pork, and dried beef. Bacon received a great deal of attention because it had the highest levels. Food processors used nitrates and nitrites extensively to give cured meats a pink, fresh look and to protect against botulism, a potentially deadly bacteria. While the government never banned these substances, they have been regulated much more tightly in recent years, and the food industry has moved toward phasing them out. When nitrites are used, they must appear on the labeling.

Researchers have also found that vitamins C and E inhibit the formation of nitrosamines in the body; and some manufacturers are now adding these vitamins to their products during the curing process. Alternatively, you can boost your intake of vitamin C- and E-rich foods when eating nitrite-laden meats, for example, by drinking a glass of orange juice when you eat bacon.

In addition to these vitamins, there are at least two other substances in many fruits and vegetables—p-coumaric and chlorogenic acids—that interfere with the tendency of nitric acid to combine with amines and form nitrosamines. Garlic, laboratory studies suggest, may also block formation of these compounds.

The nitrosamines in beer are formed during malt-kilning, a drying process which is part of beer manufacture. Dark beers have the highest levels of nitrosamines. Here, too, manufacturers are reducing carcinogens. There are fewer nitrosamines in most of today's beers than in those you drank a couple of years ago.

Nitrates also occur in drinking water. Sometimes run-off from excessive use of fertilizers contaminates water supplies with very high levels of nitrates. Most state health departments closely monitor nitrate levels in public water supplies. However, if you drink well water, you should have your water checked periodically for nitrates and other contaminants.

Smoked foods, like cured, have long been implicated in cancer. Population studies have found elevated cancer rates among groups who consume large quantities of this type of food. Stomach cancer, in particular, is higher than average.

The smoking process deposits polycyclic aromatic hydrocarbons (PAHs) on the surface of the food, and PAHs have been shown to be carcinogenic. (PAHs also result during charring—for example, on a barbecue.) However, because most Americans eat relatively little smoked food, intake of these compounds is not considered a problem.

Danger on the Barbecue?

Cooking any meat—beef, pork, lamb, poultry, fish, or game—at high temperatures adds extra flavor. No wonder, then, that charcoaling, grilling, and broiling meat—and sometimes vegetables—have become American institutions.

Unfortunately, the same chemical reaction that gives such special flavor to your grilled steak also creates a group of substances known as heterocyclic amines (HCAs). HCAs, first identified in 1976, appear when high heat is applied to creatinine, a compound found in the blood and muscle of all animals. They have been found to cause genetic mutations in cells that leave them vulnerable to cancer. HCAs are most often associated with cancers of the gastrointestinal tract; and some laboratory studies have suggested a connection to breast tumors.

HCAs are thought to work together with dietary fat to promote cancer growth. There is also evidence that certain enzymes in the liver activate HCAs. Different people produce different amounts of these enzymes, so it's possible that these compounds are more dangerous for some people than for others. One interesting study found that the HCA-activating enzymes are the same substances that metabolize the caffeine in coffee, and that people with high levels of these enzymes tend to be heavy coffee drinkers, compensating for their body's rapid breakdown of caffeine. If you're a heavy coffee drinker, you therefore might be more susceptible to the cancer-causing threat of HCAs. (No need to throw away the coffee pot yet, however. This theory is still unproven.)

If you like your meat rare, you're in luck. HCAs do not form instantaneously when meat is cooked on a high flame. It takes time for the creatinine to move to the surface of the meat, the better to be scorched into HCAs. Protracted searing at high temperature is therefore the cooking method most likely to present you with high levels of HCAs. If you must have your grilled hamburgers, at least don't make them well done.

Broiling and grilling at extremely high temperatures near an open flame (as on charcoal grills) also results in the deposit of PAHs on the surface of the food being cooked. You can scrape most PAHs from the surface of charred food. HCAs, however, are more likely to be embedded in the meat where they can't be removed.

All is not lost for meat-eaters who love the taste of charcoal broiling. You can decrease the impact of HCAs by consuming antioxidants, such as vitamins E and C and beta-carotene. Nutritionists also suggest pre-cooking meat for a couple of minutes in a microwave oven before putting it on the grill. This removes juices, thus decreasing creatinine content and reducing the amount of HCAs that can be produced.

Additives and Pesticides: No News Is Good News

Red dye number two. Alar. DDT. DES. Dioxin. The list of toxic—or reputedly toxic—chemicals that have found their way into our food supply is well-known to us all. And even though drastic measures have been taken to assure the safety of what we eat today, a hint of suspicion always remains: could this food contain cancer-causing chemicals?

The average American diet includes literally thousands of additives that have been put into food to retard spoilage, enhance flavor, and improve appearance. Foreign chemicals can also get into the food you eat in many other ways. For example, farmers feed dietary supplements to animals and dust crops with pesticides.

An astonishing amount of pesticides is used in this country: In the past 30 years their use has doubled. Any pesticide thought to be carcinogenic has been banned in the U.S. However, these chemicals can still turn up on foods imported from other countries, leaving many concerned Americans suspicious, frustrated, and worried.

Most scientists feel that the risk of cancer from food additives is minimal. The Food and Drug Administration and the Environmental Protection Agency both monitor additives; the Delaney amendment to the Federal Food, Drug, and Cosmetic Act prohibits the addition of any known carcinogen to food. Unfortunately, however, there are no absolute guarantees. "Realistically we are constrained by budgets as to how much can be done," says Carolyn Clifford of the National Cancer Institute. "And there is still a great deal to be learned from research with new pesticides, to discover what levels are safe."

Even old pesticides may continue to pose problems. DDT, once widely used, has been banned for decades; but traces of it still show up in soil, water, and produce. The same is true of other chemicals that have been

IRRADIATION: NO CAUSE FOR ALARM

Irradiation, a process that treats foods with gamma rays, can be used to kill salmonella and other organisms that cause disease, get rid of insects in spices and produce, and delay ripening and sprouting of fruits and vegetables. In this country, it has been used for food preservation only since 1992, although it has been employed for years as part of the sterilization process for medical supplies, tampons, and condoms.

Although irradiated food does not become radioactive, gamma rays can break chemical bonds in cells, loosing the unstable molecules known as free radicals—which in large quantities are suspected of promoting cancer. Some critics also charge that irradiation creates new compounds that may be carcinogenic. Indeed, among the byproducts of irradiation are benzene and formaldehyde, both considered carcinogens.

Nevertheless, the levels of irradiation used in food processing are so low that only a tiny percentage of the chemical bonds within a food are broken; and tests on animals have failed to reveal any harmful effects, even when heavily irradiated foods are given to them routinely. As a result, most experts have concluded that the process poses no real danger.

banned. Diethylstilbestrol (DES), a drug that pregnant women once took to prevent miscarriage, caused gynecological cancers and other abnormalities in their daughters. But it remained in use as a poultry and cattle food additive for years after the cancer connection surfaced. (Today, it is no longer in use.) Conversely, some substances that were withdrawn from the market because of supposed carcinogenic effects—the apple preservative Alar, for example—were found in subsequent testing to have no cancer-causing effects.

Some scientists have theorized that industrial and agricultural chemicals may bear some of the blame for the increasing rates of breast cancer in this country. Some of these chemicals are "xenoestrogens"—estrogen-like substances that are thought to share natural estrogen's reputed cancer-causing potential. However, these theories are both controversial and unproven; in fact, some studies have concluded that there is no such connection.

Researchers have recently begun investigating food packaging materials to find out if any of their components can get into foods and produce negative effects. For example, exposure to benzene, a chemical sometimes used in packaging, has been linked to blood disorders and possible leukemia in the rubber-making and gasoline-related industries. Although work in this area is still preliminary, tests have shown that benzene from packaging can migrate into meat, poultry, cheeses, and other packaged foods. Using plastic wraps for microwaving can also release chemicals into the food. Many wraps contain plasticizers to increase flexibility; one of these substances, di(ethylhexyl)adepate (DEHA), is a suspected carcinogen.

Manufacturers and regulators have become increasingly aware of the necessity to monitor our foods for contaminants. Government regulations prohibit the sale of many substances, and others are under investigation. Meanwhile, you can take a few simple steps to protect yourself:

- Use waxed paper rather than plastic wrap when microwaving.
- Wash or peel all fruits and vegetables. Use a vegetable brush for washing.
- Buy local produce whenever possible. It is less likely to have been treated with chemicals to prevent spoilage than fruits and vegetables that travel a long distance to the market.

The Latest on
Artificial Sweeteners

Americans have been using artificial sweeteners for more than a hundred years, and they've been controversial for just about as long. Saccharin had become popular by the turn of the century, and sugar shortages during the world wars boosted its popularity. Cyclamate sweetened many foods and beverages in the 1950s, and aspartame—known commercially as NutraSweet—became a diet staple in the early 1980s.

The treatment of artificial sweeteners by the agencies that monitor the food supply in our country shows how subjective the process of food regulation can be. Twenty years ago, saccharin was implicated in the development of bladder cancer in laboratory animals. At the time, the evidence was thought to be so compelling that in 1977 the FDA proposed banning the substance. However, strong consumer opposition to the ban forced Congress to impose a moratorium that has been in effect ever since. Saccharin remains on the market, and is still an ingredient in many products such as soft drinks and sugarless gum. However, products containing saccharin must bear a label warning that it causes cancer in laboratory animals.

Meanwhile, recent research indicates that the mechanism that allows saccharin to form bladder tumors in rats has no parallel in humans. Rat urine has much higher concentrations of certain proteins that react with saccharin, forming crystals that then help cause healthy cells to become malignant. Since no similar action occurs in human bladders, most researchers feel that it is unlikely that saccharin causes cancer in humans, especially with moderate use.

Cyclamate, on the other hand, has not fared as well. Despite a lack of conclusive evidence linking it to cancer, it has been banned in the U.S. Cyclamate, widely used both by itself and combined with saccharin, also produced bladder cancer in laboratory animals. While panels of both the FDA and the National Research Council agreed that cyclamate alone is unlikely to cause cancer in humans, they expressed concern that it might enhance the cancer-causing effects of other substances. So the ban remains standing, even though cyclamate is widely used in other countries, and the World Health Organization and United Nations Food and Agriculture Organization have declared it safe for human consumption.

If all this weren't enough to sour our view of sweeteners, some research purports to show that sugar itself may be involved in chemical changes in the body, causing cellular mutations that could pave the way for cancer. While no one is yet suggesting that sugar is a carcinogen, this type of report illustrates the level of speculation that still swirls around the topic of cancer-causing foods. While the current state of science provides us with an abundance of hints, definitive answers remain notoriously hard to come by. It's always wise to keep a wary eye on the latest reports; but revising your diet on the basis of a single study rarely makes sense. □

CHAPTER 14

Food That Fights Cancer: What Science Knows Today

t sounds like science fiction: "designer foods" that halt the growth of tumors; "chemoprevention" diets to keep malignancy at bay; potent protective agents on sale in every grocery store. Yet all these miracles are the subject of serious, sober investigation sponsored by the National Cancer Institute.

Although it seems too good to be true, evidence is mounting that certain substances in our diet really can shield us from cancer. We're only beginning to learn how these compounds work, but scientists have already discovered natural chemicals that can defeat malignancy at all three stages of development: initiation, promotion, and progression.

Often, the first clue to a cancer-fighting agent is a conspicuous lack of cancer in a certain group of people, leading researchers to look for something extra in their diet. In other cases, the opposite holds true; people who have developed cancer are found to be missing a particular nutritional element.

That was the story with the trace element selenium, for instance. While measuring levels of various chemicals in the blood and tissues of cancer patients, researchers discovered that patients with certain cancers had very low levels of selenium, a mineral present in fruits and vegetables grown in selenium rich soil. This led to speculation that correcting selenium deficiency might be cancer-preventive—a theory that is being borne out by current testing.

Once a cancer-fighting ingredient has been identified, it's only logical to seek ways of boosting its presence in the food supply. Hence the "Designer Foods" program, a term coined by the National Cancer Institute in 1989.

Take that idea one step further and you have "chemoprevention," or the use of concentrated supplements to cut the odds of developing a cancer. When scientists noticed the anticancer effects of beta-carotene-rich foods, for example, they mounted major long-term tests with beta-carotene supplements in an attempt to confirm the substance's ability to reverse, suppress, or prevent the growth of cancer. Many such studies are currently in progress to test the cancer-fighting properties of hundreds of substances, both naturally-occurring and synthetic. Early results show that a number may indeed discourage oral, skin, colon, cervical, stomach, lung, and head and neck cancers.

Despite these exciting prospects, however, it's important to remember that we are still a long way from guaranteed protection against cancer. The disease takes hold in many ways, most of them not fully understood; and what works for one individual may not work for the next. Chemoprevention promises to improve your odds of safety, but it's not an impenetrable shield.

Additionally, scientists still have much to learn about the way nutrients interact. Even though certain foods can be singled out as cancer-fighters, it's quite likely that they work most effectively in combination with others. For this reason, nutritionists still stress the need for a varied diet. The so-called "Mediterranean Diet," for instance, is believed to help prevent heart disease and certain types of cancer. It combines large amounts of complex carbohydrates from vegetables, beans, and whole grain products with minimal amounts of saturated fat and red meat. But by themselves, not one of these ingredients is likely to protect you from anything. It's only in concert—and in the right proportions—that they begin to work their magic. "Variety is the key," says Carolyn Clifford, chief of the diet and cancer branch of the National Cancer Institute. "There is no one perfect food that can supply all the necessary nutrients and save us from disease."

The Cancer-Fighting Dividends of Fruits, Vegetables, and Grains

The data are compelling and consistent: Population studies that examine the relationship between diet and cancer link generous intake of fruits, vegetables, and whole grains to reduced risks of cancer. In 1991, based on the overwhelming scientific findings, the National Cancer Institute began a national "5 A Day for Better Health" campaign to encourage consumption of 5 or more servings of fruits or vegetables daily. Nevertheless, most Americans do not eat even half that amount. (One serving is measured as half a cup of fresh fruit or cooked vegetables, 1 cup of leafy vegetables, a quarter cup of dried fruit, or three quarters of a cup of juice.)

Fruits, vegetables, and grains owe their cancer-preventing benefits to a host of specific nutrients—many of them unknown until recently. Here's an overview of the key players.

Fiber

The best known of the cancer-fighters, fiber has been a favorite nutritional recommendation for nearly two decades. In the mid-1970s, researchers found that some groups of people in Africa with high fiber consumption (more than 10 times greater than American averages) had extremely low rates of colon cancer. More recent studies have linked high fiber consumption with reduced rates of breast cancer.

It is important not to draw the wrong conclusions from these studies. For example, diets high in fiber are often also very low in fat, and the low fat level may play a significant role of its own in reducing cancer rates. Nevertheless, nutritionists believe that fiber itself can help prevent malignancy, especially in the colon and rectum.

We get fiber in our diet from a variety of sources; fruits, vegetables, and grains—especially whole grains. Fiber is the indigestible (or partially indigestible) part of the food we eat: the bran in grain, the pulp of fruit, the crunchy skin of vegetables, the stringy filaments of beans. Some fiber is soluble (that is, it dissolves); while other fiber is non-soluble.

The fiber you eat affects your digestion in several ways. Fiber helps move food and digestive by-products efficiently through the large intestine (colon) and out of the body. The faster food and digestive by-products travel through the gastrointestinal tract, the less time there is for potential cancer-causing agents to do their damage. Fiber is also thought to dilute potential carcinogens, thus lessening their impact. It also helps alter the metabolism of certain bacteria in the digestive tract, promoting healthy digestion.

There are four major types of fiber: cellulose, pectin, lignin, and gums. They have different qualities and they act in somewhat different ways:

Cellulose, the most prevalent type of fiber, softens the stool, prevents constipation, and dilutes bile acids in the colon that are thought to promote cancer growth. Cellulose is found in apples, whole grains, some nuts, carrots, and other fruits and vegetables.

Pectin, a gelatinous substance, also offsets bile acids. It complements the function of cellulose, encouraging healthy digestion by preventing diarrhea. Pectin comes from apples, bananas, beets, carrots, potatoes, and citrus fruit.

DIETARY FIBER SAMPLER

Apple, with skin (1)	2.8 grams
Avocado (1)	4.7 grams
Banana (1)	1.6 grams
Bran muffin (1)	2.5 grams
Cauliflower, cooked (1/2 cup)	1.0 gram
Figs, dried (1/4 cup)	8.0 grams
Lima beans (1/2 cup)	3.6 grams
Oatmeal (1/2 cup)	1.3 grams
Pinto beans (1/2 cup)	4.8 grams
Peas, cooked (1/2 cup)	3.0 grams
Potato, baked with skin (1 medium)	3.7 grams
Prunes, dried uncooked (1/2 cup)	13.0 grams
Rice, brown long-grained (1/2 cup cooked)	5.4 grams
Whole wheat bread (1 slice)	2.2 grams

Lignin acts as a binder for cellulose. It does not appear to have a major role in preventing constipation or diluting bile acids. However, it has been found to have anti-cancer effects in laboratory animals. Lignin is found in whole grains, nuts, tomatoes, peas, and some fruits.

Gums are sticky fibers derived from plants. Manufacturers use them to thicken many processed foods. Gums lower cholesterol and have anti-cancer effects, although scientists are not sure why. They are found in dried beans, oatmeal, and oat bran.

The National Cancer Institute estimates that Americans now eat an average of 11 grams of fiber daily and recommends doubling that amount. Consuming between 20 and 30 grams of fiber a day could cut your risk of cancer. But eating more than 35 grams daily may cause digestive problems, such as bloating and flatulence. You can avoid these problems by increasing the amount of fiber in your diet gradually. While supplements may furnish some benefits, researchers believe that fiber-rich foods pack a healthier punch.

Antioxidants

These health-boosting vitamins form one of the hottest areas in nutritional research—and fruits and vegetables are their primary source. Antioxidants counteract the oxidizing (burning) effects of free radicals, harmful molecules that can cause cellular damage throughout the body. Besides leading to heart and coronary artery disease by promoting the build-up of plaque in the walls of blood vessels, oxidation may increase your risk of developing health problems as diverse as cataracts and Alzheimer's disease. And oxidation can cause cellular damage that may eventually result in malignancy. Antioxidants can interrupt this process, potentially conferring protection from cancer.

The body produces its own antioxidants that combine with free radicals to help keep the oxidation process in check. But you cannot always count on these internally produced antioxidants to do the whole job, especially when you are exposed to such environmental contaminants as cigarette smoke and polluted air. Several familiar vitamins serve to augment the body's own antioxidants.

Beta-carotene

The more we discover about antioxidants, the more remains to be learned. For example, one of the best known nutrients in our diet is beta-carotene, the pigment that gives the characteristic color to carrots, cantaloupe, and sweet potatoes and is also abundant in leafy green vegetables, such as kale and spinach. But beta-carotene is only one of a number of substances called carotenoids that work in different ways to resist cancer. There are thought to be more than 500 carotenoids. Of these, some 10 percent are converted by the body into vitamin A.

Besides their antioxidant properties, many carotenoids seem to have positive effects on immune function, which can be critical in stopping cancer. Recently, researchers have been focusing on the carotenoids alpha-carotene (in carrots), lycopene (in red fruits and vegetables, such as tomatoes and red peppers), beta cryptoxanthin (in oranges), and lutein and zeaxanthin (in broccoli and leafy green vegetables). People with deficiencies of these substances are more likely to develop certain kinds of cancer, particularly lung cancer, supporting the theory that increased consumption of these carotenoids might protect against cancer. Although much research data gives cause for optimism about the carotenoid's cancer-fighting ability, scientists are still getting mixed signals. For example, the National Cancer Institute announced in 1994 that a study of nearly 30,000 male cigarette smokers had found slightly higher rates of lung cancer in those who took beta-carotene supplements than in those who did not. These unexpected results have sent researchers back to the drawing board to investigate the possibility that some other compound in beta-carotene-rich food is responsible for the protective effect noted in several other studies. (Some researchers feel, too, that this particular study was flawed because the length of time that participants took the supplements was too short to interfere with the development of cancer in long-term smokers.)

Vitamin A

As we have seen, the body turns beta-carotene and some of the other carotenoids into vitamin A. This may explain some of their anti-cancer activities. Vitamin A has been found to be an effective treatment for some cancers, both in the laboratory and in humans. It is only in recent years however, that researchers have begun sorting out the individual effects of vitamin A, beta-carotene, and the other carotenoids.

Because vitamin A plays an important role in normal cell growth, its use in the prevention or treatment of cancer—which is characterized by abnormal cell growth—is quite plausible. Additionally, it's known that vitamin A deficiency can result in decreased production of antibodies to certain diseases and in a decrease in the number of T-lymphocyte cells—the frontline defenses of the immune system.

Vitamin A is a retinoid, a category of drugs that has shown much promise in a number of current chemoprevention studies. Physicians often prescribe retinoids in ointment form to treat acne, and have noted an inhibiting effect on some skin cancers. Experiments with synthetic retinoids are showing protective action against lung, oral, cervical, and skin cancers as well as leukemia.

Beef, liver, eggs, and dairy products contain vitamin A. However, since these are foods generally high in fat and cholesterol, it is probably healthier to get most of your vitamin A via the carotenoids in fruits and vegetables.

Vitamin C

This vitamin—also known as ascorbic acid—has been associated with reduced risks of lung, breast, esophagus, stomach, colon, cervical, and bladder cancers. It also interferes with the formation of potent carcinogens called nitrosamines, and destroys or neutralizes a number of other substances that promote cancer. It works to regenerate vitamin E—another antioxidant—and enhances the immune system. And vitamin C is necessary for the production of collagen, which gives structure to bones, cartilage, muscles, and blood vessels and may help protect the body from cancer by forming a wall around malignant cells.

Although researchers have studied the effects of vitamin C on health for years, much remains unknown about the exact way it works. Recent studies have found that vitamin C alone may not be responsible for anti-cancer properties of certain foods. For example, tomato juice was found to inhibit the formation of nitrosamines even after the vitamin C was removed. Other studies have found that tomato, green pepper, pineapple, strawberry, and carrot juice all have a greater ability to prevent the formation of nitrosamines in the body than the amount of vitamin C they contain would suggest. Two other compounds—p-coumaric and chlorogenic acids—may play an important supporting role as anti-cancer agents. These acids are found in many fruits and vegetables—but not in vitamin C tablets.

Vitamin E

Sometimes referred to as the "premier antioxidant," this vitamin helps protect against cell damage caused by free radicals, interferes with production of nitrosamines, and stimulates the immune system. All three of these actions are important in fighting cancer.

Low levels of vitamin E have been linked to breast, colon, and lung cancer. Researchers have found it may have an especially potent effect against prostate cancer when taken in combination with Adriamycin, a drug commonly used for cancer chemotherapy. In laboratory animals, vitamin E and beta-carotene seem to enhance each other in the treatment of malignancies.

Vitamin E is found in grains, seeds, nuts, and oils made from seeds and nuts (for example, sunflower and peanut oil). Wheat germ is an excellent source of vitamin E.

Synthetic Antioxidants

BHA, BHT, Propyl gallate: If you're a careful reader of ingredient listings, you may have noticed these preservatives on the labels of many packaged foods. One of their primary functions is to prevent the oxidation that takes place when food spoils.

Although synthetic antioxidants are manufactured in a laboratory and do not occur naturally in food, they are still a part of our diet; and it's good to know that these substances that preserve our food may also be preserving our health. As science learns more and more about the behavior of antioxidants and the specific chemical reactions they trigger inside the body, manufacturers may be able to incorporate ever more effective protective agents into our processed foods.

The Facts about Phytochemicals

Although the word "phytochemical" gained recognition with the discovery of certain cancer-fighting compounds, it is actually a global term for all the hundreds of chemicals that are found in plants. Included among the phytochemicals are such scientific tongue-twisters as dithiolthiones,

isothiocyanates, limonene, glycerrhetinic acid, phenols, and protease inhibitors.

Some phytochemicals are common to a wide range of plants. For example, flavinoids, a group of compounds with antioxidant properties, are found in carrots, tea, citrus fruits, berries, broccoli, peppers, squash, tomatoes, soybeans, eggplant, and a variety of other fruits and vegetables. Besides their antioxidant activities, flavinoids seem to be able to inhibit the action of certain hormones such as estrogen, and may help prevent hormone-based malignancies such as breast cancer and prostate cancer.

Likewise, chlorophylls—the chemicals that make green vegetables green—have shown the ability to block the action of certain cancer-causing substances, particularly those that develop when meat is cured or charred.

Research on phytochemicals is pointing to certain vegetables and groups of vegetables that may be particularly valuable cancer fighters. Among the most significant:

Cruciferous Vegetables

No sooner had President George Bush revealed to the American public that he hated broccoli than scientists announced the discovery of a chemical in broccoli called sulforaphane that had a strong preventive effect against cancer in laboratory animals.

Meanwhile, other researchers began reporting that substances called indoles—again, isolated from broccoli and related vegetables—also showed anti-cancer effects in the lab. Specifically, a chemical called indole-3-carbinol changes the way the body processes

IT'S NOT JUST BROCCOLI

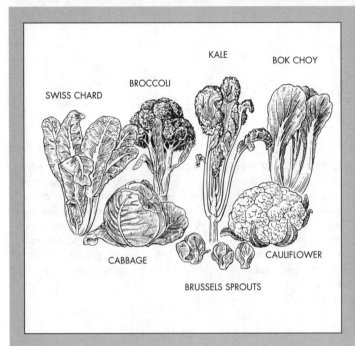

SWISS CHARD

BROCCOLI

KALE

BOK CHOY

CABBAGE

BRUSSELS SPROUTS

CAULIFLOWER

If you're one of those people who can't abide broccoli, don't despair: It shares its beneficial features with other members of a class of plants called cruciferous vegetables. Although their protective power has yet to be firmly proven in humans, laboratory research has shown these vegetables to be richly endowed with compounds that discourage the development of cancer. One, in particular, renders estrogen (suspected of promoting breast cancer) harmless.

Though broccoli and Brussels sprouts are positively loathed by many people, cabbage and cauliflower may be more to their liking. Give bok choy a try, too. This oriental vegetable has a pleasing, un-broccoli-like flavor. Try stir-frying it with mushrooms, garlic, and oyster sauce.

estrogen, a hormone associated with breast cancer, causing it to break down into a more benign substance.

And that's not all. Isothiocyanates—other chemicals present in the broccoli family—have shown the ability to trigger the formation of enzymes that can protect cells against damage from potential carcinogens. Cyanohydroxybutene (CHB) is yet another in the list of chemicals in broccoli that seems to play a role in ridding the body of cancer-causing agents.

Much to the chagrin of our former president, Americans learned that broccoli is even better for us than we had previously thought.

Broccoli is one of a class of vegetables called *brassica*. Other vegetables in this class include cabbage, Brussels sprouts, cauli-

flower, bok choy, Swiss chard, and kale. They are known as cruciferous vegetables because of their cross-shaped flowers. Besides their rich endowment of phytochemicals, cruciferous vegetables are also excellent sources of fiber, beta-carotene, vitamin C, and other vitamins and minerals.

All cruciferous vegetables are not created equal: the amount of sulforaphane and other chemicals they contain varies from vegetable to vegetable and within different batches of the same vegetable. Growing conditions—including weather and soil composition—influence the chemical composition of the

IS THERE A PHYTOESTROGEN IN YOUR FUTURE?

By shouldering aside human estrogen and working in its place, the less harmful phytoestrogens (plant-based estrogens) may cut your risk of estrogen-dependent tumors such as breast cancer. There's also a chance that they could reduce the severity of the symptoms that many women suffer at menopause.

Although the class of phytoestrogens called coumestans can be found in such foods as bean sprouts and sunflower seeds, your best source is soy-based products, which contain the phytoestrogens called isoflavones. Among the leading soy-based foods are:

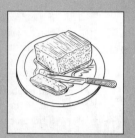

■ **Tofu.** This rubbery substance takes on the flavor of everything around it. You can add it to sauces, casseroles, and soups. It has no cholesterol, little saturated fat, and almost no sodium. A 3-ounce serving weighs in with 50 calories.

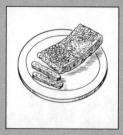

■ **Tempeh.** A nutty-flavored soybean cake, tempeh can be barbecued, added to spaghetti sauce or sloppie joes, or included in stuffing. A 3-ounce serving has 150 calories.

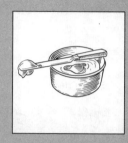

■ **Miso.** This tasty, salty paste adds unique zest to sauces, soups, dressings, and marinades. Fat is no problem, but sodium is high: 600 milligrams per tablespoon.

plants. But even if you can't be certain of the exact levels, you can be assured that cruciferous vegetables provide your body with a variety of tools to help protect you from cancer.

Soybeans and Green Tea

The cancer-fighting prowess of these two staples of the oriental diet derives from isoflavones, a form of flavinoids that occurs in a variety of vegetables, but is particularly concentrated in soybeans and green tea. In

green tea they can account for about 30 percent of the dry weight of the tea leaves. Isoflavones work in two ways against cancer: as antioxidants and as antimutagens, preventing cell mutations which can become malignancies. In animal studies, some isoflavones—called phytoestrols—have also been shown to inhibit production of the estrogen that is thought to stimulate breast cancer.

In soy products, the isoflavone that may pack the greatest punch is a substance called genistein. Laboratory tests show that genistein has the ability to modify cell proliferation and to curb angiogenesis—the process by which tumors grow the new blood vessels that supply them with oxygen and nutrients.

Studies indicate that people who eat a lot of soy-based products decrease their risk of developing certain kinds of cancer. In some Asian countries where soy-based foods are common, rates of breast and prostate cancer are far below the American norm. Now, soy products are becoming popular in the American diet as well. You can find tofu (soy-bean curd) in the produce department of most supermarkets; in the baking goods aisle there is soy flour and soybean oil; and soy-based desserts fill the freezers. Not all soy products may be equally protective, however. Fermented products, such as soy sauce, have a different chemical composition than non-fermented soy and we do not yet know whether this affects the food's anti-carcinogenic properties. Likewise, researchers have yet to establish the exact isoflavone content of the various soy-based products, nor do we know what levels are needed to confer a protective effect.

Garlic and Onions

Like soy, garlic seems to offer a variety of benefits. Although results are still preliminary, researchers are finding that in addition to promoting cardiovascular health, garlic and other members of the allium family (onions, scallions, chives, leeks, shallots) may offer protective benefits against cancer.

A study in a region of China where stomach cancer is unusually common found that the rate among the people who had eaten the most garlic and onions was less than half the rate found among those who rarely consumed these foods. Other studies have shown a link between high consumption of garlic and reduced rates of breast, stomach, and colorectal cancers.

Garlic and its close relatives contain allyl sulfides, which in laboratory tests have been found to increase the production of enzymes that help rid the body of carcinogens. Allyl sulfides also depress the growth of human cancer cells; and garlic has shown the ability to block the production of nitrosamines as well. Both garlic and onion oil have proven beneficial in treating some cases of skin cancer.

Although people have sung the praises of garlic for centuries, serious scientific research is still in its infancy. The many forms of garlic supplements on the market complicate the issue because they are not regulated and vary widely in composition. In addition, depending on growing conditions and individual strains, different batches of fresh garlic differ in their chemistry.

Other Cancer-Fighting Vitamins and Minerals

Although fruits, vegetables, and grains pack the greatest anticancer potential, they are not the only protection that diet affords. Researchers are hard at work investigating several other common dietary elements.

Selenium

Selenium, a mineral resembling sulfur, is essential to our health in small amounts, though potentially toxic in large doses. Since the 1960s, dozens of studies have linked selenium deficiency to cancer. Others have found that groups with high levels of selenium (as measured in blood and other tissue tests) have low cancer rates. Breast, prostate, skin, lung, and gastrointestinal cancers are all inhibited by selenium.

The selenium in our diets comes from fish and shellfish, organ meats, such as liver, and some whole-grain cereals. It is also present in very small amounts in fruits and vegetables grown in selenium-rich soil. Unfortunately it's hard to tell how much selenium you are getting in your diet because levels in selenium-bearing foods can vary widely. There is also a difference of opinion among nutritionists about how much selenium is necessary to protect against cancer. Scientists do agree, however, that there is a large gap between the several hundred micrograms of selenium per day that could have a role in cancer prevention and the several thousand micrograms that would cause toxicity.

Selenium works against cancer in several different ways. It is, first of all, a potent antioxidant. It also helps protect cells from damage, aids damaged cells in repairing themselves, and strengthens the immune system. In addition, selenium seems to boost the antioxidant activities of vitamins A and E.

Calcium and Vitamin D

Calcium is one of the most important minerals in our diet. It is an essential factor in processes ranging from bone formation to transmission of chemical messages within the brain, and regulation of the heartbeat. Vitamin D is necessary for the absorption of calcium. We get vitamin D from sunlight, fortified dairy products, and other food sources, such as oily fish, beef, liver, butter, and eggs. Calcium comes from milk and other dairy products, dark green leafy veg-etables, broccoli, and oily fish such as salmon and sardines.

Population studies have linked high rates of colon and breast cancer to low levels of calcium and vitamin D. These cancers occur less frequently in sunny cities such as Miami and San Antonio, than in northern cities such as Boston and Chicago, where exposure to sunlight is particularly low in winter months, when tall buildings block most of the sun's slanting rays.

Scientists theorize that calcium binds bile and other fatty acids, thereby reducing irritation in the lining of the colon and impeding the rapid growth of cancer cells. Some laboratory tests have shown that vitamin D itself slows cell growth and thus may have cancer-fighting properties of its own.

Most nutritionists insist that food and sunlight are the best sources of calcium and vitamin D. However, exposure to sunlight carries its own skin cancer risks. You must also be careful not to consume too much vitamin D; very high doses can be toxic. Taking antacids with calcium carbonate is one way to supplement calcium in your diet.

B Vitamins and Folic Acid

Some of the B vitamins—particularly B_2 (riboflavin), B_6 (pyridoxine), and pantothenic acid—strengthen the immune system and may play a role in fighting the early development of malignant cells. In some studies, people deficient in riboflavin have developed cancer of the esophagus. In laboratory tests, folic acid, another of the B vitamins, has a protective effect against precancerous cells from the colon and cervix; and women with low levels of folic acid are more likely to develop cervical cancer.

The B vitamins are available in a variety of foods. Citrus fruits are high in folic acid. Red meat, dairy products, asparagus, and broccoli contain riboflavin. Vitamin B$_6$ comes from white meat chicken and fish, whole grain cereals, egg yolks, potatoes, and bananas.

Zinc

Zinc, a metal necessary for many of the chemical reactions that take place in our bodies, helps support immune function. People with throat and prostate cancers are often deficient in zinc. Zinc supplements help fight cancer cells in laboratory animals. Meat, seafood, grains, and vegetables are good sources of this mineral.

Fats Can Be Protective Too

Dietary fat is receiving a great deal of bad publicity. We are constantly told that it is bad for us, that it leads to obesity, heart disease, cancer, and a host of other health problems. Nevertheless, *some* fat is a necessity if our bodies are to function properly. And now there is evidence that certain types of fats may have a protective effect against cancer.

Omega-3 fatty acids from fish oil have an anti-carcinogenic effect in the laboratory. These are the same fats currently under study for their role in preventing heart disease. While fatty fish, such as salmon, mackerel, sardines, herring, anchovies, and bluefish, are the best-known sources for omega-3, our bodies can also manufacture them from linolenic acid, an essential fatty acid found in rapeseed (used to make canola oil), soybeans, spinach, and mustard greens. Research on the role of omega-3s in cancer prevention is still in its early stages.

Oleic acid appears in olive oil, a monounsaturated fat. In laboratory tests, it has been found to have some protective effects against cancer. Several population studies also conclude that people who consume diets high in olive oil have low rates of cancer. The Mediterranean diet, which includes a large daily intake of olive oil, is linked with low rates of both heart disease and cancer.

Conjugated Linoleic Acid (CLA), a form of an essential fatty acid that comes from dairy products and meat, has demonstrated a strong anticarcinogenic effect against breast tumors in a number of laboratory studies. These results have confounded researchers because CLA is an animal fat, ordinarily considered exactly the thing to avoid.

An Extra Boost from Yogurt

Yogurt, like garlic, seems to have mythical health-promoting properties. Yogurt is basically milk fermented by adding bacteria that convert milk sugar (lactose) into lactic acid. Different types of yogurts vary in fat content. A cup of yogurt can contain anywhere from 0 to 11 grams of fat.

Some population studies link high yogurt consumption to reduced risks of cancer, particularly of the breast and colon. Some researchers have also observed that people whose diets include large amounts of yogurt have better immune systems. In animals, *Lactobacillus acidophilus,* a bacteria used to make some brands of yogurt, slows the growth of cancer-causing cells in the colon.

Like all the other cancer-fighting substances in our diet, yogurt offers no guarantees. Still, if colon or breast cancer tends to run in your family, you could do worse than to develop a taste for this increasingly popular food. □

CHAPTER 15

Targeting Specific Cancer Risks

After decades of research, papers, conferences, and head-scratching, scientists have concluded that what we eat contributes to about 60 percent of the cases of cancer in American women and 40 percent in American men. As scary as this may sound, it also provides a wonderful opportunity for prevention, since the reverse is also true: By eating wisely, we can reduce our odds of contracting this most dreaded of diseases.

Researchers have now learned enough about the role that nutrition plays in many forms of cancer to make some very specific recommendations on ways to fend them off. If a certain type of cancer runs in your family, a few highly targeted changes in your diet could, in years to come, literally save your life. Remember, a genetic vulnerability to cancer doesn't make it inevitable. Any nutritional measures you can take against it are well worth the effort.

Basic Rules of Thumb

Whatever type of cancer concerns you, there are a handful of simple guidelines for prevention that apply across the board: Eat more fresh fruits and vegetables, more whole grains, and much less fat than most Americans eat today—and keep your weight in check. (A study of more than a million men and women by the American Cancer Society has shown that obesity leads to higher death rates from cancers of the gallbladder, bile duct, breast, uterus, and ovaries.)

It seems that America's parents were ahead of their time in urging kids to eat their vegetables: Most experts do agree that consuming a lot of vegetables may be one of the best ways to prevent cancer. Those vegetables, though, shouldn't lie on the plate leaking water like a wet bathing suit. They need to be steamed, microwaved, stir-fried, or otherwise cooked in little or no water and served crisp, perhaps with a tasty low-fat sauce.

Scientists continue to debate the value of specific ingredients in foods. For example, some observers of the effects of nutrition are convinced that ingesting more antioxidants

DIETARY RECOMMENDATIONS FROM THE AMERICAN CANCER SOCIETY

■ To reduce your risk of colon cancer: Eat more high-fiber foods (whole grains, fruits, vegetables).

■ To reduce your risk of cancers of the larynx, esophagus, and lung: Eat foods rich in carotene.

■ To reduce your risk of cancers of the esophagus and stomach: Eat foods rich in vitamin C and eat salt-cured, smoked, and nitrite-cured foods only in moderation.

■ To reduce your risk of gastrointestinal and respiratory system cancers: Eat cruciferous vegetables (broccoli, cabbage, Brussels sprouts, cauliflower, kohlrabi).

■ To reduce your risk of cancers of the oral cavity, larynx, and esophagus, and of cirrhosis of the liver (which can lead to liver cancer): Drink alcohol only in moderation.

■ In addition: Cut down on your total fat intake and keep your weight in check.

such as vitamins A, C, and E—in food and in supplements—is the best available answer to preventing cancer and fighting its spread in the body. (Antioxidants combat the oxidation of molecules in cells. For more on these substances, see Chapter 14, "Food That Fights Cancer.")

Other experts remain cautious, pointing out that the benefits of eating fruits and vegetables may be derived from something else they contain. "The jury is still out on antioxidants," says Carolyn Clifford, Ph.D., chief of the Diet and Cancer Branch at the National Institutes of Health. "Some studies have found a slight *increase* in cancers, such as lung cancer, among people taking supplements."

More than 1,000 compounds that may discourage cancer have already been identified; one or more could conceivably be found to pack more anti-cancer power than antioxidants. The bottom line is that in more than 100 research studies, people who ate a lot of fruits and vegetables were only about half as likely to develop cancer as those who rarely ate those foods.

In general, the key to cutting your odds of cancer through nutrition seems to have two components: avoiding foods that help tumors grow and concentrating on foods that fight such growth. Neither route alone is enough. Here's a summary of ways to work toward preventing specific types of cancer with every meal and snack.

Breast Cancer

Breast cancer is greatly feared, and rightly so, as the most common cancer among American women. Your chances of contracting the disease are greater if a close female blood relative has had it. In addition, although breast cancer strikes more women after age 50 than before, thousands of women under 50 are diagnosed with it each year. But whether there is a history of breast cancer in your family or not, you can definitely improve your chances of avoiding it by following a few nutritional rules.

Among the surest findings in decades of research on the relationship of diet to cancer is the specific connection between a high-fat, low-fiber diet and breast cancer. Fat is bad news for a number of reasons that are still being studied. Dietary fat easily becomes body fat; and body fat produces extra estrogen. In turn, high levels of estrogen circulating through the blood can apparently help tumors grow in the breast and reproductive tract.

Fiber interacts with fat as well. It may reduce the body's absorption of fat, in turn reducing it's production of estrogen. Fiber also helps speed cancerous substances that have reached the intestines through and out of the body before they can cause serious damage. (For more on fiber, see the box "Fiber: There's More to the Story than Bran.")

Women who eat extra fiber also rid themselves of more of their excess estrogen in bowel movements rather than in urine. This is important because estrogen in the urine can be reabsorbed into the bloodstream and eventually reach the breasts and other organs vulnerable to hormone-related cancer. Dietary fiber "binds up" estrogen as it enters the small intestine, and may do the same with other cancer-causing agents, preventing them from being absorbed through the intestinal wall into the bloodstream where they can be carried to the breasts.

Other foods defeat the harmful effects of estrogen by displacing it within the body. Plant-based estrogen-like substances in soybeans and soybean products (including tofu) are believed to have a protective effect. Additional foods that seem to deter breast cancer in one way or another include green vegetables, omega-3 fatty acids in oily fish, omega-9 fatty acids in olive oil, wheat bran, and cruciferous vegetables, such as cabbage, bok choy, and Brussels sprouts.

Some studies have found lower rates of breast cancer in geographic areas where the water and food contain ample amounts of selenium. But the authors of *The Doctors' Anti-Breast Cancer Diet,* among many others, advise against taking selenium supplements as a hedge against breast cancer, because it can be toxic in large amounts. Do

consider taking a daily multivitamin, however, containing a modest amount of selenium. The best sources of selenium are foods such as fish (especially sardines), whole wheat, wheat germ, whole grains, mushrooms, asparagus, and garlic.

Vicki L. Seltzer, M.D., writes in *Every Woman's Guide to Breast Cancer,* "At present, dietary modification appears to be in the vanguard of our attempt to decrease the risk of breast cancer, as well as other malignancies and a variety of other serious illnesses."

Here are five ways to protect yourself:

1. Eat a low-fat diet, ideally no more than 20 percent of total calories but certainly no more than 25 percent. Remember that total calories are important, not just fat. Exercise to burn off the excess.

2. Eat foods rich in antioxidants. Consider taking antioxidant supplements as well, especially if you smoke or are under considerable stress. (But beware of overdose.)

3. Keep your waist trim. Studies indicate that the *location* of body fat matters. A waist-to-hip ratio above 0.8 may increase cancer risk. Aim for a "pear shape" rather than an "apple shape."

4. Monitor estrogen levels. Be sure your doctor does periodic blood tests, especially if you take birth control pills.

5. Limit alcohol intake. Alcohol has been linked with breast cancer.

The number of new cases of breast cancer has finally begun to decline. In addition, in January 1994, the National Cancer Institute announced that the death rate from breast cancer in the United States had dropped by almost 5 percent between 1989 and 1992. Experts say that the increased use of cancer drugs and radiation was the main reason for that improvement, but they also cite the contribution of dietary changes. Much of this information was identified through the Surveillance, Evaluation, and End Result (SEER) study, a long-term project of the National Center for Health Statistics. SEER findings are expected to provide a tremendous amount of information about cancer for many years to come.

WHERE DIETARY CHANGES MAKE THE MOST DIFFERENCE

For people at higher-than-average risk of a particular type of cancer, nutritional science now offers specific menu items that can help fend it off.

If breast cancer runs in your family, for instance, consider increasing your intake of fiber, soybean-based foods like tofu, and vegetables in the cabbage family. The fiber helps flush cancer-promoting estrogen from the body; harmless chemicals in the soy products displace estrogen; and the vegetables supply other cancer-inhibiting agents.

Likewise, if the possibility of colon cancer is a special concern, you should boost your intake of fiber and calcium. The fiber binds with potentially cancer-causing chemicals and hurries them through the colon; calcium helps maintain the health of the colon's delicate inner lining.

Other threats that can be discouraged by specific dietary improvements are cancers of the lung, liver, stomach, esophagus, and oral cavity.

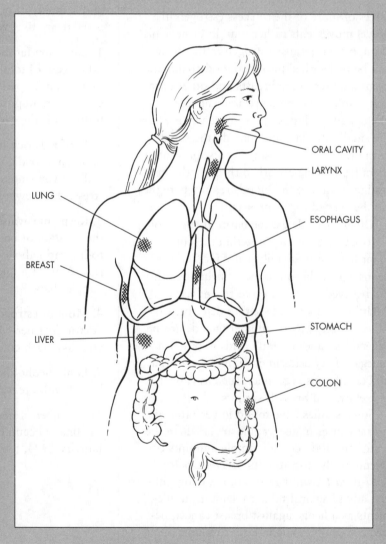

ORAL CAVITY

LARYNX

LUNG

ESOPHAGUS

BREAST

LIVER

STOMACH

COLON

Prostate Cancer

Once unmentionable in public but now much in the limelight, prostate cancer is often fatal unless it's diagnosed in its early stages. The prostate gland, which secretes male seminal fluid, is strongly affected by hormones, so dietary prevention strategies against prostate cancer are similar to those for breast cancer, although research is far from complete.

Some studies suggest that eating foods low in fat and high in antioxidants (especially vitamin A, selenium, and possibly fish oils) and vitamin D provides the most likely nutritional route for lowering the odds of prostate cancer. Fat doesn't seem to *cause* the cancer, but it does promote the growth of tumors once cancer gets started. In particular, keep to a minimum saturated fats such as beef, processed meats, butter, and whole milk.

Since the risk of developing prostate cancer increases if you are overweight, remaining trim and fit should also help reduce your risk. Men who weigh at least 20 percent more than is standard for their height, body type, and age, have a four times greater risk of prostate cancer than men of standard weight. See Chapter 5 for Height/Weight tables.

Colorectal Cancer

The last 5 or 6 feet of the intestine—the colon—join with the 5- to 6-inch rectum to create the large bowel. This is the area referred to in the term "colorectal cancer."

Along with the breast, the colon ranks high among the organs in which the odds of cancer can be dramatically reduced by nutrition. In a field noted for caution and hedging,

a 1991 report by researchers at the University of Southern California, Los Angeles, stated outright, "Dietary changes can reduce the risk of developing large bowel cancer."

As with breast and prostate cancers, a high-fat diet (especially one high in animal fats) increases the risk of colorectal cancer. When a high-fat diet is combined with a low intake of fiber, the risk becomes even greater. Some scientists estimate that if Americans reduced their consumption of animal fats by 50 percent, the number of cases of colon cancer would decrease by the same amount.

A high-fat diet increases the amount of bile acids and bacterial enzymes in the colon, where bacteria can convert them to cancer-causing chemicals. Increasing the amount of fiber in the intestines helps to reverse this effect by diluting or inactivating the chemicals and reducing the level of bile acids and bacteria.

Another important function of fiber is to keep wastes and their cancer-causing byproducts flowing quickly so that they'll leave the body before they have much time to come in contact with the sensitive cells that line the inner walls of the bowel. In a typical American diet, food takes three days or more to pass through the bowel. Eating even less fiber can allow food to remain in the body still longer. With a high-fiber diet, food is eliminated in a day or two.

Most experts recommend about 20 to 30 grams, or just under an ounce, of fiber each day. Most Americans consume only half that amount. One way to get your fiber is to eat a bowl of high-fiber wheat bran cereal every day, or its fiber equivalent. But read labels carefully; most cereals are not high in fiber. You should also increase your consumption of fruits, vegetables, peas, beans, and nuts, all of which supply fiber. Try eating a raw or cooked cruciferous vegetable (cabbage, cauli-

FIBER: THERE'S MORE TO THE STORY THAN BRAN

Most substances in food are digested before they leave the small intestine. The parts that continue through the large intestine undigested are fiber—what earlier generations called roughage.

Once it became clear that eating fiber could apparently help prevent cancers of the colon and breast, cereal companies seized the opportunity to promote their products' cancer-fighting properties. As a result, consumers began to believe that only bran cereals and grains contain fiber. If the Cauliflower Council had had millions to spend on advertising, the public impression of fiber might have been different.

Actually, fiber is present to some degree in a huge variety of plant products. There are two major types, and both can help prevent cancer.

Soluble fiber is found in legumes (peas, peanuts, lentils, and beans, for example), barley, oats, and fruits. Beans and oat bran work particularly well in clearing out the digestive system.

Insoluble (non-dissolving) fiber, which passes through the gastrointestinal tract in more or less its original form, is particularly effective against colon cancer. Excellent sources include vegetables, whole grains, baked goods made with whole wheat, and especially wheat bran.

What's required, as always, is to eat a smorgasbord of produce: not only bran but also whole vegetables, to be sure of gaining all the beneficial compounds waiting inside the fiber.

flower, Brussels sprouts) two or three times a week, as well.

Calcium, in the form of low-fat or nonfat dairy products or in fish with soft, edible bones, such as salmon and sardines, provides another hedge against colon cancer. Calcium is important because it allows the cells that line the colon to reproduce normally. Without enough calcium, the same cells multiply abnormally. Calcium inhibits malignant processes in the bowel in another way, too. When calcium meets with food-derived fats that have reached the bowel, the two materials combine, creating a harmless substance. Be sure to get *at least* the Recommended Daily Allowance of 1,000 milligrams calcium in a combination of food and pill form every day.

Another strong risk factor for colon cancer is the presence of polyps in the large bowel. These small growths on the inner walls, visible through a colonoscope, can turn cancerous over time. If you have polyps, you should try to stick to a low-fat, high-fiber, high-antioxidant diet. Even late in life, modifying your diet can help prevent polyps from becoming cancerous.

One other risk factor that should be noted is alcohol. Heavy drinking may double or triple the risk of colorectal cancer. The higher your risk, based on other factors, the less alcohol you should drink.

Lung Cancer

Lung cancer is a major killer of men and women alike. In fact, it now causes more deaths in American women than breast cancer, partly because breast cancer is being identified early and because treatments for it have grown more successful.

Over and over again, smoking has been shown to be the greatest risk factor for developing lung cancer, though air pollution might also have a role. The surest way for a smoker to cut the risk is to quit. Failing that, however, the next best move is to get plenty of the antioxidant vitamins that are thought to provide some degree of protection to both smokers and nonsmokers. Researchers believe that the most effective antioxidants are vitamin A and the "provitamin" beta-carotene, which becomes vitamin A in the body; other antioxidants are vitamin C, vitamin E, vitamin B_{12}, folic acid, and selenium.

Good food choices to discourage lung cancer include very dark green leafy vegetables (spinach, broccoli, kale), dark orange and yellow fruits (apricots, oranges, cantaloupes) and vegetables (pumpkin, squash, sweet potatoes, carrots), other citrus fruits (grapefruit, limes), soybeans and foods made from them (but not soy sauce), dried beans, tomatoes, and low-fat dairy products. The longer you have smoked, the more fruits and vegetables you need to even begin to offset the cancerous effects on your lungs. Supplements can also help, though not in megadoses that can easily become toxic. Check with your doctor before radically increasing your intake of antioxidant vitamins.

Stomach Cancer

Over the years, scientists have discovered a number of links between diet and stomach cancer. The most notorious dietary culprit is salt. Researchers say that there is a direct connection between stomach cancer and eating a large amount of salty, pickled, or smoked foods (such as smoked meats) as well as foods preserved with salt. The salt irritates the cells in the stomach lining, causing them to reproduce more rapidly than they normally would; salt may also make cancer-causing chemicals even stronger.

It seems that the incidence of stomach cancer in the U.S. dropped as canning and freezing replaced salt-based preservation as the preferred way of keeping food. Unfortunately, the processed foods we've adopted more recently contain so much salt that it once again presents a problem. The risk is heightened by eating too much vitamin-poor junk food and too little fruit and vegetables. Smoking has also been implicated in stomach cancer.

Dietary best bets to help prevent stomach cancer include lots of the following: citrus fruits and other foods containing vitamin C; liver, sweet potatoes, spinach, carrots, and other foods containing vitamin A; cabbage and other cruciferous vegetables; and onions. Those foods have been shown to reduce the risk of cancer by countering cancer-causing chemicals in the stomach, although the reasons aren't clear.

Studies in Italy and China have strongly suggested that garlic is another shield against stomach cancer. A chief biostatistician at the National Cancer Institute says, "The weight of evidence is making it look like garlic really is protective against cancer." One possible reason is that one or more chemical compounds in garlic prevent bacteria from growing in the stomach. Some of those bacteria, if left unchecked, convert food into cancer-causing compounds called nitrosamines.

Other Cancers

When cancer develops in the pancreas, treatment is extremely difficult. Prevention is therefore crucial. Moderate to heavy smokers are two to four times more likely than nonsmokers to get pancreatic cancer. Don't let your food smoke, either: Avoid red meat and cured pork products, such as ham, bacon, and cold cuts.

Eat plenty of fruits, vegetables, beans, peas, and nuts. Citrus fruits, tomatoes, carrots, and dried beans have reaped tremendous praise from researchers for warding off pancreatic cancer. Keep your alcohol intake low and your diet low in fat.

The Oral Cavity, Larynx, and Esophagus

The oral cavity includes the lips, the insides of the cheeks, the gums, the soft palate, the tonsils, and floor of the mouth, and the tongue. The larynx, or voice box, lies just above the windpipe (trachea). The esophagus is the tube leading from the mouth down to the stomach. Esophageal cancer is rare but often fatal when it strikes.

Drinking alcohol and smoking both increase the risk of oral, laryngeal, and esophageal cancers. The two habits together multiply the influence that each has separately. If you chain smoke *and* drink heavily you are many times more likely than a nonsmoker to develop oral and throat cancers.

Deficiencies in vitamin A and the B-complex vitamins, more common among heavy drinkers than among nondrinkers, have been associated with oral cancers. Vitamin C helps protect the cells that line the mouth, larynx, and esophagus against cancer. Eating a balanced diet full of vitamins and minerals while avoiding smoking and drinking is the best known nutritional way to keep these delicate tissues healthy.

PREVENTION AND TREATMENT: SAME MENU?

Nutritional recommendations for cancer prevention and cancer treatment often go hand in hand because they are based on the same clinical findings. "Prevention is just treatment, early," said Daniel Nixon, M.D., director of Cancer Prevention and Control at the Medical University of South Carolina, Charleston. Dietary patterns that promote tumor growth should simply be reversed: If fat intake encourages cancer, for example, then cutting down on fat should "starve" it.

Other experts disagree. They suggest different diets altogether for cancer patients—more fat, for example, to "build them up."

One close observer of the debate is Michael Lerner, president of Commonweal, a health and environmental research institute in Bolinas, California. Lerner, who has studied both mainstream and unconventional views of cancer, has served as a special consultant to the federal Office of Technology Assessment for a congressional study of complementary cancer therapies. In his book *Choices in Healing: Integrating the Best of Conventional and Complementary Approaches to Cancer,* Lerner summarizes the major overlapping recommendations of experts in traditional and nontraditional cancer therapies:

- Eat no more than 30 percent fat (preferably less), including vegetable and polyunsaturated fats;
- Keep your weight within normal range;
- Eat fresh fruits and vegetables every day;
- Eat plenty of fiber in both its major forms: cellulose (typically found in fruits and vegetables) and wheat bran;
- Don't smoke; and
- Drink little or no alcohol.

The Liver

Cancer of the liver has been linked with cirrhosis, a chronic liver disease in which normal tissue is replaced by fibrous tissue, leading to a loss of function. Cirrhosis is a common result of heavy alcohol consumption. One contributing factor may be the additives used in processing alcohol. Another is that people who drink heavily tend to have poor appetites. They don't eat very well and can develop nutritional deficiencies that weaken the liver and many parts of the immune system.

Taking Stock

According to Dr. John Potter, director of the Fred Hutchinson Cancer Center in Seattle, the best evidence available today indicates that vegetables and fruits are the nutritional stars in prevention of most major types of cancer. What benefits most, he says, are the epithelial (surface) cells that line many parts of the body: the lung, bladder, cervix, mouth, larynx, throat, esophagus, stomach, pancreas, colon, and rectum. Ongoing studies are expected to highlight some of those effects more definitively.

Some types of cancer were not included in this chapter because scientific findings are too limited to justify making any claims. Nevertheless, research into dietary culprits in endometrial and cervical cancer, skin cancer, and others is well underway, and could turn up some life-saving information in the coming years.

While studies continue, the best way to prevent cancer is to eat a variety of foods, never concentrating too much on any one kind. Even the noble broccoli, he points out, contains substances that have *stimulated* the growth of tumors in laboratory experiments. If you restrict your diet to a single small group of foods you will run the risk of missing out on important, perhaps still unknown, anti-cancer elements found only in others. □

Fine-Tuning Your Diet for the Stages of Your Life

CHAPTER 16

The Changes to Make When You're Pregnant

As recently as ten years ago it wasn't easy to find good advice on nutrition during pregnancy. It was assumed that a mother's diet would be adequate and that women didn't need to know the details. For generations, when people routinely cooked at home and a typical meal delivered a rich assortment of nutrients, that was probably true. But now that microwave dinners and fast food have become the routine menu for a great many busy families, excellent nutrition can no longer be taken for granted. Developing babies, unfortunately, refuse to fall in with this trend. They still prefer a good, plain, home-cooked meal. Pregnancy provides women with a wonderful incentive to return to the basics.

What does this mean in terms of your daily meal-planning? Here's a quick overview of the major dietary guidelines you need to keep in mind.

Eating For Two in More Ways than One

The primary dietary rule during pregnancy is to eat healthfully *every day*. Quality in the appropriate quantity will never be as important as it is now. You will "eat for two" (or more!) not by doubling your usual amount of food but by accepting primary responsibility for nourishing the two of you.

During pregnancy, your body will work hard to help the baby grow. You'll often feel tired and need the natural boost that an excellent diet can provide. In fact, you'll be doing a lot more than eating for two; you'll be living for two. That's an awesome job. In addition, the growth of your uterus and the extent of its muscular strength during labor will depend in large part on how well you have nourished it. Fuel your engine with the highest octane that's available.

A toddler rejecting food will throw it on the floor or spit it out. The baby in the uterus eats whatever is served. From the moment of conception, your baby's growth and development rely entirely on what you provide. If you eat fresh, well-prepared foods, so will your baby. If you fail to take in crucial vitamins and minerals, the baby will miss them—at a time of development when such a loss can never be corrected. If you smoke, drink, or take medications or drugs, your baby will, too.

Although major body parts exist more or less from the beginning of the baby's development, certain organs and other components take shape at different times: the heart, brain, teeth, and facial features, for example. Some of this growth takes place during the first weeks of pregnancy, before most women even realize they're expecting. That's why it's wise to think carefully about the implications of pregnancy before you conceive. If you want to stop smoking, there will never be a better time. If you drink a fair amount of alcohol, cut down *before* you start the baby.

It takes time to establish the strength you'll need for pregnancy, labor, and the first weeks after delivery. If you plan to breast-feed, you can help insure success by laying in stores of nutrients and fat during pregnancy to aid milk production later.

Where Your Diet Needs a Boost

Our understanding of why it's vital to eat an adequate diet during pregnancy comes from studies showing what happens when women don't. Many

YOUR BABY'S SPECIAL DIETARY DEMANDS

- **The Placenta** inhibits the transportation of fat to the fetus.

- **Vitamin D** helps the mother absorb higher amounts of **calcium** needed for the baby's bone growth.

- **Carbohydrates** are the primary source of energy for development.

- **Iron** stored in baby's liver is needed several months after birth. **Vitamin C** increases absorption.

- **Folic acid** prevents head and spinal cord defects.

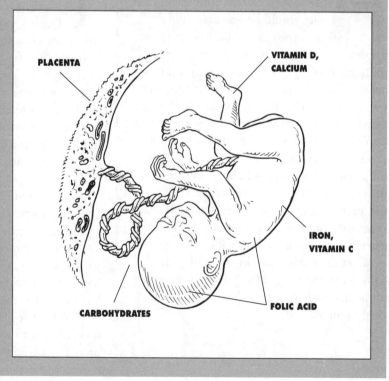

PLACENTA

VITAMIN D, CALCIUM

IRON, VITAMIN C

CARBOHYDRATES

FOLIC ACID

such studies have taken place during times of famine or economic deprivation or among societies where certain foods weren't available at all. Poor nutrition can lead to miscarriage, high blood pressure, and a condition in which the placenta separates from the uterus too early (often requiring an emergency delivery).

From your baby's perspective, a constant influx of nourishing food is crucial. If severely deprived of needed nutrients, the baby's organs might not develop properly. That could lead to potentially serious problems, perhaps persisting for life. Abnormalities in the baby's body at birth may require surgery or even be impossible to correct. Abnormal development can also continue long after birth if the developing baby received an inadequate diet.

If you are pregnant, your diet must include:

Protein. Pregnancy increases your protein requirements, but by how much is controversial. Some say you need 27 percent more protein than usual; others, 50 percent more. One standard pronouncement is to eat 50 grams a day during the first trimester (three months) and 60 grams a day for the rest of your pregnancy.

Contrary to what many people tell pregnant women, protein should still represent no more than 15% of their total diet, according to Dr. Judith B. Roepke. Roepke, a registered dietitian and professor of home economics at Ball State University, is also a consultant to the board of La Leche League International, a breastfeeding advocacy group. She notes that most sources of protein are high in fat, and therefore detrimental to your own health. Since fat is not transported well across the placenta, she observes, most of the fat you eat won't benefit the baby either.

For the protein you do need to take in, the best sources include beans, grains, meat, milk, yogurt, and tofu. Two small cubes of cheddar cheese contain the same amount of protein as a small glass of milk.

Carbohydrates. Whole-grain breads, cereals, pasta, rice and other carbohydrates provide the primary source of energy for the developing baby. Carbohydrates also insure that the body uses protein efficiently. Roepke recommends keeping your diet high in carbohydrates, modest in protein, and low in fat.

Vitamins and minerals. Pregnancy increases the body's need for vitamins and minerals. But, as with other supplements and medications, more is not necessarily better. Large amounts (megadoses) of many vitamins and minerals can be worse than taking none at all. Check with your doctor about any supplements you plan to take.

Iron. The baby draws on the mother's iron reserves, storing enough in its liver to last for several months after birth. This protects the baby against iron deficiency while living on breast milk, which contains very little iron. Most prenatal vitamin tablets contain more than enough iron to meet your needs. Another good way to add it to your diet is to use iron cooking pots. Some of the iron is absorbed by food as it cooks, increasing iron content by 3 to 30 times. Because vitamin C helps your body absorb iron, taking an iron pill with a glass of orange or grapefruit juice increases its effectiveness. Don't take iron with milk, though, which has the opposite effect.

VITAMINS AND MINERALS: YOUR DAILY NEEDS

Vitamins	During Pregnancy	During Breastfeeding	
		First 6 months	7-12 months
Vitamin A	800 (micrograms)	1300 (micrograms)	1200 (micrograms)
Thiamine (B₁)	1.5 (milligrams)	1.6 (milligrams)	1.6 (milligrams)
Riboflavin (B₂)	1.6 (milligrams)	1.8 (milligrams)	1.7 (milligrams)
Niacin (B₃)	17 (milligrams)	20 (milligrams)	20 (milligrams)
Vitamin B₆	2.2 (milligrams)	2.1 (milligrams)	2.1 (milligrams)
Vitamin B₁₂	2.2 (micrograms)	2.6 (micrograms)	2.6 (micrograms)
Vitamin C	70 (milligrams)	95 (milligrams)	90 (milligrams)
Vitamin D	10 (micrograms)	10 (micrograms)	10 (micrograms)
Vitamin E	10 (milligrams)	12 (milligrams)	11 (milligrams)
Folate	400 (micrograms)	280 (micrograms)	260 (micrograms)
Minerals			
Calcium	1200 (milligrams)	1200 (milligrams)	1200 (milligrams)
Iron	30 (milligrams)	15 (milligrams)	15 (milligrams)
Magnesium	320 (milligrams)	355 (milligrams)	355 (milligrams)
Phosphorus	1200 (milligrams)	1200 (milligrams)	1200 (milligrams)
Zinc	15 (milligrams)	19 (milligrams)	16 (milligrams)

Recommended Dietary Allowances during normal pregnancy and breastfeeding

Source: Food and Nutrition Board, National Research Council, Institute of Medicine, Recommended Dietary Allowances, 10th ed, 1989

Folate (also called folic acid or folacin). Inadequate folate during the first 4 weeks of pregnancy (before many women even realize they're pregnant) appears to produce neural tube defects in the fetus. These are serious, even fatal problems, to be avoided if at all possible. The baby's head may not develop, so that the baby is never really alive. Or the baby may have spina bifida, which is an incompletely closed spinal cord. The U.S. Centers for Disease Control and Prevention recommend that *all* women old enough to become pregnant should consume 0.4 milligrams of folate every day, either through diet or with a vitamin pill. The protection supplied by folate is especially important before conception and during early pregnancy. Folate isn't stored in the body for very long, so it must be replaced every day. Pregnant women need to be make sure they keep getting enough because they excrete four to five times the normal amount. To get enough folate in your diet, eat plenty of greens, remembering that the word "folate" comes from the same Latin root as "foliage:" *folium,* or "leaf." The many other good sources include orange juice, brewer's yeast, soybeans and other beans, cauliflower, and whole-grain breads and cereals.

Calcium. All women need calcium, and pregnant women need more. During the second and third trimesters, you need to increase your body's calcium stores to draw on while breastfeeding. At the beginning, the baby's calcium requirement is small, but teeth and bones need calcium when they start to form at 4 to 6 weeks after conception. By week 25, when the baby's bone growth is in full swing, your calcium requirements will have more than doubled. To absorb calcium, the body needs vitamin D. You get it from the sun, from fortified milk, and from vitamin supplements.

You don't like milk or can't digest it? No problem. Rich sources of calcium include broccoli, leafy vegetables (spinach and collard greens), legumes (soybeans, peanuts, pinto beans, black beans), and certain fish. A cup of cooked broccoli has two-thirds the calcium content of a glass of milk. A cup of cooked salmon, sardines, or garbanzo beans (chickpeas) contains more calcium than a glass of milk. Half a cup of ground sesame seeds contains twice the calcium of a glass of milk! Try cooking with tahini, a sesame paste used in such tasty Middle Eastern dishes as hummus, a chickpea dip or spread.

Fiber and fluids. Eating whole grains and raw vegetables and fruits will help prevent constipation. Drink a lot of fluids, especially water. You'll flush out your system and aid digestion and elimination.

A note about salt. The greatly increased amount of fluid carried around inside a pregnant woman dilutes the salt in her body. While eating a tremendous amount of salt is never wise, especially in anyone with high blood pressure, concentrating on low-sodium foods is not necessary during pregnancy. It might even be harmful if taken to an extreme. Experts now recommend that you salt food to taste during your pregnancy.

What Your Diet (Probably) Shouldn't Include

If it's important to keep your diet as healthy as possible while you are pregnant, it's just as vital to avoid those contaminants, additives, and harmful environmental effects that can hurt your baby. You must also watch out for certain foods that might be perfectly okay when you're not pregnant, but are a good idea to avoid when carrying a child.

Additives and Contaminants
There's no firm evidence that the additives in processed foods cause any harm to a developing baby. But if there's even a remote possibility, why gamble? Eating basic, natural food for nine months really isn't that much of a hardship. If you want to be absolutely certain of your baby's safety, avoid chemicals, dyes, and additives.

To dispense with surface contaminants, such as pesticides, wash and wipe dry all fresh fruits and vegetables just before preparing them. Peel off any waxed coverings on cucumbers and other fruits and vegetables. Seek greater variation in the foods you eat.

Fresh foods at farm stands are less likely to have been sprayed for a long shelf life than those in supermarkets.

Don't eat fish that may have been caught from lakes or rivers contaminated by PCBs (polychlorinated biphenyls). Avoid exposure to industrial chemicals and pesticides. Be alert for substances at your workplace that might cause birth defects. Under federal law, a pregnant woman in such a situation must be reassigned at her request.

Alcohol

Alcohol ranks third among the congenital conditions associated with mental retardation—and it is the only preventable one. Babies of mothers who consume too much alcohol, especially six or more drinks a day, are prone to fetal alcohol syndrome (FAS), sadly found in one out of every 750 babies born in the U.S.

Signs of FAS besides mental retardation include:

- Too little growth before birth (intrauterine growth retardation)
- Premature birth
- Low birthweight
- Growth deficiencies in infancy and childhood
- A combination of certain facial features: small eyes, flat nose, drooping eyelids, and crossed eyes
- Ten times the number of babies born with FAS have other problems caused by their mothers' drinking of alcohol. The Institute of Medicine sets as a maximum daily amount 2 to 2-and-a-half ounces of alcohol, 8 ounces of table wine, or 2 cans of beer. A *one-time binge can be as harmful as steady drinking throughout the pregnancy.*

Because the effects of alcohol are most serious in the first 2 months of pregnancy, when the baby's organs are developing, women who are even considering becoming pregnant should take no more than an occasional glass of beer or wine or a very small mixed drink—if that. Many doctors and nutritionists feel strongly that the safest route is to avoid alcohol completely, even for cooking, during pregnancy and for months before it might occur. Drinking heavily while pregnant can also trigger a miscarriage.

All this doesn't mean that having indulged in a few isolated glasses of wine before you learned you were pregnant should ring loud alarm bells. If you're concerned, tell your doctor exactly how much you drank to find out whether it could have made any difference.

Tobacco

Babies tend to be small if their mothers smoked during pregnancy. Breathing the smoke puffed by others (passive smoke) is almost as bad—and the developing baby breathes it as much as the mother. Smoking doubles the risk of miscarriage, especially in the first trimester. It also doubles the chances of third-trimester bleeding. Nicotine speeds up the baby's heart, interrupts its breathing and interferes with its nutrition. As blood vessels constrict in the placenta, less oxygen and fewer nutrients reach the fetus. Every cigarette preempts 250 milligrams of vitamin C as well as smaller amounts of folate, thiamin, and calcium. It has been estimated that if no

COUNTING UP YOUR CAFFEINE LOAD

	Number of milligrams of caffeine
Coffee (5 fluid ounces)	
Drip, automatic	137
Drip, nonautomatic	124
Percolated, automatic	117
Percolated, nonautomatic	108
Instant, regular	60
Instant, decaffeinated	3
Tea	
Black, imported, brewed 5 minutes (6 fluid ounces)	65
Black, U.S., brewed 5 minutes (5 fluid ounces)	46
Green, brewed 5 minutes (5 fluid ounces)	31
Decaffeinated, brewed 5 minutes (6 fluid ounces)	1
Chocolate	
Baker's brand baking chocolate (1 ounce)	25
Sweet dark chocolate candy (1 ounce)	20
Milk chocolate candy (1 ounce)	6
Chocolate milk (8-ounce glass)	5
Cup of cocoa (6-ounce cup)	5
Soft drinks (12 fluid ounces)	
Mountain Dew	54
Coca-Cola	45
Pepsi-Cola	38
RC Cola	36
Nonprescription drugs (standard dose)	
Weight-control aids	168
Diuretics	167
Alertness tablets	150
Analgesic and pain relief tablets	41
Cold and allergy remedies	27

Adapted from "Caffeine: How Little, How Much for You and Your Family?", American Dietetic Association, (booklet) 1988.

one smoked, there would be 10 percent fewer infant deaths and 25 percent fewer low-birthweight babies in the United States each year. Quitting smoking—even toward the end of pregnancy—will benefit your baby.

Caffeine

The Food and Drug Administration recommended in 1980 that women avoid caffeine during pregnancy. That pronouncement still hasn't convinced all experts, some of whom say you'd have to drink inhuman amounts to make a difference. Yet caffeine is a drug that provides no benefits to the developing baby and may do harm. The continuing question revolves around how much you'd have to drink (in coffee, tea, or cola), eat (in chocolate), or otherwise swallow (in "wake-up" pills or candies and certain headache remedies) before anything bad happens.

Possible effects of large amounts include premature birth and stillbirth. Drinking more than 400 milligrams (four cups) a day—that's virtually every day, not just once—may prevent the fetus from growing properly. One recent study suggests that the risk of having a miscarriage can be increased by drinking as little to one to three cups of coffee a day. Caffeine can also interfere with conception, so cutting back is important for women who want to become pregnant, too.

Many doctors will say it's okay to drink up to two cups (not mugs) of regular coffee (not espresso), or the equivalent amount of caffeine in another form (see table nearby), each day. That's around 200 milligrams of caffeine daily. To be sure, relishing an occasional cup of coffee or tea or a small chocolate bar won't do your baby any harm. But if you're accustomed to drinking coffee or tea all day long, it is advisable to switch to the decaffeinated type (slowly, to prevent withdrawal symptoms). Consider these reasons:

- Non-diet colas and other sodas containing caffeine also contain sugar, which fills your body with empty calories and temporarily reduces your interest in eating something nutritious.
- Many diet sodas contain an artificial sweetener called aspartame, sold under the brand name NutraSweet. There's no proof that this is harmful, except in huge amounts in rats; but why take *any* risk?
- In both mother and baby, caffeine speeds up the heartbeat. The possible effects of very large amounts include heartbeat irregularities, ulcers, and high blood pressure.
- Caffeine has physical effects similar to some natural symptoms of pregnancy, such as anxiety, sleep disturbances, headache, and stomach ache. Pregnant women need as many good nights' sleep as they can get. With a jittery baby, rest becomes harder to achieve.
- Coffee and tea are diuretics, causing the body to lose fluids rather than retain them. Yet the pregnant body needs increased fluids.
- Sensitivity to caffeine may increase during pregnancy.
- Sensitivity may also grow with age, so that the two factors together may increase the wallop a cup of coffee packs for older pregnant women.
- Coffee creates acid in the stomach, an environment already ripe for nausea and vomiting during pregnancy.

What about herbal teas? Most standard brands are fine, but watch what you sip. Caffeine isn't the only potential culprit. Some teas sold in health food stores contain plant matter that might be harmful to the baby or to you. Examples are sassafras and mistletoe. If the tea is suspect or its contents are poorly labeled, don't drink it.

How Much Weight to Gain

Doctors have flip-flopped for generations about how many pounds a pregnant woman should gain. It is generally agreed that both too little and too much weight should be avoided. Just what that means is subject to interpretation.

The current thinking is that if your weight is normal for your height you should gain 25 to 35 pounds during pregnancy. If you were underweight to begin with, you should gain more (28 to 40 pounds); if overweight, less (15 to 25 pounds). Women carrying twins may gain 35 to 45 pounds, averaging a gain of 1-and-a-half pounds a week in the last 6 months. Twins and triplets are usually born 2 to 3 weeks before the due date and should be helped to grow as big as possible, within reason, before delivery.

The usual breakdown for weight gain is 2 to 4 pounds in the first trimester and three-quarters to 1 pound a week in the second and third. The fastest weight gain usually takes place from weeks 24 to 32, when your appetite increases.

More than half of your total gain consists of the baby, enlarged uterus, placenta, and extra fluids. At delivery, about 10 1/2 pounds will come out: 7 1/2 pounds for the baby, 1 pound for the placenta, and 2 pounds for amniotic fluid—the liquid surrounding and protecting the baby in the uterus. The remaining weight you put on includes 4 to 6 pounds of fat and nutrient

WHERE THOSE EXTRA POUNDS RESIDE

Just prior to delivery, a typical mother has put on 25 to 35 pounds. Here's where the extra weight is found.

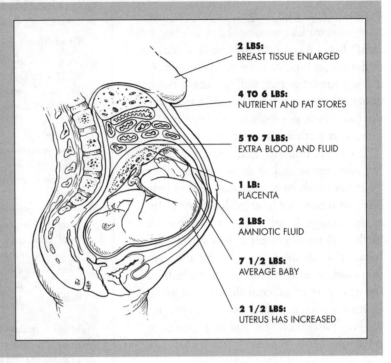

2 LBS:
BREAST TISSUE ENLARGED

4 TO 6 LBS:
NUTRIENT AND FAT STORES

5 TO 7 LBS:
EXTRA BLOOD AND FLUID

1 LB:
PLACENTA

2 LBS:
AMNIOTIC FLUID

7 1/2 LBS:
AVERAGE BABY

2 1/2 LBS:
UTERUS HAS INCREASED

stores, 5 to 7 pounds of extra blood and fluid accumulated during pregnancy, a uterus that has grown to 2 1/2 pounds in giving the baby a home, and 2 pounds of enlarged breast tissue.

By 6 months after delivery, you typically will retain about 3 extra pounds. Breastfeeding, which burns lots of calories and fat, can help melt away some of the pounds. A word on breastfeeding follows later in this chapter.

If you need to lose weight. Women for whom excess pounds are a problem should make a real effort to lose weight before becoming pregnant. Being overweight increases the risk of developing certain problems during pregnancy, such as high blood

pressure and gestational diabetes (discussed later). These conditions in turn may cause the baby to grow too large to be born vaginally or may trigger other potentially dangerous situations. Too much weight can prolong labor and even lead to a cesarean section in a woman who might otherwise not have needed one. Medical experts speculate that fat accumulated between the muscle fibers of the uterus, blocks them from contracting hard enough to expel the baby.

Nevertheless, *do not diet during pregnancy.* A developing baby can't "live off its mother's fat," but requires an ample supply of fresh foods in order to grow. Advance planning and dieting are best. During pregnancy, follow your doctor's advice about weight gain or ask for the name of a professional dietitian if you think that would help.

If you need to gain weight. Maybe a pregnant woman, like anyone else, can't be "too rich," but she can definitely be too thin. An underweight mother is more likely to have a small baby, but that will *not* make delivery easier for you; it just makes life harder on the baby. Infants weighing less than 5 1/2 pounds at birth are subject to many ills.

If you are underweight, you are more likely to be anemic and to deliver prematurely. Your baby will be at increased risk of being born with heart or lung problems or even brain damage. Death within a few weeks of birth is 30 times greater in low-birthweight babies than in larger ones. If you are a very thin woman who intends to start a baby in the next year or so, consult a doctor and gain some weight before becoming pregnant. Adding a little body fat will help you conceive, too.

Best Ways to Deal with Your Diet

A nonpregnant woman of average height and weight needs about 2,200 calories a day. During the second and third trimesters (last 6 months) of pregnancy, her energy requirements increase by about 15 percent, creating the need for an additional 300 calories a day.

Those extra calories are not a "bonus" to add thoughtlessly. Nearly every bite you take should be calculated to create a strong, healthy baby and fortify your own body. If you don't watch your food intake from the beginning, you may gain too much weight by

GETTING 300 CALORIES EXTRA: HERE'S A FEW OF THE WAYS

Food Item	Calorie Count
1 cup cooked pasta	155
1 2 1/2-inch tomato	23
1/2 cup 1 percent milk	51
1 medium apple	81
Total	**310**
4.5-ounce salmon steak, cooked	233
1 cup cooked asparagus	44
1/2 cup strawberries	22
Total	**299**
1 large boiled egg	80
1 cup shredded raw carrots	48
1 medium orange	62
1 baked potato	98
1/2 cup cooked green beans	22
Total	**307**
1/2 cup cooked brown rice	116
1/2 cup blueberries	40
1/2 cup low-fat cottage cheese	102
1 slice fresh pineapple	41
Total	**299**
1 cup orange juice	110
1/2 cup cooked lentils	106
1 medium banana	100
Total	**316**
2 slices pork shoulder	275
1/2 cup cooked cabbage	10
1 cup Romaine lettuce	10
Total	**295**
4 ounces cooked lean beef	230
1/2 cantaloupe	92
Total	**322**

the end of the second trimester and be instructed to start eating more thoughtfully. Instead, do it from the start.

You don't have to install a calculator next to your plate to monitor your calorie intake. Just remembering which of your favorite foods can be enjoyed in large quantities and which must be restricted is sufficient to keep your weight at acceptable levels while making sure you never go hungry or feel deprived.

Nutritional value is a vital consideration. Here's an example. White bread contains 70 percent to 80 percent less of the important B vitamins than whole-wheat bread. In addition, whole-wheat bread contains lots of fiber, which promotes digestion, aids bowel movements, protects against some forms of cancer, and at 67 calories per slice is a relative dietary bargain. Which will you choose?

As for those 300 extra calories a day, consider the combinations shown in the nearby box. Each group represents about 300 calories (the numbers aren't precise). As you can see, they add up to approximately one meal or two or three snacks each day.

Letting Yourself Go (a Little)

Your body is changing, your life is changing—why not your eating habits? Listen attentively to your body's signals. As soon as you feel hungry or thirsty, eat or drink. Having small, frequent meals improves bowel regularity, reduces morning sickness, and sends a constant flow of nutrients to the baby.

Stash nourishing, nonperishable tidbits wherever you spend time, including at work or even in the car. Good choices include small

WHAT TO EAT, CUT BACK, AND CUT OUT

Foods to focus on:	Have at least this many servings per day:
A full rainbow of fresh fruits and vegetables, sometimes raw and never overcooked; each color represents at least one important nutrient	
Dark green, dark yellow	1
Rich in vitamin C (citrus, tomato)	2
Other	2
Whole-grain breads and cereals	4
Milk and other dairy products	4
Other sources of protein (poultry, meat, eggs, fish)	2
Nuts, seeds, beans	2
Water, juices (not sugared juice drinks)	Eight 8-ounce glasses

Take in moderation:

Alcohol	Fat
Caffeine	Sugar

Avoid altogether:

Nicotine and smoke, including passive smoke (from other people)

Any drugs not prescribed or approved by your doctor

Food additives (chemicals, dyes) to the greatest extent possible; read food labels carefully

boxes of raisins and packets of other dried fruit. People instinctively make allowances for pregnant women's eating habits. Have fun taking advantage of your special time. You may not want to wolf down a slab of cold meatloaf during a business meeting, but you can nibble a few grapes or crackers with peanut butter at your desk before it starts.

TRY THESE VITAMIN-RICH SNACKS

■ **Sesame seeds,** which contain vitamins B2, B6, and E as well as a remarkable amount of calcium.

■ **Baked potatoes,** each of which provide an ounce of protein; fiber, especially in the skin; minerals such as calcium, iron, Vitamins B1, B2 and B9; and seven times the vitamin C of an apple.

For a warming, filling meal or snack at any time of day, bake a few potatoes and store them in the refrigerator. Steam and refrigerate some fresh chopped broccoli as well. When hungry, sprinkle broccoli over a potato and heat. Then plop some plain yogurt on top for a power-house potato plate that is low in calories!

Know what times of day (or night) hunger tends to strike, and be prepared.

Don't hesitate to be different. Breakfast on vegetable soup, hot or cold, if it appeals to you. Pour out two big bowls of whole-grain cereal with fruit and lowfat milk for your supper. Don't force yourself to eat anything that repels you; alternatives exist for every necessary nutrient.

The Right Way to Snack

Probably because of its overuse in commercials for junk foods, snacking has gotten a bad name, but pregnant women should snack often, particularly in the latter half of pregnancy. Here's how nutritionist Roepke outlines an optimal diet for the mother-to-be: breakfast, snack, lunch, snack, dinner, snack,

snack. What makes all the difference is the content of those snacks.

Anyone who's in a snacking mood wants to grab something fast. She doesn't feel like making a salad from scratch, although she might eat one if it already existed. The key is to prepare healthful snacks in advance. It's easy to scrub carrots and cut up zucchini, broccoli, and celery while doing other things in the kitchen. Fresh vegetables, herbed yogurt dip, and fruit juices become as "instant" as cookies and soda if they stand waiting and ready. Keep a few hard-boiled eggs on hand, too.

What About Vitamin and Mineral Supplements?

A supplement is nutrition from something other than food, usually in the form of a pill. Opinions on the value of supplements for pregnant women are mixed. Some people insist that women can get all the nourishment they need from food, except perhaps iron and folic acid. But that assumes all pregnant women eat five servings of fresh fruits and vegetables a day, plenty of protein, lots of fiber, half a gallon of fluid, and so on—unrealistic for many.

It's accepted that supplements are important for women who are malnourished, severely underweight, greatly stressed, or "run down," as well as those who routinely ate an unbalanced diet before conceiving. Pregnant teenagers, who are still growing, need supplements as well. Pregnant women who have previously had twins or triplets or who have had a miscarriage or stillbirth are believed to benefit from taking supplements.

Pregnant women who drink or smoke heavily, who must take medication for a chronic condition, or who are unable to digest wheat, cow's milk, or other key foods need supplements to maintain enough vitamins and minerals to nourish their babies. Healthy women who eat no meat have certain needs during pregnancy that only supplements are likely to provide.

After considering your individual situation, your doctor will suggest—or insist—that you take vitamin and mineral supplements. This might be in the form of a prenatal multivitamin taken once a day, as is the case for some 90 percent of pregnant women in the United States; as an iron or calcium pill taken by itself; or a combination. Results of blood tests and other medical assessments will contribute to the decision.

Relief from the Problems of Pregnancy

Even normal, healthy pregnancies tend to involve at least a little discomfort. Some of this is related to eating and may be relieved by diet. Here are some cures for the most common.

Morning sickness. While most women who suffer nausea and vomiting during pregnancy—and many never do—usually feel worst in the morning, symptoms can strike at any time of day. Although that experience typically occurs during the first three months of pregnancy, it can stop sooner or, more rarely, continue much longer.

Morning sickness has accompanied pregnancy for so many centuries that women have been driven to seek their own solutions. None of the following can harm you, and most will help in other ways. Try each of them until something works.

- Eat small, frequent meals, so that your stomach never contains a huge amount of food.
- Drink a lot of liquids to keep your digestive system active.
- Stay away from whatever "trigger foods" make you gag, such as rich, creamy, spicy, or greasy foods. Try to avoid odors that repel you, such as cigarette smoke or fried food.
- Don't drink coffee, which stimulates the secretion of stomach acid, already higher during pregnancy.
- Eat a high-protein snack shortly before bedtime to stabilize your blood sugar.
- Keep dry crackers or cereal next to your bed and nibble some before you get up in the morning. The dry food will absorb stomach acid that has built up overnight.
- Get out of bed slowly. Air out your bedroom frequently.
- Take your iron supplements 1 hour before a meal or 2 hours after it.
- Pour boiling water over a slice of raw ginger and sip slowly. Or buy ginger capsules at a health food store and take one daily.
- Increase your intake of vitamin B_6, contained in wheat germ, liver, kidney, oatmeal and other whole-grain cereals and breads, bananas, nuts and seeds, bran, and green leafy vegetables.

Heartburn. As the growing baby presses against your stomach, acid can be forced up into your esophagus. The burning sensation you may feel in your chest and throat after meals—especially toward the end of pregnancy, when the uterus is at its largest—can be most unpleasant.

Eat smaller meals, eat them slowly, and chew them well, especially raw fruits and vegetables. Avoid beans and other gassy foods. Don't lie down for at least an hour after any meal, to allow enough time for the digestive process to get into gear. At night, elevate your head and shoulders with pillows.

Wear loose clothes. To pick something off the floor, bend your knees rather than bending over. Ask your doctor if you may chew or swallow ordinary antacids. Some contain calcium, needed more during pregnancy.

Constipation and gas. Large amounts of a hormone called progesterone surging through the pregnant body slow down natural bowel contractions, making bowel movements more difficult. Methods for correcting this uncomfortable problem are no different for pregnant women than for anyone else.

Eat lots of fiber, found in bran, raw vegetables, fresh fruits, prunes, and figs. Drink at least eight 8-ounce glasses of fluid a day. Prune juice is a time-honored friend of the constipated. Another remedy: Boil water, pour it into a cup, add a slice of lemon or a few drops of lemon juice, and sip.

Walk up to 2 miles, or at least around the block, every day. Exercise flexes the intestinal muscles as well as those in the legs. Go to the bathroom promptly when nature calls, taking something to read or a crossword puzzle. Since iron tends to be constipating, ask your doctor if your iron supplements can be adjusted. Don't take any laxatives without your doctor's permission.

Hemorrhoids. As the uterus presses against the veins in the rectum, they can become sore and enlarged, especially toward the end of pregnancy. These are hemorrhoids. You're more likely to have them during pregnancy if you've had them before.

Even if a bowel movement won't move, try to relax rather than straining. Be patient; eventually, gravity will help out. Warm soaks in the bathtub are soothing. Pain-killing

creams, stool softeners, or appropriate suppositories may help, if your doctor approves.

A few of the more serious complications of pregnancy can also be helped by your diet. Seek advice from your doctor if you face any of the following:

Gestational diabetes. About 2 to 3 percent of women in the U.S. develop diabetes during pregnancy. It usually disappears after delivery, although many of those women develop diabetes again later in life.

Your doctor will test your blood throughout pregnancy for conditions such as this. If you develop gestational diabetes, you will need to follow the instructions of an expert in the field, such as a diabetologist, endocrinologist, or an internist or obstetrician-gynecologist who has special training. Women with gestational diabetes are given strict advice about their diets, especially the amount of sugar they eat. They learn to obtain and test samples of their own blood every day with a device available in drugstores.

Once the condition is under control, the doctor keeps track of the baby's size. If the child is getting too large, a cesarean section before the due date may be necessary.

Cravings. Variations on the old pickles-and-ice-cream theme have supplied millions of husbands with stories about their pregnant wives' demands for unusual foods in the middle of the night. It's true that pregnancy affects the tastebuds, making some foods and smells irresistible and others revolting. If what you yearn for is an ordinary food that won't hurt in moderation, go ahead.

Less common but far from unique is the confusing compulsion to eat substances such as white clay and laundry starch. Such a habit could signal iron-deficiency anemia. If it happens to you, don't be embarrassed—just talk with your doctor.

Bed rest. If your pregnancy is considered at high risk for certain reasons such as vaginal bleeding, high blood pressure, or a previous miscarriage, you may be told to lie on your left side pretty much all the time. This can last for a couple of days or go on for months. To deal with the lack of appetite, constipation, inability to get up and cook, and other diet-related complications of lying still, consider consulting a dietitian who specializes in such conditions. An organization called Sidelines provides advice to bed resters nationwide (see The Directory of Support Groups at the end of the book).

Breastfeeding: Nourish Yourself to Nourish your Baby

Breast milk is often called the perfect food for the baby. It's perfect for the mother, too, since she doesn't have to buy it, cook it, store it, or clean up after it. What she does have to do is create it, and that requires a healthy diet.

Human milk supplies enough carbohydrates, fat, protein, and most minerals to meet your infant's needs. You'll need a fair amount of extra vitamin A, C, and niacin and a little more vitamin E, thiamin, and riboflavin. Iron supplements are usually a good idea.

Although nature has contrived it so that even a mother who doesn't eat very well will make nourishing breast milk, she will feel fatigued, irritable, and "drained" in more ways than one. Furthermore, she's unlikely to make as much milk as if she were well-fed and relaxed. The typical result is a hungry, cranky baby whose discomfort may worry the mother into switching to formula.

The answer is to pay at least as much attention to the quality and quantity of your food as you did while pregnant. While being underweight may produce an inadequate supply of milk, being overweight can no longer harm the baby. As a new mother, your priority needs to be health, not looks. Just don't overeat to an extent you'll regret later on. You can compensate with certain postpartum exercises as soon as a couple of weeks after delivery, if you're feeling up to it. Actual dieting, however, should wait until the baby is at least 6 weeks old, and then be done in consultation with your doctor.

A vegetarian who breastfeeds needs to pay special attention to calcium, riboflavin, and thiamin. She may need B_{12} supplements to prevent anemia in herself and her baby. As always, the high-quality protein she needs can be found in grains, nuts, vegetables, beans, and dairy products.

How Much Fluid?

To make enough milk and remain hydrated herself, a nursing mother needs to drink at least 2 quarts of fluid every day—more in hot weather. Exactly what those fluids consist of is up to you, as long as they're good for you. Keep a supply of lowfat milk and a variety of fruit juices in the refrigerator and indulge often. Many women pour themselves a tall glass of milk, juice, or water on the way to each nursing session. You have to replace the approximately 23 ounces of milk your baby will drink every day.

One substance you'll need a great deal of is calcium. If you can't or won't drink milk, eat a lot of other calcium-rich foods (listed elsewhere in this chapter). The table "Vitamins and Minerals: Your Daily Needs" lists recommended vitamin and mineral requirements for nursing mothers during the first and second 6 months of breastfeeding. If your diet doesn't provide enough vitamin D (dairy products), vitamin B_{12} (meat), or iron, your doctor may prescribe a supplement. Many nursing mothers continue to take pre-natal vitamin and mineral supplements that provide approximately the recommended dietary allowance. That certainly can't hurt; only huge amounts (megadoses) are harmful. Taking a pill, however, isn't enough to boost the quality of your milk. Only good food can do that.

How Many Calories?

Nursing mothers secrete 420 to 700 calories into their breast milk every day. To make those calories, they must eat even more. (Mothers nursing twins or triplets need professional advice about how much to eat.)

The standard advice for women who breastfeed is to eat about 500 extra calories a day, or about 2,700 altogether—a little more than during pregnancy. The idea is that weight loss will follow naturally as your breast milk passes along lots of those calories to the baby. If you gained weight during your pregnancy within a normal range, your 8 pounds of fat reserves will be depleted by breastfeeding within 3 months.

While that's a reasonable rule of thumb, it doesn't work equally for everyone, warns dietitian and mother Eileen Behan, the author of *Eat Well, Lose Weight While Breastfeeding*. Behan notes that some women must hold their intake to far fewer calories in order to lose weight. If you have stopped exercising, for example, 2,200 calories a day may be sufficient, as long as those calories are packed with excellent nutrition. If you jog every day, you may need many more.

Age, body size, and metabolism all affect your ability to lose weight. If you're concerned about your weight, monitor what you eat and what you weigh. Eliminating sugar, which contains about 15 calories per teaspoon, and keeping fat to a reasonable proportion of daily calories will lower your calorie count without affecting the baby.

Of your total calories, 50 to 60 percent should be carbohydrates, 20 percent protein, and no more than 30 percent fat. Babies eat about 45 calories per day per pound of their weight. A 10-pound baby (at, say, two months of age) will swallow about 450 calories of breast milk a day. That's directly subtracted from what you eat yourself.

What to Avoid

Be guided by essentially the same principles you followed during your pregnancy. Avoid additives, dyes, and chemicals, including artificial sweeteners, and stay away from tobacco smoke.

Drink alcohol in moderation or not at all. Although fetal alcohol syndrome affects only fetuses, alcohol is thought to "turn babies off" by giving breast milk a flavor they don't like.

Sipping beer while nursing used to be a standard recommendation. A small glass of beer every once in a while might be all right, but don't let yourself become woozy or rely on it to relax. While beer is a source of carbohydrates and fluids, other liquids and a bounty of nutritious foods provide the same benefits.

As for coffee, tea, and other substances containing caffeine, drinking more than a little is still not a good idea. Caffeine leaves your bloodstream within 3 to 5 hours but remains in the baby's for 80 to 97 hours. That means even 3 cups of coffee a day can make a baby irritable. Don't drink coffee just so you can remain awake as you and baby pace the floor—that might be the reason you're pacing!

Among the foods often listed as potentially causing gas or colic in babies are garlic, onions, cabbage, turnips, broccoli, prunes,

beans, and very large amounts of fruit. These effects are entirely individual. If you suspect that any particular food disagrees with your baby's digestion, which is still developing and pretty gassy anyway, try leaving it out of your diet for a couple of weeks and see if the situation improves. In one study, babies consistently remained at the breast *longer* and drank more milk after their mothers had eaten garlic. You never know.

When you pass along the essence of certain foods in your breastmilk, there's a chance of causing an adverse reaction. Signs of allergy include frequent greenish stools, gas, stuffy nose, rash, and vomiting. Foods most likely to produce a reaction include eggs, dairy products, peanuts, soybeans, wheat, and fish.

If strong food sensitivities or allergies run in your family, consult a pediatric allergist about whether omitting certain foods from your diet might prevent the baby from developing allergies to them. But don't avoid a wide range of nourishing food "just in case." Always act on an expert's advice. □

CHAPTER 17

Giving Your Baby an Ideal Diet

You won't need a cookbook to help you feed your new baby, at least not for the first six months. For complete nutrition, your newborn just needs breastmilk or infant formula whenever he's hungry. Feeding an older baby isn't complicated either: at 4 to 6 months, you'll begin a gradual process of introducing your baby to regular table foods.

Your baby's first year, divided roughly into newborn (under 6 months) and older baby (6 months to a year), is a time of tremendous change: he will double his birth weight during the first 4 months, and triple it by 1 year. Also during this first year, he will change from a helpless infant to a full participant at the table, with likes and dislikes and a habit of decorating himself, his highchair, and you with his food.

When it comes to feeding infants, guidelines about food groups, the food pyramid, fat, and cholesterol—in fact most of the rules

that shape diet choices for older children and adults—simply don't apply. Because of their rapid growth and their immature digestive systems, infants have their own unique nutritional needs.

The expert source on infant nutrition is the Committee on Nutrition (CON) of the American Academy of Pediatrics, which publishes guidelines used by pediatricians and dieticians. Because infants' needs are so specialized, the USDA (U.S. Department of Agriculture) does not issue recommendations for them and even the FDA (Food and Drug Administration) relies on the CON when setting requirements for infant formula manufacturers. Your pediatrician will use the CON guidelines as a basis for recommending what is best for your baby.

Feeding your newborn is theoretically the simplest aspect of baby care: babies come into the world ready to nurse from their mother's breast, which provides a complete diet until they are 4 to 6 months old. Your body produces all the milk your baby needs. In turn, your baby is born with a strong "rooting reflex" that directs him to seek your nipple, and suck from your breast. But like most things in modern life, it isn't always that simple.

In fact, you are faced with an important choice right from the start: will you breast-feed or formula-feed?

Breast or Formula?

The choice between breastfeeding and formula feeding is a personal one, and must be based on your own physical, emotional, and life situation. Once you've decided, don't second-guess yourself: your baby will do fine either way.

From the baby's point of view, all experts, even the manufacturers of infant formula, agree: breast is best. Clinically, breastfeeding is regarded as superior for your baby—nutritionally, developmentally, and emotionally. In practice, however, this is only true if you are comfortable with your decision to breastfeed and you can make it work based on your own personal circumstances. While a lot of people may give you advice, ultimately the decision is yours.

You may already have strong feelings about breastfeeding: some women know definitely that they want to breastfeed, and are highly motivated to make it work. Others are just the opposite: they are not comfortable with the idea of breastfeeding or can't breastfeed for medical reasons. If your mind is made up, or your health requires that you forego breastfeeding, go with your feelings—

BREASTFEEDING MYTHS

Myth: You have to prepare your nipples.
Reality: Don't. It's not needed, and may actually make nursing harder in the beginning.

Myth: Nursing ruins your breasts.
Reality: It doesn't. *Pregnancy* may affect your breasts, but nursing has no impact on them.

Myth: Women with small breasts or flat nipples can't nurse.
Reality: The size of your breasts bears no relationship to your ability to produce breastmilk. If your nipples are inverted, there are simple techniques that will help you nurse successfully.

Myth: Nursing is a lot of trouble.
Reality: It can be less trouble than preparing formula and bottles, if you want to do it, and the milk is always clean and ready.

Myth: It ties you down.
Reality: Both baby and breast are highly portable. No equipment to carry, nothing to refrigerate.

Myth: Nursing excludes the father.
Reality: There are plenty of ways to include the father in the baby's life. Nursing mothers need support to succeed: the father's role can be vital. (With expressed milk, Dad can feed the baby too.)

Myth: Some women don't have enough milk.
Reality: Very rarely true. If they are healthy, eat properly and rest adequately, most women will produce all the milk their babies need.

Myth: If you're going right back to work, it isn't worth starting to breastfeed.
Reality: Every day of breastfeeding is beneficial to the baby. If you want to breastfeed after you go back to work you can by expressing breastmilk for bottlefeeding.

in most cases, your baby will be happier, and just as healthy, if you are at ease.

However, if you are one of the many women who thinks breastfeeding is a good idea but just isn't sure how it will work for you, take the time to become informed before your baby is born. Read books, go to a nursing support and information meeting, such as La Leche League, (see box), or contact a lactation consultant (ask your obstetrician or the local hospital, or check the Yellow Pages) to get a good introduction to nursing. If you're still unsure, you may want to just give it a try. You can always switch to formula feeding, but if you start formula feeding without breastfeeding first, you'll find it almost impossible to switch the other way.

Advantages of Breastfeeding
- Breastmilk is designed by nature to feed human babies
- It changes daily to meet baby's needs
- It contains many beneficial components not found in formula and is more easily digested and better absorbed
- It may help prevent allergies
- It may help prevent constipation or diarrhea which can mean less diaper rash
- Breastfeeding may offer more sucking satisfaction and better mouth development
- It has these benefits for the mother: speeds recovery after delivery; may reduce risk of breast cancer; low in cost; high in convenience; easy for nighttime feeding; less work than sterilizing bottles and mixing formula

One oft-cited advantage of breastfeeding is the bond it promotes between mother and baby. This is certainly true but you and your baby can get the same closeness even if he is bottle fed. It's all in your approach and your attitude.

Advantages of Formula Feeding
- May mean less frequent feedings
- Makes it easy to see how much your baby has eaten
- Allows father, sitter, or siblings to feed the baby
- Makes it easy to feed baby in public or social situations
- Has these benefits for the mother: your body doesn't have the demand of producing milk; you can use any birth control method; your diet is not restricted; for some, may make lovemaking more comfortable; may be less isolating

When Not to Breastfeed
You shouldn't breastfeed if you have a medical condition that makes it a risk to your health, or if you need to take medications that, if passed through your breastmilk, might harm your baby. You should not breastfeed if you use illegal drugs or abuse alcohol.

Combining Breast and Bottle
If you want to include bottlefeeding, whether to allow someone else to be able to feed the baby or because you plan to return to work, you can express your breastmilk and then bottlefeed it to your baby. To express safely and effectively, you'll need to have a refrigerator to store your milk, and you'll have to perfect a method of expressing, either by hand or with a pump. While this can get complicated at work, many companies are

making an effort to be more accommodating to nursing, working mothers.

Most experts recommend waiting between 4 to 6 weeks to introduce a bottle, to avoid nipple confusion on the part of the baby and to insure a good breastmilk supply, since frequent nursing also helps stimulate production of breastmilk.

Zealous proponents of breastfeeding, such as the La Leche league, believe there is absolutely no benefit to the baby in supplementing breastmilk with formula. Furthermore, since the baby will be nursing less, supplementing with formula may decrease your breastmilk supplies. However, you could be in a situation where supplementing is warranted. If you have any doubts about whether your baby is eating enough and growing properly, consult your pediatrician. He or she can best advise you on your baby's health, growth, and development.

Alternatives to Breastmilk and Formula

There are *no* acceptable alternatives to breastmilk or infant formula. If you choose not to breastfeed, you should use a commercial infant formula recommended by your pediatrician.

The CON strongly recommends against using cow's milk of any kind for infants under 1 year because it does not contain enough iron, essential fatty acids, vitamin C, zinc, and other trace substances. Studies show that cow's milk can also lead to bleeding in the gastrointestinal tract, which itself may lead to iron-deficiency anemia. Cow's milk is also the most common cause of food allergy in babies under 1 year.

Just because a product is called milk does not mean it is adequate nutrition for a baby: goat's milk, soy milk, and non-dairy creamers are all inappropriate for infant diets. (Soy-based *formula*, on the other hand, is okay.)

Many people offer juice or water in bottles, but this is not recommended either. Both take up room that should be reserved for breastmilk or formula. Wait until your baby is starting solids, when he may need water, and then let him have his liquids in a cup.

What is Breastmilk?

Because we generally buy cow's milk in a package from the store, we tend to view all milk as a standardized product. But nothing could be further from the truth. Human breastmilk is not standard nor is it interchangeable with cow's milk. It is a dynamic fluid that changes in composition to meet the needs of the baby as it grows.

Breastmilk varies from woman to woman, but generally consists of water, fat, protein, sugars, vitamins, minerals, antibodies, and protective elements. More than 200 constituents have been identified, including enzymes, hormones, and growth factors. Breastmilk proteins are different from those in cow's milk; they tend to form smaller curds and may be easier for a baby to digest. The proteins in breastmilk also destroy harmful bacteria and help protect your baby against infections. None of the substances in breastmilk are known to contain harmful contaminants.

Breastmilk also looks different from cow's milk. The first milk the breast produces is colostrum, low in fat and carbohy-

LA LECHE LEAGUE

La Leche League is a worldwide nonprofit organization founded by nursing mothers to help women who want to nurse their babies. It provides educational resources, professional support, and publications for parents, medical professionals, and educators. You can attend local La Leche League meetings free and tap into this network, and you can become a member if you want to receive a newsletter and other benefits. La Leche League meetings are a chance for women to share their nursing expertise, answer questions, deal with problems, and keep up on research and new developments in infant nutrition. You'll see the meetings announced in local newspapers, and your hospital or obstetrician may be able to refer you to a local chapter. If not, call 1-800-LA-LECHE or write to La Leche League International, 1400 N. Meachum Rd., Schaumburg, Illinois 60173.

drates and high in protein. It is thick and creamy-looking, and contains the antibodies that help protect your baby against infections. After the colostrum comes transition milk, which is thinner, and then mature milk, which is thinner still and often bluish-white in color.

Breastmilk changes during each nursing session as well. As your baby begins nursing, the first milk he gets is called the foremilk, the breastmilk version of skim milk. Then comes the creamier hindmilk, richer in fat and proteins.

Getting Started with Breastfeeding

For most women, after the first few weeks breastfeeding is easy and natural. However, it helps to make preparations before birth to get off to the right start. Nursing success is often directly linked to the support you get in the first few days of nursing.

Before the Birth

If you know you want to try nursing your baby, do some research ahead of time. Be sure to discuss your plans with your partner and tell your pediatrician. When you are in labor, tell the nurses at the hospital that you plan to breastfeed, and ask them not to supplement with bottles.

Arrange for support in running your household and preparing meals for a few weeks after your baby is born. Rest is critical while you and your baby get comfortable with nursing.

The First Few Weeks

Adjust your mindset: nursing a baby is like having a full-time job, at least at first. It's not an afterthought to tack on to all your other responsibilities. Give it the time it deserves.

If you have a problem or question while you are getting started, don't wait for it to get better by itself: get help immediately from a lactation consultant or La Leche League leader. Small problems can lead quickly to big problems and you'll find nursing much harder than it needs to be.

Here are the keys to breastfeeding success:

■ Learn to position your baby properly, so he can latch on and suck correctly. Watch an experienced nursing mother, and get your lactation consultant or La Leche League

FINDING THE RIGHT POSITION FOR BABY AND YOU

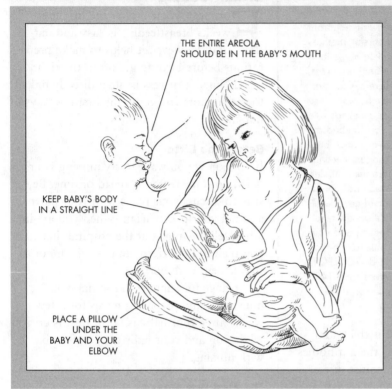

THE ENTIRE AREOLA
SHOULD BE IN THE BABY'S MOUTH

KEEP BABY'S BODY
IN A STRAIGHT LINE

PLACE A PILLOW
UNDER THE
BABY AND YOUR
ELBOW

The key lies in comfort. Find a position that gives both you and the baby relaxing support. Keep the baby's head and torso in a straight line, with the tip of the nose touching the breast.

leader to check your technique. Be sure your baby's body is in a straight line from ear to hips, nipple centered in his mouth, above his tongue, with the tip of his nose touching your breast. The whole areola should be in his mouth, not just the nipple.

■ Find a comfortable nursing position for yourself. Sitting up, propped with pillows, in bed or in a chair is good at first. Put a pillow under the baby and under your elbow, and put your feet up, too. You can also lie down to nurse or use other positions as you get more experience.

■ Give yourself time to establish the "let-down" reflex, the process by which oxytocin secreted by your pituitary gland causes milk to be released into the milk ducts. Once nursing is established, the let-down happens easily—for some women just thinking about their baby will produce it. Be aware that in the beginning, fatigue or stress may interfere so do what you can to minimize both.

■ Don't underestimate the importance of taking care of yourself. A good milk supply and successful nursing depends on you having a good diet, plenty of rest, plenty of liquids, and plenty of time to nurse in a quiet place. (For tips on the right diet for breastfeeding, turn to Chapter 15.)

How Long and How Often Should You Nurse

Your baby should nurse as long and as often as he wishes. The more a baby nurses, the more milk your body produces, so don't worry about running out. Don't try to put your baby on a schedule. It will only lead to frustration for both of you and may interfere with your milk supply and nursing success.

In general, newborns nurse every 2 to 3 hours, including during the night. Some babies nurse quickly and finish both breasts in 15 or 20 minutes. Others take their time, drifting off to sleep after a leisurely 40-minute session. Some combine both approaches, depending on the time of day. As your baby grows, he will ask to nurse less frequently; let the schedule be his choice, not yours.

How's It Going?

If you are concerned about your baby's nursing progress, talk to your pediatrician. In general, if there are 6 to 8 wet diapers and 2 to 5 bowel movements a day, your baby is nursing well. Most babies lose some weight the first week, but most will recover the weight in 2 or 3 weeks. A baby should gain about 4 to 7 ounces weekly, after the first week.

Infant Formulas

While infant formula doesn't provide the antibodies and other special components of breastmilk, manufacturers do try to match closely most of its nutritional components. Formulas are changed regularly as manufacturers refine their products to reflect current research on nutrition. Your pediatrician will be your best guide in choosing a formula.

The most commonly used products are based on cow's milk that is modified to make it suitable for infants: some examples are Enfamil, Gerber, Similac, and SMA. The formulas vary in the kind and amount of milk protein (whey and casein) they contain, as well as in the amount of iron, type and amount of fat, carbohydrates, and other nutrients in them.

For babies who can't tolerate cow's milk protein, there are formulas made from soy protein such as ProSobee, Isomil, Nursoy, and Soylac, and from hydrolyzed protein such as Nutramigen, Pregestimil, and Alimentum.

Infant formula comes in ready-to-feed, concentrated liquid, or powdered form. Your choice will probably be based on your lifestyle and budget. Ready-to-feed is the most convenient since you only have to open the can and pour the correct amount of formula into the bottle. Unopened cans do not need to be refrigerated. It is a particularly good option on trips where you may not have easy access to safe water or when you don't have time to prepare formula. Powder and concentrate both need to be measured and mixed with water, but they are less expensive than ready-to-feed.

The Equipment

There are several styles of nipples and bottles available, and you'll probably want to try them all to see which will best suit your baby. You'll also need a can opener, measuring cups, mixing spoons, tongs, a dishpan, and bottle and nipple brushes that you use only for your baby's formula preparation. For the newborn and young infant, some doctors recommend sterilizing everything; however using hot water is usually considered sufficient. Use boiled water for mixing with powder or concentrate. Ask your pediatrician about the best way to prepare the bottles.

Mixing and Storing Formula

Wash your hands and the top of the formula container before you start, and follow the manufacturer's instructions. Measure precisely.

Whatever form you choose, you should be scrupulous about sanitizing utensils and if you are using powder or liquid concentrate, about measuring and mixing the formula itself. Don't guess and don't assume that a little variance from the directions won't matter. Food contamination will make your baby sick. Over- or under-concentrated formula can harm your baby's health and growth.

Be sure that the water you use to mix the formula has not been through a water softener, which can raise sodium content to excessive levels. Also have your water checked for lead. If you use water from a well, have it checked regularly. Official recommendations call for boiling the water, even if bottled. However, some pediatricians feel this isn't necessary. If you have any questions, check with the doctor.

Keep prepared bottles in the refrigerator until you need them and use them within 48 hours. Don't keep a previously warmed bottle sitting around for later use, and don't reuse formula leftover after a feeding. Throw away whatever is left in the bottle since bacteria can grow quickly in warm formula.

Opened powdered supplies should be used within a month. All containers carry an expiration date and should not be used any later.

Giving Your Baby A Bottle

Most people warm the bottle, although there's no evidence that babies prefer it that way. If you do warm the bottle, it's best just to put in it warm water. Avoid microwaving, which can lead to hot spots. Always test the temperature by shaking a few drops onto your wrist.

Hold your baby close as though he were nursing. Bottlefeeding can give you the same opportunity for body contact and communication that breastfeeding can. Never prop up the bottle and leave him with it: babies can choke.

Traveling with Bottles

Because prepared bottles of formula must be refrigerated until you use them, you'll need a good insulated bag and an ice pack for quick trips and outings. Formula in the bottles should feel cold to your wrist to be safe for use. For longer trips, use powdered formula and take safe water with you to mix the bottles as needed, or take ready-to-feed formula. Don't forget to take whatever you need to measure and mix properly—it's just as important away from home.

Feeding Schedules

Just as if you are nursing, if you are giving your baby formula, he should have a bottle whenever he is hungry. A formula-fed baby may require fewer feedings than a breastfed baby, but in general a newborn will have about the same need for feedings: about every 2 to 3 hours, around the clock. You will soon come to know your baby's typical schedule. Bottlefeeding may go more quickly than nursing, since the baby does not have to work as hard to get the milk. Most babies will finish their bottles in a 15 to 20 minute session.

Because you can measure the baby's intake with bottle feeding, it's easier to tell whether he is eating adequately. But you should still check that there are 4 to 6 wet diapers and 2 to 5 bowel movements each day. Formula-fed babies should also gain about 4 to 7 ounces each week, after the first week, though it is not unusual for them to gain more.

Is My Baby Getting Ideal Nutrition?

Because of our culture's concern with weight and body image, some parents get worried when they see a chubby baby. This is a concern that simply does not apply to infants. While some formula-fed babies may gain excess weight if the formula is not mixed properly, healthy babies will eat appropriately if they are given the opportunity. In fact, you can compromise your infant's health by trying to keep his weight down.

The important thing is that your baby is growing normally, as determined by your pediatrician, who will chart your baby's growth at each well-baby visit and is your best guide for insuring that things are going well.

Supplements

While the CON finds that healthy breastfed or formula-fed babies don't need supplements, (the exception is very dark-skinned babies who may need vitamin D), many pediatricians recommend them as a kind of nutritional insurance.

The supplements your baby may need during the first year are iron, vitamin D,

vitamin C, and fluoride. These are often provided in multi-vitamin drops. Two common combinations are vitamins A, D, and C, with or without fluoride and iron; or A, D, E, C, and B vitamins with or without iron or fluoride. Since these combinations contain vitamins that your baby may not need, you may want to discuss alternatives with your pediatrician.

Iron: The iron supplies in newborn infants are used up by the time they are about 4 to 6 months old. The iron in breastmilk should be adequate for a while thereafter, and iron-fortified formula has enough for your infant's first year. Since iron-fortified cereal is usually introduced at about the time a breastfed baby needs more iron, supplemental iron is generally not needed, although it is often given after 6 months.

Keep drops containing iron out of the reach of children—an overdose can be toxic.

Vitamin D: Unless your baby is very dark-skinned, his skin can make vitamin D if he gets enough sunlight. In addition, infant formulas contain vitamin D, so supplements are not usually necessary. When needed, the usual recommended dose is 400 International Units a day.

Vitamin C: Your baby needs 35 milligrams of vitamin C each day, which he will get from breastmilk if you have an adequate diet, or from infant formula. When he is older, an adequate mixed diet ordinarily supplies enough. When you offer juice to an older baby, be sure it has vitamin C, either naturally or added. Baby apple juice, for example, has added Vitamin C, but regular apple juice may not.

Fluoride: Breastmilk has little fluoride, and infant formulas do not contain it. If your drinking water is not fluoridated, you will probably be advised to give a supplement of .25 mg of flouride daily. Be careful not to overuse fluoride, because it can cause spotting on your baby's permanent teeth. If you mix dry formula with fluoridated water, for example, your baby may be getting enough already. Fluoride is highly effective in preventing cavities—studies show that children who have fluoride from birth (or from six months if breastfed), have up to 65 percent fewer cavities than children who do not get fluoride.

Starting Solids

A diet exclusively of breastmilk or formula becomes inadequate to support a baby's growth at about 4 to 6 months. At the same time, your baby will begin showing you that he is ready to add solid food to his diet. He can sit up, chew, and swallow, and he will take a spoon when it's offered. He can also move food from the front of his mouth to the back with his tongue and grasp it with his hand.

Internally, his body is ready as well. His intestinal tract has developed and can protect him from foreign proteins. He is able to digest and absorb foods without stressing his kidneys.

First Foods

The first food for babies is usually an iron-fortified infant cereal—whether rice, oats, or barley—mixed with breastmilk or formula. Next usually come pureed fruits, such as banana, peach, pear, and apple, followed by pureed vegetables, usually green beans, carrots, squash, or sweet potatoes. You can introduce breads at about 6 to 8 months, and at about a year, meats and milk.
Be guided by your pediatrician's advice and don't rush to introduce new foods. One a week is the usual pace, which allows you to monitor for allergies.

For children under 6 months, the CON recommends avoiding use of home-prepared spinach, beets, turnips, carrots, or collard greens, because they could possibly contain enough nitrate to cause "blue baby syndrome" (methemoglobinemia). Symptoms are blue skin and difficulty in breathing; and the condition can be fatal. Commercially prepared baby foods contain only a trace of nitrate and are acceptable.

Mealtime

Mealtime is not just for putting food in your baby's mouth: he needs to see, smell, and feel the food, too. Don't be fussy about neatness, and don't hurry. Eating is both recreation and education for your baby. You'll get good mileage out of the right equipment: baby spoons, cups with lids, bibs with pockets, plastic plates, and a sturdy high chair with a plastic mat under it.

The beginning eater will still get most of his nutrition from breastmilk or formula, and solid foods will mainly be a supplement. As your baby gains proficiency in eating during the second half of his first year, he will get more nutrition from meals and less from nursing or formula. The beginner may need only a taste of solids twice a day with nursing or formula as needed. An older baby will probably be on a three-meal-plus-two-snack schedule, with nursing or formula for comfort only, by the end of his first year.

Choosing Baby's Food

You can cook regular table food and mash it with liquid for your baby, buy commercial baby food, or use a combination as budget and time permit. By the time your baby is a year old, a good mixed diet will include:

- 2 or 3 tablespoons of protein (cheese, fish, chicken, meat, tofu, yogurt, cooked egg yolk)
- 2 cups of a calcium-supplying food (milk in some form, whether cheese, yogurt, breastmilk, or formula)
- 2 to 4 servings of grains, pasta, whole-wheat bread or cereal, beans or dried peas
- 2 or 3 tablespoons of vegetables and fruits (leafy greens, yellow vegetables, and yellow fruits)
- one or two tablespoons of other fruits and vegetables

Keep serving sizes down to baby scale: about a fourth of a cup of cereal or pasta or half a slice of bread is a serving. Avoid giving your baby salty, fried, or high-fat, empty-calorie foods: he doesn't need them.

A beginner's food will be pureed, but as he gains eating skills, his food can be thicker and lumpier, and can begin to resemble regular table food. If you make your own baby food, a food processor, blender or baby food grinder can be a big help. It's also best to peel fruits and vegetables unless you know

they are pesticide-free, and wash thoroughly those you can't peel.

If you use baby food from jars, wash the lids and check the safety seals and expiration dates before opening. Use a serving bowl: don't feed your baby directly from the jar unless you plan to throw away what's left when he's done. Similarly, if you make your own food don't save the leftover portion from the baby's dish: it's contaminated with his saliva.

At about six months, you can begin to offer liquids in a cup. Babies this age are usually eager to learn, and starting now means they will be comfortable drinking from a cup when they are ready to be weaned later.

Weaning

Weaning means the end of nursing or formula feeding from a bottle, and can happen as soon as your baby can take the nutrition he needs from solids and a cup. Even so, most babies continue to like to suck for comfort well past their first birthday. While they may not need it for nutrition, many babies will still take a bottle (or have nursing sessions) during their second year. Check with your pediatrician for advice on weaning. Many babies wean themselves when they feel ready, if they are offered alternatives to the bottle or the breast.

Allergies

Most infant allergies are food allergies. If you have a family history of allergies, discuss your concerns with your pediatrician, who may modify the typical diet recommendations for your baby. Allergies in babies may appear as as a runny nose, cough, rash, gas, vomiting, or diarrhea.

The best protection against food allergies is believed to be breastmilk for the first 6

FIRST AID IN A CHOKING EMERGENCY

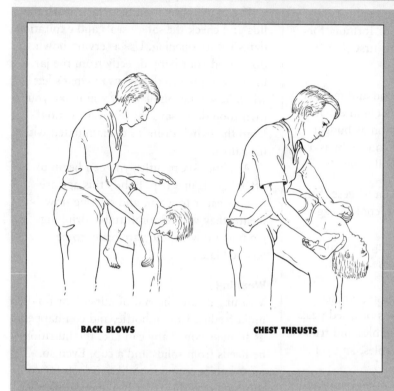

BACK BLOWS

CHEST THRUSTS

Fix these maneuvers firmly in your mind. In an emergency, there'll be almost no time for deliberation. For practice with these procedures, sign up for a Red Cross course in infant first aid.

Back Blows
Slap the baby four times between the shoulder blades while holding the baby's jaw with the other hand. Keep the baby's head lower than the rest of the body.

Chest Thrusts
Place the palm of the hand (2 or 3 fingers for a newborn) below the internipple line on the breastbone. While keeping the baby's head lower than the rest of the body, push in and up four times.

months and then a slow introduction of each new food, one per week. In general, don't rush to introduce those foods that are typical troublemakers for allergic babies, including cow's milk, nuts, wheat, eggs, corn, fish or shellfish, berries, peas and beans, and chocolate. And remember that if you're breastfeeding, these same foods could affect your milk and cause problems in the baby. If your family is allergy-prone, check with your pediatrician about modifying your own diet.

Vegetarian Diets

If you are a vegetarian and want your baby to be one, discuss your plans with your pediatrician so you can make the best diet choices and monitor your baby's growth properly.

Babies can do well on a vegetarian diet, especially if you include milk and eggs. If they are not included, your baby may suffer from shortages of protein; vitamins B_{12}, B_2, and D; calcium; or zinc. Your baby may also need iron supplements, because iron in plant food is poorly absorbed. You will also have to take special care to insure that the baby gets enough food for growth, since a vegetarian diet relies heavily on bulk foods that can be filling but short of calories.

Safety Issues

Babies are particularly vulnerable to eating hazards that would not cause problems for adults or older children.

Choking

Choking is the major cause of fatal injury in infants and children. Some foods simply should never be given to infants because they pose too great a choking hazard. These include: peanuts, grapes, popcorn, marshmallows, potato and corn chips, raw vegetable morsels, dried fruit or raisins, hard candies, fruit pieces with pits, and hot dogs.

To learn how to deal with a choking emergency, sign up for a course that includes infant CPR and first aid. These courses are sponsored by hospitals and local Red Cross chapters, or can be found in continuing education classes at high schools and community colleges.

Food-borne Illnesses

Cleanliness in preparing and storing baby food is critical. Keep hot things hot, cold things cold, and throw away any partially eaten food after a meal. Use insulated bags and cold packs when you travel. Diseases carried by raw eggs and undercooked meat are much more serious for babies.

Honey contains botulin spores, which are dangerous to infants because their bodies can not properly handle them. Do not feed honey or honey products to children under one year.

Lead can also be transmitted through food and through water that flows through leaded pipes. Eaten in high enough quantities, it can lead to serious health and developmental problems. Check your water supply, and don't feed your baby imported canned food:

lead from seams in the cans may enter the food. Also avoid ceramic, leaded crystal, pewter or any antique dishes or utensils for baby's food unless you have had them checked for lead.

Dining Out

Your baby can go with you to restaurant meals, but a little planning will make it more enjoyable for everyone. Choose a noisy, family-style restaurant where other children are eating. If your baby is not yet sitting up, take a baby seat or your removable car seat into the restaurant with you. Since a young baby probably won't be eating, bring some quiet toys to amuse him while he's awake. If you need to nurse, a shawl or blanket over the shoulder should take care of any privacy needs.

If your baby is older, take a booster seat (or use the restaurant's), and bring your own cup, plate, and spoon, as well as toys. It's a good idea to bring food too, since you may not find what you want on the menu. Yogurt travels well, or try apples, bananas, or crackers and cheese. You can order for your baby, or he can share your meal, eating whatever he has tried and liked at home. Be alert for choking, since there will be many distractions. □

Chapter 18

What's Right—And Wrong—for the Kids

If you're a parent, you probably tend to question yourself every time you make a decision about your child's care. Bringing-up-baby questions start swirling around like tornadoes well before your baby is even born. And it's quite likely that many of these questions center on how you'll feed your child.

This subject produces more questions than do many other aspects of child care, and sometimes even a few guilty feelings. Your very first choice, breast milk or formula, (see the preceding chapter) will be followed by other nutrition decisions: How much sugar? How much fat? How much milk?

This chapter covers these and other important nutritional issues for kids, based on their needs during the toddler, school age, and teenage years. It also covers such topics as allergies, food-related behavioral problems, the young athlete, and helping an overweight child.

Feeding Your Children: A Guilt-Free Approach

Every time you buy a breakfast cereal, you may wonder about sugar, about added colors, and if it's even possible to find a nutritious cereal that your kids will eat. If you find that a fast-food restaurant is your most convenient lunch option, you'll worry about how much fat is in that burger, how much salt is on those fries, and what in the world is in those shakes.

Making decisions about feeding your children is further complicated by experts who have inflexible and often contradictory points of view. And, for every conflicting theory you read, there seems to be another medical study to prove it right...or wrong.

Some experts will suggest that you impose severe limits on your children's fat intake, making them virtual vegetarians. Others mention that you can significantly improve your child's intelligence and concentration by following a specific, restrictive diet plan. You'll read that behavior and behavioral problems can be directly linked to diet. Some blame food allergies for everything from earaches to hyperactivity.

There are even a few pediatricians who will actually admit that you can become too stressed-out about feeding your kids. They'll tell you to take a deep breath, relax, and stop worrying. In moderation, they'll say, even junk food can be nutritious.

The most reliable friend you have for guiding your child's nutritional path is your own well-informed common sense. Educate yourself about what's new; be cautious about extreme theories. Whenever an "expert" advises you to completely overhaul your child's diet, think twice, unless there are compelling reasons, for a change, such as food allergies or serious behavioral disorders. Finally, weigh the nutritional benefits of a particular philosophy against how it will make your child *feel*. Even if a drastic, restrictive diet plan is physically healthy, it could inflict an emotional toll on your child that could undo all of its nutritional benefits.

Avoiding Extremes

Your child's nutritional needs are best met by a *balanced* diet with a broad variety of foods from the basic food groups, served in age-appropriate portions. (See Daily Menu Plans throughout this chapter.) The proportions needed from each food group are the same as for adults:

Number of Servings	Food Group
6 to 11	Bread, cereal, rice, pasta (many whole grains)
3 to 5	Vegetables
2 to 4	Fruits
2 to 3	Milk, yogurt, cheese
2 to 3	Meat, poultry, fish, dry beans, eggs, nuts
sparingly	Fats, oils, sweets

What To Do, Now that Your Child is Two, Three, or Four

As your child approaches the age of 2, it's up to you to set the stage for a lifetime of healthy eating habits. Start at the top—with you and the other adult members of the family serving as good examples. Don't expect your child to eat right if you don't: If you munch on potato chips, you can't possibly elicit your child's interest in carrot sticks.

Two is the delightful age of contrariness, the age when it might seem as if your child has a vocabulary of one word: NO. And this is the time when you might easily resort to using sweets as a reward or an enticement. One day, you may hear yourself saying, "Sweetie, get in your stroller and you can have a Twinkie." Or, "If you finish all those carrots, you can have a candy bar."

Is it wrong to use food as a reward? Not completely—but be careful about rewarding the eating of one food with another. In fact, most experts agree you should think twice about rewarding eating, period.

Be especially careful about rewarding toddlers and pre-schoolers with food. They really don't think the same way you

DAILY MENU PLAN FOR PRE-SCHOOLERS

Milk and dairy products (3 to 4 servings):

One serving equals
- 3/4 cup low-fat, or skim milk
- 1/2 to 3/4 ounce low-fat cheese
- 1/2 cup low-fat yogurt or cottage cheese
- 2 tablespoons powdered skim milk

Fruit (2 or more servings):

One serving equals:
- A quarter of a banana or apple
- 1/4 to 1/2 cup of canned or mashed fruit
- In addition, serve at least 1/3 cup of orange juice daily (or equivalent source of vitamin C)

Vegetables (2 or more servings; plus 1 or more servings of yellow or leafy green vitamin A-rich vegetables):

One serving equals:
- 1/4 cup cooked
- 1/2 cup raw

Meats, fish, poultry, legumes (2 to 3 ounces)

A serving at this age is 1 to 2 ounces. Limit hot dogs and lunch meats to no more than once or twice a week or switch to the new low-fat lunch meats and hot dogs.

Breads, cereals, and starchy vegetables (3 or more servings):

One serving equals:
- 1 slice whole grain or enriched white bread
- 1/2 roll, muffin, or bagel
- 3/4 cup ready-to-eat unsweetened cereal
- 1/4 to 1/2 cup cooked cereal, pasta, potato, rice, barley, or other grain
- 2 to 5 crackers

Try to use whole grains as much as possible.

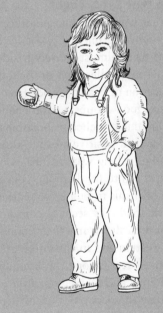

do. Here's what your toddler thinks: "A Twinkie's my prize? Wow! It must be pretty special!" Or, "A candy bar for eating carrots? Must be really good food." Those kind of messages can get a kid's food sense off to a shaky start.

A 1986 study of pre-schoolers' food preferences yielded some amusing results. The study found that kids believe that if something can be eaten at all, it can be safely consumed in any amount, and will help them grow (that is, will be healthy). So, to the very young mind, a diet consisting only of lollipops is perfectly sound, logical, and indeed, even good for you.

The study also found that little kids believe that if two foods, say, orange juice and chocolate are acceptable, than it's equally acceptable, to make a meal of them. And when an edible food touches a disgusting food (bugs) or an inedible food (paint), that may not necessarily render the edible food disgusting or inedible. (However, most kids over the age of 3 will probably avoid eating anything that crawls, although this has not been substantiated by scientific testing).

Do They Eat Enough?

What you serve your children, and what they actually eat, may be two different things—but that's almost entirely beside the point. By offering toddlers and pre-schoolers a broad selection of healthy foods from the five basic food groups, you are educating them to a lifetime of delicious possibilities. Indeed, your own positive attitude about food will go a long way toward assuring a healthy approach to food among your kids.

Bear this in mind: No matter how little food they seem to consume, or how temporarily bizarre their eating habits, starvation and malnutrition are practically nonexistent among children who, during a happy and relaxed mealtime, are offered a balanced selection of healthy foods.

Throughout the growing years, there's an easy way to tell whether your child is getting enough to eat: If the child grows and gains weight normally, looks healthy, and stays active, you can be fairly certain that he or she is consuming enough food.

Remember, though, that "normal" growth for a pre-schooler takes place at a slower pace than it did during infancy: During the first 12 months of a baby's life, a weight gain of 12 to 15 pounds is typical; between the ages of 3 to 5, a child will probably not gain more than four pounds a year, or about a third of a pound a month. The decreased growth rate might explain why pre-schoolers seem to have a decreased appetite and less interest in food.

Should there be any question in your mind as to what "normal" growth or weight gain means, check with your pediatrician.

Do Kids Really Need Three Glasses of Milk a Day?

Many parents are concerned about making sure their children get plenty of calcium to insure healthy bone strength and growth. Although 3 glasses of milk a day supply enough calcium to meet children's needs, other foods besides milk are equally good calcium sources, including cheese, dark green leafy vegetables, broccoli, and dried beans. Most experts agree that once a child is over the age of 2, the milk you serve should be skim, 1, or 2 percent.

The Two Golden Rules of Feeding Your Children

By the time your child is 2, you will have to learn how to relinquish a certain amount of control over the way he eats. According to Ellyn Satter, author and registered dietitian, there is one golden rule about feeding your children:

Parents are responsible for what foods are served to children and how they are served; children are responsible for how much—and even whether—they eat.

Another "golden rule" shared by many nutritional experts is:

Never, ever allow food to become a battle-ground or power struggle between you and your child.

Avoiding a battle over food is frequently difficult during a child's earlier years. One tactic you may find helpful is serve the meal, then physically leave the room for 5 or 10 minutes while the child decides what to eat. And when asking the child for a choice, don't leave it open-ended: Rather than saying "What would you like for breakfast?" present a couple of options, for instance "Would you like cereal or a bagel?"

Coping With Picky Eaters

There's no medical definition for a picky eater, but if your child is one, you'll know it. With pre-schoolers, foods can come in and out of favor with breathtaking rapidity for no apparent reason whatsoever. Sometimes, children can become attached to just a single food, or to weird combinations of foods.

Coping with a picky eater may strain your patience, but take comfort in knowing that most such kids become normal eaters in

HELPFUL HINTS FOR PICKY EATERS

- Never make food a battleground.
- Keep a food diary for your child—you may find that he isn't eating as badly as you think.
- Continue to offer a variety of nutritious foods in addition to the chosen few.
- Get the child involved in preparation. Cut food into fun shapes, serve raw vegetables and offer healthy dipping sauces—try seasoning plain yogurt.

a matter of time, and rarely does "pickiness" affect their health. Your picky eater may eat better than you realize. The book, *Let Them Eat Cake*, cites the example of 2-year old "Josh," whose insistence on a scrambled egg, catsup, and juice every night for dinner until he was about three and a half drove his parents crazy. But when they kept track of his all-day food intake, it became clear that in the course of 24 hours Josh ate a wide variety of other healthy foods, and so was in no danger of suffering nutritionally because of his strange evening meal.

Your child's pickiness may have nothing to do with food preferences and everything to do with the pre-school struggle for independence. If you accept pickiness as a temporary phenomenon and refuse to make a big deal about it, the problem, in all likelihood, will disappear in time.

In some cases, however, a picky eater is right. Some children may instinctively avoid certain foods because they know these items make them uncomfortable. If your child refuses to eat a particular kind of food, it may signal an allergy or intolerance. For example, if the child won't take milk, try substituting yogurt, cheese, or cottage cheese; cultured dairy products are sometimes better tolerated. If that doesn't work, just make certain you supply other calcium-rich foods; you may also want to have the child tested for a milk allergy or lactose intolerance.

If picky eating becomes perverse and persistent, or if your intuition tells you something is unhealthy about the way your child

DAILY MENU PLAN FOR SCHOOL CHILDREN, AGED 7–10

Milk and dairy products (4 servings):

One serving equals:
- 1 cup low-fat, 2% milk
- 1 ounce low-fat cheese
- 1 cup low-fat yogurt
- 3/4 cup low-fat cottage cheese
- 3 to 4 tablespoons powdered skim milk

Fruits (2 or more servings plus 1 or more of citrus fruits):

One serving equals:
- 1/2 cup fruit juice
- 1 small raw fruit
- 1/2 cup canned fruit

Vegetables (3 or more servings plus 2 or more vitamin A-rich vegetables)

One serving equals:
- 1/4 cup cooked
- 1/2 cup raw

Meats, fish, poultry, legumes (4 to 6 ounces)

A serving at this age is 2 to 3 ounces. Limit high-fat hot dogs and lunch meats.

Breads, cereals, and starchy vegetables (4 or more servings):

One serving equals:
- 1 slice whole grain or enriched white bread
- 1 bagel, muffin, or roll
- 1 cup ready-to-eat, unsweetened cereal
- 1/2 cup cooked cereal, pasta, potato, barley, or rice
- 4 to 6 crackers

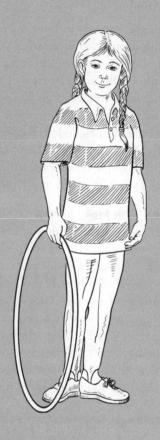

eats, consult your pediatrician. Although real eating disorders are rare in pre-schoolers, they could be an indication of more serious concerns or conditions.

Now That They're In School . . .

Call them the grazers. When your children enter elementary school, they enter an age of new independence. Now, more than ever, it's important to stock your kitchen with an assortment of healthy foods and snacks, for most children this age always seem to be hungry.

Make healthy eating easier for your children by keeping healthy foods handy. When kids want to snack, they'll grab whatever is most available:

- Pre-cut celery and carrot sticks
- Washed fruits in season
- Microwaveable popcorn (watch fat and salt content)
- Low-fat milk
- 100 percent real fruit juices
- Low-fat "string" cheese (individually wrapped) or mozzarella
- Raw, unsalted nuts—almonds, cashews, peanuts (unless the child is overweight)
- Sunflower or pumpkin seeds (if weight isn't a problem)
- Dried fruits

What About School Lunches?

The need for improvement in some school meal programs made headlines recently when the USDA convened "Healthy Kids: Nutrition Objectives for School Meals," a series of hearings in Washington, D.C. The hearings were held to explore new ways to upgrade the nutritional content of school meals. Seventy experts testified.

Of particular interest to concerned parents were four food manufacturers who make healthier food products than those now being served in school cafeterias. One was Lucille Farms, Inc., a Vermont maker of traditional Italian cheeses. Their new low-fat cheeses could make pizza—the number one school lunch choice—healthier.

Since parental involvement is a factor that directly affects whether or not a specific school district serves nutritious meals, find out what your kids eat at school. If you don't like what you learn, become involved, ask questions, and demand healthier foods.

Do They Still Need Their Vitamins?

Of course! But the consensus among professional medical and dietetic associations seems to be that vitamin and mineral supplementation is unnecessary for children who eat well-balanced diets. It's far healthier to encourage your child to eat properly than it is to suggest that a pill can take the place of sound eating habits—especially since vegetables, fruits, and other nutritious foods contain a wide variety of health-promoting substances that aren't found in vitamin supplements.

Children who subsist on high amounts of "junk food" however, may suffer ill effects, notes Dr. Derrick Lonsdale of the Cleveland Clinic in Ohio. He treated 20 such children whose diet produced a vitamin B_1 deficiency. As a result, the children exhibited the classic symptoms of beriberi, including neurotic tension, diarrhea, nausea, and excessive sweating—symptoms that might not be immediately obvious to parents. The children improved when they were given vitamin B_1 supplements.

Does vitamin supplementation in excess of RDAs have any beneficial effects for children? Medical studies show conflicting results: One study reported improved reasoning ability in children who received vitamin and mineral supplementation; another study, specifically designed to confirm or refute the first, did not corroborate the findings.

Nevertheless, if you're unsure how adequate your child's diet really is, providing a daily multivitamin is something to consider.

The Teen Years

Despite their increased nutritional needs—teenagers gain the final 20 percent of their adult height and the final 50 percent of their adult weight during this period—these kids are the least likely people to eat a balanced diet. And it is at this point in their life that you are least able to impose your dietary guidance.

How can parents make sure their teenagers eat well? If you've instilled your child with a sense of healthy eating during early childhood, he is likely to continue eating well as a teenager—and lapses are likely to be temporary.

Teens' bodies are changing rapidly and dramatically, and they often react to the changes with confusion, especially when it

DAILY MENU PLAN FOR ADOLESCENTS AND TEENS, AGED 11-17

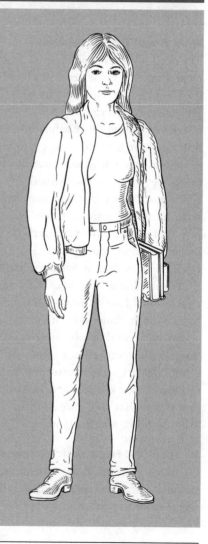

Milk and dairy products (4 servings):

One serving equals:
- 1 cup low-fat, 2% milk
- 1-1/2 ounces low-fat cheese
- 1 cup low-fat yogurt or low-fat cottage cheese
- 4 tablespoons powdered skim milk

Fruits (2 or more servings plus one or more of citrus fruits):

One serving equals:
- 1 cup fruit juice
- 1 medium raw fruit
- 1 cup canned fruit

Vegetables (3 or more servings plus 2 or more vitamin A rich vegetables):

One serving equals:
- 1/2 cup cooked
- 1 cup raw

Meats, fish, poultry, legumes (6 to 8 ounces)

A serving at this age is 2 to 6 ounces.
Keep limiting high-fat meats.

Breads, cereals and starchy vegetables (4 or more servings):

One serving equals:
- 2 slices whole grain or enriched white bread
- 1 large bagel, muffin, or roll
- 1 to 1-1/2 cups ready-to-eat, unsweetened cereal
- 1 cup cooked cereal, pasta, potato, barley, or rice; 4 to 6 crackers

comes to their appearance. One study indicates that 70 percent of teenage girls want to lose weight, but only 15 percent of them are too heavy. The same study indicates that 59 percent of teenage boys want to gain weight, although only 25 percent of them are too thin.

This is the time of life when, in girls, such eating disorders as anorexia or bulimia begin; some athletically-inclined boys, trying to "bulk up," may turn to the very dangerous use of steroids.

Does Puberty Affect a Teen's Nutritional Needs?

Early puberty can seem like a time of non-stop eating for teens, as they constantly seek to fuel their unprecedented growth.

Most boys begin puberty somewhere between the ages of 10 and 14. Other than consuming a well-balanced diet that provides adequate energy and nutrients to accommodate their adolescent growth spurt, boys have no additional nutritional demands at puberty.

Girls who are deficient in iron and vitamin A may experience a delay in the onset of menstruation, as may girls who are very athletic or very thin. Studies have shown that when a girl reaches a certain "critical body mass" of about 105 pounds (in girls of average height), menstruation will shortly follow. A girl's percentage of body fat may also be a factor determining when menstruation begins; a certain amount of fatty tissue may be needed for the hormonal changes that initiate its onset. This is supported by the fact that young female athletes and girls who have a low percentage of body fat generally begin to menstruate later than normal.

How to Buy a Breakfast Cereal Your Kids Will Eat

The new "Nutrition Facts" labels make comparison shopping easier. They list nutrient values based on a 2,000 calorie-a-day diet, showing the share of total and saturated fat, cholesterol, sodium, potassium, carbohydrates, dietary fiber, and protein a serving supplies.

But if the task of picking a nutritious breakfast cereal is made easier by the new labeling, it certainly isn't helped by cereal manufacturers, who aim directly at children their most intriguing TV commercials and print advertisements for artificially-colored and flavored, highly-sugared cereals.

So, when you're shopping the aisles looking for a nutritious cereal, your kids are liable to be begging for the one with the free toy, or the one that's a spin-off of their favorite cartoon show, or the one with the new wild colors. It's up to you to deliver the message that what the cereal contains is more important than the ads.

According to the Center for Science in the Public Interest, here are tips for choosing a good breakfast cereal:

- Ingredients are listed in descending order by amount. If sugar is listed first, reject the cereal.
- Look at the grams of sugar per serving: 6 to 9 grams a serving is about the maximum amount you want your child's cereal to have. (The American Dietetic Association recommends 6 grams). Note: Cereals containing real dried fruits are exempted from the 6 to 9 gram rule; they boost a cereal's sugar content, but provide nutritional benefits, including fiber.

- Don't be lured into buying a sugary cereal with lots of vitamins. Cereal manufacturers add vitamins as a sort of consolation prize to parents who believe that the supplements will compensate for a cereal's high sugar and additive content.
- Look for the words "whole grain" before ingredients like wheat, rice, corn, or barley.
- Check out the fat content. Most breakfast cereals are low-fat, but some granolas and cereals with coconut or nuts can contain as much as 8 grams in a one-ounce serving.

How Much Sugar is Too Much?

Unfortunately, there's no easy answer to this question. The issue of exactly how much sugar you should allow your child is confusing for two main reasons:

- There is no recommended daily value for sugar intake.
- "Natural" sugars occur in a variety of wholesome foods, including fruit and milk.

According to Bonnie Liebman, director of nutrition for the Center for Science in the Public Interest, the issue is not how much *naturally-occurring sugar* your child eats, but rather how much added sugar your child takes in.

"When children eat lots of sugary foods, like candy, soda, or sweetened snacks, they eat empty calories that contain little nutritive value. They then have no room left to eat healthier, nutrient-rich foods."

This is especially noticeable when it comes to a child's drinking habits. Notes Liebman, "the biggest source of sugar in our diets is soft drinks." She concurs with children's nutritional experts who say that when children drink soda, all they get is a fast dose of sugar, maybe caffeine and artificial flavors or colors.

But when children slake their thirst with orange juice, they get a healthy blast of vitamin C along with their sugar; with milk they get a hefty protein and calcium dividend.

The answer to the how much sugar question is basically: Don't let the child ruin his appetite. The USDA Food Guide Pyramid puts sweets in the category of fats and oils, and recommends a "sparing" amount of servings each day.

Still, there are plenty of healthy ways to satisfy a sweet tooth: You can serve your child at least 5 servings of fruit a day. There are also many cookbooks chock-full of deliciously sweet snacks that pack a nutritional punch.

Try reading: *Eating For A's*, by Alexander Schauss, Barbara Friedlander Meyer, and Arnold Meyer (Pocket Books, 1991).

Feed Me, I'm Yours, by Vicki Lansky (rev. ed., Meadowbrook, 1986).

What About Fat?

If you read the literature on nutrition, a strong voice emerges, urging us to sharply reduce the amount of fat in our diet—and our children's diet.

The generally accepted consensus among most experts, and the standard adopted in 1988 by the National Institute for Health, calls for an adult diet in which no more than 30 percent of total caloric intake is supplied by fat. This 30 percent figure is also recommended for children by the American Heart Association; and in 1992, the American Academy of Pediatrics also adopted 30 percent.

However, some experts, notably Dr. Charles R. Attwood and Dr. Michael F. Jacobson, the executive director of the

DAILY FAT TARGETS IN GRAMS

Age	2-3	4-6	7-10	11-18 Girls	11-14 Boys	15-18 Boys
Average Calorie Intake	1,300	1,800	2,000	2,200	2,500	3,000
Fat Grams (30% of calories)	43	60	67	73	83	100
Fat Grams (25% of calories)	36	50	56	61	69	83
Saturated Fat Grams (10% of calories)	14	20	22	24	28	33
Saturated Fat Grams (7% of calories)	10	14	17	17	19	23

Calorie data taken from Recommended Dietary Allowances, National Academy of Sciences, 10th Ed. (1989).

The Center for Science in the Public Interest puts these figures in perspective by noting that a typical hot dog has 13 grams of fat; one ounce of potato chips has about 11 grams; a McDonald's Big Mac has 26 grams; and a KFC Original Recipe chicken thigh has 20 grams.

Center for Science in the Public Interest, believe this figure is too high.

They argue that since coronary heart disease begins in childhood, prevention with low-fat diets should also begin in childhood. They point to studies showing the appearance of fatty deposits in the coronary arteries of children as young as three years (when they consume high-fat diets and have elevated levels of cholesterol). Fatty deposits become much more common in children as they approach their teens.

Dr. Attwood, one of the most vociferous opponents of dietary fat, argues that powerful political lobbying by the Beef Industry Council and the National Dairy Council has indoctrinated practically every adult, including physicians and dietitians, in the healthful benefits of red meat, milk, and cheese. He believes that no more than 20 percent of calories in anyone's diet should come from fat; a better amount, he says is 10 to 15 percent.

CAUTION: **All experts agree that under no circumstances should fat be reduced for children under the age of two. Restricting or limiting fat or caloric intake for infants under 24 months severely inhibits normal growth and development.**

The Center for Science in the Public Interest is more moderate in their recommendations about dietary fat, suggesting that 25 percent of calories come from fat.

Saturated vs. Unsaturated, Polyunsaturated vs. Monounsaturated

For children over the age of 2, limit saturated fats to no more than about 5 to 10 percent of their daily calories. Saturated fats are those that are usually solid at room tempera-

IDEAL WEIGHT FOR BOYS

Age (in years)	8	9	10	11	12	13	14	15	16	17
Height (in inches)	Weight (in pounds)									
43"	40									
44"	43									
45"	45	45								
46"	47	47								
47"	49	49	49							
48"	52	52	52							
49"	54	54	54	54						
50"	57	57	57	57	57					
51"	60	60	60	60	60					
52"	63	63	63	63	63	63				
53"	66	66	65	65	67	67				
54"	68	68	69	68	69	69	70			
55"	71	71	72	72	72	73	73			
56"		75	75	76	76	77	77	78		
57"		78	79	80	80	82	82	82		
58"			82	83	84	84	85	85		
59"			86	87	87	88	88	89	89	
60"				90	91	92	93	94	96	
61"				94	95	96	97	98	101	105
62"				99	100	101	103	103	107	111
63"					106	105	107	108	111	115
64"					109	110	111	113	115	119
65"						114	116	118	120	125
66"						117	121	123	126	129
67"							127	127	131	134
68"							131	132	135	139
69"							135	136	138	141
70"							140	142	143	145

ture; they come primarily from animal sources (although palm and coconut oils are saturated fats). These fats can raise cholesterol levels and contribute to heart disease.

Polyunsaturated fats, found in vegetables, fish, corn, cottonseed, sesame, soybean, and safflower oils (and margarine if it is made mainly from a liquid vegetable oil) are less harmful; and polyunsaturated fatty acids found in fish may help to *lower* blood fat levels. Countries like Japan, where people eat less meat and more fish, have lower rates of heart disease. Fish especially high in "good" fatty acids are salmon, mackerel, herring, anchovies, trout, catfish, and sardines. Still, it's wise to limit your child's intake of polyunsaturated fats to no more than 8 to 10 percent of the day's total calories.

Monounsaturated fats are found in olive oil, peanuts, avocados, some nuts, and canola oil. These fats help to lower the low-density lipoprotein (LDL) cholesterol that can build up in the blood vessels and contribute to heart disease. These should make up about 10 percent of your child's daily calorie intake. (Watch out for peanut *butter*: It often contains large amounts of added saturated fat.)

What if Your Child is Too Heavy?

We live in an age of TV, multi-media computers, and video games. Perhaps partially as a result of their inactivity, our children constitute the "fattest generation of kids and teens in the entire history of the United States," according to Dr. Peter M. Miller, author of the Hilton Head Diet for Children and Teenagers.

Dr. Miller, executive director of the Hilton Head Health Institute, reports that recent studies show that over the past 20 years, obesity in children aged 6 to 11 has increased by 54 percent; in teens, the increase is 39 percent. Twice as many children now fall into the "super-obese" category and weigh over 40 percent more than they should.

An obese child is almost certain to become an obese adult. Worse, the kid who's too fat is likely to carry an additional burden—disapproval from teachers, friends, and sometimes even members of his or her own family. This can be onerous: Studies show that even very young children perceive fat people to be less intelligent, sloppy, dirty, untrustworthy and less likable than other people. Having this kind of image among friends and even strangers is a heavy burden for a youngster to carry.

What Can You Do for An Overweight Child?

Check the charts. If your child is significantly over his or her ideal weight, it's time to intervene. Many experts recommend a "no diet" approach, especially for children who still have a lot of growing to do. The "no diet" approach means no reduction in the *amount* of food your child eats, but it does mean changes in the *kind* of food you serve. In addition, you must make lifestyle changes that increase your child's activity level.

CAUTION: **Children under the age of eight should not be placed on diets.** *Never* **restrict calories or fat for a child under the age of 2.**

As your child gets older, he or she will grow, and eventually will weigh the right amount for his or her height—as long as you help maintain a well-balanced diet. That means serving plenty of low-fat foods, including lots of fresh fruit, vegetables, grains, and lean proteins. On an "all-you-can-eat" diet, as

IDEAL WEIGHT FOR GIRLS

Age (in years)	8	9	10	11	12	13	14	15	16	17
Height (in inches)	Weight (in pounds)									
43"	40									
44"	42									
45"	45									
46"	47	47	47							
47"	49	50	50							
48"	52	52	52	52						
49"	54	55	55	56						
50"	57	58	58	60	60					
51"	60	60	61	62	62					
52"	63	63	64	64	66					
53"	66	67	67	67	68	70				
54"	68	70	70	71	71	73				
55"		73	74	74	75	77	78			
56"		76	78	78	79	80	84			
57"			81	82	82	84	89	93		
58"			84	87	86	88	93	96	100	
59"			87	91	90	93	97	101	104	105
60"				95	96	97	101	105	108	109
61"				97	101	101	105	108	112	113
62"					105	106	108	112	114	115
63"					110	111	112	115	116	118
64"					114	115	117	118	120	121
65"						120	120	121	124	125
66"						124	125	126	128	128
67"							127	129	133	133
68"							131	133	134	136
69"						133	135	136	138	
70"						134	136	138	140	

(Charts were developed by the World Health Organization and appeared in *The Hilton Head Diet For Children and Teenagers.* Dr. Peter M. Miller. Warner, 1993).

long as you strictly limit or, better yet, eliminate all fatty and sugary foods (including most "fast food" meals), your child need not feel terribly deprived.

The best way to help your *child* lose weight is to subtly revamp your whole family's lifestyle so that *everyone* gets more fit—especially if there are other overweight family members. Since temporary diets don't give lasting results, it's wise not to refer to your family-wide fitness program as a "diet."

Instead, create ways to get your family moving again, since exercise is the best defense against extra pounds. Begin serving delicious, low-calorie meals and snacks that the whole family can enjoy. Consult Section II, "Keeping Your Weight in Check,"for specific information about weight-loss and fitness programs. Part 2 of this book, "Keeping the Fun in Your Food," offers a host of ideas for preparing healthy meals the family still can enjoy.

Consider your weight-loss program as a new team approach to family fitness and a healthier, happier lifestyle. Make sure that the elements you introduce—new foods and new activities—are fun for all. If anyone perceives them as "punishment for pounds," your program is doomed before it starts.

The Allergic Child

Food allergies are often blamed for a wide variety of children's ailments, including behavioral disorders, congestion, asthma, and skin eruptions. But, according to the American Academy of Allergy and Immunology (AAAI), *less than five percent of children are truly allergic*. Instead, says the AAAI, adverse reactions to food are usually caused by the inability to digest certain ingredients, like lactose in milk or gluten in wheat. Sensitivities to substances may also be a factor: Some children react adversely to salicylates and food additives; other children (though fewer that we've been led to expect) are especially sensitive to sugar.

It's easy to confuse food allergies with digestive intolerance—both are evidenced by some kind of discomfort after eating particular foods. However, they are caused quite differently. Food-intolerant people lack the enzymes needed for the digestion of certain foods; allergic people react to a food as though it were a foreign invader. The confusion is exacerbated because the word allergy is often used to describe food intolerance.

Putting semantics aside, if your child has a problem, how do you determine whether or not your child is sensitive or allergic to certain foods?

Behavior Problems

If your child is hyperactive, prone to temper tantrums or is generally regarded as being a "difficult child," food is only one of many possible causes. But if you've ruled out disruptions in home life (a move, new job, death of close friends, or relatives), marital tension, problems within the school, and the like, your child may have one or more food sensitivities or allergies that cause the "acting out."

In 1973, the late Dr. Ben Feingold presented his observations on diet for hyperkinetic and learning-disabled children to the Allergy Section of the American Medical Association in New York. The enormous interest in the topic led him to write *Why Your Child Is Hyperactive* and *The Feingold Cookbook for Hyperactive Children*.

Dr. Feingold spent years studying the reaction of children to various foods. His research led him to believe that some children are sensitive to salicylates (a group of organic compounds related to aspirin), certain food additives, and sugary foods. Dr. Feingold insisted that children sensitive to these substances can react with such behavior disorders as hyperactivity. For them, he devised the Feingold Diet for additive- and salicylate-free meals.

The Feingold diet is the object of considerable controversy. One independent study involving 59 children between the ages of 6 to 14 years, confirmed that some children do react badly to foods containing salicylates and additives. Of the 32 children who were able to tolerate the very rigid diet, 11 showed remarkably improved behavior. However, another study found no beneficial effect; and many experts speculate that any improvement in behavior is simply a response to the extra time and attention the diet requires. One thing is certain: the diet is extraordinarily restrictive. You must completely eliminate all foods containing artificial colors and flavors, including U.S. certified, FD&C approved, or USDA approved colors or flavors, and all foods containing vanillin or caramel coloring and flavoring. Also on the hit list are all foods that contain the common preservatives BHT and BHA, which are widely used in dairy products, cooking fats and oils, and even food packaging materials.

Finally, most fruits, all berries, tomatoes, peppers, coffee, and tea are all out of bounds at the start of the diet. These forbidden foods ordinarily supply a wealth of vitamins, but you can't make up for them with vitamin supplements, because any that contain artificial colors and flavors must also be eliminated.

Clearly, this is a diet that you'll want to discuss with your pediatrician before going

further, since many experts regard it as completely discredited. Nevertheless, according to Dr. Feingold, 60 to 70 percent of those children who follow the diet precisely will see a marked improvement in behavior. For additional information, see *Your Child's Food Allergies*, by Jane McNicol (John Wiley & Sons, 1992) which offers recipes and sample menus and details a test diet for hyperactive children. *Why Your Child Is Hyperactive* and *The Feingold Cookbook*, by Dr. Ben Feingold, (Random House, 1973 and 1979), outline the pioneering doctor's plan.

If neither you nor your child notice an improvement after you strictly follow a special behavior diet, and if your child's behavior problems are so severe that they make peaceful co-existence impossible and inhibit his or her ability to learn, then ask your doctor about scheduling your child for a comprehensive physical and emotional evaluation to determine the roots of the trouble.

Other Tip-offs of Food Sensitivity

Sensitivities to certain foods announce themselves with distinctive sets of symptoms:

Congestion; frequent runny nose, ear aches, colds; bad breath; headaches. Cow's milk—the most commonly reacted-to food—can cause upper-respiratory symptoms; a lactose-intolerant child might show an excessive love or hatred of milk. Try eliminating all milk products from your child's diet for two weeks; keep a log daily and note any changes. Then, if you see improvement, you can try re-introducing foods like yogurt, low-fat cheese, cottage cheese; very often children sensitive to milk are not sensitive to its cultured forms. If all milk products are eliminated, be sure to provide adequate calcium substitutes.

"Jitteriness" or other notable signs of hyperactivity. Your child may be reacting to chocolate or cola, second only to milk as "reactable" foods. Eliminate these, and note whether jitteriness disappears or behavior improves. Caffeine could also be the culprit. Try eliminating all caffeine, found in many sodas, chocolate, and, of course, coffee.

Extreme "sweet tooth," frequent eating, parents with a history of diabetes, hypoglycemia, or alcoholism (or low tolerance for alcohol). Your child may have a sugar reaction, or may be allergic to specific sugars, such as cane or beet sugar. The chemicals used in processing can also spark reactions. However, most experts agree that sugar has been overrated as a cause of hyperactivity, and most children will tolerate at least small amounts. Few will react to lightly sugared foods eaten with other foods or for dessert.

Repetitive behaviors, bold or aggressive behavior, family history of MSG intolerance; unexplained gastrointestinal upsets or headaches. The ubiquitous MSG (monosodium glutamate), a flavor enhancer found in many processed foods and Chinese food (hence, the "Chinese Restaurant Syndrome") is a potential cause of behavior problems. People sensitive to MSG may also be sensitive to other flavor enhancers such as hydrolized vegetable protein (HVP) and hydrolized plant protein (HPP).

These substances are difficult to eliminate from your child's diet because they are so common. However, both books mentioned above have excellent recipes and strategies for coping, should you find your child is MSG, HVP, or HPP-sensitive.

When Your Child is Sick

When your child is down for the count with a cold, flu, or intestinal bug, it's time for TLC. Here are some tips about what to feed your sick child—and what to avoid.

FIRST: If your child has a fever, has vomited more than a few times, has diarrhea that doesn't abate after a few hours, is in pain—or if your child is droopy, very quiet, and just not him or herself—call your pediatrician.

Dr. Michael Mitchell, a prominent Manhattan pediatrician and author of *The Pillbook: A Guide to Children's Medications* (Second Edition, Bantam, 1994), offers these suggestions for feeding an ailing child.

1. Eliminate all milk and dairy products while your child has diarrhea or vomiting.

2. Drown a fever with plenty of fluids. When a child has a fever, sweating and rapid breathing can lead to dehydration. "I never worry when a feverish child refuses solid foods, as long as he or she gets plenty to drink," says Dr. Mitchell.

3. When your child has a simple cold or minor gastrointestinal upset, don't rush in with over-the-counter preparations. Let your child's immune system fight off the bug as nature intended it to.

If you're uncertain as to whether your child has something serious, check with your doctor.

Nutrition for Young Athletes

Nutrition for a young athlete differs very little from nutrition for adult athletes: All should eat a well-balanced diet, high in complex carbohydrates, lean protein, and plenty of fruits and vegetables. (See specific diet suggestions in Chapters 8 and 21.)

Parents need to watch over their children when they excel at a particular sport or sports, especially if they're extremely committed to achieving winning results. These children need extra guidance to help them avoid dangerous fad diets and unhealthy food supplements.

If your son plays football, lifts weights seriously, or engages in any other activities that require special muscular strength, caution him about the dangers of anabolic steroids. (Very rarely do girls abuse steroids; however, if your daughter engages in sports that require extra muscular strength, be sure to counsel her against steroid use).

A 1993 survey by the Journal of the American Medical Association revealed that over one million Americans aged 12 and older are steroid users; nearly half are under the age of 26. It's been estimated that between 5 and 10 percent of high school students may be steroid abusers.

Steroids seriously impair normal mental function; though the popular TV show, *Saturday Night Live,* has a recurring parody about steroid abusers, in real life, there's nothing funny about these drugs: They can kill you or permanently impair your mental and physical functioning. (For more information, see Chapter 21, "Boosting Energy and Fitness.")

Easy Fat-Trimming Tips

- Switch from whole milk to skim, 1/2 percent, 1 percent or 2 percent. Take the fat content down one step at a time, changing every 2 to 3 months. If even 2 percent tastes terrible to you, mix it half-and-half with whole milk for a few weeks.
- Switch from whole-fat to low- or no-fat cheese, yogurt, ice cream and other dairy products. Experiment! New advances mean that many low- and no-fat dairy products actually taste good.
- Switch from ground beef to ground turkey or chicken, especially when making meat loaf, tacos, spaghetti sauce, and chili.
- Use turkey sausage instead of pork sausage. It's available in hot and sweet Italian flavors as well as regular sausage flavor.
- Trim all visible fat from meat. Use cuts labeled "lean" whenever possible.
- Try turkey and chicken franks instead of meat franks; switch to luncheon meats made from turkey or chicken. Check nutritional labels; some products are higher in fat than others.

What About Salt?

Although the right level of salt for adults is a subject of major controversy, salt is much less of a concern for kids. Among salt-sensitive adults, excessive amounts can lead to high blood pressure, one of the major risk factors for strokes and heart disease. However, there is no evidence of such a problem in children.

A lifelong diet high in sodium has recently been linked to an increased risk of osteoporosis, the "brittle bone" disease. According to the Center for Science in the Public Interest, eating an extra teaspoon of salt each day causes the body to lose enough calcium to dissolve about one percent of bone annually—a frightening statistic at first glance. However, since most of us reach retirement without losing two-thirds of our bone mass, it seems likely that this particular problem may be over-rated. If you keep salt at moderate levels and make sure the kids get plenty of calcium, there's no reason to be concerned.

Extremely salty foods have been implicated in stomach cancer. It is said that salt acts as an irritant to the stomach lining and causes cells to reproduce more rapidly, and victims of stomach cancer tend to have consumed high-sodium diets. However, once freezing and canning replaced preservation with salt in the U.S., the odds of stomach cancer plummeted. Moderate amounts of salt as used today seem to pose little threat.

Finally, a study reported in 1993 in the British Medical Journal linked high salt consumption with deaths from asthma in men and children. Though the results of the small-scale study were by no means conclusive, they did demonstrate a relationship between high-sodium diets and asthma that should not be overlooked by parents of asthmatic children.

Experts estimate that children probably take in between 5 and 10 times the recommended allowance of sodium each day, mostly from the sodium-containing chemicals found in processed foods. You might suspect that salty-tasting snacks like potato chips would be at the top of the high-sodium list, but they're not: One ounce of potato chips has about 135 milligrams of sodium; the average hot dog weighs in at about 500 milligrams. Currently, the National Research Council of the National Academy of Sciences recommends a daily allowance of 2,400 milligrams of sodium for everyone over the age of 2.

How to Promote Good Nutrition in an Era of TV

You now have a good idea of what constitutes a good, healthy, tasty diet for your kids. But kids, especially young ones, often get different ideas from what they see on television.

According to the Center for Science in the Public Interest, every time your child sees a food commercial on TV, it's as though you let a door-to-door huckster into your home who said, "I'd like to beguile your children and lure them into bad habits that will harm their health. Please leave the room so I can speak to them directly without your interference." The average American child sits in front of a TV set between 3 and 4 hours every day. By the time high school graduation rolls around, your child is likely to have seen well over a million TV commercials.

Of those commercials, many for sugary, artificially colored breakfast cereals focus on contests or free toys instead of the cereal itself. Fast-food restaurant commercials hype toy giveaways rather than the content of kids' meals. Snack food commercials promise a child painless popularity.

Most of these commercials focus very little of your child's attention on the nutritional content of the advertised food, and can leave children with a skewed idea of what's really good for them, food-wise.

Do you have to turn off the TV to see that kids get better balanced, healthier food messages? Not necessarily—although limiting TV time and encouraging active recreation is probably a good idea anyway. Here's a much easier way to balance the commercial food messages your kids get: Get in the habit of occasionally watching TV with your kids, especially while they're little. Make a game out of helping them sift through commercial messages for the facts. Let them decide what

is accurate, unbiased information and what is a paid-by-the-product commercial message.

You are your child's best role model. If you impart the facts about foods and other advertised products in a humorous, well-informed way, you'll go far to help your child differentiate substance from hype. Inevitably, it will be your values your child chooses to emulate, not the values he or she sees on TV. □

CHAPTER 19

Changes to Make at Menopause

Diet can't *cure* the troubling symptoms of menopause, but—for many women—it can make a significant difference. And, if you take menopause as a signal for renewal and preparation for the second half of your life, the changes you make now can yield important benefits for decades to come.

When you've gone for a full year without a period, you have officially reached menopause. Nevertheless, a woman's body begins to change starting 4 to 10 years sooner. During this time, called the perimenopause, the reproductive system prepares to retire and the ovaries gradually produce less estrogen. With perimenopause comes a variety of symptoms.

For many women, hot flashes (hot flushes) are the most noticeable result of the sharp variations in estrogen levels that mark this part of their lives. This sudden burst of heat can occur at any time and spread over your upper body, perhaps causing you to break into a sweat. The good news is that a hot flash will vanish as quickly as it appears.

And despite their reputation as a universal sign of menopause, hot flashes trouble some women for only a few months, while others have none at all.

Over a span of years (often 10 or more), you may also notice changes in your skin, such as increased dryness and wrinkling, and in hair texture. The lining of your vagina may become thinner, drier, and less pliable. Your breasts may lose some of their fullness, and the nipples become less pronounced. Significantly, although some bone loss is a normal part of aging, bone loss speeds up rapidly in women at menopause.

During or following menopause, you may find yourself gaining weight. Although it occurs at a time of dramatic hormonal changes, you can chalk up this gain to advancing age. Unless you exercise regularly, you'll begin to lose calorie-burning muscle at midlife. In addition, your metabolism will slow down, and your body will no longer need energy to support your reproductive system. To maintain your former body weight, you may need to cut your calorie intake by 10 to 15 percent while increasing your level of activity.

While most menopausal changes are physical, some women also develop such emotional problems as mood swings, irritability, and fatigue. While these feelings have not been directly linked to hormonal changes, they could easily be brought on by hot flashes, sleep deprivation, and other stressful consequences of menopause. Although diet can't solve these problems, keeping your nutritional status at peak levels is obviously a wise move during this stress-filled period.

Menopause is a highly individual experience. You may recognize many of these changes, or you may hardly notice any. If any of these menopausal symptoms become extremely uncomfortable, they can be treated medically. But whether you seek treatment or not, upgrading your lifestyle and your diet can help get you through.

Why a Low-Fat Diet is Especially Important Now

Researchers are just beginning to address the special nutritional needs of menopausal women. Still, nutritional experts generally agree that a well-balanced diet featuring a variety of nutrients is essential to good health at midlife. A diet rich in vegetables, whole grains, and fruits, with moderate servings of protein, is a wise idea at any time of life. At midlife, it's also important to increase your calcium intake to maintain

healthy bones and reduce your consumption of fat—if you haven't already—to lower your risk of heart disease, the nation's Number One killer of women as well as men.

These goals are actually easier to achieve than you might think. In fact, it may take only some relatively minor adjustments. The average American woman gets more than one-third of her calories from fat—a number that needs to be cut back to no more than 30 percent, according to many doctors and nutritionists. Some researchers believe that high-fat diets are particularly harmful to women during perimenopause, since they fuel estrogen production, thereby encouraging the exaggerated hormonal fluctuations that mark the perimenopausal years.

These dramatic variations are thought to lie at the root of many of the annoying symptoms of menopause, such as missed periods and hot flashes. Sticking with a well-balanced, low-fat diet can help smooth out the decline in your body's production of estrogen. Women are never completely without estrogen, since adrenal glands and body fat continue to produce low levels of estrogen even after menopause.

Studies comparing Asian and American women suggest that lifestyle can make a substantial difference in the way your body adjusts to menopause. Japanese women, whose diets are high in plant-derived estrogens—particularly from tofu and other soy products—reportedly have very little menopausal discomfort. They also have lower rates of two major killers of American women, heart disease and cancer.

Similar anecdotal evidence has begun to emerge among vegetarian women in the U.S. These women often glide through menopause with little reported discomfort, and their doctors are beginning to credit their low-fat

MENOPAUSE AT A GLANCE

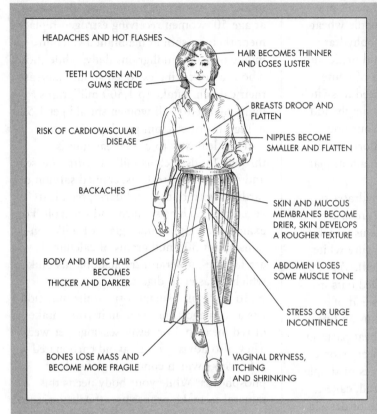

HEADACHES AND HOT FLASHES

TEETH LOOSEN AND
GUMS RECEDE

RISK OF CARDIOVASCULAR
DISEASE

BACKACHES

BODY AND PUBIC HAIR
BECOMES
THICKER AND DARKER

BONES LOSE MASS AND
BECOME MORE FRAGILE

HAIR BECOMES THINNER
AND LOSES LUSTER

BREASTS DROOP AND
FLATTEN

NIPPLES BECOME
SMALLER AND FLATTEN

SKIN AND MUCOUS
MEMBRANES BECOME
DRIER, SKIN DEVELOPS
A ROUGHER TEXTURE

ABDOMEN LOSES
SOME MUSCLE TONE

STRESS OR URGE
INCONTINENCE

VAGINAL DRYNESS,
ITCHING
AND SHRINKING

The wide array of problems shown in this diagram may seem daunting; but fortunately, few women experience every one of them. Hot flashes are the most common complaint. However, these annoying sensations pass in due course, while other symptoms may pose a much greater long-term threat. Be particularly alert for lower back pain, which may signal the onset of osteoporosis, the bone-weakening disorder that leaves older women prey to fractures. Remember, too, that menopause robs you of estrogen's protective effect on the heart, and that heart disease is the Number One killer of women.

diets. While few nutritionists advocate a vegetarian diet as a natural prescription for menopause, you can certainly arrange your meals to incorporate foods abundant in plant estrogens. These include alfalfa, apples, barley, carrots, cherries, chick peas, garlic, green beans, oats, peas, sweet potatoes, rye, and yams. These should not be eaten to the exclusion of other foods. Still, they may help moderate your body's hormonal fluctuations at menopause.

Carbohydrates provide most of the fuel for a healthy body, but it's important to choose the right ones—especially at midlife, when your body's metabolism becomes more sluggish. Complex carbohydrates, found in beans, corn, potatoes, and whole wheat, are digested more slowly and are healthier for your body than simple carbohydrates, or sugars, which enter your bloodstream directly from the digestive tract.

Nevertheless, some foods that are promoted as complex carbohydrates—including so-called "healthy" cold cereals made from whole-grain sources—actually break down very quickly in your system and don't provide long-lasting energy. Even whole wheat responds more like a simple carbohydrate when it's processed into flour and made into pasta or bread. The same is true of white rice. Remember, too, that you need to switch to complex carbohydrates—not simply add them to what you already eat. Your body converts excess carbohydrate calories into fat, which—if not balanced with additional exercise—causes weight gain.

You can add complex carbohydrates to your diet in a variety of ways. Purchase whole-grain bread instead of the usual white bread (but check the label to be sure white flour or sugar has not been added). Try brown rice instead of white, rolled oats instead of instant, rye crackers instead of saltines. Add fresh or frozen beans and peas to your diet. Look for whole-wheat pasta in the specialty section of your grocery store.

At the same time, avoid sources of simple carbohydrates such as white bread, cakes, donuts, and cookies. For a snack or dessert, substitute fresh fruit. Although fruits also are high in a simple sugar called fructose, their fiber content helps stabilize their impact on blood sugar levels.

Changes That Fend Off Disease

As the bone-maintaining levels of estrogen subside at menopause, a boost in calcium intake, along with moderate exercise, becomes absolutely essential. Without these measures, your chances of developing osteoporosis (brittle bones) rise dramatically. This debilitating disease, which affects more than 25 million Americans—most of them women—causes fractures in about half of all women over 50. In 1994, a panel of experts meeting at the National Institutes of Health recommended boosting the calcium intake for women at menopause. Beginning at age 50, women receiving estrogen-replacement therapy should maintain a calcium intake of 1,000 milligrams daily, while those who are not taking estrogen should increase their calcium intake to 1,500 milligrams daily. By age 65, all women should get 1,500 milligrams of calcium per day.

The ideal way to obtain calcium is through foods such as milk, yogurt, cheese, and other dairy products; canned salmon or sardines with bones; and dark-green leafy vegetables such as spinach and broccoli. For example, an eight-ounce glass of milk contains about 300 milligrams of calcium. If you are lactose-intolerant, try acidophilus milk which is easier to digest.

To ward off osteoporosis, some nutritionists also suggest that you limit your intake of red meat to 3 or fewer servings per week. They also advise you to avoid carbonated soft drinks which contain high levels of phosphorus. While your body needs this mineral to make proper use of calcium, too much of it can actually lead to loss of bone. For more information on preventing osteoporosis, see the Chapter 28, "Sure-Fire Way to Prevent Brittle Bones."

Estrogen has a protective effect on the heart, raising levels of "good" HDL cholesterol and lowering "bad" LDL cholesterol. It's no wonder then, that your risk of heart disease begins rising at menopause. To compensate, it's more important than ever to adopt a diet that is low in total and saturated fats and cholesterol and high in complex carbohydrates.

Breast, colon, and lung cancer are other significant risks for women at menopause and beyond. Most scientific studies that have examined the role of nutrition on cancer suggest that a diet high in fruits and vegetables—particularly those rich in vitamin A or beta-carotene—may provide some protective effect. These foods include citrus fruits and juices, cantaloupe, carrots, winter squash, tomatoes, broccoli, cauliflower, and leafy green vegetables. In addition to providing essential vitamins and minerals, these foods also are major sources of dietary fiber, which helps prevent constipation.

Fighting Symptoms with Supplements

Our ability to absorb vitamins and minerals from food becomes less efficient as we age, so it's even more important to make the right food choices—those low in calories and high in essential nutrients. Most women can get all the nutrients they require by eating a sensible, well-rounded diet. You may need supplements, however, if you have certain chronic health conditions or have developed deficiencies during an unsupervised diet or during pregnancy. Your body may also need a temporary boost during some of the major life stresses that so often coincide with menopause: career changes, children leaving home, or caring for elderly parents.

A multivitamin pill can supply the daily requirements that may be missing in your diet. Be cautious, however, about taking high doses of individual supplements; large doses of some vitamins can do more harm than good. For example, too much vitamin B_6 can cause nerve damage, and high doses of

vitamin D can cause kidney stones, constipation, or abdominal pain—particularly in women with existing kidney disease.

Some women claim that vitamins (and herbal remedies) serve as natural therapy for such symptoms of menopause as hot flashes. However, their effectiveness is unproven, because few scientific studies have been done. Before starting any supplementation program, you really should consult with your doctor or a registered dietitian.

Vitamin E is one agent that does have a proven track record: It appears to relieve hot flashes and vaginal dryness, and some women claim that it gives them more energy and an improved sense of well-being, as well. Most nutritionists believe that a diet containing whole grains, green vegetables, beans, and nuts can provide menopausal women with an adequate intake of vitamin E, but the supplement is certainly a big seller. An antioxidant, vitamin E also protects red blood cells and has other health benefits. It may not be suitable, however, if you have certain health conditions such as high blood pressure or diabetes.

Other vitamins, including B-complex and C, are also reported to relieve menopausal symptoms, including hot flashes. While the B-complex vitamins certainly promote digestion and healthy skin and vitamin C aids in wound healing and resistance to infection, any additional effect on menopausal symptoms is unproven.

Vitamins, used properly, can enhance the absorption of essential minerals in your diet. For example, vitamin D is important for calcium absorption and bone formation. Other essential minerals are zinc and magnesium. Zinc helps maintain pliancy in your genital tract, while magnesium helps prevent mood swings and insomnia. Found naturally in leafy green vegetables, nuts, and seeds, magnesium also boosts the calcium levels in your blood.

Many women swear by the benefits of herbal teas. These teas, and natural substances such as garlic, garden sage, dong quai, chamomile, catnip, hops, and passion flower have been promoted as satisfying self-help remedies for some menopausal symptoms, including hot flashes and skin changes. Flaxseed oil and evening-primrose oil have been shown to stimulate the natural production of small amounts of estrogen. Although not approved as a remedy for hot flashes, some women have found them effective.

Ginseng, another source of plant estrogen, is the natural remedy most often mentioned for the relief of menopausal symptoms. Ginseng can be taken in capsule form; as a tea or syrup; or as a root. Because no clinical studies have been done to prove ginseng's effectiveness, its use for the treatment of menopausal symptoms is not endorsed or regulated by the U.S. Food and Drug Administration. Be cautious if you try it. It is known to raise blood pressure.

Foods to Cut Down On

Overdoing a number of our favorite foods at this point in your life can not only aggravate some menopausal symptoms, but increase your risk of post-menopausal disease. And because of the complex way foods interact, certain substances can undo some of the benefits of any healthy additions you make to your diet.

TAKE THESE STEPS FOR BEST HEALTH AT MENOPAUSE. . . AND AFTER

- Follow a low-fat diet that includes generous servings of green, leafy vegetables, beans, and whole grains.
- Cut back on fat by reducing the use of heavy creams and sauces, gravy, butter, and vegetable shortening.
- Prevent high blood cholesterol levels by limiting the animal fat in your diet to three servings weekly and restricting your use of eggs.
- Take in 1,000 to 1,500 milligrams of calcium daily through low-fat, high-calcium dietary sources such as skim milk, plain low-fat yogurt, and broccoli.
- Substitute fresh or dried fruit for sugar- and fat-laden sweets.
- Get enough vitamin D to enhance calcium absorption—either through regular exposure to sunlight or via a vitamin D supplement.
- Keep caffeine and alcohol to a minimum, and try to quit smoking.

Sodium

Sodium plays an essential role in our bodies. It regulates blood pressure and transmits nerve impulses. But most of us get more than enough from dietary sources, so using a lot of salt is unnecessary and can be harmful. There is an as yet unconfirmed belief that excessive salt contributes to high blood pressure—which is a health risk as you age. And there is definitely a link between salt and osteoporosis. In fact, excess sodium leeches calcium from your digestive tract before it can be used by your bones, literally pulling it into the kidneys, where it's eliminated from the body.

Unless you prepare meals carefully, using only fresh ingredients, you probably get plenty of sodium from a variety of sources. These include baking soda, baking powder, canned and cured foods, prepackaged and convenience foods, potato chips, condiments, and flavor enhancers such as MSG. The easiest way to avoid eating too much salt is to remove the salt shaker from the kitchen table and stop cooking with salt. In addition, cut back on salt-cured and smoked foods, such as sausages, smoked fish, ham, bacon, bologna, and hot dogs.

Americans are conditioned to use salt. Your family might protest for a week or so, but they'll be surprised how quickly they adjust to the real taste of food.

Caffeine

If you're a heavy coffee drinker—and most American women are—now's the time to cut back on caffeinated coffee or eliminate it from your diet altogether.

A stimulant also found in soft drinks, chocolate, and tea, caffeine is used by most people to overcome fatigue and work harder or faster—thus, the traditional "coffee break" mentality in American business. At menopause, however, coffee and other caffeinated beverages can increase the number or intensity of hot flashes. Caffeine also has been implicated in breast changes such as fibrocystic disease, in osteoporosis, and in a rise in serum cholesterol associated with heart disease. Despite our affection for coffee, it's difficult to make a case for caffeine use at menopause.

Warning: If you're used to drinking five or six cups of coffee or caffeinated soft drinks daily, eliminating caffeine too quickly can trig-

ger withdrawal symptoms. These range from headaches and nervousness to drowsiness, nausea, and constipation. To avoid caffeine withdrawal, switch gradually to decaffeinated drinks over a period of several weeks.

Sugar

Fluctuating hormones affect blood sugar levels and can cause cravings for sugar. Refined sugars—those found in your sugar bowl and in candy, cakes, pastries, cold cereals, syrups, and a nearly endless variety of processed and prepackaged foods—are packed with calories and little else. They make it easy to gain weight, but contribute nothing of value to your nutritional status. Sugar also suppresses the body's use of calcium and phosphorus. And too much sugar can cause a vaginal discharge that can contribute to recurring vaginal and urinary-tract infections.

In general, you can suppress a craving for sweets by keeping your protein levels steady. Also, be sure to stock your pantry with healthy alternatives. Fresh and dried fruits contain the natural sugar fructose along with fiber. A small serving can quench a sugar craving and serve as a natural laxative to aid your digestive system. Scientists believe that fruit may also help protect against stomach and colon cancers. Today's grocery stores carry nearly every variety of fruit year-round—from the mundane to the sublime. Indulge your taste buds while treating your body to good nutrition.

Fats and cholesterol

Prior to menopause, estrogen helps suppress the buildup of fat along arterial walls that often results from intake of too much saturated (animal) fat and cholesterol. But as menopause drives down your estrogen levels, this extra protection vanishes, leaving you prey to the arterial buildup that often ends in cardiac disease, heart attack and stroke.

Some experts have suggested that rising rates of breast cancer may also be due to the excessive amounts of abnormal fatty acids in our diet—particularly those found in margarine, vegetable shortening, and fast foods.

Although a modest amount of fat is a recommended part of our diet, it is easily obtained from meager amounts of lean meats, nuts, fish, and poultry. Fats can be used sparingly to add taste to a menu—for example, a dab of avocado to garnish a salad or a spoonful of peanut butter on whole-grain toast. But otherwise, spare your heart by reducing or eliminating your intake of butter, rich sauces and gravies, fatty meats, and whole milk and ice cream. Bake, steam, or broil your food instead of frying it in fat. And serve eggs and organ meats sparingly. Though they add iron and protein to your diet, they have extremely high concentrations of cholesterol. For more information, see Chapter 10, "What to Do About Fat."

Alcohol and smoking

Numerous studies have confirmed the negative effects of alcohol and smoking on a woman's health at midlife. Although recent studies have touted a modest intake of alcohol to boost "good" HDL cholesterol levels, and guard against heart disease, you should be aware that much of this research was conducted on men. Generalizing the benefits to women—particularly during the midlife transition—could be unwise.

In any event, alcohol is thought to aggravate hot flashes in menopausal women, and heavy use of alcohol is a known risk factor

for osteoporosis. Some studies have also linked alcohol to increased risk of breast cancer and high blood pressure; and its high sugar content adds empty calories to your diet that can easily cause weight gain. Most experts agree that minimizing or eliminating your alcohol consumption, including beer and wine, boosts your overall health at midlife and beyond.

As for tobacco, lung cancer now causes more deaths in American women than breast cancer. Heavy smokers also tend to have an earlier menopause, which has been linked to higher rates of heart disease and osteoporosis.

Several new studies have confirmed that cutting out smoking even in midlife or old age—cuts your chances of developing cancer of the lung, mouth, esophagus, kidney, stomach, and colon. It also helps the heart, lung, and circulatory systems and reduces the impact of emphysema or chronic lung disease. By giving up cigarettes, you'll unquestionably improve the health of your heart and lungs and decrease your risk of developing osteoporosis. (For more, see Chapter 30, "What Smokers Need to Know About Diet.")

Remember that variety and moderation are the keys to good nutrition during this exciting, though occasionally turbulent, period. At midlife—even more so than in your younger years—you are what you eat. Embrace a healthy diet for its boost to a robust heart, strong bones, and radiant skin. Maximizing your intake of nutritious foods and minimizing your reliance on empty calories will prepare you to appreciate the joys of menopause without suffering its sorrows. □

CHAPTER 20

Dietary Targets for Your Senior Years

Scientists have yet to discover the silver bullet that will reverse the effects of aging. But there are still plenty of common-sense measures you can take to keep your health and well-being right where you want them. The retirement years are a time when you need fewer calories, but as much—if not more—nutrition; so you have to build a dietary strategy that makes every calorie count. This is also a time when a few basic changes can help fend off the ravages of heart disease, high blood pressure, brittle bones, and other disorders that frequently—but not inevitably—accompany our later years. The dietary tactics for fighting these "diseases of maturity" are covered in chapters of their own. Here we're examining the best ways to optimize your overall health.

The Obstacles We Face

No matter what we do, advancing years make it harder to stay in shape. As we age, the rate at which we store and burn energy slows down. We begin to lose muscle mass, while the percentage of fat in the body gradually rises. As aging continues, the heart muscle becomes taut and pumps blood less efficiently, making healthy physical activity more difficult. The bones grow porous and stiff, eventually posing the danger of fractures. The liver and kidneys begin to shrink—ultimately to little more than half their original size—diminishing the body's ability to handle alcohol, medications, and minerals. The stomach's capacity to produce the acid needed for digestion also declines, sometimes leading to hidden malnutrition.

Compounding these problems, many people begin to have trouble with their teeth and gums as their later years approach—ultimately losing their ability to enjoy a healthy meal. At the same time, the senses of taste and smell tend to decline. Bitter tastes begin to prevail over more pleasing sweet and sour flavors; and food becomes less appealing just when the body could benefit from a

IS YOUR DIET UP TO PAR?

This quick self-test for people over 65 was developed by the Nutrition Screening Initiative, a consortium of three dozen medical and government organizations led by the American Academy of Family Physicians, the American Dietetic Association, and the National Council on the Aging.

Circle the number of each statement that applies to you; add up your points, then check your total against the nutritional scores.

1. An ongoing illness or current condition has made me change the kind or amount of food I eat. (2 points) _____

2. I eat fewer than two full meals per day. (3 points) _____

3. I eat few fruits, vegetables or milk products. (2 points) _____

4. I have three or more drinks of beer, liquor or wine almost every day. (2 points) _____

5. I have tooth or mouth problems that make eating hard for me. (2 points) _____

6. I don't always have enough money for the food I need. (4 points) _____

7. I eat alone most of the time. (1 point) _____

8. I take three or more different prescription or over-the-counter drugs a day. (1 point) _____

9. Without meaning to, I have lost or gained ten pounds in the past six months. (2 points) _____

10. I can't always shop, cook or feed myself. (2 points) _____

Total _____

NUTRITIONAL SCORES:

0-2: No problem. Recheck your status in six months.

3-5: Your diet could stand some improvement. Check with your local Office on Aging for information on available programs. The National Association of Area Agencies on Aging Eldercare Locator can assist in finding help. Call (800) 677-1116 toll-free. Recheck in three months.

6 or more: You have a real problem. Don't hesitate to tell your doctor, registered dietitian or local social worker about this test and see what can be done to help.

nutritional boost. Together, all these changes conspire to make a carefully planned diet more important than at any other time of life.

Barriers to a Decent Diet

Despite the greater importance of nutrition, many older people wind up eating *less*. Nearly half of all older hospital patients and two-fifths of nursing home residents are believed to suffer from malnutrition. Even retirees with full Social Security and pension benefits often lack proper nutrition.

The problem stems both from eating the wrong kinds of food and from simply not eating enough. As the biological clock winds down and the body begins to lose mass, many older people find that their interest in food—and, sometimes, their appetite for it—has also diminished. Even though the demand for calories declines as we age, our intake may drop too low to meet even these reduced requirements. Add to this the fact that the body's need for some nutrients actually increases with age, and it's easy to see how malnutrition can develop.

Some researchers suspect that the biological mechanisms controlling our food intake become less responsive as we age. Consequently, when elderly people are recovering from an illness or injury, their normal appetite may not return as quickly as a younger adult's. In this way, a temporary illness can set off a long-term nutritional problem. The array of medications that many older people must take on a continuing basis can also lead to a deficiency if one of them suppresses the appetite or alters taste sensations. It's true, too, that for many older people, shopping and cooking becomes too much of a chore. Their mobility is more limited. Labels are harder to read. Big supermarkets, with their sprawling aisles and busy parking lots, present a growing challenge.

The loss of a spouse can be an especially damaging blow at this point—in terms of physical health as well as emotional well-being. Loneliness and depression, which seem to strike older men particularly hard, can easily destroy the appetite. Indeed, the weight loss, lightheadedness, disorientation, lethargy, and loss of appetite that are often diagnosed as illness in the elderly are actually the consequences of clinical depression.

Robbed of the motivation of cooking for two, and daunted by the demands of the big shopping centers, too many older people find themselves subsisting on convenience-store items—canned soups, candy, and snack foods. Fortunately, there are plenty of ways to break out of this rut.

If you suspect you're depressed, talk to your doctor about it; the problem *can* be remedied. If you think one of your medications may be affecting your appetite, see about having it changed. There are alternatives for virtually any drug you take; and even a change in dosage could have a beneficial effect.

To get more variety in your diet, you can plan shopping trips with friends. There are plenty of healthy, easy to prepare items to be had at the supermarket for far less than the cost of convenience foods. Try to dine out more frequently, either with friends or at the local community center or church. And if your budget is becoming a problem, you owe it to yourself to look into available sources of help. Contact your local Agency on Aging. You may be eligible for foods stamps and other meal programs. Don't hesitate to take advantage of them. Remember that you've been supporting them with your tax dollars long before you ever needed them yourself.

Super-Charging Your Diet For Your Later Years

As you approach retirement, your nutritional requirements definitely undergo a change. Although your demand for calories may decline slightly, your need for protein, calcium, and a number of vitamins is on the rise. To fully meet these escalating requirements, experts recommend the following menu daily:

- For men, at least three half-cup servings of low-fat milk or dairy products such as cheese, cottage cheese, or yogurt. Women should make it four. (This intake is slightly higher than the "Food Pyramid" recommendation in Chapter 1.)
- Two or three three-ounce servings of protein-rich foods such as poultry, fish, eggs, beans, nuts, or lean meat.
- Five or more servings of fruit and vegetables, including a citrus fruit or juice and a dark green leafy vegetable.
- Six or more servings of rice, pasta, bread and cereal products made with whole grain or enriched flours.

That may sound like a lot of food, especially now that we're all so diet conscious. On balance, however, medical experts say we should be more concerned about adequate calorie intake as we grow older, rather than worrying about too many calories. Indeed, in evaluating older patients, some doctors have begun to challenge the validity of the standard height and weight tables used by insurance companies to establish "ideal" weights according to sex and body type. Originally intended for younger adults, these tables have become benchmarks for older people for lack of any other standard. Despite these tables, an average weight gain of 5 pounds per decade, beginning in your 40s, is now considered normal.

Total weight is not the only indicator of your health. The ratio of muscle to fat and the distribution of fat are believed to be just as important. Studies have found that, no matter what their total weight, older people whose body fat is concentrated around their waists, rather than at their hips, face a greater risk of heart disease, stroke, diabetes, high blood pressure, cancer, and gallbladder disease.

If you are truly overweight, it's clear that you ought to cut back on calories. Remember, though, that you must be careful to avoid shortchanging yourself of essential nutrients in the process.

Make Sure You Get Protein

Protein is the basic material in all body cells, including those in your muscles, organs, skin, bones, blood, hormones, and hair. It enables the cells to grow and helps the body to resist disease.

As the body's calorie intake declines, the share of protein needed in your diet rises. It's crucial, therefore, that you keep the protein content of your diet up to par. While an extra high-protein diet can leech some of the calcium from your bones and weaken them, too little protein will impair your body's ability to maintain and repair tissue.

Meat, fish, dairy products, and eggs are rich sources of protein. Although many contain fat and cholesterol, some foods from this group should be part of your diet every day. Plant foods such as dry peas and beans, grains, nuts, and seeds also contain protein and are especially valuable in combination with animal or other plant proteins.

Boost Carbohydrates and Fiber

Carbohydrates are the body's main source of fuel. Between 40 and 50 percent of your daily calories should come from carbohydrates, and most of these should be complex carbohydrates, or starches, which are digested more slowly and provide more sustained energy. Sources of complex carbohydrates include whole grain breads and

SIX DIETARY TARGETS FOR YOUR RETIREMENT YEARS (AND BEFORE)

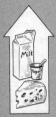

1. Get plenty of calcium.
For older women in particular, developing the brittle bones of osteoporosis is a major threat. Go heavy on dairy products, making sure they're low-fat; and ask your doctor about taking a calcium supplement. Even if you're a man, you can't afford to short-change yourself on calcium. Osteoporosis doesn't strike men as often as women, but it is still a risk.

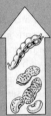

2. Eat more low-fat protein.
As a share of your diet, your protein requirement goes up as you grow older. However, you still need to keep a tight lid on fat and cholesterol. The solution: increase your intake of beans, peas, lentils, nuts, and grains. These plant products supply extra protein without blowing your budget for fat.

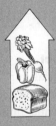

3. Boost your intake of fruit, vegetables, and grains.
The need to emphasize the complex carbohydrates found in these foods doesn't change as you age—and the fiber many of these products supply is an important dividend for older people. A little extra fiber helps keep the digestive system in good order, and can lower your cholesterol levels as well.

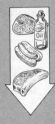

4.Go easy on fat and cholesterol.
For some people in their middle years, excessive fat and cholesterol can lead to heart disease. Although recent research suggests that if you survive into your 70's, this may no longer be a threat, it's probably wise to hedge your bet and keep fat at moderate levels anyway.

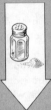

5. Keep an eye on your salt intake. As you grow older, your sensitivity to salt increases. This can aggravate high blood pressure, kidney disease, and congestive heart failure—all of which become more likely as you age. If you don't have high blood pressure, you can be a little more relaxed; but it's still a good idea to keep salt intake to a minimum.

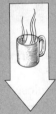

6. Cut back on alcohol and caffeine. Older bodies have less tolerance for both. "Overdoses" of caffeinated coffee could be the root of a number of problems, ranging from sleep problems to irregular heartbeat. Too much alcohol can lead to high blood pressure, liver disease, and increased odds of several cancers.

cereals, pastas, potatoes, and vegetables. Fruits and milk products are the only simple carbohydrates, or sugars, that you should include in your diet on a regular basis. Cut down on sweet desserts, candy, honey, and other sugary foods, which boost your calorie intake but not your nutrition.

Many sources of complex carbohydrates also provide dietary fiber, or roughage, which offers additional health benefits to seniors. Although its role is not yet fully under-

MANAGING THE DIGESTIVE PROBLEMS OF THE LATER YEARS

Disorders of the digestive tract cause more hospital admissions than any other group of diseases, and they strike middle-aged and older adults the most.

Constipation becomes more of a problem as we grow older, and diet is often to blame. Seniors who have difficulty chewing may shun needed high-fiber foods in favor of a soft, processed diet. Lack of exercise and inadequate fluid intake make the problem worse. But rather than reaching for a laxative, which can interfere with the absorption of minerals and other nutrients, consider new ways of getting fiber into your diet.

Some whole grain products can be tough on the teeth, but there are plenty of softer alternatives including oatmeal, stewed or canned fruits, beans, steamed vegetables, brown rice, and salad. A boost in your intake of these foods will also reduce your risk of developing diverticulosis, in which small sacs form on the wall of the large intestine—often causing abdominal pain.

The stomach's ability to produce the acid needed to digest food also decreases with age, leading to additional digestive problems. Heartburn, which results from a backflow of gastric juices into the esophagus, also becomes more likely. It can be minimized by avoiding rich or spicy foods such as tomato products, fried foods, and chocolate. Eating small, frequent meals, using antacids judiciously, and sitting up for several hours after eating also help to control the problem. (Check with your doctor, however, before assuming the problem is heartburn—it could be your heart! For more on this and other digestive problems, turn to Chapter 25.)

Milk, or lactose, intolerance is also more common in older adults. It is caused by an age-related decline in levels of lactase—the intestinal enzyme that digests the sugar found in milk. Symptoms include cramps, gas, bloating, and diarrhea after consuming milk or a milk product. You can often manage the problem successfully by mixing milk with food or other beverages, eating processed cheeses and yogurt, or eating smaller and more frequent servings. As an alternative, acidophilus milk, sold in grocery stores, contains an additive that makes the milk easier to digest. For more on lactose intolerance, see Chapter 24.

stood, dietary fiber helps to prevent constipation and may reduce the risk of other intestinal disorders, including diverticulosis and cancer of the colon and rectum. Recent research suggests that a diet high in fiber helps to control blood sugar and lower blood cholesterol levels.

While natural sources of fiber certainly aid the digestive process and may provide other benefits, fiber is not a tonic for old age. If you eat the recommended amounts of whole grain cereals and breads, vegetables, and fruits, there's no need to take a supplement.

Cut Back on Fats and Cholesterol

Despite all the claims and commercials for "light," "lean," and "reduced fat" foods, fat is not all bad. In fact, it contains essential nutrients and allows your cells to function properly.

Fats have many important functions. They make food more appetizing by adding flavor, aroma, and texture. They help to maintain healthy skin—a major concern for older adults, whose skin can become thin and fragile. Fats also carry the fat-soluble vitamins—A, D, E, and K—and are needed to help the body absorb these important nutrients.

The problem with fat is that we generally get too much of a good thing. In older adults, as in the young, no more than 30 percent of total calories should come from fat. Of the various types of fat, the most beneficial are the mono- and polyunsaturated fats found in plants. These include corn oil, safflower oil, soybean oil, sunflower oil, olives and olive oil, peanuts and peanut oil, and peanut butter. Saturated fats and cholesterol are less desirable. To cut down on them limit your intake of eggs and organ meat, as well as butter, cream, lard, mayonnaise, salad dressings, gravies, sauces, and snack foods such as potato chips.

A great deal of confusion exists about the relationship between dietary fat and cholesterol—particularly in older adults. Cholesterol is essential for proper nerve function and other vital processes, but our bodies are quite capable of producing all that we need. The American Heart Association advises adults to limit cholesterol consumption to about 300 milligrams per day, or about the amount in one egg yolk. For some people, intake above that level can lead to accumulations in the blood that build up inside the walls of the arteries, a principal cause of heart attacks and strokes.

Although half of the four million U.S. adults with heart disease are over 65, medical experts have become deeply divided over the impact of cholesterol in senior citizens. While many continue to insist on low-cholesterol diets for older people with other health risks, some now maintain that cholesterol levels in the mid-200s—considered relatively high for younger adults—pose little risk among the elderly.

The reason for the disagreement is conflicting research. Numerous long-standing studies have indicated that elevated blood cholesterol is associated with an increased risk of heart disease in people over 65. Several more recent studies, however, have failed to confirm this link in otherwise healthy adults over the age of 70. Reducing cholesterol levels may not make much sense for people in their 80s and 90s, these researchers suggest.

To cut your blood cholesterol, you not only must reduce your dietary intake, but must cut back on saturated fats as well. Although these fats are *not* cholesterol themselves, they can increase the amount of cholesterol in your blood.

As most recovering heart patients have already learned, reducing the fat and choles-

DIABETES: YOUR RISK INCREASES WITH AGE

Up to one-fifth of adults over 65 may have some impairment in their ability to utilize blood sugar (glucose). Levels of unused glucose in the blood gradually increase in everyone after age 50, but outright diabetes—the inability to convert enough blood sugar into needed energy—is much less common. Most older adults have type II diabetes, which can be treated in several ways.

If you develop a mild case of diabetes, you may be able to control your blood sugar with nothing more than strict adherence to a special, low-sugar diet. If that doesn't work, your doctor will prescribe a glucose-lowering drug or, if need be, insulin. In any event, the condition is not something to take lightly since numerous studies have shown that people with even mildly elevated blood glucose levels face a greater chance of heart disease, stroke, blindness, and loss of limbs due to poor circulation. For more on the latest treatments for this dangerous disease, see Chapter 23.

MEETING THE CHALLENGE OF ALZHEIMER'S

Trying to upgrade the diet of someone with Alzheimer's disease or another form of memory impairment may be an unrealistically ambitious project. Remembering or understanding dietary instructions or preparing a new dish may be nearly impossible for an older adult with this tragic condition. Even early in the disease, when normal body functions remain intact, people with memory loss may resist changes to their routine. If you attempt to change their diet, they may become agitated or simply refuse to eat.

Instead of playing by strict—and sometimes controversial—nutritional rules, focus on the individual's food preferences. If maintaining weight is a problem, try serving milk shakes and custards with regular meals. The keys to meeting the nutritional needs of someone with Alzheimer's are kindness, patience, and persistence.

terol in your diet is rarely easy. Nevertheless, there are a number of relatively painless strategies for cutting back as outlined in Chapter 10, "What To Do About Fat."

If your health is generally good, and you decide that the opportunity to enjoy your favorite foods outweighs the possible benefit of a lower cholesterol profile, you do have some research on your side.

Remember, however, that cholesterol is only one of the culprits in heart disease. For greatest safety, you still need to get regular exercise, stop smoking if possible, and keep your weight under control.

Go Heavy on the Calcium

Unlike the debate over cholesterol, scientists vehemently agree that older people should pay extra attention to their calcium intake.

Postmenopausal women and older men are faced with the threat of osteoporosis, which thins the bones and can lead to crippling—even fatal—fractures of the wrist, spine, and hip. Aging interferes with your body's ability to absorb calcium, and reduced physical activity further impairs calcium absorption. A diet extra high in protein, fat, and fiber, excessive consumption of alcohol and caffeine, and smoking also heighten your risk.

To build and maintain bone in later life, calcium-rich foods are essential. Lowfat milk, yogurt, cheese, and other dairy products are ideal sources of calcium. If you're unable to drink milk because you're lactose-intolerant, other calcium-rich foods include tofu, green leafy vegetables such as broccoli and kale, and pinto and kidney beans. You may also want to consider a calcium supplement. For more information, see Chapter 28, "Sure Fire Way to Prevent Brittle Bones."

Consider Extra Vitamins and Minerals

Conventional wisdom argues that a healthy, well-balanced diet will provide all the vitamins and minerals you need to meet the extra demands of aging. For the many older people who don't eat enough, however, this assurance is somewhat beside the point. For them, a balanced, moderate vitamin/mineral supplement can make a lot of sense. Special situations may also call for supplementation. We've already looked at the need for calcium. In addition, people recovering from illness or surgery may need extra vitamin C and zinc to promote the healing of skin wounds. Dieters and heavy drinkers can also benefit from supplements.

Even more significantly, several recent medical studies and an endorsement from the Alliance for Aging Research in Washington, DC, support sharply higher amounts of daily antioxidant supplementation—specifically, 250 to 1,000 milligrams of vitamins C,

YOUR MEDICATIONS: HOW MANY DO YOU REALLY NEED?

More than three-fourths of Americans 65 and older take at least one prescription drug, and many take several. The more drugs you take, the greater your risk of drug interactions, which can ruin your appetite, cancel the effects of a drug, and cause dangerous side effects such as dizziness, confusion, fatigue, memory loss, and depression. Moreover, as one specialist after another writes prescriptions, an estimated one in four older adults winds up taking too many, or the wrong kinds, of medicine.

Many drugs can alter your nutritional status. For instance, if you take a water pill (diuretic) for high blood pressure or congestive heart failure, you may be losing excessive amounts of potassium, calcium and other important minerals—losses you can ill afford if your diet contains inadequate amounts of these nutrients to begin with. For other potential conflicts between drugs and your diet, see Chapter 29, "Foods to Watch Out For When Taking Medication."

Although it's dangerous to suddenly stop taking certain medications—particularly blood pressure drugs and heart medication—you should schedule annual "brown bag" reviews of your drugs with your doctor. Gather all of your medications—including over-the-counter medicines such as cough syrups and pain relievers—dump them in a bag, and sit down with your doctor or pharmacist to see whether some should be changed or discontinued altogether. It's not unusual to find that you're taking two different drugs that do the same things, or two that cancel each other out.

100 to 400 International Units of vitamin E, and 10 to 30 milligrams of beta-carotene—in the hope of improving immunity, reducing coronary artery disease, and decreasing the risk of infection in old age. In studies conducted in the U.S. and Canada, older patients who received a multivitamin supplement with higher levels of these nutrients showed significant improvement in their immune systems and a reduction in infection-related illnesses.

On the other hand, there's no question that megadoses (10 or more times the Recommended Daily Allowance) of vitamin and mineral supplements can be dangerous, since the aging kidneys or liver may not be able to get rid of the excess. Whenever you take a nutrient in amounts that exceed what your body can handle, you court the risk of side effects. For example, too much vitamin A can cause headaches, nausea, diarrhea, and eventually liver and bone damage. High doses of vitamin D can cause kidney damage and even death. When taken in excessive amounts, supplemental iron can build up to toxic levels in the liver. And taking too much of one mineral can upset the delicate balance of others. For instance, excess phosphorus interferes with the body's ability to absorb calcium.

It's true, too, that totally unfounded nutritional claims abound. Claims that fish oils can reduce the risk of heart disease are clearly exaggerated—though they do appear to reduce the likelihood of blood clots. Likewise, assertions that vitamin B_{15} reverses the aging process lack much scientific justification. As a rule of thumb, it's wise to be cautious about sharply jacking up your intake of any individual vitamin or mineral without first consulting your doctor. He or she can recommend supplements at a dose that is safe and sensible, making allowance for your age, medical condition, and any medications you take. Remember, too, that a hodgepodge of pills and potions will never work as a substitute for a complete, balanced diet.

Put a Lid on Salt

As we grow older, salt becomes more of a problem for us. The sodium in table salt is a necessary part of life. It helps to maintain blood volume, regulate water balance, transmit nerve impulses, and perform other vital functions. It appears naturally in a variety of foods, including cheeses, eggs, meat, and fish, yet many of us continue to pour on additional sodium in the form of table salt.

As taste sensations diminish with advancing years, it's tempting to compensate by adding even more salt. However, this can be harmful, particularly for older adults. Excess sodium is normally pulled from the body by the kidneys. But aging kidneys are notoriously liable to malfunction; and if they cannot process all of the salt, your body compensates by building up fluid. This can lead to high blood pressure which increases your risk of heart disease, stroke, or kidney failure. Excessive sodium intake also can worsen the consequences of existing kidney disease and congestive heart failure.

Removing the salt shaker from the table and avoiding salt during food preparation are two of the best ways to reduce your sodium intake. In addition, check the labels on the foods you buy. Federal laws require commercially prepared foods such as soups, frozen dinners, and other processed items to list their sodium content in the "Nutrition Facts" box, and you'll find that there are large amounts of sodium hidden in processed foods—everything from breakfast cereals to canned goods. Replace these prepackaged

SOME TIPS FOR SHOPPING AND PREPARING MEALS

- Plan major shopping expeditions with a friend.

- If a package is too big, ask for help. Meat or produce employees can repackage items for you in smaller servings.

- Watch out for sodium if you have a blood pressure problem. Manufacturers list the sodium content of their products on the labels. If sodium is one of the first three ingredients listed, the product is high in sodium. When preparing fresh meat and produce, use lemon, pepper, herbs, spices, powdered mustard, or finely chopped garlic to flavor foods, rather than salt.

- Always keep several days-worth of canned or frozen fish, meat, fruits, vegetables, and soups on hand so you can prepare a good meal even when you can't get to the grocery store.

- Switch from red meat to veal, poultry, fish, seafood, and meat substitutes and increase the number of meatless main dishes on your menu to 3 or more per week. Reduce egg consumption to no more than 2 egg yolks per week.

- Use vegetable oils such as safflower, sunflower, corn, soybean, and olive oils instead of butter, lard, and other animal fats.

- To cut your workload in the kitchen, prepare large amounts of dishes such as chicken casserole or spaghetti sauce and refrigerate or freeze the leftovers for later use.

- Eat with friends. Start a potluck club where each member takes turns hosting the group for dinner, and everyone brings a dish. Everyone gets more variety with less trouble.

foods with fresh fish and poultry, fresh vegetables, fruits and grains.

Be especially suspicious of packaged snacks—potato chips, pretzels, crackers, and nuts. They normally contain large amounts of salt. Fresh or dried fruits such as raisins and figs make healthier snacks. Remember, too, that sodium is found in many beverages, such as soft drinks and beer, and in a wide variety of medications. Reducing the sodium in your diet without completely ruining your meals is no easy trick. Nevertheless, it can be done. A liberal dollop of garlic during cooking, a spritz of lemon juice, or a pinch of herbs can repair much of the damage. See Chapter 35 on herbs and spices for more ideas.

Cut Down on Caffeine

Like salt, caffeine turns up in unexpected places: chocolate, soft drinks, tea, some aspirin compounds, and other over-the-counter medications. And as we grow older, our tolerance of caffeine declines.

Although caffeine is a stimulant usually consumed precisely for its "kick," its unpleasant side effects are more likely to surface in our later years. These range from anxiety and irritability to sleep disorders, migraine headaches, diarrhea, indigestion, and irregular heartbeat. Caffeine also can exaggerate the symptoms of older people with muscle tremors, such as those with Parkinson's disease, and increase the agitation of individuals with dementia.

If you're used to drinking several cups of coffee, tea, or caffeinated soft drinks daily, consider gradually switching to decaffeinated drinks. You may find that a cup of soup is just as satisfying as tea in the evening or on a cold winter day. And whenever you need a medication, be sure to ask your health care professional or pharmacist to help you select one that doesn't contain caffeine.

Keep Alcohol to a Minimum

It's estimated that one of every four older Americans has two or more drinks a day. The ramifications are numerous. Alcohol is a diuretic that can deplete your water volume. Consuming even modest amounts increases your chance of developing osteoporosis, kidney and liver disease, and inflammation of the pancreas. Several studies have linked alcohol to an increased risk of high blood pressure and even cancer. Its high sugar content makes it a bad choice for diabetics. Its empty calories make losing weight more difficult. And nearly half of all prescriptions written for the elderly also interact with alcohol.

With age, the liver's ability to deal with alcohol declines. Even if you have only 1 or 2 drinks a day, you tend to burn the alcohol more slowly, so higher concentrations remain in your blood over a longer period of time—an important point to remember if you need to drive. Most experts agree that, by minimizing or eliminating your alcohol consumption, including beer and wine, you can boost your overall health profile during your later years.

Remember, though, that the key to maintaining a really good diet is to think in terms of addition, not subtraction. Cut fat and cholesterol by *adding* whole grains and vegetables to your diet. Cut salt by *adding* new flavors like garlic, lemon, herbs, and spices. Add excitement to your meals with new colors and textures to make your plate more eye-appealing. Add more fun to your meals by dining with friends. You worked hard all your life; enjoy your later years to the maximum, and enjoy in good health. □

Special Problems, Special Diets

CHAPTER 21

Boosting Energy and Fitness: Which Foods Really Work?

Astroll through the aisles of any health food store will reveal a dazzling array of sophisticated and seductively packaged fitness foods, dietary supplements, vitamins, minerals, herbal con- coctions, organic derivatives and scores of other ingestibles. These products tempt those who dream of effortless weight loss, acceler- ated muscle-building, or fail-safe protection against aging. Their very names attest to their claims: "Fat Burners." "Brute Strength." "Longevity."

But instead of pushing your "buy me" button, products that promise "easy" fitness should sound shrill alarms.

By 1996, sales of fitness foods will top $4 billion dollars and will account for more than half of all health food store revenues. What exactly are these products?

Miracle Foods or Money Wasters?

Nowadays, almost any substance you ingest in hopes of improving your level of nutrition is called a dietary supplement or "fitness food." Once you achieve optimal nutrition by using supple- ments—so the theory goes—you will perform better, have boundless energy and strength, be able to burn fat and calories more rapidly, and have a body that looks and acts young well into old age.

For many people, dietary supplements, including vitamins and minerals, may have a place in a healthy diet plan. Products such as nutritionally complete formula meals are indispensable for the ill or the elderly, and for people otherwise unable to consume enough nutrients to meet daily needs.

But there are thousands of products whose health and fitness claims cannot be scientifically proven—and some of these could be harmful.

Promises, Promises

Promises made by so-called fitness foods run the gamut from speedy, effortless weight loss to efficient, muscular weight-gain. Other products claim to grow hair, reduce the risks of birth defects, lower stress, improve athletic performance, combat osteoporosis, and heighten sexual prowess.

How do you know which preparations will fulfill their promises? The truth is, you really don't, and, in many cases, unless you're an expert on nutrition or chemistry, it is unlikely that reading the label will help you choose a product that does what it says it will do.

One of the problems consumers face is that regulations governing health claims made by manufacturers of dietary supplements are in a state of flux.

In 1990, the federal Food and Drug Administration passed the Nutrition Labeling and Education Act, which required food makers to back all explicit and implied health claims—even those suggested by the product's brand name—with scientific documentation. It also set standards for the meaning of "low," "light," and "free".

Now, for example, each serving of a "low-fat" product must contain no more than three grams of fat in each serving or 100 grams of the food. Products labeled "low-cholesterol" must contain a maximum of 20 milligrams of cholesterol, per serving or per 100 grams.

So far, only two health claims are allowable under the law. Foods high in calcium can now be labeled "aids in preventing osteoporosis;" foods rich in folic acid can claim to help prevent birth defects when taken by pregnant women. Other claims are being considered for approval.

Supplement labels printed after July 1, 1994, cannot make unproven health claims. However, Congress is considering a bill that could lower the standard for substantiating health claims made by dietary supplements.

According to some experts, no matter what the regulations eventually say, consumers will still have to be wary of dietary supplements' health claims. It's estimated that the supplement industry spends about $500 million each year on advertising, while the U.S. Food and Drug Administration's health-fraud fighting budget is only about $1.5 million a year. Enforcement of any regulations will be difficult, so before you buy, be sure you are well informed.

Which Fitness Foods Keep Their Promise?

The good news is that some products that make fitness claims can and do deliver on their promises. Certain packaged food mixes and diet supplements actually can help you lose weight and reduce body fat.

But there is a caveat. No preparation is effective alone; to achieve fitness you must also follow a well-balanced diet and stick with an exercise plan.

Fitness foods and supplements come in many forms: metabolism-boosting capsules; combination plans consisting of various nutrient-containing capsules along with powdered meals; or simply powders you mix with water, juice or milk to make meal-in-a-glass shakes.

One of latest of these products, MET-Rx™, describes itself as an "engineered food," claims to be "the most perfect food the world has ever seen," and comes with a free 40+ page booklet. Scores of other products, such as Infiniti, Cybertrim, Quicktrim, make similar fitness claims.

The MET-Rx booklet cautions that the product works best in conjunction with an exercise program (one is provided; it includes daily weight training alternating with aerobics) and a diet plan. Calories and foods are limited; suggested menus, recipes and portion sizes are provided.

The diet recommendations made by MET-Rx's manufacturers are sound; the exercise plan is similar to one a personal trainer might recommend. But given calorie limitation, a well-balanced diet, and a daily 30 minute workout, almost anyone would lose body fat, increase muscle mass, and enjoy the energizing benefits that come with regular exercise.

It is estimated that a year's supply of products such as MET-Rx costs around $2,500. The question is, are they really worth the money? The answer is up to you.

Some people do well on prepackaged plans that eliminate food choices and guesswork. If you're one of these people, choose your muscle-building or weight-loss/muscle-toning product carefully to make certain it is well-balanced (or that you're allowed to get the nutrients you need from whole foods). Double-check with your doctor to be certain that the preparation you've selected is a healthy one and that the exercise program is safe for you. Then follow the manufacturer's recommendations and directions carefully.

Which Fitness Foods Don't Deliver?

Be wary of any fitness food or dietary supplement that makes miraculous claims. If a claim sounds unbelievable, it probably is. Pharmaceutical companies and medical researchers spend billions of dollars each year seeking solutions to obesity and cures

WHEN BUYING DIETARY SUPPLEMENTS OR FOODS TO INCREASE FITNESS...

Check out all claims and benefits carefully. And ask these questions when deciding whether a health claim is legitimate:

- Are claims substantiated by reputable experts who have no financial interest in the company?

- Are research results available? A scrupulous retailer will have the supporting material, or will know where to get it.

- Are claims based on results of scientific tests—or merely on testimonials from users?

- Does the product promise fast, dramatic, or miraculous cures or results?

- Does the company have a real address—or just a post office box number?

- Is the company well-established and respected in the industry; does it have a full line of mainstream products?

for life-threatening diseases. When a discovery occurs, it makes headlines.

Think back to the end of 1994, for instance, when researchers working at Rockefeller University announced they had isolated a gene in mice that appeared to govern body weight. Though the scientists cautioned that a medical solution to obesity was still at least five to ten years away, the story was the day's leading news in major media across the country.

Rest assured: When science finds a genuine cure for obesity, impotence, or AIDS, you'll have heard about it on the evening news. If a spectacular claim on the label of a dietary supplement seems unfamiliar, that's probably because it's false.

Vitamin and Mineral Supplements: Which Ones Aid Your Fitness Regime?

Athletes, take note: There is no scientific evidence to indicate that vitamin supplements work as ergogenic (performance-enhancing) aids for healthy, well-nourished individuals, nor is there any evidence to suggest that using vitamins can boost normal energy or strength.

However, research does suggest that deficiencies of certain nutrients may lead to significantly impaired performance. Even short-term deficits of B vitamins, especially thiamin, riboflavin and niacin, can hamper aerobic endurance. Female runners with iron deficiencies are also at risk for endurance problems. In these cases, athletic function returns to normal as soon as the deficiencies are corrected.

Some studies suggest that antioxidant vitamins—C, E, and beta-carotene—can limit or repair the stress that can cause muscle damage during exercise. While hard scientific study has yet to prove that antioxidant supplements can improve athletic performance, some researchers believe that these supplements can guard against damage during training and competition.

Endurance athletes, especially those who are vegetarians or who consume fewer than 2,000 calories a day, may want to consider taking supplements containing E, C, B-complex and iron.

For more information on these and other vitamins, see "Nutrition, A to Z," later in this book. For female athletes—in fact, for all women—a bone-strengthening calcium supplement is advisable, too.

Some Promising News . . . These May Work

Caffeine. Studies have shown that caffeine may improve endurance and possibly even strength. Caffeine, the central nervous system stimulant found in coffee, tea, cola drinks, chocolate and many over-the-counter energy aids, is one of the substances most commonly used by athletes.

There is some evidence to indicate that caffeine may increase the muscles' fuel-burning abilities, and extend the amount of stored sugar available for energy use. Runners and cyclists have reported being able to achieve greater-than-normal-distance after a couple of cups of coffee.

But beware: Caffeine can also speed muscle contraction, which can lead to cramps. It may increase heart rate and cause palpitations in susceptible individuals. It also heightens the risk of heat stroke. In fact, in excessive amounts, it is on the list of drugs banned by the International Olympic Committee. Don't forget, too, that caffeine increases your need to urinate and drink extra fluids, which might be highly undesirable during competitive events.

Chromium picolinate. This mineral has gained recent popularity for its abilities to improve glucose (blood sugar) tolerance and reduce blood serum cholesterol levels. The jury is still out on its real value. According to the *Medical Tribune,* a few studies have suggested that supplementing the diet with this mineral may help reduce body fat without cutting caloric intake. In a study of young athletes, those given chromium picolinate lost 22 percent of their body fat in 6 weeks, compared to 6 percent lost by a control group. In another study, subjects who were given from 200 to 400 micrograms of chromium picolinate a day averaged a loss of 4.2 pounds of fat and a gain of 1.4 pounds of muscle. Yet the majority of studies have failed to show any benefit at all.

Less controversial is the need for chromium supplements. At least one study indicates that the average, well-balanced diet may provide too little chromium to meet even basic needs. The diets studied provided only 13.4 micrograms per 1,000 calories. Although the exact RDA for chromium has yet to be established—estimates range from 50 to 200 micrograms a day—the National Academy of Science recommends 130 micrograms a day.

Carnitine. There is still much controversy about this vitamin-like amino acid. Though there's no question that carnitine aids in the metabolism of fat, can it also improve stamina?

According to one proponent, Brian Leibowitz, M.S., author of *Carnitine: The Vitamin B-T Phenomenon,* the answer is a resounding yes. One of carnitine's benefits, says Leibowitz, is that it can provide athletes with added strength and endurance.

Indeed, one study does show that carnitine supplementation improves athletic performance by 6 to 11 percent. However, another indicates that it had no effect on performance. *The Journal of the American Dietetic Association* suggests that there are "insufficient research data" available for using carnitine as a performance enhancer. And the French government recently took action against the makers of dozens of dietary supplements containing carnitine after a commission concluded that it neither enhanced athletic performance, nor was effective in assisting weight loss.

You can easily prevent carnitine deficiency by eating beef steak and ground beef, bacon, cooked fish, chicken breast, whole milk, cheese, and whole wheat. Vegetarians can combine rice, corn, or wheat with beans, to make certain they get an adequate supply.

Should you also use supplements of carnitine? Many experts say no. Others say that supplemental carnitine will produce no negative side effects, and that 100 milligrams, taken on an empty stomach 3 times a day, may help speed weight loss.

What Doesn't Work

Alcohol. Theoretically, alcohol could enhance endurance by literally making you forget that you're tired. However, it is far more likely that drinking before a workout or competitive event will impair rather than improve your performance. Alcohol acts on the liver to decrease the release of glucose, which can lead to low blood sugar and fatigue. Drinking alcohol diminishes your capacity to think and reason and lowers your body temperature, an especially dangerous—even fatal—condition for skiers and swimmers. Drinking alcohol slows your reflexes and impairs your balance, increasing the risk of injuries. It can also lead to dehydration and heart illness.

Bee pollen has long been touted as a panacea for everything from impotence to memory loss. Though it is rich in many essential vitamins, minerals, and amino acids, studies have been unable to link it definitively to the enhancement of performance or athletic ability.

Bee pollen can cause life-threatening allergic reactions in some people. It should be avoided by those suffering from gout or kidney disease; and should never be given to infants. Although makers claim benefits for its "pure protein" content, it is ineffective as an energy booster, and at up to $45 per pound, is a wildly extravagant protein supplement.

Vitamin B$_{15}$ (calcium pangamate). Although animal studies conducted in the Soviet Union suggested that vitamin B$_{15}$ may enhance metabolism, at least four major studies in the U.S. found no connection between its use and an increase in fitness. Indeed, this product is so suspect that the Food and Drug Administration forbids its sale.

Coenzyme Q$_{10}$. A fatty substance with the characteristics of a vitamin, coenzyme Q$_{10}$ plays an essential role in heart functioning and metabolism. It has been used therapeutically in cardiac patients to increase the amount of oxygen the body can use and to improve their exercise performance.

However, both the *Journal of the American Dietetic Association* and the *International Journal of Sports Nutrition* warn that research does not support the value of coenzyme Q$_{10}$, either alone or as part of a commercial supplement, for boosting athletic performance.

One company, Swanson Health Products of Fargo, North Dakota, responding to pressure from the FDA, agreed to stop making

therapeutic claims for its coEnzyme Q$_{10}$, which it had marketed it as a digestive aid.

However, others have called coenzyme Q$_{10}$ an effective free radical fighter that has promise for use as a fitness-enhancing supplement.

Spirulina. This substance is, quite literally, pond scum—a blue-green algae that forms on the surface of ponds and lakes. The hype surrounding spirulina touts it as an energy and immunity booster that cleanses and detoxifies the body. Claims have been made for its effectiveness in treating Alzheimer's disease, alcoholism, herpes, diabetes, arthritis, certain cancers, mood swings, jet lag, and drug addiction.

Spirulina's food value is similar to that of the highly nutritious soybean, but with spirulina going for as much as $300 a pound, soybean products are a far better buy. The commonly recommended dosage contains little protein and fewer vitamins and minerals than are found in broccoli. Worse still, some products sold as spirulina contain none of the substance at all.

Choline. is present in many foods and is readily manufactured by the body. There is no scientific evidence to indicate that choline can help counter the aging process or that it has any other special benefit. However, studies are being conducted to determine whether it is effective in treating certain brain disorders.

Ginkgo Biloba. Because this substance is found in the oldest living trees on the planet, some people have speculated that ginkgo biloba may be useful in treating a variety of disorders, such as Alzheimer's disease, circulatory problems, anxiety, and memory loss. There is no proof whatsoever to back any of these health claims. Although it is an essential nutrient for trees, ginkgo biloba has no known value to humans.

Ginseng. The Chinese believe ginseng to be a panacea for almost all diseases; it is also widely used by millions as an aphrodisiac. Its popularity and use in this country soared when news stories revealed that Russian athletes and cosmonauts swore by its energizing properties.

There is much lore and legend surrounding ginseng, but very little in the way of hard scientific data to prove its health benefits. On the contrary, it may cause harmful side affects, such as high blood pressure.

If you are one of the five to six million who choose to use this very costly substance, purchase it only from reputable companies: A study that analyzed 54 ginseng products found a quarter of them to be completely ginseng-free.

Shark cartilage. This trendy substance is cropping up in many supplements marketed as anti-inflammatory agents and in those promising to reduce muscle discomfort. It has also been touted as a remedy for cancer.

Does it work? No clinical tests confirm the claims of shark cartilage as an anti-inflammatory. As for its cancer-fighting benefits, even the manufacturers of shark cartilage admit that no links between the substance and the disease have been scientifically proven.

Read the Label! Ingredients to Avoid

In addition to having no scientifically proven benefits, there are some supplements that may actually be dangerous. For example, some nutritional supplements containing *desiccated porcine or bovine thyroid* may, if taken in excess, contribute to an overactive thyroid (hyperthyroidism). In general, products that contain substances derived from the glands of animals should be approached with caution; they may cause allergic reactions in some people, or could contain impurities that could be harmful.

Be Safe

How can you be certain that a dietary supplement is completely safe? Follow the suggestions in the box on choosing dietary supplements. Make certain you're dealing with reputable, well-established companies. Avoid products that make wild, unsubstantiated claims. If someone recommends a product to you that contains unfamiliar ingredients, such as yohimbe bark or orchic, ask to see scientific proof of their efficacy.

For the best advice, start by asking your doctor. Although most doctors lack specialized knowledge of nutrition, they can usually refer you to a registered dietitian (RD), or they may be part of a medical group that has an RD on staff. There are 63,000 RDs across the country. Unlike "nutritionists," each registered dietitian has gone through an approved course of study and testing; each is required to keep his or her credentials— and knowledge—up-to-date.

To locate a registered dietitian in your area, or to get more information, you can call the American Dietetic Association's Hotline at 1-800-366-1655. Up-to-the-minute recorded information is available, as are free brochures. RDs are also listed in the Yellow Pages under "Dietitians."

Although they claim to be experts, some fitness publications may not provide the soundest or safest nutritional advice. While many of these publications are scrupulous about accepting advertisements only from reputable manufacturers, others are not.

If you see a big ad for a dietary supplement close to an article praising its benefits, ask yourself this: If a publication relies on advertising money from supplement makers for its revenue, how objective will it be when it writes about its advertisers' products?

Carbohydrates— The Real Fitness Foods

What about the *real* fitness foods— those foods that aren't engineered or designed, and that do not resemble edible chemistry sets? Which natural foods most enhance your energy and your fitness level?

Overwhelmingly, experts say that a diet rich in complex carbohydrates—fruits, vegetables, and grains—and low in fats is the surest way to overall health, energy, and fitness.

The U.S. Department of Agriculture recently revised its "Food Guide Pyramid" and now suggests that your daily diet should contain six to 11 daily servings of foods from the bread, rice, cereal, grain, and pasta group. Clearly, complex carbohydrates should form the foundation of a healthy eating plan.

What Is a Carbohydrate?

There are two basic types of carbohydrates: starches (complex carbohydrates) and sugars (simple carbohydrates). Both simple and complex carbohydrates occur naturally in foods and can be chemically processed and refined.

Simple carbohydrates circulate in your body as "blood sugar," or glucose. This type of sugar is essential for supplying the body with energy.

The most common complex carbohydrate is starch, which is made up of hundreds of glucose units linked together. Because starch must be broken down before use, it provides a longer-lasting source of energy.

Your body converts both simple and complex carbohydrates into glycogen, a substance stored in the muscle and the liver as an energy reserve. While it is essentially true that the more carbohydrates you take in—whether simple or complex—the more energy you'll have, it is better to choose foods rich in complex carbohydrates than foods rich in simple carbohydrates.

Foods rich in complex carbohydrates generally contain large amounts of other essential nutrients, such as vitamins and minerals. In addition, they are often excellent sources of dietary fiber, and are often low in fat.

In other words, foods such as starchy vegetables, pasta, whole-grain bread and cereals, barley, and rice provide plenty of long-lasting energy and offer lots of valuable nutritional benefits, while excess calories from sugary treats, which quickly shoot up your blood sugar level, can leave you feeling listless later on.

Carbohydrates and Weight Loss

Until recently, most weight loss programs advised dieters to eat plenty of lean protein while limiting fats, starches, and sugars. Converting protein to energy is more difficult for the body than converting carbohydrates to energy. As a result, dieters on high-protein, low carb diets often complained of feeling tired, weak, and exhausted.

The latest thinking has changed all that. Now the American Dietetic Association recommends making 55 to 60 percent of your diet complex carbohydrates. Though some "insulin-resistant" people need to go easy on carbohydrates in order to lose weight, for the majority of us, this percentage works best. In addition, keep fat to about 30 percent or less of your daily calorie intake; protein should make up the rest.

By limiting calories and following an exercise program that includes aerobics as well as strength training, dieters can expect to lose, on average, over a pound a week. In addition, they can expect to gain increased stamina, endurance, and energy. (For more detailed weight loss guidelines, turn to Chapters 6 and 7.)

Top Energy Foods

Complex carbohydrates are excellent energy boosters. Grain products and fruits are your best sources; and many offer a host of extra benefits. For example:

- **Amaranth:** This unfamiliar but highly nutritious grain is high in calcium. Like brown rice, whole wheat, buckwheat, and barley, it is a rich source of fiber and trace minerals.
- **Bananas, cantaloupes, oranges:** These fruits are loaded with vitamins, fiber and carbohydrates, and one banana contains as much as 25 percent of a day's supply of potassium, a mineral needed for healthy blood pressure.
- **Carrots:** By far the richest natural source of beta-carotene, carrots are high in fiber and minerals. Enjoy carrots frequently in all forms: cooked, raw, and as juice.

- **High C Fruits:** A single serving of citrus fruit offers a day's supply (or very nearly so) of vitamin C; and so do kiwis, pineapples, persimmons, and honeydew melons. In addition, many of these are loaded with potassium and other valuable nutrients.
- **Beans:** All beans are high in iron and other minerals, high in fiber, and can be good sources of protein when combined with other vegetable proteins, such as rice.
- **Potatoes:** A good source of vitamin C, copper, magnesium, phosphorous, potassium, iron, and fiber, and low in calories. Eat them plain or with low-fat dressing.

When's the Best Time to Eat for Energy?

Recent studies at the University of Texas Exercise Science Labs indicate that your body uses carbohydrates most effectively within 2 hours after a workout. John Ivy, Ph.D., who conducted the tests, suggests that a good way to fight fatigue and feed muscles is to eat a protein and carbohydrate meal shortly after exercising. Doing so, he says, will maximize absorption of essential nutrients.

Why Do Athletes "Carbo-Load?"

"Carbo-loading" is a dietary regimen that some marathon runners and other endurance athletes use to increase their stamina for races and other rigorous competitions.

The theory behind carbo-loading is that by "starving" skeletal muscles of their primary source of energy, glycogen, for a few days (by eating high-carb foods in much smaller amounts than normal), you can coax the muscles into soaking up glycogen when foods high in carbohydrates are eaten shortly before competition.

Studies have shown that a meal heavy in carbohydrates can indeed boost muscle

DRINK MORE WATER WHEN...

- **Flying**—Drink 8 to 20 ounces between 30 to 60 minutes before your flight; continue sipping water during the flight.

- **You are at elevated altitudes**—The higher you go, the lower the water content in the air. Drink extra water to compensate.

- **The temperature is high**—When heat makes you perspire, drink plenty of extra water.

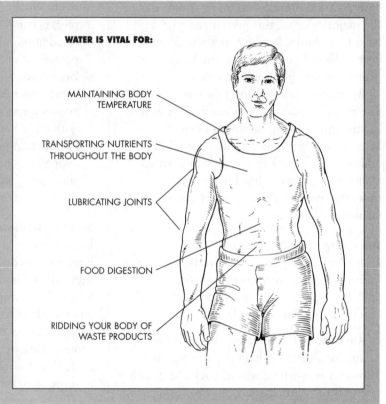

WATER IS VITAL FOR:

MAINTAINING BODY TEMPERATURE

TRANSPORTING NUTRIENTS THROUGHOUT THE BODY

LUBRICATING JOINTS

FOOD DIGESTION

RIDDING YOUR BODY OF WASTE PRODUCTS

glycogen by nearly 80 percent and enhance endurance, if not necessarily speed.

If you're a well-trained athlete in generally good physical condition, it is probably safe to carbo load. Studies haven't as yet turned up any negative effects from eating this way. As a matter of fact, the very low levels of blood sugar that result from carbo-loading may contribute to the good feeling called "runner's high." Be aware, however, that classic carbo-loading can also cause cramping, diarrhea, and extra water weight. Experts now recommend moderation.

All About Fluid Replacement

As we go through our daily activities, we are constantly losing fluid through perspiration and urine. Exercise increases this water loss. Doctors and nutritionists agree that you must drink liquids to replace those you lose, but which should you choose—and when should you take them?

Water

For most of us, the best way to replace fluid is to drink plain, pure water. Even though water has no nutrients, it is one of the body's most essential components.

In fact, our bodies are more than half water. Even our bones, the body's densest components, are nearly one-third water. The brain is 75 percent water. The blood is 90 percent water. We can only survive about four days without water, although we can go for a couple of weeks or more without food.

Whether or not you are athletic, drink plenty of water. Start your morning with eight to 16 ounces, and take time for water breaks throughout the day, especially when exercising. Try to drink at least a half cup (four ounces) of water each hour—more if the air is dry or if it is hot. Don't forget that caffeinated and alcoholic beverages are diuretics; consume a glass of water along with your coffee, tea, or wine.

Sports Drinks vs. Juice

When do you need more than water to replenish the body's fluid losses? Unless you're very serious about your exercise, the answer is rarely.

If you work out vigorously for over an hour, or at a moderate pace for over two hours, then it's time to add energy (carbohydrates) to your drink. Otherwise, you are apt to suffer from fatigue or loss of endurance.

Diluting fruit juices half and half with water will give you a refreshing drink that serves up about the same amount of carbohydrates as most sports drinks—about 6 to 8 percent by weight. Drinking higher-carb fluids—whether juice or sports drinks—will slow absorption and may cause cramping.

Avoid sports drinks high in fructose, which can cause nausea and diarrhea at concentrations of 10 percent or higher. Most athletes tolerate simple sugar beverages well at concentrations higher than 10 percent; some

can take beverages with glucose-polymers (maltodextrin or Polycose) at carbohydrate concentrations of up to 15 percent with no ill effect. However, it's wiser to water the sweeter drinks down to the 8 percent level.

What About Electrolytes?

What many sports drinks provide that most diluted juices do not is a variety of electrolytes such as sodium, magnesium, and potassium. Do you need them?

Electrolytes may improve a beverage's taste and lead to increased fluid consumption. But most sports physiologists agree that the main point is to slake thirst and provide your body with needed fluid by drinking before and during exercise, and drinking beyond your thirst when you've finished working out. Precisely what you drink is of secondary importance.

(On the other hand, adding electrolytes to a beverage may improve water and glucose absorption. Some studies have shown that beverages with glucose and electrolytes are more efficient for maintaining your body's fluid balance.)

Look beyond the complicated chemistry of sports beverages and here's the bottom line: Drinking is essential to maintaining your energy and endurance; and a limited carbohydrate intake is needed to keep up your strength when you're engaged in activities that require lots of endurance.

If you work out hard for less than an hour, or not so hard for less than two hours, water is just fine for you. If you're a more dedicated athlete, a more serious sports beverage may be a better choice. But no matter how vigorously, or for how long, you exercise, drink well beyond your level of thirst, and you will fulfill your body's fluid needs.

WHAT SPORTS BEVERAGES CONTAIN

Beverage	Serving Size	Carb. (Grams)	Carb. %	Calories	Electrolytes (milligrams)			Other
					Potassium	Magnesium	Sodium	
Carbo Force	16 oz.	100	22	400	99	*	less than 35	Vitamin C: 30 mg, Chromium: 100 mcg
Exceed	8 oz.	59	25	230	140	130	115	25% RDA for Thiamin, Niacin, Riboflavin
Gatorade	8 oz.	14	6	50	30	--	110	
Gold's All Day	10 oz.	31	11	125	--	--	--	
Fat Burning Xcelerator	18 oz.	0	0	0	--	--	30	L-Carnitine: 1000 mg, Chromium: 200 mcg, Vitamin B_6: 50 mg, Choline: 200 mg
Hydra Fuel	16 oz.	33	7	132	99	25	50	Vitamin C: 60 mg, Chromium: 25 mcg
Pro Carb	18 oz	112	22	450	*	*	*	Chromium*
Sun Bolt	11.6 oz	51	15	210	*	--	150	Caffeine: 58 mg, Vitamin C: 110% RDA
Super Tea	16 oz	100	22	400	99	*	less than 35	Vitamin C: 30 mg, Caffeine: 100 mg, Chromium: 100 mg
Ultra Fuel	16 oz.	100	22	400	99	25		100% RDA or more for: Vitamins B_1, B_2, B_3, B_6; 1000% RDA for Pantothenic Acid; 100% estimated requirement for Biotin, Chromium

* Manufacturers do not specify amount.

Body-Building Specialties: Bigger Muscles in a Can?

How can you develop the strength and musculature of a Hercules or an Amazon? "It's easy," say unscrupulous manufacturers. "Simply open a can and follow the directions."

Earlier this decade, scientists from the federal Centers for Disease Control and Prevention reviewed hundreds of self-proclaimed body-building, energy-releasing, and muscle-enhancing products. None were found to have any positive effect whatever on muscle size or strength.

Yet the market for protein- and amino acid-based products is a tremendously profitable one. Why? The answer lies in the consumer: Men and women who are avid body-builders and fitness enthusiasts are extremely susceptible to the aggressive marketing efforts of companies who promise them better bodies. In a study of competitive body-builders, 90 percent of the men and

100 percent of the women were found to use nutritional supplements.

Though no study exists to prove that using amino acid or protein supplements will enhance musculature, there are reliable studies proving that athletes and body-builders believe in the effectiveness of ergogenic (performance-enhancing) drugs and aids. As long as this misconception exists, so will the market for worthless and potentially dangerous muscle-building formulations.

Doesn't Protein Build Muscles?

According to one expert, the only way to get muscles from a protein or amino acid supplement is by lugging the can home from the store.

What, then, is behind "protein builds muscles" theory? Protein contains amino acids that trigger the release of growth hormone. As its name implies, this hormone stimulates muscle growth, thereby decreasing fat storage. So, if some amino acids are good, more must be better, right?

"Wrong," say the experts. It's true that when you eat a protein such as meat, your body uses the amino acids to make new protein in the form of hormones, enzymes, and, yes, muscle tissue. But doctors, dietitians, and physiologists now know that more protein doesn't equal more muscle formation. Extensive research proves that adequate calorie intake, combined with exercise, is what really builds and strengthens muscles.

Most of us get twice the amount of protein we need every day. Your body cannot store unused protein. The excess makes fat or is converted into energy in an unusually complicated process. Waste products from this conversion are excreted through urine, which places strain on the kidneys and liver. Excess protein consumption also slows the absorption of much needed calcium.

So adding even more protein by taking dietary amino acid and protein supplements is not only ineffective, it could harm your body over time. And if you want another good reason not to buy these supplements, check out their labels. According to the *Tufts University Diet & Nutrition Letter,* some of the *safer* ingredients in these supplements include conch grass, adrenal gland concentrate, and insect hormone.

TEN STEPS TO NATURALLY STRONGER MUSCLES

No one needs steroids, protein powders or exotic, expensive dietary supplements to build a better body. If you really want a more powerful physique, follow these steps:

1. Strength train 3 times a week—for an hour only.

2. Exercise the major muscle groups first.

3. Perform one set of exercises for each muscle group.

4. Generally, don't do less than 8 or more than 12 repetitions per exercise.

5. Lift until you can't lift again.

6. Increase your calories. Add 500 from carbohydrates. Include 1.5 grams of protein for each kilogram (2.2 pounds) of body weight.

7. Make carbohydrates 60 to 70 percent of your diet.

8. Eat carbohydrates two hours before you exercise and immediately after you finish.

9. Drink fluids before, during and after your exercise.

10. Add one hour of rest for every hour you exercise.

A safe limit for amino acids has never been established, and it's possible that large doses could lead to harmful imbalances. William Evans, Ph.D., is director of the Laboratory of Human Performance and Research at Penn State University. He is also the nutrition and fitness consultant for the Boston Bruins hockey team. According to Evans, who has conducted extensive research on amino acid and protein supplements, "A good healthy diet takes care of dietary needs. If those supplements [advertised] in magazines had any benefit, you can be sure I'd be recommending them to the team."

The (Very) Bad News About Anabolic Steroids

Anabolic steroids are drugs that are illegally used by some athletes to stimulate the buildup of muscle tissue. Closely related to the male sex hormone testosterone, these powerful medications do have several legitimate therapeutic uses. Physicians prescribe them to treat some growth disorders, to offset the negative effects of chemotherapy and radiation treatments, and to cure certain kinds of anemia.

However, using steroids over a prolonged period, even in moderate doses, can lead to disastrous side effects with potentially fatal consequences. Steroids can compromise the healthy functioning of your liver, cardiovascular system and reproductive organs.

Steroids can harm or even destroy the mental process. Athletes who take steroids are at risk for wild mood swings, and worse:

A study of 156 steroid users found that more than 25 percent suffered from severe psychiatric disorders ranging from severe depression to episodes of wild and unwarranted enthusiasm. Steroid use can cause psychotic behavior; some people have even killed while under the drug's influence.

By taking steroids athletes put themselves and others at increased risk for serious injuries, not only because the drug fuels their aggressive tendencies, but also because their extra-large muscles put stress on joints and ligaments that aren't equipped to handle the increased strain.

Children and Steroids

A 1993 survey by the *Journal of the American Medical Association* revealed that over one million Americans aged 12 and older are steroid users; nearly half are below the age of 26. An estimated 5 to 10 percent of high school students may be steroid abusers.

Efforts by celebrities like Arnold Schwarzenegger and the late Lyle Alzado, a football star who attributed his fatal illness to steroid abuse, may help alert young people to the dangers of these drugs. It is also essential that parents, coaches, and teachers be well-informed. No win in the world, no medal, ribbon, or trophy, is worth taking a life-threatening gamble on steroids. □

Chapter 22

Best Bets When You're Stressed Out

The baby's crying. Your secretary calls in sick. A car veers into your lane. You bounced a check. Traffic's tied up for miles. You're graduating from medical school. Your mother's in the hospital. It's snowing. Your divorce is final.

Q. What does each of these scenarios have in common?
A. If repeated, combined, and sustained, situations like these can produce enough stress to make you sick.

When Does Stress Do Damage?

Stress is simply the body's response to a threat. Whether the stressful situation is physical (an impending car accident) or psychological (a down-sizing at your company), your body undergoes a dramatic reaction that readies you for "fight or flight" from the danger.

A flood of hormones courses through your system and enters the bloodstream. Your blood pressure rises. Proteins are converted to sugars to provide readily accessible energy. You may experience a surge of unusual strength.

This stress response was essential thousands of years ago, when a fast response to attack was the only guarantee of survival. These days, threats are slower and subtler, and rarely call for dramatic physical response. Problem is, our bodies never learned this. They still react . . . and react . . . and react again.

If stressful situations were rare, our bodies would be little the worse for wear. In today's world, however, we're all too frequently bombarded with situations that prompt repeated stress responses.

A string of stressful, albeit minor, problems can cause your body to build up a response that's as dramatic as a reaction to a serious threat, leaving you feeling drained and exhausted. When minor stress repeats itself over time, the feeling of exhaustion can become chronic, and you could notice a variety of other disturbing symptoms as well.

Since Dr. Hans Selye first discovered the link between stress and disease in 1936, studies have proven its connection with a va-

THE RAVAGES OF STRESS

All of the symptoms here could be related to excessive stress. They could also be the result of some other disorder. To rule out a medical problem, your first line of defense is always a visit to the doctor. Then, if stress turns out to be the culprit, consider the dietary additions and deletions summarized in the chapter below.

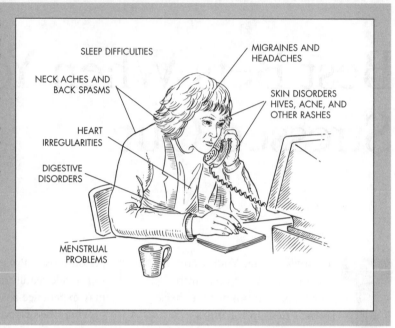

SLEEP DIFFICULTIES

MIGRAINES AND HEADACHES

NECK ACHES AND BACK SPASMS

SKIN DISORDERS HIVES, ACNE, AND OTHER RASHES

HEART IRREGULARITIES

DIGESTIVE DISORDERS

MENSTRUAL PROBLEMS

riety of symptoms. The conditions listed in the box above can be caused or aggravated by stress. Seek medical help—and be sure to give your physician a complete physical and emotional history—if you experience any of them.

The Toll Stress Takes

Certainly the physical stress of illness or injury results in increased nutrient needs. And, as you recover, your vitamin and mineral needs increase, too. However, on emotional stress the jury remains out.

Although some authorities say there's still no conclusive evidence that stress increases your body's need for nutrients, many others are convinced that stress does rob your body. When you undergo severe stress for prolonged periods, they contend, such nutrients as protein, calcium, vitamin C, potassium, zinc, and magnesium become depleted.

Additionally, since it's likely that your body uses vitamin A, the B-complex vitamins, pantothenic acid, vitamin E, and linoleic acid during the stress response, nutritional advisors often recommend getting extra amounts to ease the ravages of stress.

Nutritionists Eberhard and Phyllis Krohausen argue that the release of certain chemicals during stress leads to the production of free radicals, the highly destructive compounds that can oxidize (burn) key molecules within the cells. Many experts now suspect that such free radicals are linked to the aging process and such diseases as cancer.

Some studies now suggest that the vitamins known as "antioxidants," which include vitamins C, E, beta-carotene, and B-complex, can help prevent or repair the damage these compounds cause.

Stress definitely does deplete protein. During stress, your body converts it to fuel at a prodigious rate (one recent study indicates that in a day of severe physical stress, the body converts as much protein as you get in four quarts of milk). It's no surprise, therefore, that amino acids—protein's building blocks—are often packaged as stress-relieving dietary supplements. However, there is still no scientific proof that these supplements can actually make a difference.

Stress also indisputably, if indirectly, erodes your nutrition when it causes or aggravates destructive or unhealthy behavior patterns (such as smoking, drinking, substance abuse, or eating disorders). Still, there is no known way to calculate the exact impact of stress on your nutritional status. And there is no general prescription for repairing the damage that stress can do.

The most that can be said with certainty is that if you undergo a period of severe, protracted stress, or have symptoms of a stress-related disorder, it makes sense to pay extra attention to the way you eat. This is a time when a well-balanced diet is more important than ever. And a well-balanced multivitamin—including the antioxidant group of nutrients: C, E, beta-carotene, and B-complex—might be something to consider as well.

"LIFE CHANGE UNIT" RATINGS OF COMMON STRESSORS

Exactly how much stress are you under? Any change means stress; and the more profound the change, the greater its impact. Use the ratings below to gauge the cumulative effect of the readjustments you're currently experiencing in your life. Note that a sudden burst of relatively minor events can easily cause as much stress as a major loss or disaster.

Stressful event	LCU
Child leaving for college	28
Major change in eating habits	29
Vacation	29
Job promotion	31
Major change in sleeping habits	31
New romantic relationship	32
Breaking up	35
Troubles with co-workers	35
Changing jobs	38
Major change in living conditions	39
Major purchase	39
Troubles with boss	39
Major dental work	40
Injury or illness that hospitalized you or kept you in bed a week or more	42
Marital reconciliation	42
Accident	44
Marriage	50
Major change in health or behavior of family member	52
Miscarriage or abortion	53
Marital separation	56
Job demotion	57
Loan or mortgage foreclosure	57
Decreased income	60
Pregnancy	60
Divorce	62
Death of brother or sister	64
Getting fired	64
Death of parent	66
Death of spouse or child	105

How Your Diet Can *Contribute* to Stress

A healthy diet is often the first casualty of severe stress. The nagging feeling of, "so much to do, so little time," can send you racing from one thing to another without a relaxed, well-balanced meal. It seems like a small sacrifice—but the real sacrifice can be your health.

You can actually intensify the level of emotional stress you experience by eating incorrectly. If you stop eating or eat less, you won't fulfill energy demands or meet nutrient requirements. And if you eat everything in sight, you'll gain weight, which for many people is in itself a source of stress.

The worst possible diet plan for those under stress is no plan at all. When you have difficult times, it's easy to skip meals, eat junk food, and fill up on sweet or salty snacks. But in times of stress dietary vigilance is more important than ever, because adding a bad diet to your other problems is a prescription for disaster.

Any of the following routines is taboo—and can have serious health consequences—for anyone under prolonged stress:

- Crash diets
- Extreme overeating
- Skipping breakfast (or any meal)
- Sugary breakfast pastries and donuts, in place of meals
- Any diet that doesn't deliver minimum Recommended Daily Allowances
- Excessive alcohol consumption

A Note about Cadmium

Cadmium is a heavy metal that enters the food chain via sewage sludge that is converted to fertilizer by agricultural companies. Cadmium has been found in high concentrations in tobacco and lettuce.

A 1987 study found that rats on high-cadmium diets displayed increased anxiety and an inability to cope with stress. And given a choice between water and water

SOME FACTS ABOUT CAFFEINE

Caffeine's action occurs from 30 to 60 minutes after ingestion

200 milligrams of caffeine (about 2 cups of coffee) can:
- Increase alertness and reduce fatigue
- Temporarily increase heartbeat and blood pressure
- Interfere with sleep
- Increase flow of urine

300–1,000 milligrams of caffeine (3 to 10 cups of coffee) can cause:
- Insomnia
- Shaking and nervousness
- Irregular heartbeats
- Increased feelings of anxiety

Caffeine Counts in Common Sources

Product	Caffeine (in milligrams)
Brewed coffee, 1 cup	50–150
Instant coffee, 1 cup	30–120
Sweetened coffee mix, 1 cup	40–80
Decaffeinated coffee, 1 cup	2–8
Brewed tea, 1 cup	20–100
Instant tea, 1 cup	30–70

For caffeine content of other foods, beverages, and medications, see the box on "Counting Up Your Caffeine Load" in Chapter 16.

laced with alcohol, cadmium-fed rats preferred the latter, while cadmium-free rats chose pure water every time. When placed in stressful situations, the cadmium-fed rats drank twice as much alcohol as they did in non-stressful situations.

In 1992, the Occupational Safety and Health Administration, reduced by 95 percent the permissible exposure limit for cadmium, which has been linked to lung cancer and kidney disease. Vitamin E has been found to reduce cadmium-induced biochemical reactions in experiments on rats. The researchers concluded that vitamin E's antioxidant properties might help protect against oxidative damage caused by cadmium.

Watch Out for Caffeine

It seems only logical that people already overstimulated by stress should avoid the extra stimulation of caffeine. In a study conducted at Duke University, the blood pressure of men who consumed caffeine prior to doing math problems rose 20 percent, and their adrenaline levels escalated 160 percent. Men in the control group, who thought they might be getting caffeine but actually didn't, experienced increases of just 10 and 40 percent, respectively.

For most people, caffeine in moderation (2 or 3 cups of coffee a day) seems perfectly harmless. And some people may even experience beneficial feelings.

Studies conducted at M.I.T. showed that caffeine improves performance; those given caffeine demonstrated increased reaction speed, better concentration, and greater accuracy than those given caffeine-free substitutes. Other research suggests that caffeine may increase athletic endurance.

But many people are caffeine-sensitive and can feel nervous, shaky, or "overstimulated" after drinking just 1 cup of coffee. Many people avoid caffeine at all costs from late afternoon on, as it interferes with their sleep. (If insomnia troubles you, *never* drink coffee after 4:00 PM.) In short, some people find that caffeine is essential as a morning eye-opener and for maintaining a "clear" head; others are affected negatively. Think twice about your caffeine intake if your blood pressure is already elevated. And if caffeine bothers you—don't use it.

Should You Consider a Supplement?

If the claims of diet supplement manufacturers were true, no one would ever have to suffer the ill effects of stress. Health food and nutrition shops are jammed with products claiming to cure, prevent, or repair the ravages of stress. There are stress vitamin combinations, herbal preparations, and amino acid concoctions. In traditional drugstores, several over-the-counter preparations promise stress relief.

There may be valid reasons to take some of these supplements. But you have to remember that none of them can banish the *source* of stress from your life. A supplement might improve your health, but it won't diminish your problem.

Meals in a Can

When stress is particularly severe and unremitting for a period of time, you must take special action. Perhaps a family member has a chronic or life-threatening illness, or you're the new mother of twins or triplets. Maybe you're engaged in a protracted legal battle or you're renovating your house from top to bottom. At times like these, it's easy to skip meals and ignore your own health and nutrition.

If you're going through this kind of stress, make the time to check with your doctor. Be certain to explain your circumstances and ask about recommended stress therapies. Seeking the advice of a support group or a counselor could be especially helpful at a time like this.

If you're skipping meals, eating on the run, or are too upset to eat, this is also the moment to consider enriching your diet with a well-balanced dietary supplement. Many "meal-in-a-can" or powdered products contain a complete day's supply of nutrients. It's far better to down a healthy shake than to skip a meal or grab a fast-food burger.

When selecting a supplement, read the label carefully to be sure it's well-balanced and doesn't contain any harmful or unnecessary additives. Ask the retailer about the taste, too—this isn't the time for anything that isn't pleasantly palatable. Does it need to be mixed, or can you drink it straight from the can? Can it be mixed with milk? With fruit juice? Can you add flavor and nutrition-boosting ingredients? Follow package directions carefully, add healthy snacks, and resume a regular diet as soon as you can.

Vitamin Supplements

In spite of everything we're learning about

FIGHT OR FLIGHT

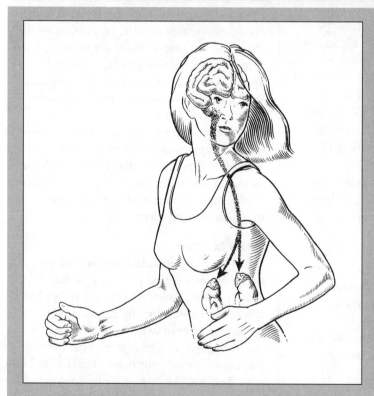

Faced by a threat, your body responds with a complex cascade of chemicals. The hypothalamus, alerted by the brain, pumps out a specialized hormone that ultimately prompts the two adrenal glands (perched atop the kidneys) to release the energizing hormone known as adrenaline. The result — faster pulse, higher blood pressure, sharpened awareness — is the "fight or flight" response we call stress.

the physical toll of stress, researchers have failed to find any stress-relieving benefit in extra doses of vitamins an minerals. However, when you're too distracted to eat a well-balanced diet, stress can prevent you from getting your Recommended Daily Allowances of necessary nutrients. This can lead to nutrient insufficiencies, which are unhealthy and can amplify the harmful effects of stress. Taking a well-balanced vitamin supplement insures that your daily needs will be adequately met even if your diet falls below par.

Megadosing on vitamins to relieve the symptoms of stress is not only unnecessary, say the experts, it's probably unhealthy, too. When nutrients are taken in isolation or in very high amounts, the effects of other equally valuable nutrients can be altered or even negated. Here are just two examples of the way that increasing a single nutrient can backfire:

- Taking more than 1,000 milligrams per day of vitamin C can decrease the availability of copper and selenium.
- When iron and copper are taken together, they compete for absorption. Copper is absorbed; iron is not and accumulates in the colon. Bacteria thrive on the iron, resulting in water and mineral loss.

Amino Acid Supplements

In her book, *Managing Your Mind & Mood Through Food,* M.I.T. researcher Judith J. Wurtman, Ph.D., notes that amino acids—the building blocks of protein—are prime ingredients of natural mood-modifying chemicals in the brain, including dopamine, norepinephrine, and serotonin. She contends that one amino acid, tyrosine, stimulates the production of "alertness" chemicals,

while another, tryptophan, increases levels of serotonin, a calming chemical.

But before you rush out to buy amino acid diet supplements, remember that Dr. Wurtman and many other nutritional experts agree that the best sources of amino acids are the foods you eat. She cautions, as do others, against buying supplements for several reasons:

- No safe levels have been established for amino acids; large doses could lead to harmful imbalances.
- Synthetic tryptophan is still not approved for use in diet supplements. Tryptophan is harmless when obtained naturally from foods such as dairy products and turkey.
- Excessive amounts of concentrated tryptophan can cause drowsiness or dizziness.
- Excessive amounts of concentrated tyrosine can affect blood pressure.

In the 1980's a tryptophan supplement was implicated in an outbreak of a rare, painful, and debilitating blood disease which struck more than 1,000 people—and killed over 30. The culprit ultimately proved to be impurities associated with processing, rather than tryptophan itself; but the potential for disaster still lurks in any dietary supplement. Exotic ingredients come to market daily, it seems, all making extravagant, seductive claims—with stress relief among the most prominent. No one can be sure that these unfamiliar substances are safe and effective. In fact, you can't even be certain that a product contains what it claims. Your safest course when approaching any kind of supplement is to stick with well-known manufacturers and recognized, established brands—though even this confers no guarantee of efficacy.

Stress-Beating Diet Plans

The best stress-fighting diet plan is one that ensures general good nutrition and health—one that builds a "bank account" of nutrients to deal with the damage of stress. Aim for a high-carbohydrate, low-fat mixture of foods like that in the USDA's Food Pyramid, or go even further with a Mediterranean-style diet that virtually eliminates red meat (See Chapter 1 for details).

Many experts now recommend getting two-thirds or more of your daily calories from complex carbohydrates found in grains, vegetables, and fruit. A case in point: the "Optimum Diet For Optimum Health," a proposal based in part on a mid-1980's study of 6,500 people in 65 counties across China. One of the findings of the study, published in 1990 as *Diet, Lifestyle and Mortality in China*, was the fact that the closer a specific region's diet came to the Western model—high in animal protein and fat, low in fiber—the more people suffered from the "diseases of affluence:" coronary heart disease, various cancers, leukemias, and diabetes. The healthiest diets in the study, on the other hand, included minimal amounts of meat and dairy products, boasting overall percentages like these:

Food	Percentage of Diet
Grains, beans, seeds, nuts	50%
Vegetables	30%
Fruits	10%
Dairy Products	6%
Protein (meat, fish poultry)	4%

Food Group	Percentage of Diet
Complex carbohydrates	70 – 75%
Fats	15 – 20%
Protein	10%

COPING WITH STRESS

Eliminating the source of your stress is, of course, the best way of coping. Often that's simply impossible, however. If you can't head off stress at the source, investigate ways of controlling it. Try learning a stress management technique such as relaxation exercises, yoga, or meditation. Biofeedback has shown excellent results in moderating reactions to seriously stressful conditions. One of the most effective of all stress-fighters is regular exercise, which has the added benefit of providing a host of other healthy advantages as well (see Chapter 8).

Remember that you don't have to suffer through a difficult time alone, and so doing may be harmful to your health. When troubles threaten to overwhelm you, don't hesitate to consult a good mental health professional or join a support group. Sharing your problems with others can be the start of true stress relief.

Three Squares A Day?

Some experts suggest that eating enough of the right foods isn't sufficient to alleviate the symptoms of stress. *When* you eat, and *how* you combine food, may be just as important in counteracting the effects of stress. For example, rather than eating three large meals a day, it's probably better to eat three smaller meals, supplemented by one or two "power snacks," says nutritionist Joan Horbiak.

This eating strategy is said to be a good stress fighter because it keeps blood sugar at a constant level. And when you're under severe stress, your digestion may be upset to the point where eating a larger meal produces discomfort. Power snacks are complex carbohydrates like bagels, cereals, and fruits. Try low-fat muffins or fig bars—easy to find and eat on the run. Pop a container of low-fat yogurt in the freezer for a mid-afternoon treat. Here are a few good menu ideas for stressful times, drawn from nutritionist Wurtman's book, *Managing Your Mind & Mood Through Food*. These combinations are designed to provide you with the energy you need to stand up to stress.

Best breakfasts

1 serving fresh fruit
1 egg, cooked without fat
2 slices whole wheat toast with
   2 tablespoons fruit preserves

or

6 ounces fruit juice
1-1/2 cups high fiber cold cereal
1/2 cup berries or 1/2 sliced banana
1/2 cup low-fat milk

or

6 ounces fruit juice
8 ounces low-fat yogurt (plain, lemon, vanilla)
1/2 cup granola, mixed with 2 tablespoons raisins, chopped dates or apricots

Mid-morning snacks

4 to 6 ounces orange juice
2 rice cakes
1 slice low-fat cheese

or

8 ounces low-fat chocolate milk
   (skim or fat-free)
1 slice raisin bread
2 teaspoons cottage cheese

or

1 ounce turkey or tuna
1 slice bread or 3-inch pita
1 carrot

Lunch

3 ounces of low-fat protein
   (tuna, lean roast beef, skinless poultry, etc.)
2 slices whole grain bread
   (or 1 pita, bagel, or roll)
1 salad of lettuce, broccoli, carrots, etc., with 2 tablespoons low-calorie dressing
1 piece of fruit or cup of fruit salad

WHERE TO GET EXPERT ADVICE

Start by asking your doctor. He or she may refer you to a registered dietitian (RD), or may be part of a medical group that has an RD on staff. There are 63,000 RDs across the country. Each has gone through an approved course of study and testing. Each is required to keep his or her credentials—and knowledge—up to date.

To locate a registered dietitian in your area, or to get more information, call the American Dietetic Association's Hotline at 1-800-366-1655. Up-to-the minute recorded information is available, as are free brochures. RDs are also listed in the Yellow Pages under "Dietitians." Nutritionists may or may not be licensed nutritional experts; check credentials before you become a client.

Mid-afternoon snacks

5 graham crackers *or*
15 Ritz crackers *or*
15 jelly beans *or*
1 English, bran, or corn muffin with
  1 teaspoon jelly *or*
1-1/2 cups Cheerios without milk

Dinner

4–6 ounces lean protein (broiled fish, skinless, boneless poultry, lean beef)
1 baked/steamed potato (or 3/4 cup pasta, rice, or other grain)
2 servings raw, steamed, or microwaved vegetables
1 serving fruit

Foods to Emphasize

When you're undergoing a stressful time, choose foods that make few demands on your body yet provide the energizing nutrients you need. The following are especially good choices. They digest quickly and easily, are dense in essential nutrients and/or fiber; leave little residue for the liver to detoxify, and don't cause toxic build-up in the bowel and vascular systems.

apples, apricots, bananas, beets and beet greens, buckwheat, cabbage, carrots, cantaloupe, cauliflower, celery, chard (Swiss), dates, grapefruit, grapes, kale, millet, nectarines, oranges, pears, peas, pineapple, potatoes, rutabaga, sprouts, sweet potatoes, and tomatoes. □

CHAPTER 23

Coping with Diabetes: The Basic Rules to Remember

Though the mere mention of the words cancer or AIDS continues to strike fear in the hearts of almost everyone, few of us react that way to diabetes. We tend to view a diagnosis of cancer or AIDS as a death sentence, while diabetes is regarded as just another chronic condition. The frequent urination, abnormal thirst, and weight loss that signal the onset of the disease are bothersome, but once you begin treatment, life goes on pretty much as always.

Or so it seems. In reality, the nearly 14 million Americans who have diabetes face the danger of several serious complications, including heart disease, kidney failure, blindness, and damage to their nervous system. Many others must undergo limb amputations as the disease plays havoc with their circulation. Clearly, diabetes is not the minor ailment some people imagine it to be.

In fact, according to the American Diabetes Association, the disease is the fourth leading cause of death in this country, claiming 160,000 lives each year while exacting a heavy financial toll. Estimates of treatment costs combined with lost productivity hover near $100 billion annually.

Despite these disheartening statistics, there's still room for optimism. Recently, a major 10-year study offered new hope for diabetics. The Diabetes Control and Complications Trial (DCCT) found that an intense, tightly orchestrated treatment plan can reduce the risk of long-term complications by 50 percent or more.

While the DCCT results apply mainly to insulin-dependent diabetics (those who produce little or no insulin), most experts say the treatment may also benefit people with non-insulin-dependent diabetes (those in whom insulin simply fails to do its job). There are, however, a few drawbacks to consider. The program can be expensive. It demands steadfast commitment. And it requires a basic understanding of how your body processes sugar. To weigh the benefits of this latest approach to diabetes against its demands, here's what you need to know.

How Carbohydrates Keep Us Going

Most of the energy our bodies need to keep running comes from the carbohydrates in our food. Carbohydrates come in two forms: starches and sugars. Starchy foods include potatoes, rice, bread, and pasta; among the sugars are honey, molasses, and table sugar (sucrose). Other sugars are found in a variety of foods, including milk (lactose) and many fruits (fructose).

The digestive system breaks down starches and most food sugars into glucose, the form of sugar that's burned by our cells. The glucose is then absorbed into the bloodstream and carried to all the body's organs and tissues, where it powers brain activity, muscle action, nerve transmission, and other life-sustaining functions.

If blood levels of this vital fuel drop *too low*, the organs—especially the brain—start to malfunction. By the same token, if there's *too much* glucose in the blood, there are equally serious consequences, as we'll see in a moment.

It takes an "orchestra" of hormones to keep blood sugar levels within normal range. One of the key members of this orchestra is insulin, a substance normally secreted into the bloodstream by the pancreas. By assisting in the transfer of glucose from the bloodstream to the cells, insulin assures the body of a steady supply of fuel while clearing the blood of excess amounts.

THE BODY'S TINY, VULNERABLE INSULIN FACTORY

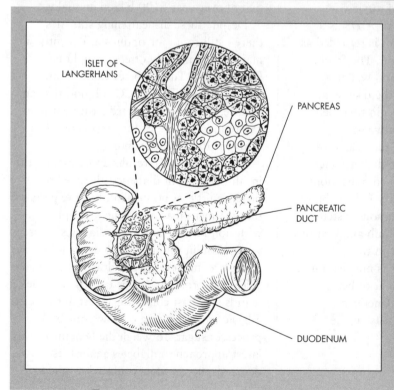

ISLET OF LANGERHANS

PANCREAS

PANCREATIC DUCT

DUODENUM

Nestled just below the stomach at the upper end of the intestines (the duodenum), the pancreas plays two distinct roles, pouring digestive juices into the intestines while it secretes insulin into the bloodstream. The insulin is manufactured in little clumps of cells—the Islets of Langerhans—tucked within the tissue of the pancreas. If the body's immune defenders mistake the Islets for invaders and destroy them, insulin production fails and Type I diabetes results. In Type II diabetes, the Islets survive and continue to produce; but for reasons we don't fully understand, the body's cells fail to use the insulin efficiently.

What Goes Wrong in Diabetes?

One of two things happens in diabetes. In insulin-dependent diabetes—most often seen in children and young adults—the pancreas fails to do its job, producing little if any insulin. In non-insulin-dependent diabetes—most often found in the middle-aged and elderly—the pancreas continues production, but the body either requires more than it can make or fails to respond properly to the available supply—a condition called insulin resistance.

In either case, blood sugar levels continue to go up and up as the intestinal tract converts carbohydrates into sugar and pours it into the bloodstream. Without insulin to speed sugar into the cells the body's energy level declines, resulting in the tired, listless feeling that often marks diabetes. Then, as unused sugar continues to mount, it begins to "spill" out of the bloodstream into the urine.

Faced with a syrupy concentration of sugar, the kidneys draw extra fluid from the body to dilute the urine. Unfortunately, this only makes matters worse, leading to increasingly serious dehydration. As the situation continues to unfold, a complex series of biochemical changes takes over, causing a dangerous acid condition to develop in the body. Left unchecked, this condition leads to coma and death.

How It All Starts

Although scientists understand a great deal about the way insulin- and non-insulin-dependent diabetes develop, they still don't know the exact causes. Insulin-dependent diabetes—also called Type I—is thought to be the result of an autoimmune reaction in which the body mistakes its own tissues as foreign proteins and begins to attack them as if they were an invading bacteria or virus. In Type I diabetics, the theory goes, the immune system misreads the insulin-producing cells of the pancreas as an invader and mounts an all-out attack, destroying the organ's ability to produce insulin.

The insulin-resistance encountered in non-insulin dependent, or Type II, diabetes is probably the result of a genetic flaw, but researchers also believe that overeating and overweight are contributing factors. In fact, between 80 and 90 percent of Type II diabetics are obese. It seems that the fat cells of an overweight person are not as sensitive to the insulin as they should be. That prevents cells from taking up sugar.

A Range of Treatment Options

If unusual thirst or hunger, frequent urination, fatigue, or muscle weakness lead you to suspect you have diabetes, your first move is to see a physician for a complete diagnostic workup. To determine whether you really have the disease, the doctor may measure your blood sugar levels after a short period without food, or order a glucose tolerance test. If you have to take the tolerance test, you'll be asked to drink a sugar solution on an empty stomach. You'll then have several blood samples taken (usually every hour for 2 or 3 hours) to see how your body handles the load. Ordinarily, your blood glucose level would rise quickly, then gradually drop to normal. If you are diabetic, however, the level will still be somewhat elevated at the end of the test.

If you do have diabetes, you have several options. The treatment plan used in the DCCT study is one. Since it reduces long-term complications so dramatically, many diabetes specialists are extremely enthusiastic about it. Unfortunately, without the help of a team of specialists that includes an endocrinologist, nurse educator, nutritionist, and maybe even a behavioral psychologist, the program is hard to follow.

An insulin-dependent diabetic on the DCCT program usually must take 3 to 4 injections of insulin daily. Someone with the non-insulin-dependent form of the disease usually starts out with a special diet and exercise program. If that fails to work, the doctor may prescribe oral medicine or insulin injections. The DCCT approach also requires you to test your blood sugar levels several times a day with an electronic glucose meter, then carefully schedule meals and exercise based on the results of the tests.

The aim of this intensive program is to keep your blood sugar to near-normal levels, which range from 80 to 120 milligrams per deciliter on an empty stomach. At bedtime, the numbers to aim for are 100 to 140 milligrams per deciliter.

Diabetics on more traditional, less rigorous regimens may take only one or two insulin shots a day and test their blood sugar levels less frequently—if at all. In fact, some diabetics continue to rely on urine test strips to check their sugar levels instead of using a glucose meter. Most diabetes specialists advise against relying solely on urinary sugar testing, however, because it's not sensitive enough.

Since the intensive program requires so much work, many people are choosing a middle ground between the DCCT approach and traditional care in the hope that they can still reduce the risk of chronic complications.

Diet Therapy: The Latest Thinking

Regardless of which options you choose, one of the cornerstones of treatment for all diabetics is good nutrition. And that means more than a standard diabetic diet. What you really want is an individually tailored plan that explains what to eat, how much to eat, and when. Since a registered dietitian has the expertise to give you this information, you need to enlist one for planning your strategy. If your doctor has no dietitian on staff, you can contact the local affiliate of the American Diabetes Association or the national office of the American Association of Diabetes Educators for the name of a qualified consultant.

Even if you have the help of a dietitian, you and your families still need to understand the basic diet strategy. The latest nutrition guidelines from the American Diabetes Association (AOA) stress the importance of achieving reasonable weight. This is especially important for Type II diabetics in whom excessive numbers of fat cells may be one of the sources of the problem.

As a rule of thumb, anyone who needs to shed unwanted weight can expect to lose about a pound a week by reducing his usual daily food intake by 500 calories. A weight-loss diet should not drop below 1,200 calories for women and 1,500 calories for men. Anything less than this could leave you with vitamin and mineral deficiencies.

How you divide up these calories depends upon your treatment goals and any complications you may have. If you are seriously overweight, but otherwise healthy you should probably get about 20 percent of your calories from protein, less than 30 percent from fat, and about 50 percent from carbohydrates.

When choosing carbohydrate-rich foods, you don't necessarily have to restrict simple

THE BOTTOM LINE ON DIET

Latest guidelines from the American Diabetes Association stress the same factors that everyone should watch for:

- Keep your weight normal; lose extra pounds if you have to.
- Boost your carbohydrates to 50 percent of your calories.
- Cut fat to 30 percent of your calories.
- Make sugary foods part of a balanced meal.
- Back up your diet with regular exercise.

sugars, according to the latest ADA guidelines. Researchers have failed to prove that sugar, when included as part of a "mixed meal," is any more likely to raise blood sugar levels than are starches. This is true, in part, because the other elements of such a meal—protein, fat, starches, and fiber—blunt the effects of the sugar.

That doesn't mean you can eat all the cake, candy, and ice cream you want. Adding sweets to a meal that already provides the right number of carbohydrate calories can raise blood sugar levels. (And, of course, the extra sugar raises total calories, making it that much harder to lose weight.)

It's also important to keep in mind that while many diabetics now have some freedom with simple sugars, if you fall within a group considered "sugar-sensitive" you won't have that luxury. Sugar-sensitive diabetics have to limit foods that rapidly enter the bloodstream, such as table sugar, honey, molasses, and candy. They may also need to cut down on fruit or eat it at the end of a meal; some diabetics may have to avoid fruit juices altogether because of their almost immediate impact on blood sugar.

How can you tell which foods work best for you? That takes a lot of experimentation and blood-sugar self-monitoring. The only sure-fire way to create a diet plan that keeps blood sugar at near normal levels is to get in the habit of testing your blood sugar both before and one to two hours after meals. By seeing how various foods affect these readings, you can adjust the timing and ingredients of your meals and snacks.

Your diet should also help control abnormal levels of fats in your blood, a common problem among diabetics. In practical terms, that means limiting your intake of saturated fat and cholesterol. Among the worst offenders are fatty cuts of beef and pork, egg yolks, whole milk, cheese, and baked goods made with coconut and palm oils. (For more information, see Chapter 10, "What to Do About Fat.")

Regardless of the type of diet you need, you shouldn't try to change all your eating habits at once—or get discouraged if it seems like you're taking two steps forward and one step back. Almost everyone finds it difficult to give up deeply ingrained habits.

It helps to try to understand as much as you can about *why* you eat what you do. Many of us harbor subtle, often half-unconscious attitudes toward food that can hinder our ability to adapt to a new diet. Uncovering these attitudes can help you stay on course. (For tips on analyzing your approach to food, see Chapter 31, "Fitting Health into Your Everyday Meals.")

Success Is In the Details

Even if you find it relatively easy to master the basics of your new diet, there are still a lot of details to consider. For instance, is it okay to drink alcohol? Should you take vitamin or mineral supplements? Are there any advantages to replacing sugar with artificial sweeteners?

What About Alcohol?

The American Diabetes Association says that moderate use of alcohol should not create any problems for most diabetics, assuming their blood sugar levels are under control. That means no more than two drinks a day for men and one for women. (A drink is defined as a can [12 ounces] of beer, a glass [5 ounces] of wine, or one and one-half ounces of 80-proof hard liquor.)

This advice comes with several caveats: You should only drink alcohol with a meal; it can cause low blood sugar in a person who has fasted for more than 5 hours. The risk is even greater for anyone taking insulin or oral drugs that lower blood sugar levels, such as Orinase or Tolinase.

And people who have had a problem with alcohol abuse, as well as those with pancreatitis, gastritis, certain forms of kidney and heart disease, frequent bouts of low blood sugar, and neuropathy—a form of nerve damage common in many diabetics—should probably not include alcohol in their diets at all.

Do You Need a Nutritional Supplement?

Unfortunately, there's no simple answer to that question. A lot depends on your body's reserves. For instance, studies have shown that if you have a deficiency of the trace element chromium, your body will have a harder time handling sugar. Although there is no hard evidence, researchers suspect that chromium deficiency may be more of a problem among the elderly and the poor than among other diabetics. Good sources of chromium include whole-grain breads, brewer's yeast, and cheese.

There is more evidence to suggest that some diabetics need extra magnesium. Experts say magnesium deficiency in diabetics is probably due to loss of the mineral in the urine. A lack of magnesium may contribute to insulin resistance, making it harder for the body's cells to take up sugar.

The threat of magnesium deficiency is greatest among pregnant women, those with congestive heart failure, and anyone taking diuretics, digoxin, or a group of antibiotics called aminoglycosides (gentamicin, streptomycin, tobramycin).

Before considering a magnesium supplement, however, you should talk with your doctor. High doses can be harmful in anyone with abnormal kidney function—a common problem for those with diabetes.

Studies have also shown that the levels of zinc in a diabetic's blood are generally lower than normal. If you develop diabetic leg ulcers, zinc supplements may help to heal them.

Are Sugar Substitutes a Good Idea?

Since the American Diabetes Association guidelines no longer limit dietary sugar, there's less need to be concerned with sugar substitutes. But because there are now so many of these products, and so many conflicting claims about their value, you still might want to review their advantages and disadvantages.

The sweeteners sorbitol, mannitol, and xylitol (called sugar alcohols) all contain calories, which means they have to be counted toward your carbohydrate allowance. The good news is that they don't raise blood sugar levels as much as sucrose (table sugar) and most other sugars. Keep in mind, though, that too much of these sugar alcohols can cause diarrhea.

The advantage of sweeteners such as aspartame (NutraSweet) and saccharin, is that they do not add calories to the diet. Nor do they affect blood sugar levels. Some research suggests, however, that they may produce side effects.

The Food and Drug Administration has received hundreds of complaints about aspartame saying that it causes headaches, anxiety, depression, irritability, insomnia, dizziness, abdominal pain, diarrhea, and rash. Careful scientific studies, however, have failed to verify any of these claims beyond a reasonable doubt.

Some experts want saccharin banned because in animal studies it appears to have caused cancer of the bladder. Others point out that the doses used in the studies were huge—much higher than a normal person would ever consume. Whatever the truth is, the specter of cancer, plus the fact that saccharin can reach a developing baby, has prompted some experts to urge pregnant women to avoid it.

Why Exercise Is Crucial

While adjusting your diet is a crucial part of your treatment for diabetes, it won't be very effective without enough physical activity. Exercise can help lower your blood sugar levels by making the cells more responsive to insulin and by increasing the number of calories your body burns. Aerobic exercise is most effective because it has the greatest impact on overall blood sugar control. If possible, you should exercise at least 3 days a week for at least 20 minutes a day.

Regular exercise is also an indispensable part of any weight loss plan and allows you to be a little more liberal with your diet. But remember: in order to determine how much liberty to take, you need to test your blood sugar levels before and after exercising.

For a diabetic, it's especially important to get a complete physical before starting an exercise program. Because diabetes can be accompanied by so many complications, your doctor will have to determine whether there are any signs of heart, eye, kidney, or nerve disease. If there are, you may have to modify the type, duration, and intensity of activity.

Someone with eye disease, for example, needs to avoid exercises that raise blood pressure, which can further damage the eyes. That means replacing sit-ups, calisthenics, and weight lifting with low-impact aerobics and non-jarring activities such as walking. (See Chapter 8, "Exercise: The Other Half of Weight Control," for more information.)

Diabetes is clearly a more dangerous problem than some imagine it to be. If ignored, it can cause serious, and sometimes life-threatening consequences. But if you follow a basic healthy diet, watch your sugar levels, exercise, and take medication as prescribed, you can do much more than *cope* with the disease: You can feel better and be healthier than ever. □

CHAPTER 24

When Good Food Makes You Feel Bad: Living With Allergy

Some of the most basic and wholesome foods—milk, eggs, or bread—can have very *unwholesome* effects if you are one of the millions of people who are painfully sensitive to them. Immediately after eating—or hours or even days later—you may break out in a rash or hives (itchy, red, raised patches of skin), have grinding stomach aches and diarrhea, go to bed with a headache, or experience any number of other symptoms, from leg cramps to choking. While many foods can cause reactions ranging from mild to severe, some are much more common culprits than others (see the "Common Offenders" box nearby).

Most people just don't recognize or understand the dangers. Tell a food server in a restaurant that you can't eat peanuts, and you may be served a dish cooked in a pan that held another customer's peanut-laden meal—

a potentially lethal mistake for a person with a peanut allergy. Tell a friend who's making you dinner that lobster is a no-no, and you may find it has been used anyway in preparing a sauce. They aren't trying to hurt you, they just can't imagine it making a difference.

When a person is highly sensitive to a type of food, even the tiniest amount may trigger a reaction; for example, as little as one 5,000th of a teaspoon of peanut, according to the Food Allergy Network, a respected consumer information group. In fact, some people even feel mild symptoms come on if they touch such a food or enter a room where it's being prepared. The odor, fumes, or microscopic pieces in the air will do it. "Some people wheeze when they walk past the nut store at the mall," notes Dr. Jeffrey Factor, an allergist in West Hartford, Connecticut.

Anyone who has ever had a strong allergic reaction to food knows just how serious a problem it can be. Yet not everyone takes the necessary precautions to prevent it from happening again or to handle it when it does. You should know that most of the people who experience life-threatening reactions to

COMMON OFFENDERS

Most Common In Adults

Peanuts, peanut products (these are legumes, like beans—not nuts)

Nuts from trees (Brazil nuts, hazelnuts, walnuts, pecans, others)

Shellfish (shrimp, crayfish, lobster, crab, snails)

Other fish

Most Common In Children

Cow's milk, dairy products

Eggs, especially the whites

Soybeans, soy products

Wheat

Peanuts, peanut products

Fruits, especially citrus (oranges, lemons, limes, grapefruit, tangerines) and berries (especially strawberries)

Less Common (But Just as Potent)

Corn

Tomatoes

Legumes other than peanuts, including peas, soybeans, lentils, pinto beans, lima beans, and licorice

food have previously been "warned" by milder symptoms produced by the same foods.

True food allergies are rare, occurring in only about 1 or 2 percent of adults. It's also unusual for an individual to be allergic to more than one or two foods. Allergic reactions range from severe and even fatal *anaphylaxis* to milder forms of sensitivity and hypersensitivity. A true allergic reaction is a misdirected attack by the body's immune system against an ordinarily harmless substance.

Other forms of food-related discomfort don't involve the immune system, but can be just as real and troubling. Some involve an intolerance or inability to digest certain foods. Others are a response to a specific chemical or additive found in the food, much like the side effect of a medication.

Whether the problem is an allergy, an intolerance, or a chemical side effect, the bottom line is the same. You need to find out what's causing the reaction and make sure it stays out of your diet.

What Happens During an Allergic Reaction

A real allergic reaction is a case of mistaken identity. The body's immune system identifies a protein or related substance in the offending food as the enemy and sends out a battalion of defenses to destroy it, just as it would attack a virus or bacteria. In both types, the immune system also marshals overeager soldiers called histamines, which produce painful sensations in the skin, eyes, and throat (see box, "When the Immune System Goes on the Attack").

The entry of an **allergen,** (any substance that causes an allergic reaction), into the body of a susceptible person triggers a chain of events in the immune system. In one type, antibodies are created after one exposure to the food in order to fight the "invaders" next time. These antibodies are called immunoglobulin E (IgE) and can usually be identified by a blood test (see the section on diagnosis, later in the chapter). In another type of reaction, cellular allergy, immune cells called lymphocytes become sensitized over time by exposure to certain chemicals

WHEN THE IMMUNE SYSTEM GOES ON THE ATTACK

Mast cells containing granules or small "packages" of chemicals, are located throughout the body tissue, especially near the lung, nose, and stomach. Clinging to the outside membrane of each mast cell are up to 100,000 immunoglobulin E (IgE) molecules of various kinds, that can respond to individual foreign substances called antigens.

When an antigen traveling through the blood comes into contact with a type of white blood cell called a plasma cell, the plasma cell produces an antibody to fight the antigen. These antibodies begin to flow through the bloodstream. As soon as they touch at least two "receptor" IgE molecules on a mast cell, the cell explosively degranulates (discharges granules) into the bloodstream. There, the granules break open, releasing histamine and other substances (mediators) meant to attack the antigen. A flood of these substances can simultaneously cause adverse reactions in the body. Other white blood cells (basophils), which travel through the blood, respond similarly to antibodies by spraying histamine and serotonin at them.

When an ordinarily harmless foreign substance such as food comes to be viewed as an antigen by the body, it's considered an allergen, the cause of an allergic reaction.

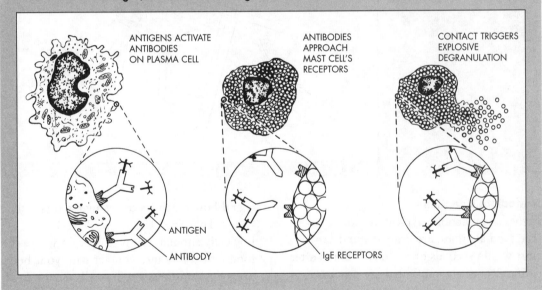

ANTIGENS ACTIVATE ANTIBODIES ON PLASMA CELL

ANTIBODIES APPROACH MAST CELL'S RECEPTORS

CONTACT TRIGGERS EXPLOSIVE DEGRANULATION

ANTIGEN

ANTIBODY

IgE RECEPTORS

and proteins in food. When next they meet, the lymphocytes overreact, expelling the foreign material just as they would reject an organ transplant.

The effects of exposure to a food allergen range from a little tingling in the mouth or swelling and redness of the skin to life-threatening difficulties. Symptoms may include difficulty breathing, hives, vomiting, and diarrhea (see box on "Typical Symptoms of True Food Allergy"). In many children, the first red flag is eczema, a rash that may appear anywhere on the body, especially the cheeks and buttocks (often severe in infants).

TYPICAL SYMPTOMS OF TRUE FOOD ALLERGY

The first signs of an immediate allergic reaction may be itching and swelling in your mouth. This may be followed by progressive difficulty breathing, with coughing, wheezing, chest tightness, and a feeling that your throat is closing up. The worst reactions end in anaphylaxis (see accompanying box).

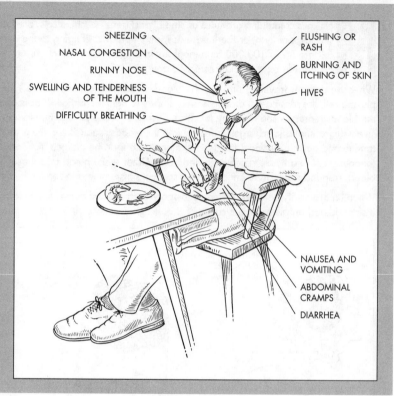

SNEEZING
NASAL CONGESTION
RUNNY NOSE
SWELLING AND TENDERNESS OF THE MOUTH
DIFFICULTY BREATHING

FLUSHING OR RASH
BURNING AND ITCHING OF SKIN
HIVES

NAUSEA AND VOMITING
ABDOMINAL CRAMPS
DIARRHEA

Immediate Reactions

Immediate reactions, typical of most true food allergies, are dramatic and can start within seconds or up to two hours after eating. Routinely implicated are peanuts, tree nuts such as walnuts, eggs (especially the whites), and shellfish with outer skeletons, such as shrimp and lobster.

The especially severe reactions called anaphylaxis start quickly, from a second after eating the offending food to 15 minutes later, depending on how severe the person's allergy is and how much food was ingested (see the "Signs That Spell Emergency" box). Logically enough, symptoms begin where the food first comes into contact with your body. Your lips and tongue will swell, the inside of your mouth will start to itch, and you may feel a sense of impending doom. Something is telling you to get help. Ignoring that extremely useful warning is a big mistake, and can be a fatal one since death can occur within two hours of exposure. Fortunately, of the 1,000 or so Americans who go into anaphylactic shock each year, all but about half a dozen survive.

Here's a standard scenario. George munches a shrimp cocktail at a party. The inside of his mouth itches, but he hardly notices it and makes no connection with the food. Not long afterward, he cooks a shrimp dish. His lips tingle and he develops a rash. *Now is the crucial time for him to see a doctor and learn about his allergy,* but it doesn't occur to him. A month later, one spoonful of shrimp bisque at a restaurant makes him gasp for air and nearly collapse as painful hives pop up all over his body. Fortunately, the restaurant proprietors know what to do. In the hospital emergency room, George is told never to eat shrimp again.

Delayed Reactions

Delayed reactions, such as headache, lethargy, mood swings, loss of concentration, possible skin involvement—may not appear for a day or even longer, making the source of the problem difficult to diagnose. In one sort of delayed reaction, symptoms begin 12 hours after the food is eaten and peak in 24 to 48 hours. A more protracted type doesn't produce symptoms for 18 to 24 hours; they're most severe in 72 hours. Foods typically causing delayed reactions, which may not be true allergies, include dairy, wheat, corn, and all kinds of chemicals (although some people may have immediate reactions from ingesting them). There is some speculation that chronic conditions such as irritable bowel syndrome, colitis, and rheumatoid arthritis are delayed allergic reactions to specific foods. This contention remains speculative and highly controversial.

Cross-Reactivity: When a Reaction "Runs in the Family" ... of Foods

You could very easily have a reaction to one food, and then sometime later have a reaction to a different food. You might think there is no connection. But even very different foods from the same family share the same troublesome substances. Lectins in various types of legumes, are one example. The resemblance isn't always obvious—except to your immune system, which responds as though the foods are the same. A person who is allergic to ragweed, for example, might develop an itchy mouth after eating melons.

One nurse who constantly wore latex gloves (made from the rubber tree) had a life-threatening reaction to chestnuts after ignoring a previous mild reaction to the gloves. (She might also have reacted badly to avocado or banana, which grow on related tropical trees.) Fortunately, she recovered.

Dietitians and allergists can explain which "plant cousins" might affect your hypersensitivities. Books on allergy also provide such lists. Related foods that you might not think of include apple, pear, and quince; beet and spinach; buckwheat, rhubarb, and sorrel; cashew nuts, pistachio nuts, and mango; avocado, bay leaf, cinnamon, and sassafras; allspice, and guava.

People who are allergic to foods in unrelated food families have **coincidental allergies.** Some such combinations are more common than others—grains, citrus fruits, and legumes, are one example. An allergy to eggs, however, isn't necessarily accompanied by an allergy to chicken, or a milk allergy by one to beef.

It is all too common for people with stomach aches, headaches, or other complaints for

SIGNS THAT SPELL EMERGENCY: ANAPHYLAXIS

The most dangerous form of allergic reaction is anaphylaxis, literally "without protection." Without fast treatment, the throat swells enough to close off the airway, leading to suffocation. Meanwhile, blood pressure falls until the person goes into shock. Foods that cause anaphylactic reactions most often are peanuts and peanut products such as peanut butter; tree nuts; shellfish, especially shrimp and crab; and other fish. Other reported incidents have involved milk, soybeans, wheat, barley, rice, corn, potatoes, spinach, bananas, melons, tomatoes, citrus fruits, and chocolate. Any severe food allergy could trigger the condition. People with asthma are at greatest risk.

Anaphylaxis can also result from insect stings or from aspirin and a few other medications, especially penicillin. In rare cases, someone goes into anaphylactic shock while doing strenuous aerobic exercise such as running (exercise-induced anaphylaxis). The exercise-induced attacks are prompted by foods that prove allergenic only when combined with exercise. When primed by these foods, the blood vessels' natural response to physical activity triggers mast cells into releasing their potent inflammatory chemicals.

Anyone who has ever experienced an anaphylactic reaction should always carry a preloaded syringe of epinephrine (adrenaline). Popular brands include EpiPen (one dose) and Ana-Kit (multiple-dose package). You should also wear a special bracelet that describes the problem and provides a doctor's name and phone number. If you should

BE ALERT FOR ANY COMBINATION OF THESE EARLY SIGNS OF GRAVE DANGER:

- FEELING OF IMPENDING DOOM
- LIPS TURN BLUE, STARTING AT EDGES
- TONGUE IS SWOLLEN
- MOUTH AND THROAT ITCH
- THROAT BEGINS TO CLOSE UP (IMMEDIATE DANGER OF SUFFOCATION!)
- SKIN BECOMES HOT AND ITCHY OR BREAKS OUT IN HIVES
- NOSE FEELS STUFFED; SNEEZING
- SHORTNESS OF BREATH; WHEEZING
- EYES TEAR, SWELL UP, OR ITCH
- EARS THROB
- VOICE BECOMES HOARSE OR CHANGES PITCH
- CHEST FEELS TIGHT AND PAINFUL
- RAPID HEARTBEATS
- URGENT NEED TO GO TO THE BATHROOM
- DIZZINESS OR COLLAPSE (SHARP DROP IN BLOOD PRESSURE)

LESS COMMON:

- NAUSEA, VOMITING, DIARRHEA, STOMACH PAIN, UTERINE CRAMPS (IN WOMEN)

become unconscious, people will know what's wrong and what to do. Bracelets can be purchased from Medic Alert, P.O. Box 381009, Turlock, CA 95381, 800-344-3226. Prices for different metals and styles range from $35 to $75.

Any combination of the symptoms listed here, particularly during or soon after a meal, suggests an anaphylactic reaction to food. (The symptoms are the same whatever the cause, but food causes more anaphylactic deaths per year than insect stings.) If epinephrine is not available, and the person is conscious, administering a liquid antihistamine is better than nothing. Then rush the victim to the nearest emergency room. *Do not* let him or her leave the room alone and *do not* "wait to see what happens." Seconds count.

which their doctors couldn't find an underlying disease or condition to be told, "It's all in your head." Sometimes that may be true. But, in millions of cases, the problem may be an unrecognized non-allergic reaction to one or more specific kinds of food or components of food. Anyone with physical problems that might be related to food should explore that route. Numerous books on the subject by physicians and other health practitioners are studded with convincing case histories of patients of all ages who found relief from longtime and/or severe symptoms only after learning which foods to avoid.

The Elusive Reactions: Intolerance and Chemical Side Effects

Some of these hard-to-pin-down problems result from abnormalities of the digestive system. The best known, an inability to digest milk and dairy products due to an enzyme deficiency, is explained in detail in the box on "Lactose Intolerance."

Another, involving a rare inability to digest the gluten in wheat and some other types of grain, is discussed in Chapter 25, "Dealing with Digestive Disorders."

Many problems, however, are triggered not by digestion, but by chemicals found naturally in food or inserted as additives. These substances can produce side effects resembling those of a drug. An example is caffeine. When someone who becomes jittery and anxious or gets a headache from drinking regular coffee finds he has no symptoms from the decaffeinated brew, the problem isn't with the coffee itself, it is with the caffeine. This common type of dietary problem is called a pharmacologic reaction.

Among the Offending Chemicals Found Naturally in Food:

Serotonin, found in tomatoes, plums, avocados, and pineapple. It can cause headaches and nausea and can raise blood pressure. **Histamine** is found in Swiss and other fermented cheeses, wine, dried sausage, anchovies, sardines, tomatoes, spinach, tuna and mackerel that weren't sufficiently chilled before canning or cooking, and fermented foods such as sauerkraut. Reactions include gastrointestinal distress, headache, flushing and reddening of the skin, and itchy eyes. Histamines are formed naturally in food by the action of non-disease-causing bacteria.

Methylxanthines, including caffeine and theobromine, are found in coffee, tea, cola drinks, chocolate, and cocoa. They may induce headache, stomach pain, diarrhea, nervousness, rapid heartbeats, restlessness, insomnia, mood swings, and an inability to concentrate.

Some people's reaction to chocolate is more likely pharmacologic than allergic. Chocolate is, in fact, "one of the most misunderstood foods," and true allergy to it is extremely rare, says Dr. Jerry Shier, an allergist and immunologist in Silver Spring, Maryland. The jittery, irritable feeling it provokes may result from a chemical in chocolate called phenylethylamine. If a true allergic reaction strikes, says Dr. Shier, it's likely to be the fault of other ingredients in the candy, such as milk, peanuts, or various nuts from trees.

Tyramine is found in wine and cheeses, especially hard cheeses such as Stilton, blue cheese, and aged cheddar. It produces symptoms like those of the methylxanthines.

LACTOSE INTOLERANCE: NOT QUITE AN ALLERGY

Many people assume they're allergic to milk because whenever they drink it or eat ice cream, cheese, or other dairy products, they have gassy stomach pain, bloating, and diarrhea. Some of those people are indeed allergic to milk, as an allergist can discover, and they should avoid it. But others have a digestive problem called lactose intolerance.

What they have is not an allergy but the most common form of **enzyme deficiency.** The missing or insufficient intestinal enzyme is lactase, which is needed to break down the natural sugar in dairy foods (lactose) into smaller parts to complete the process of digestion.

When people with lactose intolerance drink milk or eat a dairy product, the lactose remains in the intestines, where it is prey to natural bacteria. The resulting bubbly fermentation causes gas and diarrhea, usually starting from 15 minutes to several hours after eating. (To those symptoms, someone with a true milk allergy might add nasal congestion, headache, frequent urination, and hives.)

Lactose intolerance is far more common among some ethnic groups than others. According to the National Center for Nutrition and Dietetics of the American Dietetic Association, the condition is found in about 80 percent of Asians and Native Americans, 75 percent of blacks, 50 percent of Hispanics, and 20 percent of whites.

Diagnosis

Considering the symptoms, it's easy to see why lactose intolerance can be misdiagnosed as an ulcer, irritable bowel syndrome, or some other gastrointestinal disorder. Taking a **lactose intolerance test** can determine whether lactase deficiency is causing your problem. In the doctor's office, you're given 50 grams of lactose to drink. Lactose intolerance is diagnosed if diarrhea, abdominal bloating, and discomfort result within 20 to 30 minutes, and if blood tests demonstrate little or no sugar has reached your blood.

If even that is uncertain, the diagnosis can be confirmed without question if little or no lactase is found in a laboratory analysis (biopsy) of a small piece of tissue taken surgically from the jejunum, which is part of the small intestine.

A safe, inexpensive, and fairly reliable way to diagnose the problem is with the **hydrogen breath test.** After being given a certain amount of milk to drink on an empty stomach, you'll breathe into a device that traps and measures exhaled air at timed intervals. If your small intestine fails to break down the lactose from the milk, excess carbohydrates will reach your colon and undergo fermentation by bacteria there. This will increase the level of hydrogen in your blood and in your exhalations.

With your doctor's permission (to make sure you won't be triggering a serious milk allergy) you can test yourself at home. Avoid all dairy products for two weeks. If formerly frequent pains fade away, you may be on the right track. Now drink a glass of milk. If the pains come back, lactose intolerance may be the culprit. If you have no such reaction for a few days, eat some dairy products and drink a little more milk until you're eating a fair amount at one time. If no symptoms appear, the problem probably lies elsewhere.

Some Common Additives, Which Include Preservatives, Flavorings, and Colorings: MSG. Monosodium glutamate, used to enhance flavors in cooking, and in prepared foods, causes headaches and other symptoms in some people. Studies are inconclusive about its effects, and the Food and Drug Administration (FDA) has placed no restriction on its use. If MSG seems to affect you, don't patronize restaurants that use it.

A milk product called Lactaid is available in the milk section of many supermarkets. Another way to cope is to swallow lactase tablets before eating dairy products or to add lactase drops to milk before drinking it. Depending on the extent of your reaction, you may be able to eat dairy products that are low in lactose, including cheddar and other hard cheeses. Plain (not flavored or frozen) yogurt that contains active cultures may work for you, too.

If you have to avoid all milk products, your doctor will advise you to take calcium tablets, since milk is a major source of that important mineral. Eat heartily from the large group of nondairy calcium-rich foods, such as potatoes; broccoli; dark green, leafy vegetables, such as collard greens, kale, and spinach; legumes, including soybeans, peanuts, and beans (assuming they agree with you); sesame seeds; and certain oily fish, such as salmon and sardines, especially the canned kind containing edible bones.

When shopping, watch for these words on food labels, all of which indicate dairy: the obvious, such as milk, cream, butter and most margarines; and the less obvious, including nonfat milk solids, lactose, lactoalbumin, casein (which represents 80 percent of the protein of cow's milk), sodium caseinate, and whey (20 percent of the protein in cow's milk).

For a meal out, try an Asian restaurant such as Chinese, Japanese, Korean, or Thai. Not surprisingly, milk is not a staple of these cuisines, which were developed by people with a very high rate of lactose intolerance.

Sulfites keep food looking fresh and retard spoilage. They're used on dried fruits and dried potato products such as mashed potato flakes. Sulfites are sometimes sprayed on raw shrimp while they're still on the boat. A rash of bad experiences at salad bars, including deaths, led the FDA to clamp down about 10 years ago, forbidding sulfite spray on fresh fruits and vegetables sold or served raw. In addition, sulfites must be included on the ingredient list when used as preservatives in packaged or processed foods.

Eating anything that contains sulfites causes mild to severe breathing difficulties in about 5 percent of people with asthma, or over a million Americans, according to the Center for Science in the Public Interest, an advocacy and research group in Washington, D.C. Sulfite symptoms include flushing, faintness, weakness, cough, and turning blue—as well as loss of consciousness and death. Nonasthmatics may also have bad, though typically less severe reactions to the chemical as well. The reason isn't clear, but may be metabolic: a deficiency of sulfite oxidase, the enzyme that breaks down sulfites in the body. If you think sulfites may make you feel unwell, avoid foods that contain sodium sulfite, sulfur dioxide, or sodium or potassium bisulfite or metabisulfite.

The best-known source of sulfites in food is wine (see the box on "Complex Effects of Wine"). Some wine labels now declare their bottles' contents to be sulfite free, and people with mild adverse reactions to sulfites might try those.

Benzoates. These preservatives include benzoic acid, sodium benzoate, BHA (butylated hydroxyanisole), and BHT (butylated hydroxytoluene). The benzoates can cause chronic skin problems and severe asthmatic reactions in adults. They're found in bread, milk powder, potato powder, fat, oil, margarine, mayonnaise, jam, chocolate, soft drinks, and instant drink powders.

COMPLEX EFFECTS OF WINE

Plain wine constitutes a cocktail of natural drugs. **Tyramine** can induce symptoms like those of caffeine: headache, stomach ache, anxiety, and rapid heartbeats. Nearly all wines contain **sulfites,** used to stop the fermentation process and stabilize the wine. Some brands have been advertising their freedom from that chemical on the label. **Molds** and **yeasts** trigger many allergic reactions. Red wines in particular also contain **histamines,** the major chemical mediator responsible for allergic symptoms, including migraine attacks. Other possible ingredients are **sulfur dioxide** and **egg white.**

Champagne processing starts with a mixture of different grapes, any of which might provoke a reaction in susceptible people. Techniques for aging and fermenting wines vary from one vineyard to another and are traditionally kept secret. You may find that only certain types, nationalities, brands, or even years of wine bother you; take note and avoid them. Newer vintages may give you more headaches than older ones. And like any form of alcohol, wine can increase the risk of developing an immune allergic reaction to other foods.

FD&C Yellow Dye #5 (tartrazine), a widely used food coloring, induces itching, hives, nasal congestion, and/or headaches in sensitive individuals. The best proof is the label rather than the food itself, which could be any of a variety of colors; green, orange, purple, or another mixed color. Read the labels of orange drinks, pies, gingerbread, butterscotch chips, instant puddings, gelatins, hard candies, cake mixes, processed cheese, refrigerated rolls, and even shampoo and toothpaste.

Phenolphthalein. Related to tartrazine and derived from coal tar, this chemical is used to make candy pink. It can produce headaches, breathing difficulties, and other physical problems.

When Food Allergy Starts

Allergies and other adverse food reactions can begin at any time in your life. Whether or not you develop food allergies depends on heredity, your ability to absorb nutrients in the intestine, your immune response, the types of food you eat, and the amount of a particular food that you eat at one time.

Any tendency you may have towards allergies is with you from birth. A child who has one allergic parent has roughly a 20 to 40 percent chance of developing some kind of allergy, twice as likely as a child with nonallergic parents. If both parents have allergies, the risk is about four times as great (40 to 60 percent). When both parents have the same allergy, the likelihood rises to 60 to 80 percent.

People who are born with a general vulnerability to allergies usually have their first reactions early. For instance, an allergy to milk, the most common allergic problem in infants, often appears in the first days of life.

In any case, children are far more susceptible to food allergies than adults. The lining of their gastrointestinal tract is still immature, allowing substances to more easily stream out into the blood and trigger reactions. Up to about 8 percent of children in the United States have true food allergies. The proportion with an intolerance or chemical sensitivity is a great deal higher. Fortunately, at least 80 percent of food allergies that begin in childhood are outgrown by the age of 5. Most persistent are some of the fiercest allergies: to peanuts, tree nuts, shellfish, and other fish.

MINIMIZING ALLERGIC REACTIONS IN YOUR BABY

There is nothing you can do to prevent allergies in infants, but there are ways to minimize the risk of an allergic reaction. If your family has a history of food allergies, and you plan to breastfeed, you may be advised not to eat the foods that are most likely to upset your baby's digestive system, particularly milk and wheat. Waiting until your baby is six months old before starting solid foods can also delay the baby's direct exposure to possible allergens. If you are bottlefeeding and your baby has a reaction to cow's milk-based formulas, you should know that there are soy-based formulas and other substitutes as well. (See Chapter 17 for details.) (A child with an allergic older sibling has about a 25 to 35 percent chance of being allergic as well.)

You may be given similar advice if your baby is colicky. Colic is generally defined as inconsolable crying for more than 3 hours a day, more than 3 days a week, for 3 or more weeks. Providing additional feedings—a time-honored way to soothe a cranky baby—only intensifies the problem if it happens to be related to food (not always the case). Such babies are crying because their stomachs hurt.

You should consult your pediatrician or family doctor before you make any changes on your own in your baby's diet, to make sure that both of you remain well nourished. If milk is abandoned, calcium supplements will be needed.

Avoiding allergenic foods during pregnancy does not seem to prevent allergies in the baby. And avoiding foods while breastfeeding won't necessarily prevent the baby from developing allergies after weaning. For all this advice, you may have to consult an allergist.

Your First Move: Seeing a Doctor

Identifying and dealing with food allergies, especially when their cause is far from obvious, can take a long time. You might explore the subject with your family doctor. If you aren't getting anywhere, consider consulting an allergist. These specialists need several years of additional training after medical school to obtain board certification in allergy and immunology. To find an allergist near you, call the nearest large medical center or hospital affiliated with a medical school.

The first thing your doctor will do is take a comprehensive medical history, followed by a careful physical examination. You want to be sure that the source of your problems isn't a disease before you and your doctor begin searching for foods that could be bothering you.

Certain symptoms you've had at any time, even in infancy, are red flags to an allergist. These include rashes, scratching, runny nose, itchy eyes, a sense of choking, and asthma-like symptoms, even if you've never had asthma. Atopic dermatitis, a form of eczema (skin rash), is considered a telltale sign, especially in children. So is flushing under the skin. Abdominal pain, nausea and vomiting, diarrhea, and low blood pressure may also suggest allergies.

Because the tendency to allergy and hypersensitivity is so closely related to heredity, your doctor will want to know as much as possible about present or past symptoms in your close blood relatives. Find out what you can before your appointment.

Why Diagnosis Is Difficult

Other than anaphylactic reactions to food, which are swift and consistent, symptoms from unwelcome foods can vary not only from one person to another but from one day to another. Depending on the individual, the many factors involved (besides the type of food eaten) include its amount; how ripe it was (tomatoes, for example, become increasingly likely to cause a reaction as they ripen); whether it was raw or cooked, and how it was cooked; what other foods you ate at the same time; the status of your immune system; and other triggering factors such as whether you were sitting in a room full of smoke or perfume.

In people with multiple hypersensitivities, it's often a combination of events that precipitates the reaction, such as eating a candy bar before cutting the grass, then devouring a tub of movie popcorn swimming in additive-laden fake butter. Some people do better in summer than in winter.

Stress also affects the power of an offending food to impose physical symptoms. And hypersensitivities can appear or disappear suddenly, without any apparent reason. Other than anaphylaxis, symptoms of allergy can be confused with those of many other conditions—peptic ulcer, hiatal hernia, arthritis, thyroid deficiency, sinus infections, and exhaustion. Furthermore, while an immediate reaction to a food usually leaves no question of its cause, the source of a delayed reaction is extremely hard to identify, especially if the problem is a combination of foods. Tests may fail to pin-point any of the foods. No wonder many doctors (and patients) are skeptical or give up.

In addition, doctors who don't happen to have a special interest in allergy may not even think of food as the culprit unless you suggest the possibility yourself. Medical schools have always given short shrift to all aspects of nutrition, food allergy included. While that may be changing in some places, many doctors still belittle or ignore the potentially significant role of food in their patients' ill health.

Compounding the problem is doctors' justifiably low opinion of individuals and organizations that capitalize on people's pain and confusion. Some such practitioners and groups may be downright unscrupulous, while others well-meaningly offer unproved tests, products, and services for high fees. Physicians have been trained to reject any scientifically unsound practice.

The Diagnosis: Tests You Can Try

The most important goal is to learn whether you have a food allergy in the first place. You don't want to ban a food without good reason. But because food allergies come in such variety—multiple, cumulative, delayed—you'll have to proceed slowly.

Allergists use several tests to confirm suspicions of specific food allergy. These tests are far from absolute but can be helpful in making a diagnosis.

Skin Tests

In these tests, the doctor places a few drops of a commercially prepared liquid extract of a food on your back or arm. A needle is either gently drawn through the liquid along the top layer of skin (prick test) or scratched a little deeper into the skin (scratch test). If a red bump and surrounding rash (wheal and flare reaction) appears after about 10 to 20 minutes, you've had a positive response. That food can then be checked into further.

Skin tests provide a high rate of false-positives, in which the result says you are allergic but you're really not. When the test is negative, however, you are highly unlikely to be allergic to the food. Skin tests work about 30 percent of the time for genuine food allergies; for allergies to airborne particles, such as pollen, they are about 95 percent accurate.

Although your regular internist or family practitioner may be able to provide good advice about your reactions to food, have any skin testing done by a board-certified allergist, suggests Dr. Martha V. White, director of research at the Institute for Asthma and Allergy, Washington Hospital Center, Washington, D.C. Such specialists are trained to know the difference between a true-positive result and a false-positive one induced by hives or strongly reactive skin. They're aware of reasons your skin might not respond to the test; for example, if you're taking an antihistamine. Most important, they're best equipped to handle the rare case of a bad reaction, such as shock.

Blood Tests

In the radioallergosorbent (RAST) test, done in a laboratory, a small sample of serum (the liquid part of blood) is mixed with a food extract in a glass dish. If the white blood cells release a large amount of IgE antibodies in an effort to fight the intruder, you're supposedly allergic to that food. The problem with RAST tests is that they cost two or three times as much as skin tests, take much longer, and are not as reliable. You may also hear about another blood test called the enzyme-linked immunosorbent assay (ELISA). It is a respectable test but has a comparably poor accuracy record for detecting allergies.

Open Challenge

After a negative skin test result, indicating that you're not likely to have a severe reaction to a suspected food, you'll swallow capsules containing a small amount of the food, or eat it in another form, and then see what happens. If you can eat increasing amounts, up to a normal portion, with no reaction, the food is probably safe for you. This is done in the doctor's presence. Open challenge is also used to confirm a positive skin test—provided your allergic sensitivity isn't severe.

Closed Challenge

In this procedure you are given unmarked foods to eat, disguised by being freeze-dried and placed in an opaque capsule or stirred into another mixture, as the doctor watches for a reaction. This method is considered foolproof, especially if done as a double-blind test—the procedure used in the best scientific studies. Double-blinding means that neither you nor the person handing over the pill (or other form of disguised food) knows its contents, which were previously coded by someone else. Preconceptions therefore can't color the outcome for either of you. For young children, small amounts of suspected allergenic food are hidden in foods they can tolerate.

Challenges are done in the doctor's office. If your doctor believes that the food being tested could provoke a severe reaction, however, the site may be a hospital emergency room—just in case. The greater the likelihood of a life-threatening reaction, the less likely it is that a challenge will be risked.

The Elimination Diet

One good way to identify allergens is an elimination diet. You'll temporarily remove offending foods from your system, then cautiously reintroduce them *in pure form* (without additives) one at a time. If symptoms disappear in a food's absence, then return in its presence, you have probably found your problem. Follow-up testing can help make sure.

In a general elimination diet, the most common allergens (and your favorite foods) are removed for as long as it takes to clear out your system. Instead, you'll eat foods that you don't consume regularly, perhaps lamb, rice, and pears, and that are therefore unlikely to have caused your symptoms. You may be asked to temporarily stop taking vitamin and mineral supplements and even prescription drugs, (with the prescribing doctor's permission) in case a pharmacologic reaction is involved. Heavy coffee or tea drinkers are advised to wean themselves gradually before starting the diet, to prevent uncomfortable symptoms of caffeine withdrawal.

Some doctors advise cleansing the system with a five-day fast, eating or drinking nothing but distilled water. However, this is very difficult—even dangerous—and is not generally recommended. Most people follow a specific diet written out for them by an experienced health professional. Having a doctor or dietitian oversee your plan will keep your diet balanced and healthy. And no cheating, or it's back to square one.

Before you change your menu, you'll keep a food diary. Each day, you'll write down every bite you eat, when you felt symptoms, how long they lasted, and how intense they were, on a consistent scale (such as 1, mild; 2, moderate; 3, severe). You'll list any other precipitating factors, such as stress, as they occur.

Avoiding an offending food for a while permits your body to "calm down" so that consuming a small or even a moderate amount later may have no ill effects. Eating large quantities of the offending food again,

however, is likely to rekindle the hypersensitivity. The best route is moderation.

If eating a certain food makes you feel a little bit sick, but you can't imagine life without it, stop eating it for at least three months, or in extreme cases for a couple of years. Then eat a small amount no more than once or twice a week and see if the situation has improved. *Note:* This strategy may help with pharmacologic reactions and intolerance, but won't work with a true allergy. In fact, if you're truly allergic, symptoms upon suddenly reintroducing the food could be dangerous. *Any food that has ever caused symptoms of early anaphylactic shock must be avoided for life.* To be sure, consult a physician.

Don't attempt an elimination diet without a doctor's supervision if you have asthma, heart disease, diabetes, Crohn's disease (a bowel disorder), or any other serious chronic condition. For children, the entire procedure should be overseen by an allergist since a poorly designed diet could lead to severe nutritional deficiencies.

The Diagnosis: Tests to Avoid

Cytotoxic testing. This lab test has fallen into disrepute for its notorious lack of accuracy. It works like this: a small amount of blood is placed in a glass dish and a food extract is added. The sample is not checked for IgE, as in a blood test. Instead it's studied for a strong reaction in the white blood cells. The variables are so many and the rate of accuracy is so low—with the test either identifying a harmless food as harmful or vice versa—that this method is now generally considered useless.

IS SUGAR-INDUCED HYPERACTIVITY JUST HYPE?

About 20 years ago, many parents of hyperactive children eagerly accepted a physician's hypothesis that what made their kids bounce off the walls was sugar and the chemical flavorings and colors added to food. Since then, a number of studies have essentially debunked that proposition. Nevertheless, some families have insisted that removing those items from the children's diets improved their behavior.

Many pediatricians dismiss the idea. Others believe as strongly that children's antisocial, even bizarre and sometimes self-destructive behavior often stems from food hypersensitivity. The precise foods in question vary with each child; there may be one or many. In any case, trying an elimination diet with the advice and strong support of a sympathetic pediatric allergist may be worth a try when other medical conditions have been ruled out and nothing else is working.

Off-the-wall testing. Just laugh at ads in newspapers promising to identify all your allergies by using magnets or by analyzing your hair. The diagnosis is hard enough with *real* tests.

Clinical ecology. This well-meaning group tends to see chemical hypersensitivity lurking behind every disorder. You owe yourself a more reasonable approach.

How to Cope with Food Allergy

How much effort you decide to expend on finding out what's wrong and taking steps to correct it will depend on how uncomfortable your symptoms are. If you have reason to believe that eating a peanut or shrimp could kill you, your desire to eat peanuts will quickly subside. If a slice of bread baked with wheat flour gives you stomach problems, you'll munch on rice cakes with relish.

As these two examples illustrate, the best way to treat adverse food reactions is prevention: avoiding the food. When that isn't possible, or until the correct foods can be diagnosed, certain symptoms (especially respiratory ones) can at least be improved.

Drugs

Medications can only relieve symptoms, not remove the allergy. Still, prescription drugs can be extremely helpful. Great caution is used in prescribing these medications to pregnant and nursing women.

Decongestants, like those used to reduce cold symptoms, can reduce swelling and congestion.

Antihistamines. For sneezing, runny nose, itchy skin or hives, the doctor may prescribe an antihistamine such as hydroxyzine (Atarax), diphenhydramine (Benadryl), astemizone (Hismanal), or terfenadine (Seldane). These drugs are not strong enough to counteract an anaphylactic reaction.

Nasal sprays. Cromolyn (Nasalcrom) and steroids such as Vancenase, Beconase and Nasacort discourage release of irritating histamines and the slow-reacting substance of anaphylaxis (SRS-A).

Bronchodilators in tablet or aerosol form aid breathing by opening air passages in the lungs. This is especially important for people with asthma who experience bronchospasms—spasmodic contractions of large air passages (bronchi) in the lungs. Examples are metaproterenol (Alupent, Metaprel), and albuterol (Proventil).

WATCH OUT FOR HIDDEN PROBLEMS

Once you've realized you shouldn't eat something, you'll find it in unexpected places. Here are a few examples. Not all brands apply.

Corn shows up in:

Antacids	Chewing gum	Salt
Aspirin	Frozen turkey	Soft drinks
Bacon	Glue on stamps and envelopes	Toothpaste
Baking powder	Instant coffee	Vitamin pills
Breath spray	Marshmallows	
Candy	Paper cups and cartons	

Milk can be found in:

Candy	Processed lunch meats	Soup (canned)

Wheat can be part of:

Baked beans (canned)	Gin	Soup (canned)
Beer	Gravy, canned or powdered	Soy sauce
Bouillon cubes	Ice cream cones	
Bourbon	Salad dressing	

Yeast lurks in:

Dried fruits	Mushrooms
Fruit juices in bottles or cans	Vinegar (as an ingredient of mustard, ketchup, relish,
Grapes	horseradish, pickles, sauerkraut, mayonnaise)
Miso soup	Wine

Steroid creams such as hydrocortisone (Cortaid) can relieve itching.

Side effects are an occasional byproduct of these medications. They may include dry mouth, drowsiness, anxiety, frequent or painful urination, nausea, vomiting, loss of appetite, stomach pain, constipation or diarrhea, and headaches. New antihistamine preparations such as Seldane, Claritin, and Hismanal are much less likely than older ones to dry out the mouth and nasal passages and cause overwhelming sleepiness.

Unconventional methods

You may hear of people who swear by unconventional treatments. But you should remember that they are called unconventional because either there is insufficient evidence to show that they work, or the evidence clearly shows that they are harmful.

In *sublingual treatments,* small amounts of the allergenic food are placed under the tongue. The idea is to "inoculate" the body against the food. This could be extremely dangerous if you were to have a strong allergic reaction during the treatment; and there's no proof that it works.

Provocation/neutralization (P/N), or symptom provocation testing, calls for giving the person troublesome foods, in diluted form, in increasing increments until a reaction is provoked. Applications designed to neutralize the allergy follow. This method is questioned by many, although not all, mainstream physicians. *Injections* of the offending substance, useful for respiratory allergies, are not recommended for food as they could incite a severe reaction. Unsafe *autogenous urine immunization,* injections of your own urine, can lead to nephritis, a serious kidney disease.

Modifying Your Diet

To maintain good nutrition, if you must omit important foods indefinitely, consult a professional for personal diet planning and advice. A registered dietitian (R.D.) is certified and listed by the highly respected American Dietetic Association (see the Directory of Support Groups at the end of the book for details.) Ask your doctor or hospital to recommend someone, or find out if your allergist or pediatrician works regularly with one. In some states, an equivalent title is Licensed Clinical Nutritionist. "Nutritionists" in general don't necessarily have the same education or training.

Learn the many names for whatever ingredients you must avoid. Wheat may be listed as gluten, egg white as albumin. Your allergist or dietitian can provide a list of alternates.

Study the labels on food as well as on every commercial product that enters your mouth (see box, "Watch Out for Hidden Problems"). The new federal guidelines on food labeling helps make the list of contents easier to find and understand. Don't assume you know what's in a food just because you have read the label before; ingredients

change. The more severe your symptoms, the more scrupulous you must be. And don't hesitate to call the company directly. If a consumer information number isn't listed on the label, call the company directly and ask to speak with a customer service representative.

Find out what foods can be substituted nutritionally for the ones you can't eat. Many excellent books on allergy and nutrition provide such suggestions. Allergy associations can supply book lists.

Seek out the many cookbooks that provide tasty allergy-wise recipes. Enjoy the imposed adventure of exploring new foods and unfamiliar ethnic cuisines. Browse at health food stores, where you'll find recipe books and helpful advice as well as food.

After educating yourself, educate others:

- Before dining at a friend's home, call and discuss your situation. If enough of the menu can't be adjusted to provide you with a full meal, offer to contribute a dish. Or eat something at home before you go. When you can help it, don't eat troublesome foods for social reasons or just because you're hungry.

- Waiters are casually asked the ingredients of dishes on the menu every day. Make it clear why your questions are important. If your food server seems bored or unsure about the contents of a dish, ask to speak with the chef or order something else. Or, call the restaurant in advance to discuss your needs with the chef. In general, simple dishes, simply cooked, are safest.

- Obtain a card from the Food Allergy Network (800-929-4040) listing your allergy or hypersensitivity. Show it to food servers for official-looking proof that your food "preferences" are a matter of health—and possibly life or death. □

CHAPTER 25

Dealing With Digestive Disorders

The fact that bad food can cause an upset stomach is not exactly a news flash. But the way in which diet affects a *chronic* digestive problem is a bit more of a mystery. Scientists are still at work unraveling many of the connections. However, it's quite clear that the disorders discussed in this chapter are profoundly influenced by what you do or do not eat, or can be helped by adding or eliminating certain types of food. Changing your diet as a first step in therapy is usually a wise choice and is certainly more cost effective than waiting until the problem puts you in the hospital. In the United States alone, 5 million people each year are hospitalized with digestive disorders, and some $500 million is spent on medication.

Fortunately, drugs and surgery are available for severe conditions. And for some problems, seeing your doctor is the best course from the start. Most gastric ulcers for instance, can now be easily cured with antibiotics; so why condemn yourself to a bland diet instead?

Touring the Digestive Tract

The digestive tract is really just a long, winding tube. Rings of thick muscle, or sphincters, cordon off different sections of the tube: the esophagus, stomach, small intestine, and large intestine. Each section has its own role to play in digestion; and each can fall victim to its own set of ailments.

Stretching some 40 feet in adults, the digestive tract receives nine to 10 quarts of internal secretions daily to aid the digestive process. The salivary glands add a little over a quart of saliva each day to change starchy foods to sugars. Saliva mixes with food to create a ball of slippery material called a bolus. As the bolus makes its way down the esophagus, the sphincter connecting the esophagus to the stomach—the lower esophageal sphincter (LES)—relaxes, allowing the bolus to enter.

TROUBLE SPOTS ALONG THE TRACT

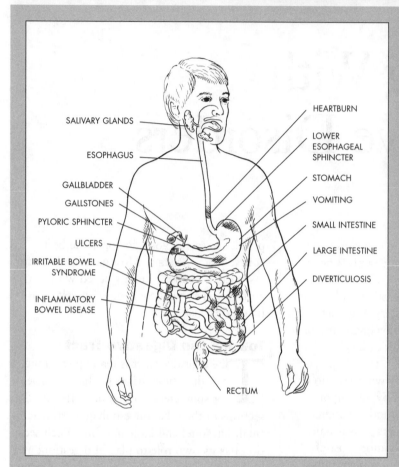

SALIVARY GLANDS

ESOPHAGUS

GALLBLADDER

GALLSTONES

PYLORIC SPHINCTER

ULCERS

IRRITABLE BOWEL SYNDROME

INFLAMMATORY BOWEL DISEASE

RECTUM

HEARTBURN

LOWER ESOPHAGEAL SPHINCTER

STOMACH

VOMITING

SMALL INTESTINE

LARGE INTESTINE

DIVERTICULOSIS

With 40 feet of tubing in which things can go wrong, it's no wonder that the digestive tract is the source of so many woes. Some areas are more trouble-prone than others. The juncture of the esophagus and the stomach—source of all our heartburn—is one. Another is the zone where the lower end of the stomach meets the small intestine, a favored haven for ulcers. Finally, towards the end of the tract, the large intestine is victim to more than its share of irritation and inflammation.

Although dietary changes can relieve some of our digestive problems, a surprising number seem unaffected by the food we eat. For instance, while the (often ineffective) prescription for ulcers used to be a bland diet, we now know that antibiotics are usually a sure cure.

When the LES relaxes at the wrong time, and gastric juices are "refluxed" back into the esophagus, *heartburn* occurs.

The stomach is a bulge in the digestive tube about the size of your two fists together. It can expand to twice its size after a large meal. If you eat too much food, or if you

swallow some dangerous compound (like poison), *vomiting* can ensue.

Most food stays in the stomach for three to five hours as the stomach muscles churn and squeeze it. The stomach is lined with glands that secrete about two quarts of gastric juice daily to aid this part of the digestive process. Gastric juice consists primarily of water, pepsin (an enzyme to break down protein), and hydrochloric acid.

Some people cannot break down proteins properly. They are *intolerant* to certain proteins, most often those found in the gluten of wheat, rye, oats, and barley. Other people have low levels of the intestinal enzyme lactase—which is responsible for breaking down lactose (milk sugar)—and are therefore intolerant to milk. Such intolerance can lead to diarrhea, gas, and cramps, but it also can be responsible for more serious conditions, such as malnutrition and iron-deficiency anemia, and can aggravate a digestive disorder called *celiac sprue*.

Hydrochloric acid kills some of the bacteria you ingest with food and also breaks down the complex sugar sucrose into the simpler glucose that the body uses for fuel. It was once believed that this acid was solely responsible for *ulcers*, but it's now agreed that a bacteria is the primary culprit. A deficiency of hydrochloric acid is also suspected of causing common indigestion and gas, and bacterial infections.

A system of rhythmic contractions known as peristalsis moves the bolus (now a more soupy mixture known as "chyme") from the lower end of the stomach, through a sphincter called the pyloric valve, and into the small intestine in a series of small, spoon-size squirts.

The small intestine is small only in its diameter (being about one inch). In length it runs about 23 feet. Food takes from two to nine hours to move through the winding passage.

The small intestine needs three quarts of watery fluid every day to make absorption of nutrients easier. Absorption then continues in the large intestine, or colon. Half-way through the colon digestion is complete. In the second half, water is reabsorbed, leaving a mass of solid waste, consisting of undigested fibers, fat and bacteria. In all, the colon itself is five feet long and looks like an upside-down "U." When a section of the intestinal wall is weak, there is a tendency for a bulge or pouch to form, resulting in *diverticulosis*.

Many beneficial bacteria live in this section of the digestive tract. They are essential for a healthy digestion, but are also the main cause of gas.

Some common problems, like persistent diarrhea and constipation, can be symptoms of diseases such as *irritable bowel syndrome* and *inflammatory bowel disease*. These two digestive disorders can occur anywhere in the digestive tract, but show up most often in the intestines. Inflammatory bowel disease includes disorders such as *Crohn's disease* or *ulcerative colitis*, both of which still defy lasting cures.

The food we commit to the daily journey through the digestive tract can aggravate many of its problems; and a simple change in diet can sometimes provide substantial relief. If you suffer from one of the following problems, these suggestions may prove helpful.

LEADING PERPETRATORS OF HEARTBURN

If you suffer attacks of heartburn, try cutting back on the foods below. Some, like spicy foods, seem obvious. Others you might never suspect.

- Alcohol
- Chocolate
- Caffeinated foods, such as coffee or tea
- Fatty foods
- Orange juice
- Peppermint and spearmint
- Spicy foods
- Sugar
- Tomato juice

Heartburn

If you've ever had a really bad case of heartburn, you may have been surprised and thankful to learn you weren't having a heart attack. The gripping pain can spread into the arms, neck, face, and back, mimicking the symptoms of heart disorders such as angina. But despite its name, heartburn has nothing to do with the heart; it's merely the result of "reflux" or backwash of acidic stomach contents into the esophagus.

Normally, the lower esophageal sphincter (LES), which separates the esophagus from the stomach, opens and closes on schedule. When food is swallowed and needs to enter the stomach, it relaxes; once the food has passed by, it tightens again. Reflux occurs when muscle pressure in the LES is relatively low. Pressure can be raised by protein and lowered by fat, alcohol, caffeinated beverages and smoking. Because LES pressure drops during pregnancy, scientists believe that fluctuating estrogen and progesterone levels also play a role.

The LES relaxes after certain foods are eaten. While this is no problem to most people, it causes painful symptoms in those prone to heartburn. When the condition becomes chronic, the inflamed lower esophagus becomes sensitive to even more types of food, which is probably the reason many people react badly to spicy food.

To manage heartburn, try the following:

- Drink plenty of water to soothe irritated esophageal tissues and flush acidic stomach contents back where they belong.
- Eat small meals to avoid distention of the stomach.
- Don't eat within 3 hours of bedtime.
- Reduce your weight to relieve pressure on the abdomen.
- Avoid constricting clothes.
- Stop smoking.

You can use gravity to alleviate some of the pain of a heartburn attack:

- Avoid bending over.
- Stand up rather than lie down; don't lie down for 3 hours after eating.
- Use a 6- to 10-inch wedge under your pillow so your esophagus is higher than your stomach while you sleep.

Heartburn can be a symptom of monosodium glutamate (MSG) allergy or sensitivity. Other symptoms include headache, warmth, stiffness, weakness, tingling, pressure, light-headedness and general stomach discomfort. A flavor enhancer used in many Chinese dishes and sold under the trade name Accent (among others), MSG has been the culprit in many vague and annoying food reactions.

Food Poisoning and Vomiting

Sudden abdominal pain, nausea, vomiting, and diarrhea can occur in as few as four hours or as many as 30 hours after consuming tainted food. Headaches, cold sweats, shivering and, occasionally, double vision can accompany the problem.

The most common form of food poisoning is caused by toxins released by bacteria. In badly canned foods, the bacterial invasion called botulism can cause a life-threatening emergency. In fresh foods, *Salmonella* organisms are usually the culprits. Bacteria get into food from infected animals, from animal excretions, or from infected humans preparing the food.

The best first aid for food poisoning is to rid yourself of the offending material by vomiting, then replace lost water and salt.

However unpleasant it may be, vomiting can save your life or at least bring relief in times of extreme digestive distress. If you swallow a poisonous substance, if you've eaten too much for your stomach to handle, or if the food you ate was tainted with harmful bacteria, the upper part of your stomach sends messages to the medulla of your brain. The brain then orders the pyloric valve between the stomach and the small intestine to relax. Churning in this area sends the digesting food back up into the upper stomach, and the muscles of the abdomen force the contents out of the stomach.

The mechanism of vomiting is a clear example of the close connection between the mind and the digestive system. Nerves from various parts of the body can cause vomiting when you get seasick or carsick; or when you see, smell, taste, hear or touch something unpleasant. If you have a chronic digestive disorder that is difficult to manage and you regularly experience nausea and vomiting when facing emotionally charged issues, you may benefit greatly from psychiatric counseling for your disorder.

Lactose Intolerance

If milk gives you discomfort, you may have a deficiency of the digestive enzyme *lactase*, which is responsible for processing *lactose*, the natural sugar in milk. Lactase splits lactose, a "disaccharide," into the two "monosaccharides" glucose and galactose. For those people who don't have enough lactase, the milk sugar remains undigested, or *malabsorbed*, and passes to the large intestine. Once here, it draws excess water and yet more sugar. The beneficial bacteria that live in the colon then rapidly ferment these sugars. Because this process produces gas and acids, lactose intolerance can cause cramps, bloating, flatulence, and diarrhea.

The process of making yogurt and cheese breaks the lactose molecule, so people who are lactose intolerant can usually eat these calcium-rich dairy products without experiencing the same painful symptoms. This biological process probably accounts for the belief that cheese and yogurt are "binding;" when people who are lactose intolerant switch to cheese or yogurt, they notice that their stools become firmer. Unfortunately, some manufacturers of soft cheeses and yogurt now add milk back into their products, bringing the levels of lactose back up. Before buying these foods, check the labels to see if the products contain active cultures, since live bacteria break down the lactose. For more on this common food sensitivity, see Chapter 24.

Gluten Intolerance

Another intolerance—to the gluten in wheat, rye, oats, and barley—can lead to the inflammation of the intestines, called "celiac sprue." Gluten consists of water-insoluble glutenin and soluble gliadins. The gliadins are toxic and in some people can damage the soft, gland-lined tis-

GLUTEN LURKS IN UNLIKELY PLACES

You'd expect to find the wheat protein gluten in baked goods, cereal, and pasta. But in tomato sauce?! Here are a few of the products in which gluten hides.

- Nondairy creamer
- Yogurts with fruit
- Hot chocolate mixes or cocoa
- Chocolate
- Bouillon cubes
- Soup mixes and canned soups
- Cheese spreads
- Chip and dip mixes
- Lunch meats
- Processed meats, such as sausage and canned meat products
- Meat sauces (such as soy, Worcestershire)
- Tomato sauce
- Peanut butter

sue of the intestinal lining (the mucosa), although the reasons for this are unknown. The damage makes it difficult for the mucosa to properly absorb nutrients.

About one of every 2,500 people has celiac disease. It is more common in women than men, and occurs most frequently in people hailing from northwestern Europe. In fact, the highest prevalence of celiac sprue is in Galway, Ireland, where one of every 300 people has the disease. It is rare among people of African, Asian, Jewish, and Mediterranean origin.

Symptoms of gluten malabsorption include diarrhea or constipation, gas, weight loss, and fatigue. Serious cases can lead to iron-deficiency anemia or osteomalacia, a disorder of the bones caused by vitamin D deficiency. A bloated abdomen, a greasy stool, and an increased appetite are also signs of this disorder.

Nutritional therapy calls for the elimination of all gluten-containing foods—a tall order in our society, where so many processed foods contain wheat. Wheat flour can be found in everything from ice cream, salad dressings, canned foods, instant coffee, and tea, to catsup, mustard, and most candy bars. Get into the habit of reading all food labels and checking the ingredients of processed foods. Additionally, beware of food additives, emulsifiers, or stabilizers when cooking or when dining out.

Flours made from rice, soybean, buckwheat, potato, tapioca, and corn are nontoxic and can be used by people who are gluten-intolerant. Cookbooks that can help you prepare gluten-free meals include *Gourmet Food on a Wheat-Free Diet* and *Easy Rice Flour Recipes* by Marion Wood.

Peptic Ulcers

Researchers have recently disproved almost all of our most long-standing beliefs about peptic ulcers—those of the stomach and upper small intestine (the *duodenum*). It was once thought that people under extreme stress produced more stomach acid and were therefore more prone to ulcers. Once the lesions in the stomach or intestinal wall established themselves, physicians recommended eating a bland diet and drinking milk. Now we know that an S-shaped bacterium called *Helicobacter pylori (H. pylori)* causes most of these ulcers. Ulcers have been shown to heal as fast on a liberal diet as on a traditional bland diet. And although drinking milk can lower stomach acid concentrations briefly, acid secretion then comes on stronger than before.

The link between bacteria and ulcers came as quite a shock to the scientific community, which held to the precept that no such organism could live in the highly acidic environment of the stomach. But the crafty *H. pylori* can produce a substance called urease, that breaks down urea and produces ammonia, creating a nonacidic area in which the bacterium can thrive. It is the ammonia that eats away at the mucosal layer of the stomach to produce gastric ulcers and of the upper small intestine to produce duodenal ulcers.

Experts believe that *H. Pylori* causes 80 percent of all gastric ulcers. Other causes include genetic predisposition, smoking, and overuse of pain killers such as aspirin and ibuprofen that can weaken the mucosa and make it more susceptible to stomach acid.

Not everyone who has *H. pylori* in their digestive tract will get ulcers. Worldwide, an estimated three billion people are infected with the bacteria, and of this number, one in four to one in eight will get an ulcerative disease.

For most people, a course of antibiotics will cure the ulcer. But if you're among the unlucky minority for whom this doesn't work, there are some nutritional steps you can take to at least manage the condition. You should also find out if you are allergic or sensitive to any foods. (See Chapter 24 on food allergies.)

Avoid any foods or beverages which increase acid production. Even if stomach acid didn't start the ulcer, it can make it worse

and interfere with healing. Refined sugar can stimulate acid production, as can alcohol, caffeine, and even decaffeinated coffee. Contrary to popular belief, spicy foods and citrus fruits do not seem to be harmful to the majority of ulcer sufferers.

Bismuth (the active ingredient in Pepto-Bismol), a mineral that has been used for over 200 years for the treatment of indigestion and gastric problems, was recently shown to be as effective as the newest class of anti-ulcer medications, with a lower rate of recurrence. However, since regular use may cause damage to the nervous system, doctors recommend that people with ulcers take no more than 120 milligrams of bismuth four times a day before meals and at bedtime, and limit their course of treatment to six to eight weeks.

Animal studies of zinc have shown that this mineral can prevent the release of chemicals that weaken the mucosa, and that zinc can promote ulcer healing.

Licorice root with an acid removed (deglycyrrhizinated licorice) has also shown to be as effective as new anti-ulcer drugs, and it appears to protect against aspirin-induced damage to the stomach lining.

Gallstones

Removal of the gallbladder is the most common abdominal surgery among American adults. On average, 500,000 of the 15 million Americans with gallstones require hospitalization every year.

Gallstones, small rock-like balls of crystallized cholesterol, are formed when the delicate balance of ingredients in bile is disrupted. Bile is made by the liver and stored in the gallbladder. It is made up of bile salts, lecithin, cholesterol, and various byproducts of dead red blood cells. When the concentration of one of these elements changes, gallstones can develop. They become a real problem when they lodge in one of the bile-carrying ducts and cut off the supply of bile to the small intestine. Bile is essential for the digestion of fat.

Diets high in fat and sugar and low in fiber are most likely to promote gallbladder problems. Food sensitivities also play a role. When 69 people with gallbladder problems were placed on a diet that eliminated suspect foods, all saw their symptoms disappear. Ninety-three percent of the people experienced a return of their symptoms after they ate eggs; 64 percent after they ate pork, and 52 percent after they ate onions.

In general, if you suffer from gallstones you should:

- Stick to a low-fat, low-sugar, high-fiber diet
- Lose weight (if you are overweight)
- Always eat breakfast
- Avoid any foods that you notice cause your symptoms to flare up

Diverticulosis

The large intestine is a smooth-walled muscular tube that contracts three to four times a day, usually during or just after eating. This contraction moves the intestinal contents towards the rectum for eventual disposal. Fiber in the diet strengthens the contractions and keeps muscular walls in tone.

When the diet lacks sufficient fiber, the walls of the lower intestine thicken, the passage narrows, and the relative pressure on the walls becomes greater. If pressure is high and certain sections of the walls are weaker

than others, they may begin to bulge. The outpouchings that occur in this way are called diverticula, and the condition which arises is called diverticulosis. When the diverticula become inflamed, as they do in roughly five percent of patients, a life-threatening condition known as diverticulitis can occur.

The cause of diverticula is unknown, but much evidence points to diet. Diverticula were medical curiosities until the early 1900s, when the milling of wheat—which removes much of the fiber from flour—became widespread and the fiber content of most breads plunged 80 percent. Refined sugars also became commonplace during this period, as exports made their way throughout the world. Since then, the incidence of diverticulitis has risen dramatically. To illustrate, consider what happened in England during World War II: As imports declined, the people had to eat only what they could produce locally—more grain and less refined sugar. The forced change in diet then put a halt to the rising rate of diverticulitis-induced death.

Diverticula occur most often in older people; they are uncommon in people less than 40 years old. One in every four people over 60 has the outpouchings; once past 80, one in every two people has them. Scientists presume either that it takes many years for the diverticula to develop or that the colons of older people are less likely to withstand the intestinal pressure without herniating, or both.

Diverticulosis does not lead to colon cancer, but recent studies show that the chances of both rise together—probably because both are promoted by a low-fiber diet.

Symptoms of diverticulitis include alternating constipation and diarrhea, pain and

MEDICATIONS THAT CAUSE DIARRHEA AND CONSTIPATION

Certain medications can disrupt the efficient balance of the digestive system, causing diarrhea and constipation, or holding food in your stomach longer than usual. Antibiotics can kill beneficial bacteria in your large intestine, allowing the unrestrained growth of a bacterium called *Clostridium difficile*. This bacterium inflames the intestinal wall making it "weep" excess water and mucous, resulting in watery stools. Antibiotics known to cause this problem include ampicillin, clindamycin, and the cephalosporins.

Overuse of magnesium antacids and laxatives can also cause chronic diarrhea. In fact, surreptitious laxative abuse has been found to be one of the major causes of diarrhea, especially in women who presumably are taking them to control their weight. (All for naught, apparently. A study of Correctol tablet use, found that the laxative decreased calorie absorption by only five percent.)

Oddly enough, overuse of laxatives can have the opposite effect. By damaging the nerves of the colon, they can cause chronic constipation. In addition to laxatives, other common drugs known to cause constipation are:

Antacids (containing calcium or aluminum)
Antidepressants
Barium
Bismuth (Pepto-Bismol)
Blood pressure drugs
Drugs for Parkinson's disease
Major tranquilizers
Medications for the blood (especially iron)
Pain killers (narcotic drugs)
Pain relievers (over-the-counter analgesics)
Seizure medications
Water pills (diuretics)

Adding beneficial bacteria back into your system can be helpful, and can be achieved by supplementing your diet with Lactobacillis Acidophilus, sold over the counter at most drug stores.

Antidepressants and drugs used to treat Parkinson's disease can also slow down stomach activity, causing a feeling of fullness, bloating, heartburn, or indigestion, pain in the mid-abdomen, nausea, and vomiting of food eaten hours before. To help prevent these side effects, don't recline for at least an hour after eating, eat small meals frequently, and consider asking your doctor to change the dosage of your prescription.

---

tenderness in the colon, and gassiness. If you have this disease, you should eat a high-fiber diet to thwart its progression, but antibiotics or even surgery may become necessary. A high-fiber diet may also prevent the disease from occurring.

Gas

Gas may be a social embarrassment, but it is both a necessary part of the digestive process and an important warning sign of various disorders. About two pints of gas are normally produced in the human gastrointestinal tract daily, more when carbohydrate-rich foods (like beans)

are eaten. If you are plagued by excessive gas without eating such foods you may have a malabsorption disorder in which the starches and sugars you eat are not sufficiently digested in the small intestine and reach the colon in large amounts.

By the time food enters the large intestine, most of it has been digested. Bacteria inhabiting this segment of the digestive tract then break down what remains—usually indigestible cellulose and other carbohydrates. As the bacteria go about producing food for themselves, they are also releasing nutrients such as vitamins B and K for their human host. When they act upon carbohydrates, however, the fermentation that takes place produces gases such as hydrogen, carbon dioxide, and methane. It makes sense, then, that a diet high in sugar, starch, and fiber can cause excess gas and even abdominal discomfort.

If you have excess gas due to malabsorption or some other disorder, it is usually because food is being rushed from the small to the large intestine, where undigested carbohydrates are being broken down too quickly for the colon to absorb. Pain and bloating with accompanying gas are the result. To remedy the problem, try these measures:

- **Sugar:** Avoid non-absorbable sugars such as those found in beans and peas. Also, avoid lactose (milk sugar), if you think you might be lastase-deficient.
- **Fructans:** Avoid carbohydrates found in artichokes, onions, leeks, and chicory, because the small intestine cannot digest them.
- **Starch:** Try to eat starches that are cooked and still hot, and stick to white bread. Rice starch is almost completely digestible. Avoid unmilled grains and seeds, unripe bananas, incompletely cooked potatoes, and cooked and cooled starches other than cereal starches.
- **Fiber:** Keep your intake of fiber at the average or even below-average level. Since fiber is so beneficial to other digestive processes, however, you may want to try doing without this step.

Diarrhea and Constipation

When food residue is rushed through the intestines, as when the lining is irritated or inflamed by infection, the colon does not have sufficient time to absorb excess water. As a result, runny stools may occur several times a day. Diarrhea can also develop when too much fluid is drawn into the intestines, due to illness outside the digestive system. Conversely, when food residue stays in the large intestine for extended periods of time, too much water is absorbed back into the body, and hard stools result every few days.

The only nutritional therapy for diarrhea is simply to replace water and electrolytes, a process called rehydration therapy. The World Health Organization developed a liquid preparation to treat cholera and tropical diseases, but the principles apply to anyone suffering from acute diarrhea. Here is a home brew you can try: Dissolve 1/4 teaspoon salt and four heaping tablespoons of sugar in 150 milliliters (2/3 cup) of boiling water. Add 150 milliliters of fresh orange juice and 200 milliliters (7/8 cup) of tap water. This brew will provide needed amounts of sodium, potassium, and sucrose. Avoid anti-diarrheals, such as Lomotil, Donnagel—PG, and Imodium.

There seems to be a clear association between diet and constipation. Dietary fiber, while it is no panacea for all cases of constipation, can increase stool weight, frequency, and water content. Different fibers have different effects; the soluble fibers containing pectin and mucilage (found in citrus fruits and bananas) have the least effect on the bowels, and fibers in foods such as bran have the most. Corn bran relieves constipation more effectively than wheat bran. Foods containing cellulose (bran, whole grain flour, some fruits and vegetables) survive the digestive process better than the noncellulose fiber in oatmeal, breakfast cereal, and sesame seeds.

If you eat a diet low in fiber, it might be advisable to add bulk slowly. The best way is to switch from white bread to whole wheat bread. You could also add half a cup of bran to your food daily, and increase your intake half a cup at a time over a few weeks until you reach two cups daily.

Irritable Bowel Syndrome

This disorder, also known as spastic colon or irritable colon, has no known cause. People whose family members have the problem are more likely to develop it. Symptoms include constipation (usually with abdominal pain) or diarrhea (usually without pain), bloating, gas, passage of non-bloody mucous, and a sensation of incomplete rectal emptying. Constipation and diarrhea can be intermittent, and the stools may be pellet-like during the constipation phase. The symptoms are similar to those of inflammatory bowel disease but no inflammation is present.

Irritable Bowel Syndrome frequently accompanies psychological disorders, leading some researchers to suspect an emotional origin. Men and women with the disorder often score high in the areas of anxiousness and depression on psychological personality tests, and tend to be more neurotic than people without the disorder. In fact, one of the most common prescriptions for the problem is for antidepressants.

Since symptoms of the disorder arise from spasms of the bowel muscles, some experts

BEST (AND WORST) CHOICES FOR INFLAMMATORY BOWEL DISEASE

Many doctors feel that diet doesn't make any difference in this puzzling, frustrating disease. However, when doctors do prescribe a special diet, it usually involves plenty of these low-residue, easily absorbed foods:

- Meat
- Fish
- Rice
- White bread
- Pasta
- Dextrose
- Gelatin
- Hard-boiled eggs

Avoid these high residue foods:

- Apples
- Oranges
- Celery
- Cabbage
- Tomatoes
- Berries
- Raw egg albumin

thought that a high-fiber diet—which increases the fecal bulk in the colon and, therefore, acts as a type of cushion—might alleviate some of the symptoms. However, in a recent study, people who supplemented their diets with fiber and those who didn't experienced the same results. Another study did find that a high-fiber diet gave relief to patients with hard stools or constipation, but not to those with diarrhea, bloating, and gas.

If you suspect that certain foods aggravate your symptoms ask your doctor about an elimination diet. Otherwise, except for adding dietary fiber to relieve constipation, there is no dietary advice for treatment of IBS.

Inflammatory Bowel Disease

There are two million Americans with either ulcerative colitis or Crohn's disease, the two major forms of Inflammatory Bowel Disease. The cause of the disorder is unknown (although there does appear to be some hereditary basis) and no specific preventive or curative measures stand out above the rest, making Inflammatory Bowel Disease one of the most difficult diseases to treat. Symptoms of both ulcerative colitis and Crohn's disease include abdominal pain and diarrhea. People suffering from these conditions—often adolescents and young adults—are sometimes malnourished since they may not have much of an appetite and may be unable to absorb sufficient nutrients from the intestines. In fact, some patients need injections of nutritional supplements in addition to the foods they eat.

Ulcerative colitis results from the development of ulcers on the lining of the large intestine. As with gastric ulcers, a bacterium might be responsible, although this is currently just a theory. Dr. Barry Marshall, the Australian doctor who upset the medical community by showing the link between *H. pylori* and gastric ulcers (he actually swallowed some of the bacteria to prove his point), suspects that ulcerative colitis is related to some infectious process because it affects only the colon and has the same characteristics as a bacterial infection.

Physicians sometimes prescribe a diet low in residue along with multivitamin supplements for ulcerative colitis. Foods to favor, and those to avoid, are listed in the box nearby.

A small study of people with mild to moderate ulcerative colitis showed recently that treatment with omega-3 fatty acids could improve symptoms. Omega-3s have known anti-inflammatory effects. Seven of 10 patients reported either moderate or marked improvement in their symptoms; this finding was borne out by a slightly larger study of both ulcerative colitis and Crohn's disease patients. The omega-3s worked only for the ulcerative colitis group, however.

Unlike ulcerative colitis, Crohn's disease can be found anywhere along the digestive tract, although it occurs most often in the lower small intestine. In the diseased areas, ulcers dot the thickened intestinal wall, often deepening to the point of perforation. Between these areas, the lining is relatively healthy. Young people are more likely to have Crohn's disease than older adults; its peak occurrence is in the 30s and 40s. It is most prevalent among white people and those of Jewish origin.

The common complaints of this disorder—abdominal pain and diarrhea—occur in 80 to 90 percent of cases. When the disease occurs in the small intestine, rather than elsewhere in the digestive tract, it may also cause weight loss, anorexia, fever, nausea and vomiting, fatigue, and intestinal obstruction.

There is no medical agreement on a specific diet for the treatment of Crohn's disease, but several small studies have uncovered certain measures that may be helpful to some individuals. For example, it is known that people with the disorder tend to eat more sugar than those who are disease-free, suggesting that a diet low in refined carbohydrates may be useful as a preventative measure. Refined carbohydrates include refined sugars such as cane, beet, and corn sugar, white (bleached, enriched) wheat flour; and white (polished)

rice. Some studies even indicate that a diet rich in fiber and unrefined carbohydrates can relieve the symptoms of Crohn's disease and reduce the number and duration of hospital stays. Researchers also suggest eating foods low in residue and high in protein, especially lean meat and liver (see the box on "Best (and Worst) Choices for Inflammatory Bowel Disease").

If all else fails—for Crohn's disease or any other digestive ailment, remember that emotions can also play havoc with the digestive system. Previously untreatable or unexplainable ailments of the digestive tract have sometimes spontaneously disappeared after seemingly unrelated personal issues were resolved. Don't hesitate to seek professional assistance. Psychotherapy, biofeedback, behavior modification, and hypnosis may all be helpful in relieving gastrointestinal disorders. ☐

CHAPTER 26

Arthritis Diet Remedies: Fact or Folklore?

Arthritis sufferers have been trying for centuries to rid themselves of their debilitating pain. They have covered themselves in cow manure twice a day, stood naked under a full moon, kept two sesame seeds in their navel overnight while sleeping, worn radioactive devices, endured scores of bee stings, tolerated venoms of snakes, and recently have even rubbed on the mechanical lubricant WD-40. If these measures helped, it was probably because the sufferers wanted them to so desperately. Some scientists today credit such a "placebo effect" with the pain relief gained from special arthritis diets. Others believe dietary manipulation can truly ease pain; but even they say we need more long-term scientific studies.

One in every seven Americans has some type of arthritis. That's about 75 million people who have symptoms of the disease from time to time, 22 million who have moderate problems with arthritis, and three million who are severely afflicted. The Arthritis Foundation has warned that, as the

average age of the U.S. population rises, arthritis could become the epidemic of the future. The Centers for Disease Control and Prevention (CDC) project that by the year 2020, the number of people with arthritis will increase 57 percent, and the number of people with arthritis-related activity limitation will increase 66 percent.

Even though "arth" means joint and "itis" means inflammation, some types of arthritis don't involve inflammation or the joints. One type, ankylosing spondylitis, involves inflamed ligaments attached to the bone. Lupus, another type of arthritis, is a connective tissue disease. Osteoarthritis, the most common type, is the result of a breakdown of cartilage in the joint; rheumatoid arthritis (RA) involves an inflamed joint membrane; and gout involves deposits of uric acid crystals in the joint fluid.

Inflammation—heat, swelling, pain, redness and/or loss of motion—is the common

HOW ARTHRITIS DISABLES THE JOINTS

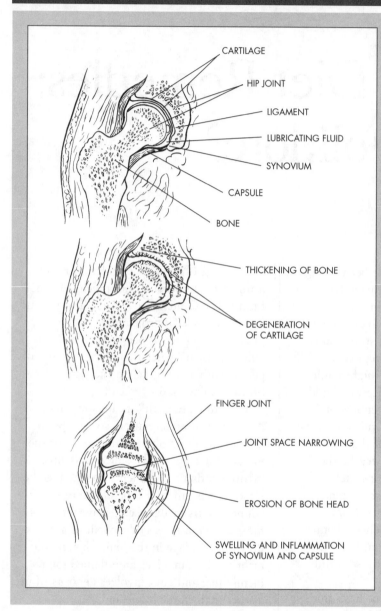

CARTILAGE

HIP JOINT

LIGAMENT

LUBRICATING FLUID

SYNOVIUM

CAPSULE

BONE

THICKENING OF BONE

DEGENERATION
OF CARTILAGE

FINGER JOINT

JOINT SPACE NARROWING

EROSION OF BONE HEAD

SWELLING AND INFLAMMATION
OF SYNOVIUM AND CAPSULE

Normal joint: Where two bones meet, our bodies normally provide a simple and effective lubricating system. Ligaments binding the bones together form a capsule within which a thin membrane called the synovium exudes a fluid lubricant. For good measure, the ends of both bones are cushioned by a smooth layer of cartilage.

Osteoarthritis: In this form of arthritis, trouble begins when the protective cushion of cartilage between the bones slowly degenerates. As it disappears, the synovium and the ends of the bones thicken within the joint, leading to the aching stiffness that characterizes the disease.

Rheumatoid arthritis: The culprit here is the synovium, which for unknown reasons becomes swollen and inflamed, leading to irreversible damage to the joint's capsule and protective cartilage. Eventually the unprotected ends of the bones themselves begin to erode.

link between most of the more than 100 types of arthritis. Scientists are just beginning to understand the inflammatory process. They know that it begins with a trigger such as an infection or tissue damage. In response to this trigger, white blood cells rush to the affected area and release chemicals to begin the repair process. Among them are **prostaglandins**—which can both reduce and promote swelling, and **leukotrienes**—which quickly intensify inflammation. The white blood cells also release digestive enzymes to remove bacteria and other foreign agents in the area. The white cells recognize these invaders as **antigens** and focus their attack on them. However, the enzymes the white cells release can also digest cartilage, bone, ligaments, muscle, and other tissues. In inflammatory rheumatic diseases like arthritis, this attack on the tissues becomes chronic.

Gut Reactions: Diet and the Inflammatory Process

So how could diet become involved in this process? Some scientists speculate that the trouble may start in the intestines, where foreign antigens can slip through the layer of mucus coating the intestinal wall, enter the bloodstream, and travel to a joint. The presence of antigens there attracts the white blood cells that launch the inflammatory process.

If these invading antigens are byproducts of a particular food to which you are allergic or sensitive, eliminating it from your diet could reduce swelling in the joint and cut down on arthritis pain. However, very few people have a true food allergy. Another explanation offered is the presence of lectins, food molecules that can act like antigens. Two researchers writing in the British Journal of Rheumatology point out that many foods commonly mentioned in discussions of food allergy, such as peanuts, beans,

peas, lentils, edible snails and wheat, are particularly rich in lectins.

These researchers also suggest that arthritis patients may experience a greater transfer of antigens through the intestinal wall because of damage to the intestinal lining from the prescription medications such as nonsteroidal anti-inflammatory drugs that many arthritis sufferers take. They say that dietary manipulation, including fasting for short periods of time, could reduce the number of antigens available to breach the intestinal lining.

The two researchers doubt that the placebo effect is the only explanation why many arthritis sufferers are helped by changing their diet. They believe that hope provided by a new therapy can buoy patients enough for them to believe their pain has been mitigated, but that it is "insufficient to explain significant improvement" seen in the available studies. Furthermore, if a placebo effect were responsible for the improvements, one would expect them to be temporary. But this, they say, is not always the case.

Other specialists take an entirely different point of view about dietary therapy for arthritis. Cody K. Wasner, MD, a practicing rheumatologist and chairman of the Arthritis Foundation's Committee on Unproven Remedies believes that while a small number of people may be helped by avoiding certain foods, altering the diet by reducing food intake—that is, fasting in some form or another—usually doesn't help the disease. He thinks that one reason arthritis may improve when food is restricted is a temporary malfunction of the immune system that for a time disables its inflammatory attack on the body's own tissues.

Confusing Advice
and What to Do About It

Specialists aren't the only ones who can't agree. A 1990 study of 21 popular books about dietary treatment of arthritis revealed tremendous confusion. Seventeen books advocated some form of dietary change, three were against it, and one was noncommittal. The advice given varied widely from book to book and was sometimes totally contradictory.

Wasner says one reason arthritis sufferers are inundated with advice on self-treatment is that people don't take the disease seriously enough. "If you had breast cancer, people aren't going to say, 'oh, you don't need therapy or radiation, what you need to do is eat more bran.'"

Perhaps the lack of awe over this chronic illness is because it isn't life threatening. It could also be due to arthritis' position as a "non-flashy" disease. Wasner points out that it has only recently begun to receive attention from the medical community, whereas "we have 2,000 years of culture that says we don't even treat it, that it's just like getting gray hair, that you just have to live with it."

Even if the few scientific studies conducted so far on the link between diet and arthritis were all clear cut, it would still take many more to wring acceptance from the medical community. Long-term side effects must be established first, says Jeffrey C. Delafuente, MS, a professor at the University of Florida College of Pharmacy. The traditional drug therapy available to treat arthritis has been studied for as long as 50 years, so doctors are bound to recommend it over any dietary therapy about which little is known.

Still, many arthritis sufferers have challenged a conservative medical community. In a nationwide survey of 1,051 people with osteoarthritis or RA, nearly half of the re-

GOUT AND FOOD: A PROVEN LINK

Gout is the only form of arthritis that is unquestionably linked to diet, although the number of people whose gout can be blamed entirely on what they eat is small. For a victim of gout, foods high in substances called purines, such as liver, kidney, fish roe, mussels, anchovies, peas, beans, pancreas and brain, add to the existing problem of elevated levels of uric acid in the blood. Drinking too much alcohol and crash dieting can also raise the level of this acid. The uric acid that the body either overproduces or can't get rid of forms into tiny crystals like shards of glass which float in the joint space. When the immune system attacks these crystals, inflammation occurs.

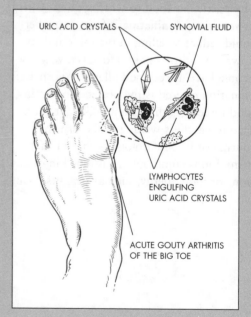

URIC ACID CRYSTALS — SYNOVIAL FLUID

LYMPHOCYTES
ENGULFING
URIC ACID CRYSTALS

ACUTE GOUTY ARTHRITIS
OF THE BIG TOE

spondents admitted to changing their diet to see if it would help their condition, even if their doctors were against the idea. Some respondents simply started eating healthier foods, avoiding fats, and increasing their intake of vegetables. Others tried systematically eliminating foods from their diet and discovered some that they thought they could associate with flare-ups of their arthritis. Still others added vitamins, minerals, and other supplements like fish oil to their diets.

Every person is unique; what works for you might not work for someone else. What follows is a brief overview of the dietary manipulations that others have tried. If you do decide to experiment with one of these changes, remember that it's still important to consult your physician, no matter how conservative he may be. Depending on your medical condition, a particular diet could be dangerous for you, or could interact badly with your medication. You're always free to make the final decision; but do it with your doctor's help.

Elimination Diets

The link between arthritis and diet first came under serious investigation in the late 1970s. The studies were small, usually involving less than 25 patients. The initial studies found improvement among subjects who first fasted and then reintroduced foods in such a way as to determine which ones had a negative effect on the disease. The offending foods usually turned out to be dairy products, meat, corn, or wheat.

Then in 1983, a completely contradictory study of 18 patients was published. It found

THE DONG DIET'S DO'S AND DON'TS

In "The Arthritic's Cookbook," Dr. Collin H. Dong blames arthritis on the typical American diet. Crippled with what seemed to be hopeless arthritis at age 35, the Americanized doctor switched to a diet from his Chinese heritage. He claims that he was "utterly amazed" at the results. Here are some of his basic guidelines:

Foods you can eat: all seafood except sardines; all vegetables except tomatoes; vegetable oil; soybean margarine; egg whites; oatmeal; cream of wheat; grits; any kind of flour; sugar, honey, maple syrup, or corn syrup; all kinds of rice; bread without preservatives; tea and coffee; and plain soda water.

Foods you can't eat: meat and meat broth; fruit; dairy products; egg yolks; vinegar; pepper; chocolate; dry roasted nuts; alcoholic beverages; soft drinks; and all additives, preservatives, and chemicals.

Foods you can eat sometimes: chicken breast and chicken broth; a small amount of wine in cooking; a pinch of spicy seasoning; and noodles and pasta.

no relation between food and arthritis symptoms. However, the study design didn't allow for systematic withdrawal of offending foods, and 13 of the 18 subjects defaulted early.

That same year, another study was published. This one had been started in the mid-70s following publication of two "arthritis cookbooks" that received wide media attention. Both books advocated diets that ruled out dairy products, fruits, meats, alcoholic beverages, and all preservatives. One of these diets was called the "Dong diet" after Collin H. Dong, MD, from China. (For details, see the nearby box.) As a placebo, the

PINPOINTING OFFENDING FOODS

If you suspect that something in your diet may be aggravating your arthritis, you need to be systematic in your pursuit of real proof. Here are a few tips:

■ Keep a diary of everything you eat, and a diary of pain and other arthritis symptoms. When you compare the two, you may see some correlation. For example, the milkshake you drank Friday night may have caused the pain and swelling in your wrists on Saturday. However, the problem and frustration come when you try to determine the specific source of the problem: Was it the fat-laden ice cream (dairy) in the milkshake or the sugar?

■ Once you suspect a certain food is the culprit, stop eating it for at least five days so you can be sure it is completely out of your system. Then add that food back into your diet and see what happens. If you follow this process twice and each time you get worse when the food is reinstated, you may be on to something. However, most researchers studying the correlation between food and arthritis say six weeks is the minimum time needed to reliably and accurately test any correlation.

■ Carefully consider the food group you are considering banishing from your diet. Dairy products may aggravate your arthritis symptoms, for example, but they also provide essential nutrients. Make sure you can get those nutrients from other foods. Work with your doctor and even a dietician if possible.

researchers tested this diet against an arbitrary diet of their own creation. Almost half of the patients on the experimental diet got better, but so did almost half of the patients on the placebo diet. The researchers couldn't explain it. Still, two of the patients taking part in that study decided to stay on the experimental diet for good; they both were convinced that certain foods initiated a flare of their arthritis symptoms.

More studies followed. The number of participants and the duration of the specific diet increased. Almost all the studies showed some correlation between diet and arthritis symptoms, and most participants noticed that they could reduce their use of medication. As the data began to arrive, the scientists conducting these studies identified certain aspects of what they saw as a link between food and arthritis. They researched food allergy and determined that very few patients actually suffered from this condition. They decided that weight loss itself—brought on by a restricted diet—didn't account for all the benefits. Then they started carefully identifying the types of foods that were most likely to be associated with a flare-up in arthritis symptoms.

Usually, the patients in the studies would fast for seven to 10 days. While fasting, they were given either water only or they were placed on some other type of fasting diet, such as a combination of fish, pears, carrots, and water. (Another fasting diet that was used was a combination of herbal teas, garlic, vegetable broth, decoction [flavor extraction by boiling down] of potatoes and parsley, and juice extracts from carrots, beets, and celery.) The researchers called this the elimination phase. If participants' symptoms disappeared, then foods would be added to the diet one at a time to discover the offending food. This was called the re-introduction phase. The patients were compared with others who were on a normal diet as controls. Most of those who fasted improved significantly during the fasting period, only to relapse when food was reintroduced. However, if each person adjusted his or her diet individually, the improvement could sometimes be sustained.

By 1987, 48 RA patients had completed a study to determine particularly troublesome foods. After six weeks of dietary elimination, 41 were able to identify foods that had caused a flare in their symptoms. Cereal foods like corn and wheat were considered a problem by more than half of the study participants. Here is a list of foods the patients found troublesome (some of which contradict Dong's recommendations), and the percentage of symptomatic patients affected by the food:

Corn	57%
Wheat	54%
Bacon/pork	39%
Oranges	39%
Milk	37%
Oats	37%
Rye	34%
Eggs	32%
Beef	32%
Coffee	32%
Malt	27%
Cheese	24%
Grapefruit	24%
Tomato	22%
Peanuts	20%
Sugar (cane)	20%
Butter	17%
Lamb	17%
Lemons	17%
Soya	17%

Participants in the national survey on arthritis also reported cutting out some foods. Of the 1,051 people who were sent detailed questionnaires in the mail, 10 percent reported being sensitive or intolerant to certain foods. Red meat turned out to be the culprit most often associated with a flare-up of arthritis pain for this group. In addition, survey respondents mentioned as triggers sugar (and sweets in general), fat and fried foods, salt, caffeine, dairy products, nightshade vegetables (tomatoes, white potatoes, eggplant, and bell peppers), pork and smoked or processed meats, alcohol, junk food, starches, additives and preservatives, acidic foods, and chocolate.

Supplementation Diets

People with arthritis often have vitamin and mineral deficiencies, but these deficiencies are thought to be a result of the disease rather than its cause. Such problems are associated with other immune system diseases as well. Studies involving vitamin and mineral supplements have shown conflicting results with few hard conclusions. If you eat poorly overall, then take vitamin supplements and see an improvement in your condition, does it mean that the lack a specific vitamin caused your arthritis? More than likely, the supplement merely boosted a taxed immune system, making you feel better overall. Still, there is some evidence that certain supplements may work directly on the inflammation that causes painful joints.

TIP-OFFS OF A BOGUS REMEDY

Bookstores abound with information on new treatments for arthritis, including new diets. Television, radio, and magazine advertisements may try to convince you that changing the way you eat will cure your disease. The Arthritis Foundation compiled this list of 10 practices typical of promotions for unproven remedies. The Foundation warns that even a doctor's testimonial doesn't always make a claim legitimate. You should be alert for these signs:

1. A cure is offered. (There is no known cure yet for any form of chronic rheumatic disease. All current treatments merely reduce the symptoms and slow the progress. When genuine cures are found, there won't be any question about it; the whole world will know.)

2. The cure or remedy is described as a "secret" formula or device—as "exclusive," or "special." (Legitimate scientists don't keep their discoveries secret or exclusive.)

3. Testimonials and case histories of people who have supposedly been helped by the remedy are offered as "proof" of its effectiveness. (A few successes—if true—still don't prove the remedy will work for everyone.)

4. The remedy or treatment is described in sensational articles in tabloids and special health-interest publications, or advertised in magazines and through mail order promotions. (The tabloids are fun; but you should never take them seriously.)

5. Quick, simple relief of pain is promised or implied. (There is nothing simple about arthritis.)

6. The treatment is promoted as "cleansing" the body of poisons or "toxins" to allow the body's "natural" curative powers to clear up the disease. (They won't.)

7. Drugs and surgery are condemned as damaging, dangerous, and unnecessary and you are advised to try a nondrug treatment. (Standard treatments can be dangerous for some people, but that doesn't mean a nondrug treatment will work.)

8. No reliable evidence or scientific proof is offered to back up claims that the advertised remedy is safe and effective. (The promoter has not had the method properly tested in clinical trials.)

9. A special diet or nutrition treatment program is promoted as the answer. (Research scientists have not found any foods or nutrients that, by themselves, cause any rheumatic disease, or can be relied on to make any of these diseases better or worse [except modestly in gout].)

10. The "medical establishment" is accused of conspiracy to thwart progress by refusing to "recognize" or "approve" the remedy being promoted. (Doctors are conservative; but they have no reason to deliberately block progress.)

Fish Oil

The latest supplement to bring hope to arthritis patients is fish oil. This oil contains what scientists refer to as omega-3 fatty acids, a type of polyunsaturated fat. Research is showing that, unlike saturated animal fat, omega-3 fatty acids may reduce cholesterol buildup, lower blood pressure, prevent blood clots, and even cut the risk of some types of cancer. Recent studies have shown that fish oil may also aid in the treatment of arthritis. Two of the acids contained in the oil—eicosapentaenoic acid (EPA) and docosahexaenoic acid (DHA)—reduce production of the prostaglandins and leukotrienes that promote inflammation.

The beneficial effect of fish oils on arthritis was seen as early as 1959, when arthritic patients taking cod liver oil showed clinical improvement in their symptoms. After several other small studies, a formal trial was launched in which some patients received fish oil capsules and others received olive oil capsules. Olive oil currently has no known role in arthritis treatment; it was used as a placebo against which to measure the effect of the fish oil. The researchers carrying out the study noted that after 14 weeks of treatment the patients taking fish oil reported significantly fewer tender joints and a delay in the onset of fatigue. A similar trial, also using olive oil as a placebo, found that patients taking fish oil supplements had fewer painful joints and increased grip strength after 12 weeks. Morning stiffness and overall pain relief improved in both groups of patients, but curiously, more so in the group receiving olive oil.

So far, only high doses of fish oil in capsule form have been studied, and only for short periods of time. Scientists are concerned about long-term toxicity. They'd also like to know whether fish oil in smaller doses will impart similar benefits. High dose fish oil concentrates are available only by prescription and can be fairly expensive. Low dose capsules are available over-the-counter in health food stores, supermarkets, and pharmacies. They have been known to cause side effects such as upset stomach, gas, and a fishy aftertaste in the mouth. Fish oils also thin the blood, which is why they are being studied in heart disease patients.

A better way to increase the amount of omega-3's in your diet may be to eat more cold-water ocean fish. Here is a list of fish (6 ounce servings) with high omega-3 content (in grams):

Mackerel, Atlantic	4.4
Mackerel, king	3.7
Herring, Pacific	3.1
Herring, Atlantic	2.9
Tuna, bluefin	2.7
Sablefish	2.6
Salmon, chinook	2.6
Sturgeon, Atlantic	2.6
Tuna, albacore	2.6
Whitefish, lake	2.6
Anchovies, European	2.4
Salmon, Atlantic	2.4
Salmon, sockeye	2.2
Bluefish	2.0
Mullet	1.9
Salmon, coho	1.7
Salmon, pink	1.7

Other oils produce similar effects for arthritis sufferers, and for similar reasons. Evening primrose oil, for example, which is high in gammalinolenic acid (GLA), has been shown to inhibit the formation of leukotrienes. Blackcurrant seed oil, rich in linolenic acid, can reduce the level of prostaglandins in the body. Both these oils, however, need more study before we can be certain of their value in arthritis treatment.

Vitamins and Minerals

Deficiencies of a single substance, as opposed to an overall nutritional deficiency, are uncommon. Some studies have shown improvement in arthritis patients given supplements of individual vitamins or minerals, while other studies have disputed those findings. Research with animals has shown that vita-

ALCOHOL AND (ARTHRITIS) DRUGS DON'T MIX

Not only do alcoholic beverages add troublesome extra pounds because of their high calorie content, they can also affect how well some arthritis drugs work. If you drink while you are taking nonsteroidal anti-inflammatory drugs, aspirin, or gout medication, you're more likely to experience stomach problems. Acetaminophen combined with large amounts of alcohol can cause liver damage. Alcohol can also increase the level of uric acid in the blood, making gout medication less effective.

Here are a few of the drugs that don't mix with alcohol:

Generic Name	Brand Names
acetaminophen	Datril, Panadol, Tylenol
allopurinol	Lopurin, Zyloprim
colchicine	Colchicine
diflunisal	Dolobid
fenoprofen	Nalfon
ibuprofen	Advil, Motrin, Nuprin, Rufen
indomethacin	Indocin
ketoprofen	Orudis
meclofenamate	Meclomen
naproxen	Naprosyn
piroxicam	Feldene
Probenecid	Benemid
salicylate (aspirin)	Anacin, Bayer, Bufferin, Ecotrin, Empirin, Zorprin
sulfinpyrazone	Anturane
sulindac	Clinoril
tolmetin	Tolectin

mins A, B, C, D, and E are all related to immune system functions, either by supporting immune response or otherwise regulating the system. Iron deficiency can seriously impair the immune system, reducing its ability to digest bacteria and produce enough of the "T cells" that direct immune response and attack infection. Zinc, copper, magnesium, and selenium also play a role in immune response.

Since rheumatic diseases are often characterized by abnormal immunologic activity as the body "turns on itself," attacking healthy cells, it's natural to assume that strengthening the body with added nutrients could

blunt these responses. Unfortunately, supplementation doesn't work on the principle that "if a little is good, more is better." In fact, you can *damage* your immune system if you take some supplements at too high a dose. So if you choose to add selected supplements to your diet, always consult your doctor first. Here are a few of the vitamins and minerals that have been studied in arthritis sufferers:

Vitamin B. Studies have shown that some people with arthritis are deficient in the B vitamins, including B_6, thiamin (B_1), riboflavin (B_2), niacin (B_3), pyridoxine (B_6), cobalamin (B_{12}), folic acid, pantothenic acid, and biotin. In 1983, a group of researchers studied the diets of 24 patients with rheumatoid arthritis and 12 with osteoarthritis and found that most were consuming far less B vitamins than they should. In 1987, the diets of 52 people with rheumatoid arthritis (RA) were also found to be vitamin B-deficient. Some foods rich in B vitamins, like liver and kidney, are off limits to arthritis sufferers because of the high levels of purines they contain. Other foods containing vitamin B, such as whole-grain cereals, fish, and green leafy vegetables, are recommended for arthritis sufferers. One reason why arthritis patients may be deficient in B vitamins is that the drugs they use, including aspirin, can actually deplete the body of B vitamins.

Vitamin C. The body's stores of vitamin C are often depleted by inflammation. Taking 500 milligrams a day of this water-soluble vitamin has been known to improve the spontaneous bruises which often accompany RA, and it may also improve the effectiveness of aspirin in the body. At the two extremes, the Food and Drug Administration sets the recommended daily allowance (RDA) for adults at 50 milligrams, while the well-known scientist Dr. Linus Pauling recommended 18 grams a day as a preventive measure. You can get vitamin C naturally by increasing your dietary intake of citrus fruits, melons, green leafy vegetables, tomatoes, and green peppers.

Vitamin D. Osteoarthritis can cause thinning of the bones, so patients with this disease may need additional vitamin D and calcium. In addition, steroid medications, like prednisone, which are often given to arthritis sufferers because they are powerful anti-inflammatories, can cause bone deterioration. In 1974, some British scientists published information about 17 elderly women with RA. Five of the women had suffered fractures in their leg bones, while the other 12 had not. Upon interviewing the study subjects, the researchers found that the women with the fractured bones all had diets deficient in vitamin D. These five women were also housebound and therefore unable to spend time in the sunshine, which produces vitamin D.

Vitamin E. Several small studies have been conducted with arthritis patients who took vitamin E supplements. They experienced improvement in their symptoms, but the researchers conducting the study weren't sure why. It is known that vitamin E also works in tandem with vitamin C to fight the chemicals that destroy joint cartilage, so it may be helpful in slowing osteoarthritis. Corn oil, sunflower seeds, wheat germ, nuts, whole grains, and legumes are sources of vitamin E.

Calcium. If you're worried about your bone density, you should increase your intake of calcium along with vitamin D. In addition to natural aging, drugs often given to arthritis patients can reduce calcium levels. Supplements can help fight osteoarthritis, but they shouldn't take the place of foods high in calcium. Make sure you add some of these calcium-rich foods to your diet: low-fat milk, yogurt; calcium-fortified juice; sardines, salmon and mackerel (canned with bones); tofu (with calcium sulfate); cheese (cheddar, Muenster, American, part-skim mozzarella).

Copper. The ancient Greeks believed copper had mysterious powers to heal aches and pains. Some arthritis sufferers wear copper bracelets as a folk remedy; and small traces are actually absorbed into the body. But those with RA usually have higher than average levels of copper in their blood, not lower. This is important because high levels of copper can make you feel sick. Most experts believe that copper has no place in causing or treating the disease.

Selenium. Patients with RA seem to have lower levels of the trace mineral selenium than people without it. Selenium deficiency does cause a type of arthritis known as Kashin-Bek disease, which is more common in areas where the soil is particularly low in the mineral. Generally though, studies of selenium supplementation have been contradictory. If you choose to enrich your diet with selenium, eat more fish, organ meats, whole grains, beans, and nuts.

Zinc. Too much copper in the body can lead to zinc deficiency because the two minerals balance each other. In some studies patients taking zinc supplements have seen improvement. Half of the 24 people involved in a study conducted in the 1970s took 220 milligrams of zinc 3 times a day and found they experienced less morning stiffness, less swelling, and felt better overall, compared to the other half of the patients who were given placebos. Unfortunately, other studies conducted since then have had conflicting results. If you choose to increase zinc in your diet, good sources include oysters, ground beef, veal, pork, fish, soybeans, granola, cheddar cheese and tofu.

The Importance of a Well-Balanced Diet

Some studies have suggested that an unbalanced diet could be one of the triggers for the development of rheumatic diseases such as RA. Although we don't know this for sure, we do know that a balanced diet provides nutrients essential to your well being. Naturally, it's important for everyone to eat properly, but it's especially

SEVEN GUIDELINES FOR A HEALTHY DIET

The Arthritis Foundation suggests following these seven rules to maintain a healthy diet.

- Eat a variety of foods
- Maintain ideal weight
- Avoid too much fat and cholesterol
- Avoid too much sugar
- Eat foods with enough starch and fiber
- Avoid too much sodium
- Drink alcohol in moderation

ARTHRITIS ON THE INTERNET

The nonprofit Arthritis Foundation is the only national, voluntary health organization working for people with arthritis. It is actively exploring many different options for arthritis treatment, including diet. It maintains a databank, tracks research involving all types of therapies, and is in the process of making information available through personal computers.

You can access articles from the Foundation's magazine, *Arthritis Today,* through the Internet, a network of over 20 million computer users worldwide. The Foundation is also working with *America Online* to provide arthritis-related information. You can also find articles on arthritis in *America Online's* Better Health and Medical Forum, where you can communicate directly with other arthritis sufferers. A forum is an electronic meeting place where interested parties can "talk" to one another by typing messages and posting them on a "bulletin board." *America Online* is currently negotiat-

ing a joint project with Shoppers Express to allow subscribers to purchase groceries and drug store items electronically and have them delivered to their homes.

You can also network with other computer users who have arthritis through *CompuServ* and *Prodigy,* two other popular computer networks. For instance, *Prodigy* subscribers can exchange messages through the Medical Support Bulletin Board, where many arthritis-related topics are covered.

The Arthritis Foundation has a wealth of information about the disease. Among the pamphlets available is "Diet: Guidelines and Research." It was published in 1987, but the organization says that the information is still accurate. Order this pamphlet or any other materials by contacting the Foundation at PO Box 19000, Atlanta, GA 30326 (phone: 1-800-283-7800).

important if you have arthritis because of the many barriers to good nutrition that you may face.

Arthritis pain can make hunger seem relatively insignificant and can easily interfere with food shopping or cooking, leaving you with an inadequate diet. You may pass up some necessary foods, like vegetables, because they require more effort to prepare and would therefore tax swollen and aching joints.

Your medications can also interfere with a good diet. Some drugs can upset the stomach, causing nausea, diarrhea, and other reactions that result in either a lack of appetite or an inability to digest food properly. In addition, some medications can rob your body of essential vitamins and minerals. For example, steroid medications cause the body

to lose potassium and retain sodium; if you have gout and are taking colchicine, it affects how well your body absorbs vitamin B_{12}; and penicillamine, often given to people with RA, lowers the body's levels of copper.

One of the most important things you can do is to avoid foods high in saturated fats. Such foods are high in calories that would be better coming from a wider variety of nutritious foods. Scientists in Moscow recently showed that an overall healthy diet, with only small quantities of saturated fats (but with higher levels of polyunsaturated fatty acids than many of the people in the study usually consumed), brought about improvement in many arthritis patients. Within the first two weeks of the study, more than two-thirds (67.6 percent) saw a marked decrease in painful joints, and 82 percent saw an improvement in morning stiffness. Nearly one quarter (24 percent) of the patients were able to reduce their dosage of antirheumatic drugs; for example, they lowered their intake of ibuprofen by 400 to 600 milligrams per day, and lowered their intake of prednisolone by 1.25 to 2.5 milligrams daily.

The authors of the study contend that the whole nutrient mix in the test diet, which restricted saturated fats while increasing the amount of polyunsaturated fats (including omega-3's) was responsible for the improvement in the subjects' arthritis symptoms. They believe it was also responsible for lowered blood pressure in patients who were mildly hypertensive, and contributed to weight loss in patients who were obese. Here is the nutrient content of the daily diet they followed:

total protein:	90 grams (including 50 grams animal protein)
total fats:	70 grams (including 30 grams vegetable fat)
carbohydrates:	350 grams (including 15 grams refined carbohydrates)
fiber:	25 grams
cholesterol:	0.27 grams
polyunsaturated fatty acids:	17.9 grams
calcium:	1.1 grams
phosphorus:	1.9 grams
iron:	0.27 gram
zinc:	0.016 gram
vitamin C:	0.16 gram
vitamin E:	0.03 gram
total calories:	2390

Today, you should be able to prepare nutritious foods without putting too much strain on painful joints. Prepared vegetables—raw carrots, cabbage, lettuce, cucumbers, and squash—are available already sliced, diced, and peeled in the produce sections of many supermarkets. If stores near you don't yet carry these products, speak to the manager. Frozen vegetables are almost as good as fresh ones and can be much simpler to prepare. Use canned vegetables only if fresh or frozen produce is unavailable, because canned foods often contain unwanted sodium and preservatives.

You may soon be able to select your groceries, household items, and prescription medications from your home computer, and have them delivered directly to you. (See the section on resources for more information.)

You can learn other labor-saving cooking techniques from an occupational therapist. Ask your doctor to recommend someone for you. You can also check with your local Cooperative Extension Service or local chapters of the Arthritis Foundation about cooking classes or demonstrations with helpful hints.

Why You Should Watch Your Weight

Some experts believe overweight people are more susceptible to certain kinds of arthritis. As with almost all the other aspects of this disease, however, more studies are needed to explain and verify this theory. Still, there are many benefits to losing a few pounds if you are overweight and troubled by arthritis pain. For example:

■ Those extra pounds burden joints that already protest against stress, like the knees and hips.

■ Tendons and ligaments can become separated by layers of fat. This padding can interfere with the leverage your muscles and tendons apply to your joints, helping to cause bursitis and tendonitis.

■ Many older adults with arthritis also are troubled by hypertension or heart disease. Extra weight can make these two conditions worse.

■ If you are overweight you are probably less active than you should be. Physical activity strengthens bones and muscles; lack of activity weakens them.

A healthy diet can help you shed some of those extra pounds. In addition, check with your doctor about starting an exercise program that will be right for you. For example, jogging may not be a good idea, but walking every day might be perfect. If walking is too uncomfortable, hydrorobics, a type of aerobics that uses gentle water exercises, might be the answer. Most health clubs and spas offer these aquatic programs, and local chapters of the Arthritis Foundation often set them up at swimming pools operated by the YMCA. □

CHAPTER 27

Latest Thinking on Diet and Immunity

Can vitamins cure an infection or prevent one from taking hold? Sadly, the answer is No. However, extra doses of certain vitamins do seem to reduce the severity of some infections. And there's no question that an outright vitamin deficiency is an invitation to disease.

As we all know in this era of AIDS and HIV, a robust immune system is all that stands between us and perpetual infection. And the nutrients in our diet have a definite impact on the status of the system. This was firmly established long ago, when doctors noticed that under-nourished patients were less able to fight infection. More recently, many experts have come to believe that the lowered immunity that accompanies old age is to some extent a result of poor nutrition, rather than inevitable decline.

Nutritional Mainstays of Immunity

Maintaining your immune system in peak condition may require more than the official Recommended Daily Allowances (now called Daily Values)—or so some studies suggest. RDAs were established to prevent deficiency diseases, not to help the immune system; and these values have rarely been changed. On the other hand, too much of certain nutrients can actually hamper immunity.

To be honest, this is an area of science where confusion still reigns. The immune system is complex and resilient. In some people, a vitamin deficiency may have no practical effect at all. In others, extra vitamins and other nutrients may prove to be helpful. Amid all the uncertainty, however, a few vitamins and minerals stand out. Here's a look at those that seem especially important for a strong, healthy immune system.

Vitamin A
A deficiency can increase your vulnerability to infection, but overdosing is harmful. Getting less than the Recommended Daily

Allowance of 5,000 International Units of vitamin A can:

- Reduce the size of the thymus, a gland that makes the disease-fighting white blood cells called lymphocytes
- Shrink the number of lymphocytes
- Reduce production of antibodies that fight infection
- Reduce the ability of the respiratory tract to push bacteria out of the system

Carotenoids such as beta-carotene are forms of vitamin A. They help regulate three types of immune cells: T and B lymphocytes, natural killer cells, and macrophages.

We do not yet know whether people who get too little vitamin A or beta-carotene actually become sick more easily or whether their illnesses are more serious. Some studies indicate that if you develop a bad case of measles or pneumonia, or have a long-lasting fever, you need more vitamin A than the Food and Drug Administration (FDA) recommends. Conversely, there is evidence that the body reduces vitamin A circulation as part of its response to infection. If this is true, increasing vitamin A levels during infection would be counterproductive, as long as the person had an adequate amount before getting sick.

In any case, several studies in developing countries have found that giving vitamin A supplements to children with measles significantly reduced their chance of dying. Most of these children were vitamin-A deficient before they became ill. In at least one study, children receiving vitamin A had fewer measles symptoms than those who didn't take the vitamin.

There is some evidence that supplemental vitamin A can increase the immune response of cancer patients, as well—although extremely high doses seem to suppress it. Too much beta-carotene also may impair the immune system. A recent study of smokers conducted in Finland found a slight *increase* in lung cancer among the smokers who took a daily 20-milligram beta-carotene supplement. Based on this finding, some nutritional authorities now recommend limiting your beta-carotene intake to the amount found in a standard multivitamin tablet.

Vitamin A is fat-soluble. Unlike water soluble vitamins, it is stored in your body fat, where it can build up to dangerous levels. Taking too much of it can cause headache, nausea, and possible liver problems.

Vitamin B complex

Deficiencies of the B vitamins definitely lower your resistance. Deficiencies of B_2, B_6, B_{12}, folate, and pantothenic acid have the greatest impact. A deficiency of biotin or thiamine is less significant. Oral contraceptives tend to reduce the supply of several B vitamins, including B_6. Eating foods rich in the B vitamins should be enough to overcome this effect, however.

Vitamin C

The craze over vitamin C's power to prevent and treat colds started with the Nobel Prize-winning chemist Linus Pauling's 1970 book *Vitamin C and the Common Cold*. Pauling advised taking 3,200 to 12,000 milligrams per day, far higher than the recommended 60 milligrams. Today, experts agree that smokers, people regularly using aspirin or tetracycline, and women taking oral contraceptives, may

KEY PLAYERS IN YOUR IMMUNE SYSTEM

Antibodies—elements of the immune system targeted to specific invaders that you have been exposed to before.

Macrophages—cells that kill bacteria by surrounding and, in effect, eating them.

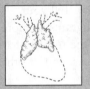

Lymphocytes—infection-fighting white blood cells. Lymphocytes play a role in making antibodies.

T-cells—a type of lymphocyte attacked by HIV.

Thymus—the gland where cells mature into lymphocytes.

Neutrophils—compose about 75 percent of circulating white blood cells.

Interleukin-2—A hormone that promotes growth in the number and power of T-cells.

need more than the RDA. However, most nutritional authorities recommend 100 milligrams a day, not several thousand. Studies testing Pauling's cold theory indicate that vitamin C probably does not prevent colds but may make them milder and shorten their duration.

How does vitamin C affect immunity?

Vitamin C has been proven to boost the bacteria-killing ability of certain immune cells called macrophages and neutrophils. Some authorities believe that vitamin C also stimulates production of interferon, an important chemical in the immune system, and that it improves the thymus gland's ability to make infection-fighting lymphocytes, a type of white blood cell.

Is the recommended amount enough? In a number of studies, megadoses have delivered only minimal benefits, producing at best minor symptomatic relief. In one study, doses of less than 100 milligrams daily were said to achieve the same results as 1 to 2 grams per day.

Other studies, however, do bear out the protective power of much higher-than-recommended doses. One well-controlled study showed that, when volunteers were deliberately infected with a cold-causing virus, those taking 500 milligrams of vitamin C four times a day (that's a total of 2,000 milligrams or 2 grams per day) had symptoms half as severe as those taking a dummy pill instead. Some nutritionists now recommend taking 750 milligrams daily during the cold season as a preventive measure, and raising that amount to 1 gram (1,000 milligrams) at the first sign of cold symptoms. If you get a cold, they advise taking 500 milligrams every two-and-a-half hours during the daytime and 1 gram of time-released vitamin C at bedtime. Other experts, however, continue to advocate sticking with the current Recommended Daily Allowance.

Can too much hurt you? Unlike vitamins that remain in your body fat, vitamin C is water soluble. Because excess amounts are rapidly flushed from the body, the danger of overdosing is minimal. Large doses, however, can lead to diarrhea, gas, and heartburn. Taking 5 to 10 grams a day can cause nausea and vomiting.

People with certain health problems may experience additional side effects:

■ High vitamin C intake can reduce the effect of warfarin, a medication used to thin the blood, and of certain drugs used to treat infections of the urinary tract. If you take these drugs you should not supplement your diet with megadoses of vitamin C.
■ Because it is an acid, vitamin C may irritate stomach ulcers.
■ If you have problems storing iron, vitamin C can cause serious problems by releasing too much iron into the blood.
■ In people with genetic blood diseases such as sickle-cell anemia or thalassemia, too much vitamin C can make red blood cells self-destruct.
■ Animal studies have also shown that megadoses can lead to spontaneous abortion.

Anyone taking megadoses of vitamin C over a long time can become dependent on it. The body may respond to uninterrupted high levels by activating an enzyme to destroy the vitamin. If you then cut your dosage too quickly, you may go through a withdrawal process that includes signs of vitamin C deficiency.

What to do. The consensus today is to take no more than 1,000 milligrams of vitamin C per day. Taking it in small doses with meals rather than all at one time increases the amount that your body absorbs. Always swallow the tablet immediately; chewing vitamin C can erode tooth enamel. Tell your doctor if you take 1,000 milligrams or more daily. Megadoses may affect the results of blood sugar checks for diabetes, and of other medical tests.

Vitamin E

There is renewed interest in vitamin E lately due to its antioxidant effect. As an immunity-booster, however, its value is debatable. In the past, some experts have recommended taking 3 to 4 times the Recommended Daily Allowance of 30 International Units to keep the immune system at its peak. However, megadoses of vitamin E have been found to suppress the function of B cells, an important component of the immune system. And in the recent study of Finnish smokers, 50 milligrams per day was associated with an increased risk of stroke (although the risk of prostate cancer declined). On balance, it seems wisest to stick with the RDA.

Iron

Many Americans lack sufficient amounts of this important mineral. Menstruating women, for example, lose iron with the blood in their periods every month. Without enough iron, the number of antibodies in the immune system are reduced, and the system's natural killer cells, neutrophils, and macrophages are unable to kill bacteria as effectively as they should. Iron deficiency may also lower both the number of white blood cells and their ability to fight infection.

Too much iron however, may be as dangerous as too little. Iron overload interferes with immune responses and reduces the number of cells that grow into lymphocytes. It also can produce an iron storage disease called hemosiderosis. There is no evidence that supplementing the diet with doses of iron exceeding the recommended 18 milligrams per day can "soup up" your immune response. You should take iron supplements only to correct a deficiency.

Because bacteria need iron to grow, some authorities have argued that iron deficiency actually reduces risk of infection. Most human studies do not support this conclusion. Reducing iron offers no protection against disease, and correcting the deficiency does not increase the number or seriousness of infections.

L-arginine

Imbalances in amino acids, the building blocks of proteins, can impair immune response. In animals, L-arginine stimulates the adult immune system and reduces the growth and spread of experimentally induced tumors. In studies with people, use of this amino acid has led to an increase in the number of lymphocytes and has shortened hospital stays after major operations. Some evidence suggests that large doses of L-arginine could help in treating AIDS and cancer. However, researchers want more information before recommending L-arginine supplementation.

Protein

Severe protein insufficiency reduces the size, weight, and function of the thymus, a small organ located in the chest. Because the thymus makes the white blood cells that produce antibodies and kill invading microorganisms, shrinkage of the gland decreases the body's ability to fight infection. Protein deficiency is uncommon in this country except among the poor, those with certain illnesses, and elderly people who may find it too difficult or expensive to prepare nutritious meals. In fact, because most of us eat more protein than we need, deficiency is rarely to blame when the immune system malfunctions.

Selenium

Although a lack of selenium is linked to an increased risk of cancer, its role in fighting infection is unclear. When levels are too low, the body cannot produce sufficient antibodies to combat illness. (Vitamin E reverses this effect.) A moderate increase in intake has been found to boost immune response in animal tests; but an overdose can do the opposite. (For men, 70 micrograms per day is an overdose; for women, it's 55 micrograms.)

Zinc

Consuming less than the Recommended Daily Allowance of 15 milligrams of zinc per day hampers the immune system in several ways:

- Shrinks the size of the thymus, where the disease-fighting white blood cells called lymphocytes are made
- Reduces number of lymphocytes
- Slows production of lymphocytes
- Impairs the function of lymphocytes and the germ-killing cells called macrophages
- Decreases antibody response
- Prevents wounds from healing properly

Zinc deficiencies can reduce immunity in both school-age children and women of child-bearing age. There is also some evidence that healthy people consuming low–normal levels of zinc have diminished immune response.

According to some estimates, fewer than 50 percent of Americans get an adequate amount of zinc. Among those most likely to be deficient are the elderly, dieters, alcoholics, pregnant women, infants, and people with injuries, burns, or infections. Zinc is found in animal-derived foods such as meat, eggs, and cheese, and restoring zinc-rich foods to your diet can bring the immune system back to par within two weeks.

When it comes to zinc supplements, however, more is definitely not better. In fact, exceeding the RDA even slightly may be harmful. Overdosage (300 milligrams a day) may actually impair immunity, while doses of 90 to 100 milligrams per day taken over a long period of time can reduce immunity, lower levels of "good" HDL cholesterol, and produce anemia.

What to Eat—and Not Eat—When You're Sick

The old saying about starving a fever was right. Starving a fever isn't much of a deprivation, either, since illness usually ruins your appetite. In fact, it appears that loss of appetite is the body's way of saying that you should eat less while it battles foreign microorganisms. As part of this strategy, the body usually withdraws iron, zinc, and other nutrients from the bloodstream and stores them in the liver, thymus, and bone marrow so bacteria can't snap them up.

Well nourished, otherwise healthy adults can deal with the nutritional depletion that results from infection. But extra care is needed for children, the elderly, and anybody who is sick more than about five days or loses five percent of their weight. A vitamin or mineral supplement or a liquid nutritional supplement taken under a doctor's supervision may be helpful. If you lose a great deal of weight during an infection, you may require extra protein to nourish your immune system.

When your fever breaks, drink lots of water and other fluids—especially citrus juice—to replace the fluid you have lost. Also, eat grapes, juicy fruits, milk shakes, broth, and whole grain breads. They can help replace the missing nutrients. Citrus and other fruit juices and juicy fruits are especially good sources of potassium.

Feeding a cold is another piece of folklore that turns out to be correct. Hot, spicy foods, such as chili peppers, horseradish, black and red pepper, garlic, and pepper sauce may stimulate mucus flow and relieve symptoms of asthma, bronchitis, sinus trouble, and colds. However, people with asthma who are taking theophylline should not feed their cold charcoal-broiled meat, broccoli, or cabbage. Research at Rockefeller University in New York has shown that protein, hydrocarbons on charcoal-broiled meat, and chemicals found in cruciferous vegetables such as broccoli can speed up liver function and rush some drugs, including theophylline, out of the system before they've done their job.

Science also is finding evidence to support the use of chicken soup as a cold remedy. In the late 1970s, researchers learned that hot liquids—including chicken soup—break up congestion, relieve sore throat, and increase the flow of nasal secretions. This may help block cold viruses from infiltrating the body. Inhaling the vapors of hot liquid through the nose seems to do the trick. In 1993, Dr. Stephen Rennard of the University of Nebraska found that a much-diluted version of chicken soup made from his wife's family recipe was capable of reducing the inflammation that causes many cold symptoms, such as a sore throat and production of phlegm. The hundreds of biologically active compounds found in the vegetables used in the soup may be the "good guys." Although soup doesn't cure the underlying problem, neither do any of the drug store remedies.

Extra Vitamins for the Elderly?

The elderly get sick more easily, take longer to recover, and are more likely to develop life-threatening illnesses. In fact, infections are the fourth leading cause of death in the elderly. Although the immune system declines naturally with age, an insufficient diet can make matters worse.

Several surveys have shown that almost one-third of apparently healthy elderly people get too little iron, zinc, beta carotene, and vitamins B_6 and C. Correcting these deficiencies with supplements has successfully strengthened immune response. Although heredity also may play a role in immune system decline, some researchers now feel that reduced immunity need not inevitably accompany aging. Indeed, 20 to 25 percent of older people maintain immune systems as

vigorous as those of younger adults even into their 70s and 80s.

Ideally, the elderly should build up their immune systems by eating more fruits, vegetables, and other nutrient-rich foods. Unfortunately, however, those who have lost a spouse or live alone are often not motivated to fix healthy meals. Some senior citizens cannot get out to shop; others have lost their teeth or have other medical problems requiring special diets. Many take several prescription drugs, some of which may interfere with absorption of nutrients from food. (See Chapter 29 for details.)

For all these reasons, extra vitamin and mineral supplements may be a good idea for some older people. The additional nutrients are not, of course, a guarantee against illness; and researchers feel that the evidence in their favor is not yet conclusive. Still, hints are accumulating that taking supplements above the Recommended Daily Allowance can indeed boost immune function in the elderly. Here are some of the specifics.

Vitamin E. Giving megadoses of vitamin E (around 1,000 International Units or more) to healthy older people for a short time boosted immune function in at least two studies. However, the research did not track the seniors' ability to avoid and fight infection over the long term, so the researchers say that further work is needed before they can recommend that older people routinely take vitamin E supplements in excess of the 30 International Unit RDA.

Vitamin B$_6$. There is some evidence that extra vitamin B$_6$ can give older immune systems a boost. In a study at Tufts University, a dosage of 50 milligrams a day (25 times the 2-milligram RDA) hiked immune response to that of much younger adults. However, there's a definite danger in large doses. Some people develop reversible nerve damage at doses of 100 milligrams per day. No conclusive research has been done in this area, so the wisest course is to stay relatively close to the official RDA.

Beta-carotene. A handful of studies have shown an increase in the number of natural killer cells in healthy elderly people taking 30 to 60 milligrams of beta-carotene daily for about 2 months.

Multivitamin and mineral supplements, with extra vitamin E and beta-carotene. One study of 95 people age 65 and older found that taking a vitamin E-and beta-carotene-rich multivitamin not only reduced infections, but also increased the protection afforded by flu shots—a vital consideration for older people, who are more likely to get sick from, and die of, the flu than are younger adults. Larger studies are needed to be sure that these findings are valid, however.

Zinc. While the recommended amount of zinc (15 milligrams daily) can increase the number of T-cells in the immune systems of older people, larger doses (less than 10 times the RDA) can cause bloating, nausea, cramps, diarrhea, and fever. Even higher amounts can lead to bleeding and anemia.

HIV, AIDS, and Nutrition

Good nutrition does absolutely nothing to prevent HIV infection. The virus is transmitted by intimate sexual contact whether you have a balanced diet or not. However, there is some reason to believe that an enriched diet can slow the progression of the disease. And because AIDS is often accompanied by malnutrition, careful attention to diet is especially important.

Nutrition is a problem for several reasons. Lack of energy or motivation to prepare meals make people with HIV more likely to eat improperly. As HIV progresses, patients are prone to develop infections that cause diarrhea and make it more difficult for the body to absorb needed nutrients from the food they do manage to eat. And many drugs used to treat HIV and its complications can cause nausea, vomiting, or weight loss: Trimethoprim can lead to folic acid deficiency; pentamidine can cause low blood sugar. People with AIDS are also vulnerable to "AIDS-wasting syndrome," a condition which produces severe, life-threatening weight loss. This complication requires nutritional supplements and sometimes, medication.

Preliminary evidence suggests that supplementing a diet rich in fruits and vegetables with a multivitamin that includes iron, vitamin E, and riboflavin may, in some cases, delay the development of full-blown AIDS. In a 6-year study of 296 HIV-infected men, researchers found a 31 percent reduction in development of outright AIDS among those on a vitamin-rich diet—far from conclusive proof, but still encouraging.

Some smaller, shorter studies have evaluated effects of a single nutrient on people with HIV. One such study of 21 HIV patients produced an increase in the immune system's T-cell activity after 4 weeks of 180 milligrams of beta-carotene daily. This dose is very high, but has been given to persons with certain skin conditions without adverse effects. Iron, on the other hand, definitely should not be taken in large doses. It may cause dormant bacterial infections to re-emerge.

Going to Extremes

People who suffer from AIDS are often desperate. Many seek alternative therapies, including nutritionally based options. Here are some of the untested, nontraditional programs they are likely to encounter.

Megadoses of nutrients. Although large doses of vitamins A, C, E, B$_{12}$ and both selenium and zinc are sometimes recommended to increase the number and activity of the immune system's T-cells, very high doses have not been proven effective, and may even be dangerous. Regular consumption of more than 50,000 IU a day of vitamin A (10 times the recommended amount) can be poisonous to the system. As little as 25 milligrams of zinc daily can cause nausea and impaired immune function.

The University of Miami School of Medicine's Biopsychosocial Center for AIDS has come up with a more moderate approach. It suggests that patients with early HIV infection should take the following nutrients daily. (The FDA's Recommended Daily Intake is shown for comparison.)

- Vitamin A, 10,000 IU (RDI = 5,000 IU)
- Vitamin B$_2$, (riboflavin), 9 milligrams (RDI = 1.7 milligrams)
- Vitamin B$_6$, more than 20 milligrams (RDI = 2 milligrams)
- Vitamin B$_{12}$, 50 micrograms (RDI = 6 micrograms)
- Vitamin C, 360 milligrams (RDI = 60 milligrams)
- Vitamin E, 60 milligrams (RDI = 30 IU)
- Zinc, 75 milligrams (RDI = 15 milligrams)

Note, however, that the use of zinc is questionable. In one study, the risk of developing AIDS was 3 times higher in men who took more than 20 milligrams of zinc daily. The risk began rising at 12 milligrams per day.

Dr. Berger's Immune Power Diet. This regimen is based on a 1985 book that blames poor health on "immune hypersensitivity" to common foods such as milk, wheat, corn, yeast, soy, sugar, and eggs. The diet has not been tested scientifically, and is too low in fat and calcium to be considered healthy.

AL 721. This product is made from soy or egg yolks, and consists of active lipids and lecithin. The Food and Drug Administration tested the preparation for use by HIV patients and found few side effects but no consistent benefit. In some studies, AL 721 increased body weight and levels of both "good" (HDL) and "bad" (LDL) cholesterol. While AL 721 may not help much, it probably can't hurt.

Macrobiotic diet. Based on Asian philosophy, this low fat, high fiber program is intended to improve health by restoring balance in the body. Up to 50 percent of the diet consists of whole grain cereals, 20 to 30 percent of fresh vegetables, 10 to 15 percent of cooked beans or seaweed, and 5 percent of miso (fermented soy paste) or tamari broth soup. Macrobiotic diets can cause protein deficiency and do not offer enough riboflavin, niacin, or calcium for adults.

Butylated hydroxytoluene (BHT). Assertions that this antioxidant food preservative kills HIV by attacking the outside coat of the virus are unfounded. The product also may not be safe.

Laetrile. Evidence indicates that treatment with this substance, originally intended to destroy a tumor enzyme in cancer patients, is not only ineffective but also potentially harmful. Proponents recommend laetrile as part of a regimen including a strict vegetarian diet that excludes milk and other animal products along with meat and vitamin supplements. This program may not supply enough calcium, iron, niacin, and vitamin B_{12}, and may include too much thiamin, vitamin A, vitamin C, and zinc.

The Gerson method. Aimed at AIDS-induced cancers, this program includes an inadequate diet of unproven effectiveness. It restricts intake of all food except oatmeal and fresh fruits and vegetables, and advocates using enemas, especially coffee enemas, to create an environment hostile to cancerous cells.

The Kelley regime excludes meat, peanuts, and milk (in all forms except yogurt) in an effort to overcome a supposed pancreatic enzyme deficiency. It substitutes almonds for meat and recommends various supplements. Possible dangers of the diet include vitamin A toxicity, protein and calcium deficiencies, and fluid losses.

Getting More Nutrients Into the Diet

When getting enough food becomes a problem, the usual caloric no-nos become a recommended diet. Consider cooking with milk instead of water, buy canned fruit in heavy syrup, and eat more than three meals a day (snacking is fine). A doctor or nutritionist may recommend a liquid food supplement, such as Ensure or Sustacal. If lesions in the mouth make it painful to eat, try soft foods, such as poached eggs and ice cream. □

CHAPTER 28

Sure-Fire Ways to Prevent Brittle Bones

t's not every day that scientists find an easy, painless way to cut your chances of a debilitating disease in half. But for osteoporosis—the brittle bones of old age—that's exactly what they've done. We now know that just by maintaining a calcium-rich diet from childhood onward, you can dramatically improve your odds of escaping the disease. Characterized by loss of bone density and strength, osteoporosis affects more than 25 million people in the United States—80 percent of them women—and is the major underlying cause of bone fractures in postmenopausal women and the elderly.

Osteoporosis-related fractures can occur in any bone, but the most common sites are the spinal column, the wrist, and the hip. Rapid loss of bone mass begins to occur in a woman's spinal column following menopause. When the loss becomes great enough, a simple action, such as bending forward while making a bed, can cause enough pressure to produce a spinal compression fracture, resulting in chronic pain, loss of height, and a characteristic "dowager's hump." Wrist fractures also occur commonly among women with osteoporosis.

Hip fractures in the elderly are one of the most serious health problems in the U.S. Broken hips are associated with more death, more disability, and higher medical costs than all other osteoporosis-related fractures combined. Up to 20 percent of older adults die within a year of breaking their hips. Of the survivors, fewer than half return to the full level of activity they previously enjoyed.

Other factors that increase your risk of osteoporosis, which can affect not only postmenopausal women but all elderly women and men, include:

Age. Although denser bones delay the onset of osteoporosis, normal aging inevitably includes some gradual loss of bone.

Gender. Osteoporosis is estimated to be six to eight times more common in women than in men because women's bones are usually

INSIDE A BRITTLE BONE

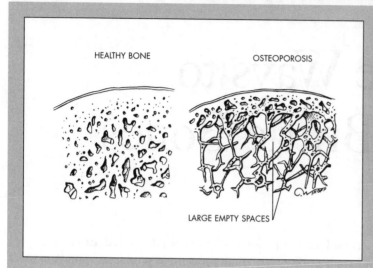

HEALTHY BONE

OSTEOPOROSIS

LARGE EMPTY SPACES

When the life-long process called bone remodeling slows, calcium leaches out faster than bone cells can restore it. The result is an increasingly porous skeletal structure given to tiny fractures you may never notice. As the disease progresses and bone density declines, major fractures of the hip, spine, or wrist become ever more likely.

less dense to begin with, and because the lower estrogen levels that accompany menopause cause women to lose bone mass much more rapidly.

Early menopause. The sooner estrogen levels drop, the greater the chances of developing osteoporosis. Either a naturally early menopause or surgical menopause (removal of the ovaries) can be at fault.

Ethnic background. Asian and Caucasian women and men are at greater risk than African-Americans, whose bone mass is generally about 10 percent greater.

Lack of weight-bearing exercise. The significant loss of bone mass in astronauts (who spend considerable time in a weightless environment) demonstrates the importance of weight-bearing exercise—particularly walking—in maintaining strong bones.

Body weight. Thin, small-boned women—particularly female athletes, such as gymnasts and runners, who exercise so strenuously

that their periods cease—face a heightened risk of developing osteoporosis even as young adults.

Heredity. A history of broken bones or stooped posture in older family members—especially women—can be a warning that you too are at risk.

Alcohol and smoking. Heavy drinkers and smokers have weaker bones. Alcohol disrupts bone formation. Smoking decreases absorption of calcium.

Osteoporosis also may occur as a side effect of prolonged use of thyroid hormones, anticonvulsants or steroid drugs. Hyperthyroidism, rheumatoid arthritis, kidney disease, and certain cancers, such as lymphoma and leukemia, can also lead to osteoporosis.

Medical researchers still don't know why, given identical chances, one person develops osteoporosis while another doesn't.

Nevertheless, they have learned a great deal about how to prevent the disease. In fact, the good news is that if your bones reach their maximum density (or mass) by the time you are 30, and if you take steps to curb the rate of natural bone loss in later life, you run little risk of developing the condition.

A vast body of research has now confirmed the need for adequate calcium intake during early life to build denser, stronger bones and during later life to slow down the rate of natural bone loss. Although everyone experiences some bone loss with age, osteoporosis and disabling bone fractures *are not* a normal part of aging.

Why the Fuss Over Calcium?

Bone is living tissue that is continually being broken down, or resorbed, and rebuilt. This process is called remodeling. Nearly all of the calcium in your body is stored in your bones and teeth. Calcium not only makes your bones hard but performs such essential functions as helping your blood to clot and enabling your heart and other muscles to contract. Whenever your dietary intake of calcium is too small to meet your body's needs, increased amounts are drawn from the bones to maintain a relatively constant supply in the bloodstream.

Human bone grows most rapidly throughout childhood and adolescence. More than one-third of total adult bone mass develops between the ages of nine and 18. During your 20s, bone growth increases by approximately 15 percent. Peak bone mass—when bones are their strongest—occurs between the ages of 25 and 35. After that, bone mass gradually diminishes and your bones begin to lose their strength.

Your bones are in constant flux. Certain hormonal signals prompt the breakdown of old bone, while others encourage new bone deposits. When you are young, old bone is replaced by new bone every 90 days. Once you attain peak bone mass, the rate of bone dissolution exceeds the rate of new bone creation, resulting in gradually decreased bone mass and density.

Millions of Americans get far too little calcium to prevent osteoporosis. One national survey found that average daily intake ranges from only 530 milligrams among middle-aged women to a high of 1,179 milligrams among teen-age boys. On average, no adult women met the Recommended Dietary Allowance of 800 milligrams per day. How much does this matter? In June 1994, a panel of experts convened by the National Institutes of Health (NIH) in Bethesda, Maryland, reviewed the latest scientific data and concluded that optimal calcium intake is most important from childhood through the mid-20s, when bones are growing at their fastest rate; in women following menopause, when rapid bone loss can occur; and in older adults.

Consequently, the panel recommended boosting the calcium intake for children, teenagers, and young adults. Children are the most worrisome because their calcium intake has actually declined over the past four decades, in stark contrast to their nutritional needs. A calcium-rich diet also is essential during the crucial bone-forming years between adolescence and young adulthood. The panel concluded that high levels of calcium (up to 2,500 milligrams daily) in a youngster's diet produce no undesirable side

HOW MUCH CALCIUM DO YOU NEED?

	amount of calcium per day (milligrams)	
	NIH Consensus Panel	RDA (Recommended Daily Allowance)
Infants, Children and Young Adults		
0-6 months	400	400
6-12 months	600	600
1-10 years	800-1,200	800
11-24 years	1,200-1,500	1,200
Adult Women		
Below 24 years, pregnant or breastfeeding	1,500	1,200
25 and over, pregnant or breastfeeding	1,200	1,200
25-49 years	1,000	800
50-64 years, taking estrogen	1,000	800
50-64 years, not taking estrogen	1,500	800
65 and older	1,500	800
Adult Men		
25-64 years	1,000	800
65 and older	1,500	800

Summary of recommendations for optimal calcium intake made by the consensus development panel convened by the NIH, June 1994. Optimal calcium intake refers to the level of calcium consumption from the diet plus supplements, if needed, that is necessary for a person to maximize peak adult bone mass and minimize bone loss in later years.

Sources: National Institutes of Health, Bethesda, MD; National Osteoporosis Foundation, Washington, DC.

effects yet have the potential of decreasing the risk of hip fracture in later life by as much as 50 percent.

A decline in estrogen levels during menopause causes accelerated bone loss in women, which lasts approximately six to eight years. After this time, the bone loss becomes more gradual—similar to that of aging men. To avoid depletion of bone mass and reduce the risk of osteoporosis-related fractures during midlife, the NIH panel recommended that postmenopausal women aim for a daily calcium intake of 1,000 to 1,500 milligrams. Because older adults have more problems absorbing calcium than do younger people, the panel also advised women and men 65 and older to boost their calcium intake to 1,500 milligrams of calcium daily.

Because there is no real cure for osteoporosis, prevention is paramount. Scientists know that, by consuming the proper amounts of calcium at the right times in life, you can minimize bone loss.

Finding Sources of Calcium

You can achieve your recommended daily allowance of calcium by eating a calcium-rich diet, choosing calcium-fortified foods, taking calcium supplements, or combining these strategies. Vitamin D enhances calcium absorption, while certain medications and foods reduce its availability.

Dietary sources of calcium are not difficult to find. Milk and milk products are naturally rich in this important mineral. They also provide vitamins A and D, protein, magnesium, and phosphorus, the other building blocks for bone. Four eight-ounce glasses of skim milk contain approximately 1,200 milligrams of calcium—roughly the recommended amount for teenagers and young adults. One study showed that 12-year-old girls who consumed just one additional glass of milk per day for 18 months developed higher total body and spinal bone mass than those who did not. Unquestionably, a glass of milk with each meal and an afternoon snack is a healthier—and often cheaper—alternative for young people than sodas, sports drinks, or powdered fruit drinks. For the lactose-intolerant, lactose-reduced milk, which contains 20 percent less lactose than the regular kind, provides a good alternative to skim or lowfat milk while delivering a comparable amount of calcium.

Calcium-rich foods need not be fattening, either. One cup of skim milk (302 milligrams calcium) has only half the calories of a cup of whole milk (291 milligrams calcium). A cup of plain lowfat yogurt (400 milligrams calcium) has fewer calories than a similar serving of lowfat fruit-flavored yogurt (314 milligrams calcium). In addition to the wide range of dairy products available in your supermarket, other calcium-rich foods—many of them low in calories—include dark green vegetables, such as broccoli, kale, and mustard and turnip greens; tofu; dried beans; and the soft bones of canned fish such as salmon and sardines.

It's important to remember that dieting and eating a calcium-rich diet are not mutually exclusive. A study of nine- to 12-year-old girls who increased their calcium intake from 750 milligrams per day to 1,370 milligrams daily for one year by consuming more dairy foods found they developed greater total and spinal bone density than girls who did not change their diets, yet they gained no extra weight.

To keep your weight down and your bones strong, boost your calcium and hold down the calories by snacking on broccoli with lowfat cheese dip—less fattening than chips—or drinking low-fat milk instead of soft drinks. For a treat, try switching from cake or cookies to lowfat frozen yogurt or ice milk. When snacking, try sprinkling Parmesan cheese on plain popcorn. Never starve yourself to lose weight, because this can increase bone loss so severely that you can begin developing osteoporosis in your 20s. Girls and teens who try to emulate the pencil-thin waifs who populate fashion magazines are setting themselves up for a future of chronic pain.

Eating calcium-fortified foods is also a valid way of boosting your calcium intake.

LOOK FOR CALCIUM IN UNEXPECTED SOURCES

Being good to your bones doesn't necessarily mean eating cottage cheese every day for the rest of your life. Many prepared foods, ranging from fortified orange juice to some kinds of tortillas, contain calcium-based food additives. In fact, a wide variety of unexpected foods contain some calcium. Depending on the quantities and combinations you consume, eating a balanced diet can provide an adequate amount of calcium without restricting your choices to dairy products. For example, just one slice of calcium-fortified bread provides as much calcium as a glass of milk.

Read food labels carefully. You may be surprised at what you find. Following are some examples of the amount of calcium present in a variety of foods

Food	Serving size	Calcium (milligrams)	Calories	Fat (grams)
Dairy Products				
Cheddar cheese	1 ounce	204	115	9
Mozzarella cheese (part skim milk)	1 ounce	207	80	5
Cottage cheese (lowfat 2%)	1 cup	155	200	4
Milk, Skim	1 cup	302	85	
2%	1 cup	297	120	5
Whole	1 cup	291	150	8
Yogurt, Plain, lowfat	1 cup	415	145	4
Fruit-flavored, lowfat	1 cup	345	230	4
Cheese pizza (1/8 of 15 inch pie)	1 slice	220	290	9
Macaroni & cheese	1 cup	200	230	10
Fish				
Salmon, pink (canned, with bones)	3 ounces	167	120	4.6
Sardines (in oil, with bones)	3 medium (3 ounces)	370	175	9
Bread and Cereal				
Oatmeal (instant, fortified)	1 packet	160	105	4
Pancakes (from mix)	one 4" pancake	30	60	2
Wheat bread (enriched)	1 slice	30	65	1
Broccoli, raw	1 spear	72	40	0
cooked, chopped	1 cup	354	45	0
Collards, fresh, cooked, drained	1 cup	357	30	0
Kale, fresh, cooked, drained	1 cup	179	42	0
Other				
Hot cocoa	6 oz	90	100	1
Tofu, 1 piece (1 1/2 x 2 3/4 x 1 inches)		100	85	5
Tomato soup (made with milk)	1 cup	160	160	6
Pork and beans	1 cup	140	310	7

Source: "USDA Nutritive Value of Foods." Washington, DC, Human Nutrition Information Services, U.S. Department of Agriculture, 1985; 72. Home and Garden Bulletins.

Since 1993, the U.S. Food and Drug Administration (FDA) has allowed food producers to claim benefits against several diseases—among them, osteoporosis. Authorized claims must meet federal standards prohibiting false or misleading labeling.

As a result, food labels now not only list the calcium content of a product but tell whether the level is high enough to reduce the risk of osteoporosis without also delivering excessive amounts of other nutrients, such as fat. For example, whole milk, though high in calcium, cannot bear a calcium-osteoporosis claim because it also delivers an excessive level of fat. Skim and lowfat milk and milk products, yogurt, tofu, and calcium-fortified citrus drinks generally qualify for the calcium-osteoporosis health claim.

Though experts strongly recommend a calcium-rich diet as the preferred source of this important mineral, supplements do provide an alternative. The calcium from most supplements can be absorbed as easily as the calcium in milk, though calcium citrate supplements may make a bit more calcium available for use by the body. Recent studies show that this type of supplement also causes less constipation than others, has fewer gastrointestinal side effects, and is less likely to cause kidney stones. Calcium carbonate is often recommended because it contains the highest percentage of absorbable calcium gluconate. Calcium-containing antacids in liquid or chewable form are a good source of calcium if you have difficulty swallowing tablets.

You don't need to get "chelated" calcium tablets. They are costly and offer no advantage over other types of calcium. Calcium supplements containing magnesium are also unnecessary, since most people get enough magnesium in their diets. Likewise, calcium plus Vitamin D is usually unneeded. You're likely to be getting enough Vitamin D from fortified foods, your multivitamin supplement, or exposure to sunlight. Avoid bone meal and dolomite. These "natural" supplements may be contaminated with toxic substances such as lead, mercury, and arsenic.

Calcium supplements are best absorbed in the presence of plenty of stomach acid, so it's better to take them with meals. Absorption is also better if you take the tablets throughout the day rather than in a single dose. To make certain a supplement will be properly absorbed, check the label to see whether it meets U.S. Pharmacopoeia (USP) standards, or test a tablet by dropping it into a small glass of vinegar and stirring occasionally. If the tablet doesn't dissolve within 30 minutes, the calcium probably won't be absorbed by your body.

Although too much calcium is suspected to increase the risk of kidney stones, the NIH consensus panel still concluded that calcium supplementation, up to a total of 2,000 milligrams daily, appears to be safe in people who are not at risk for kidney stones or high levels of blood calcium.

The NIH recommendations are generally higher than the standard. Recommended Daily Allowances (RDAs) are currently a source of considerable debate among the experts. While they are resolving the problem, remember that consuming adequate calcium—whether through diet, supplements, or a combination—remains essential to maintaining bone strength and preventing osteoporosis-related fractures. Your physician or a Registered Dietitian can provide additional information about how to meet your individual needs.

REMODELING IN PROGRESS

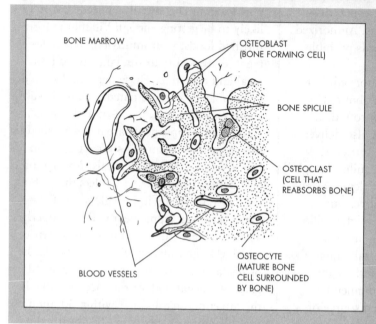

BONE MARROW

OSTEOBLAST
(BONE FORMING CELL)

BONE SPICULE

OSTEOCLAST
(CELL THAT
REABSORBS BONE)

OSTEOCYTE
(MATURE BONE
CELL SURROUNDED
BY BONE)

BLOOD VESSELS

Deep within the bones, an army of cells constantly tears down aging bone mass and builds it anew. Since estrogen fosters new growth, the reduced levels found in menopause can quickly lead to a reduction in bone density. Adequate supplies of calcium *throughout life* can alleviate the problem. After menopause, hormone replacement therapy can boost the bones' calcium absorption, preventing osteoporosis in three-quarters of the women at risk.

Other Factors with Impact on Your Calcium Levels

Your body's ability to use the calcium you consume depends on not only the total calcium content of your diet but also other dietary elements that can either boost or inhibit its absorption. For example, the absorption of calcium from some leafy green vegetables such as broccoli and kale compares favorably to the absorption of calcium from milk. (Spinach, on the other hand, is not a good source due to poor absorption.) Caffeine and salt both increase the loss of calcium through the urine; while high amounts of fiber tend to reduce calcium absorption.

Vitamin D promotes absorption of calcium from the intestines into the bloodstream. Your skin manufactures this vitamin whenever exposed to sunlight. For many people casual exposure to the sun—15 minutes to an hour per day—is enough to provide all the Vitamin D they need. It's also commonly available in Vitamin D-fortified foods, such as milk and cold cereals.

Nevertheless, Vitamin D deficiency remains a health risk for older adults—particularly the homebound elderly and those in long-term care facilities. Because adequate levels of this important vitamin are essential for proper calcium absorption, the NIH panel stressed the need for supplementation, when necessary, to achieve the Recommended Daily Allowance of 400 International Units (IU). Be careful, though, to restrict your intake to the RDA, because massive doses of vitamin D can be harmful.

Salt. The high sodium content of a vast variety of foods can play havoc with your calcium level. Sodium pulls large amounts of calcium into the kidneys, where it is subsequently lost through the urinary tract. Over the course of a decade, addition of little more than a teaspoon of salt per day to the diet of a healthy postmenopausal woman is enough to draw 7 to 8 percent of the calcium from her bones.

Protein. While it's true that protein encourages loss of calcium through the urine, it's also a fact that most protein-rich foods—including meat, milk, and eggs—contain high levels of phosphorus, which has the opposite effect. The net effect of such foods on your calcium balance is therefore of little concern, provided you eat them in moderate amounts and get enough calcium to begin with. In excessive amounts, however, both protein and phosphorus can have negative effects on your calcium status.

Caffeine. In recent years, there have been many studies on the impact of caffeine on calcium absorption. Most researchers have concluded that a lifetime daily intake of two or more cups of caffeinated coffee—the kind most American adults drink regularly—is associated with a decrease in bone density.

Caffeine-containing beverages have been found to promote the loss of calcium through the kidneys and intestines—and the more of these beverages you drink, the greater the loss. Anyone drinking these beverages should therefore be sure to increase their calcium intake proportionally.

Alcohol and tobacco. Smoking and alcohol damage your bones and additional calcium often can't compensate for it. Heavy smokers generally show significantly lower bone density than nonsmokers and tend to maintain a leaner body weight; women who smoke experience an earlier menopause. In fact, the increased prevalence of women smokers over the past three decades may be a contributing factor to the rise in osteoporosis-related fractures among older women today. Excessive drinking also can trigger the development of osteoporosis and can place people in situations where they face a heightened risk of accidents or falls. To maintain adequate bone density, avoid smoking altogether and either refrain from drinking or reduce your intake of alcoholic beverages.

Estrogen replacement therapy. Since estrogen is so important for maintaining bone density in women, physicians often recommend estrogen replacement therapy (ERT), or hor-

SEVEN EASY WAYS TO DEFEAT OSTEOPOROSIS

- Get your full allowance of calcium
- Cut your caffeine consumption to a maximum of 3 cups per day
- Keep your protein intake reasonable (If you're average, divide your weight by 2. The result is the number of grams of protein you need daily.)
- Hold your daily intake of fiber below 30 to 35 grams
- Keep your alcohol intake moderate (no more that 1 or 2 drinks daily)
- Don't smoke
- Make weight-bearing exercise part of your daily routine.

mone replacement therapy (HRT)—a combination of estrogen and progesterone—at menopause. ERT, coupled with a high-calcium diet and moderate exercise, is considered the best strategy to prevent rapid loss of bone density following menopause. Some researchers believe that, even when started later in life, estrogen provides some protective effect against hip fractures in older women.

Nevertheless, ERT is not a substitute for calcium. If you decide to begin ERT or HRT after weighing all the benefits and risks, you should continue to keep your calcium intake at recommended levels.

Other nutrients. Phosphorus is commonly believed to influence calcium absorption, but the jury is still out on its practical effect.

Researchers believe that phosphorus tends to suppress the urinary loss of calcium. However, too much phosphorus may accelerate loss of bone. To keep your phosphorous level in line, avoid consuming large quantities of foods labeled as containing sodium phosphate, potassium phosphate, phosphoric acid, pyrophosphate, or polyphosphate.

Physicians also prescribe calcitonin for women and men who already exhibit signs of osteoporosis or for postmenopausal women who are not using estrogen replacement therapy. This naturally occurring hormone helps to regulate calcium absorption and bone development and slows the natural breakdown of bone. Recent medical studies also indicate that bisphosphonates, another group of naturally occurring compounds, can slow bone loss. Researchers are giving a great deal of attention to the role that biophosphonates may play in treating osteoporosis. Someday these substances may replace calcitonin for certain kinds of cases.

Exercise. Weight-bearing exercises—activities that force bones to work against gravity—are important for preventing osteoporosis. Walking, probably the most beneficial weight-bearing exercise, can help to maintain overall body strength and stability even in very elderly people. Other desirable activities for people of all ages are racquet sports, basketball, soccer, hiking, skiing, jogging, aerobic exercise, dancing, stair climbing, rollerblading, bicycling, and rowing.

Remember that the benefits of these activities last only as long as you continue them. If you are at risk of developing osteoporosis, you should make exercise an integral part of your life.

Prevention of osteoporosis requires attention to diet and lifestyle issues throughout your life. We can make sure children and grandchildren grow up with strong bones, but what about ourselves? Are we doomed to fractures because of all those glasses of milk we never drank?

No matter what your age or the present state of your bones, it's never too late to slow the process of osteoporosis or reduce the possibility of broken bones. Don't look back; look ahead. Start now to eat a balanced diet that includes adequate amounts of calcium and no more than moderate levels of salt and caffeine. Encourage other family members—from toddlers to grandparents—to do the same. Exercise regularly, and reduce or eliminate your smoking and alcohol use. Then take advantage of the opportunity to use your strong, healthy bones for life. □

Chapter 29

Foods to Watch Out For When Taking Medication

Take three times daily with meals.... Do not take with dairy products.... Avoid alcoholic beverages. You've probably seen instructions like these many, many times on your prescription and over-the-counter medications. They are telling reminders that food and medicine can interact in numerous unsuspected ways. Some foods can reduce a medication's effectiveness; others may make it more effective (and possibly, even harmful). Likewise, certain medicines can undermine good nutrition, especially in people who had nutritional problems to start with.

Although some food/drug interactions may be quite dangerous, most don't produce any sudden or dramatic symptoms. However, they can cause bothersome side effects and minor nutritional deficiencies—problems that often

go unrecognized, according to Jeffrey B. Blumberg, Ph.D., professor of nutrition at Tufts University. "People may take a drug that doesn't seem to work—or that causes lethargy, irritability, confusion, or other symptoms—and then blame the drug or just old age," he says. "But the actual problem may be something like a drug-induced vitamin deficiency that could be easily corrected."

Doctors have trouble predicting when many of these interactions will occur. Scientists still have a lot to learn about how food and drugs affect each other and about the way the body uses trace nutrients—substances such as iron, zinc, and copper that are vital to health in very small amounts. These trace nutrients can also be affected by medicine.

Food/drug interactions also tend to be unpredictable because individuals vary considerably in their response to a particular medication, and because no two people eat exactly the same diet. We do know, however, that for some people the chance of a troublesome interaction is higher. Among those at greatest risk:

- The elderly, who are most likely to be taking one or more types of medication and to have other health and nutrition problems
- Heavy drinkers with liver or kidney disorders
- People who do not eat an adequate or balanced diet
- Men and women on special, restricted diets
- People with cancer or diseases of the stomach and intestines
- Pregnant and nursing women

If you are in any of these groups, make a special point of asking your doctor or pharmacist about food/drug interactions when you get a prescription for a new medication. And don't forget that the "over-the-counter" medications that you buy without a prescription—aspirin and antacids, for example—may also interact with food. Watch out for alcohol, too. It interacts badly with a large number of medicines.

How Food Affects Medicine

One factor couldn't be simpler: it's merely the amount of food in your stomach when you take your medicine. The size and composition of a meal determine how quickly the stomach empties its contents. That pill you swallowed will reach the small intestine for absorption into the bloodstream much faster after a light snack than after a three-course dinner. Many drugs are most effective on an empty stomach, with nothing to interfere with the breakdown of the medicine or slow its delivery to the rest of the digestive tract.

However, doctors often recommend taking medication with meals for several reasons. Mealtimes provide an easy reminder to take several doses a day. Some medicines—aspirin or nonsteroidal anti-inflammatory drugs

FOOD/DRUG INTERACTIONS THAT CAN CAUSE SERIOUS HARM

Most food/drug interactions do not have the potential for serious or permanent damage. But these do:

Potassium-rich food plus amiloride (Moduretic) or triamterene (Diazide, Dyrenium, Maxzide)

Taken together, they can result in toxic levels of potassium.

Double-concentrated grapefruit juice plus felodipine (Plendil)

This combination may result in dangerously high concentrations of the drug's active ingredient and possibly lead to heart rhythm problems.

Tyramine-containing foods plus furazolidone (Furoxone), isocarboxazid (Marplan), phenelzine (Nardil), selegiline (Eldepryl), or tranylcypromine (Parnate)

May cause dangerously high blood pressure.

Insulin and alcohol

This combination may cause a rapid worsening of low blood sugar (hypoglycemia).

Source: Red Book Database, Medical Economics

such as Advil or Nuprin, for example—can irritate the stomach lining unless they are buffered by food. Other drugs—including blood pressure-lowering medications such as clonidine (Catapres) and reserpine (Serpasil), and water pills such as chlorothiazide (Diuril)—actually work better on a full stomach.

But, while a meal can protect the stomach from some drugs and boost the potency of others, some of the things you eat can cause problems with certain medications. Difficulties with absorption head the list.

Foods can cut down on drug absorption, and vice versa. A familiar example is tetracycline, an antibiotic that binds with the calcium from dairy products in the small intestine. As a result, the gut absorbs less tetracycline—and less calcium, too. The result of this double-barreled interaction could be an infection that's slower to heal, plus a temporary loss of some bone-building calcium. To prevent this from happening, be sure to take tetracycline and several other types of antibiotics at least two hours before or after eating any dairy products or calcium-containing supplements or antacids.

MAO Inhibitor Means Caution

Some foods contain substances that react chemically with the active ingredients in certain drugs, making them more or less potent or even toxic. A prime example is the potentially deadly interaction between a food ingredient called tyramine and a class of drugs called the monoamine oxidase (MAO) inhibitors, which are prescribed for depression and, sometimes, for Parkinson's Disease. These drugs include the antidepressants isocarboxazid (Marplan), phenelzine (Nardil), and tranylcypromine (Parnate), as well as the Parkinson's drug selegiline (Eldepryl).

If you are taking these drugs, you must be careful to avoid all foods containing tyramine, including such items as hard cheese and aged soft cheeses, liver, pickled herring, yogurt, Chianti wine, and salami. (For more tyramine containing foods, see nearby box.) If you eat any of these foods while taking MAO inhibitors, your blood pressure could sky-rocket, creating the risk of a stroke or even death. (MAO inhibitors also react badly

FOODS AND BEVERAGES CONTAINING TYRAMINE

Avoid these selections if you are taking one of the antidepressant drugs such as Marplan, Nardil, or Parnate, the Parkinson's medication Eldepryl, or the infectious diarrhea remedy, furazolidone (Furoxone).

Foods

- Cheeses (except cream cheese, cottage cheese, and ricotta)
- Sour cream
- Homemade yogurt (Store-bought yogurt is all right.)
- Liver
- Smoked or pickled fish, such as herring
- Fermented sausages (salami, bologna, pepperoni, summer sausage)
- Brewer's yeast
- Canned or overripe figs
- Fava beans, broad beans (You may eat string beans and baked beans.)
- Fermented or aged foods
- Anchovies
- Avocados
- Soy sauce
- Chocolate

Beverages

- Red wine, Chianti, sherry
- Liqueurs
- Beer (including alcohol-free beer)

Clear spirits or white wines may be safe in moderation; ask your doctor how much, if any, is an acceptable amount. Your physician may also advise you to cut down or eliminate coffee, tea, and soft drinks containing caffeine; and to avoid such nonprescription medicines as cold or allergy pills and diet pills.

Adapted from: *The Over-50 Guide to Psychiatric Medications*, 1989.

with many other drugs. Make sure each doctor who treats you—and even your dentist—knows that you are taking an MAO inhibitor before prescribing any other medicines.)

Beware Licorice and Onions

Eating a lot of natural licorice, or taking herbal remedies that contain licorice, may interfere with the action of high blood pressure drugs, such as water pills. Licorice contains a substance that can cause the body to retain sodium; and this can push blood pressure up to unhealthy levels. Most licorice sold in the U.S. is artificially flavored, but some imported candies may contain the real thing.

The clot-preventing drug warfarin (Coumadin) may become too powerful—possibly causing bleeding problems—if you eat a lot of onions. Conversely, if you load up on foods rich in vitamin K (including green leafy vegetables such as spinach and Brussels sprouts) you might defeat the effectiveness of these anticoagulant drugs, because vitamin K promotes blood clotting.

Potassium: A Balancing Act

If you take drugs to lower blood pressure, it pays to keep an eye on potassium intake. This mineral may be affected by so-called water pills: thiazide diuretics such as hydrochlorothiazide (HydroDIURIL), and other diuretics such as furosemide (Lasix) and bumetanide (Bumex). These drugs help lower blood pressure by flushing out fluid and sodium, but they may also get rid of too much potassium, which is essential to the functioning of heart and muscles. Eating plenty of potassium-containing foods such as bananas and orange juice, often prevents depletion. Your doctor may also wish to test your potassium level, and might prescribe supplements if necessary.

On the other hand, some blood pressure medications do exactly the opposite, acting to block potassium loss. They include so-called "potassium-sparing" diuretics (Aldactone, Dyazide, Moduretic,) and "ACE inhibitors" (Capoten, Prinivil, Vasotec). With these drugs, the danger is an accumulation of *too much* potassium, which can slow the heart, leading to weakness and even shock. If your physician prescribes one of these drugs, avoid using potassium supplements or salt substitutes containing potassium. Moderate amounts of potassium-containing foods, however, are safe.

How Drugs Affect Nutrition

A number of common prescription and nonprescription drugs can sabotage good nutrition. People who must take drugs at high doses or for extended periods are at highest risk. The drugs can erode nutrition in several ways.

SOME FOODS THAT INTERFERE WITH DRUGS

Foods	Drugs
Dairy products	Tetracycline
High-sodium foods	Diuretics
High-fiber foods	Digitalis
High-protein foods	L-dopa
Leafy vegetables	Warfarin
Soybeans, cabbage, kale	Thyroid hormone

SOME DRUGS THAT CAN CAUSE NUTRITIONAL DEFICIENCIES

Drugs	Deficiency
Birth control pills and estrogen-replacement therapy	Folic acid, vitamin B_6
Certain water pills	Magnesium, potassium
Isoniazid	Niacin, vitamin B_6
Questran	Vitamins A, B_{12}, D, E, and K
Seizure drugs and sedatives	Calcium, folic acid, vitamins D and K
Steroid medications	Vitamins B_6, C, and D

Tough On the Taste Buds

Some medications can alter the sense of taste, either blunting flavors or making some foods taste different or "off." Among the drugs that may have this effect are penicillin, an antifungal medication called griseofulvin (Fulvicin, Grifulvin), the cholesterol-lowering drug cholestyramine (Questran), and medications used in chemotherapy for cancer.

Many other medicines can cause dry mouth, making it difficult and unpleasant to chew and swallow. These include some allergy drugs (antihistamines), high blood pressure medications, and antidepressants.

Appetite Beaters

There is a long list of drugs that cause digestive upset, including pain killers, estrogen preparations, and cholesterol-lowering medications. Some drugs take the edge off the appetite; others can make you feel miserable—nauseated, bloated, and gassy.

Constipation or diarrhea are other common causes for a loss of appetite, especially in older people. Among the drugs causing constipation are codeine, morphine, and iron supplements. If you are taking powerful painkillers, ask your doctor about using a stool softener or other preventive.

If you experience any digestive symptoms or just find yourself losing weight—especially after starting a new medication—tell your doctor. The answer may be as simple as changing the amount or timing of your dosage, or switching to a different medication in the same category. But don't try such experiments on your own, particularly with prescription drugs!

Physicians prescribe some drugs deliberately to suppress appetite for purposes of weight control. However, using appetite-controlling drugs on a long-term basis is controversial and can be dangerous. A healthy diet and exercise are the keys to weight loss; ask your doctor before taking any over-the-counter appetite suppressants.

Appetite Boosters

Some drugs stimulate appetite to such an extent that overeating becomes a temptation. These include blood-sugar-lowering medications for diabetes such as chlorpropamide (Diabinese), glipizide (Glucotrol), glyburide (Micronase), and tolbutamide (Orinase). Antidepressants and high doses of corticosteroid drugs may also trigger hunger pangs.

Absorption Problems

Certain drugs can cut down on the body's ability to extract nutrients from food in the same way as some foods can keep drugs from being properly absorbed. Antacids containing aluminum and calcium can keep the intestines from absorbing phosphorus, a mineral vital to healthy bones and teeth. Antacids can also impair the body's use of thiamin (vitamin B_1) and iron.

Both the antibiotic neomycin and certain other drugs, such as cholestyramine (Questran), impair the absorption of fat-soluble vitamins (for example, A, D and K.) Cholestyramine may also decrease the absorption of folate, cobalamin, iron, calcium, and magnesium.

The chronic use of laxatives may also affect absorption, especially when the laxatives act by irritating the lower intestines. The active ingredient in Ex-Lax can cause diarrhea; and people who use this product for extended periods of time may develop deficiencies in vitamin D and calcium. They may also run low on potassium as a result of losing a large amount of fluid in a short time. If you are troubled with constipation, ask your doctor about diet changes and fiber supplements that can help. To avoid becoming dependent on laxatives, use them sparingly and only as a last resort.

Certain drugs may include substances, such as the sodium found in many antacids and some forms of penicillin, that you may wish to avoid or eliminate from your diet. Some people are allergic to the inactive ingredients used in pills or capsules (starches, flavors, or coloring agents) and may need to take their drugs in a different form.

Alcohol

Few people think of alcohol as a drug; but it is. And alcohol, whether in cough syrup, wine, or any of its other forms, can interact with many different medications—sometimes in dangerous ways.

In large amounts, alcohol can suppress the cleansing action of the liver causing drugs to clear out of the body more slowly and thereby strengthening their effect. Watch out for alcohol in combination with:

- Sedatives, especially barbiturates (such as Nembutal or Seconal) and tranquilizers (Valium, Xanax, Ativan, and others). These medications can be dangerously potent when taken with alcoholic beverages.
- Blood-sugar-lowering drugs such as Diabinese, Glucotrol, Micronase, and Orinase, and an antibacterial drug called metronidazole (Flagyl). They can cause nausea and flushing when taken with alcohol.
- Nitroglycerin, often prescribed for chest pain. Combined with alcohol, it can dangerously lower blood pressure, causing dizziness and fainting.
- Aspirin. Taking large doses with alcohol can result in excessive stomach bleeding.
- Acetaminophen. Overdoses aggravated by alcohol can cause liver damage.

Special Concerns for Children

Children, too, are at risk for food/drug interactions. Their smaller bodies may respond to fluctuations in a drug's potency that an adult might not notice.

If your child is ill and cannot keep down food and medicine, ask the physician if there are any other formulations available (for example, a liquid instead of a pill). If a youngster regularly takes medication with meals, but illness has changed his or her regular eating patterns, check with a doctor or pharmacist before giving medication on an empty stomach, advises Leslie Hendeles, Pharm. D., professor of pharmacy and pediatrics at the University of Florida in Gainesville. This is especially important with theophylline, an asthma medication that varies widely in effectiveness depending on whether or not it is taken with food.

Children, like adults, can suffer indirect nutritional damage from drug side effects

INTERACTION QUICK REFERENCE

Taking this drug . . .	with these foods . . .	Can lead to:
Achromycin (tetracycline)	Dairy products	Reduced effectiveness of medicine
Altace (ramipril)	Salt substitutes containing potassium	Heart rhythm problems
Larodopa (levodopa)	High-protein foods (meat, fish, eggs)	Reduced effectiveness of medicine
Capoten (captopril)	Salt substitutes containing potassium	Heart rhythm problems
Coumadin (warfarin)	Foods high in vitamin K (leafy green vegetables)	Reduced effectiveness of medicine
	Foods high in vitamin E (boiled or fried onions)	Bleeding problems
Declomycin (demeclocycline)	Dairy products	Reduced effectiveness of medicine
Dyazide (triamterene)	Salt substitutes containing potassium	Heart rhythm problems
Eldepryl (selegiline)	Tyramine-containing foods	Dangerously high blood pressure
Isoniazid	Tuna, sauerkraut, yeast extract	Headache, palpitations, flushing, sweating, itching, diarrhea
Marplan (isocarboxazid)	Tyramine-containing foods	Dangerously high blood pressure
Maxzide (triamterene)	Salt substitutes containing potassium	Heart rhythm problems
Moduretic (amiloride)	Salt substitutes containing potassium	Heart rhythm problems
Nardil (phenelzine)	Tyramine-containing foods	Dangerously high blood pressure
Parnate (tranylcypromine)	Tyramine-containing foods	Dangerously high blood pressure
Plendil (felodipine)	Grapefruit juice	Disturbed heart rhythm
Prinivil (lisinopril)	Salt substitutes containing potassium	Heart rhythm problems
Sinemet (levodopa)	High-protein foods (meat, fish, eggs)	Reduced effectiveness of medicine
Vasotec (enalapril)	Salt substitutes containing potassium	Heart rhythm problems

such as nausea and diarrhea. By killing the good bacteria in the intestines, antibiotics such as amoxicillin (Amoxil) frequently prescribed for middle ear infections, can cause diarrhea; and long-lasting or severe diarrhea can result in debilitating losses of fluids and minerals. "To prevent this problem, try giving your child yogurt that contains active lactobacillus cultures," advises Hendeles. You can offer up to three servings a day, he says, but don't give your child antibiotics within two hours of serving yogurt or other dairy foods.

What You Can Do

Food/drug interactions are almost always either manageable or avoidable. It is important to recognize the signs of a possible reaction and to call your physician immediately if you suspect a problem. Your pharmacist or a registered dietitian are also excellent sources of advice when food and medication don't seem to mix. Working with these professionals and your doctor, it's usually possible to work out a medication plan that combats your health problem without undermining your diet.

Variety and moderation are the keys to a good diet. People who don't get enough calories or protein respond to drugs differently from those who are well-nourished. The problem is most serious in hospitalized or seriously ill people, but it can affect others as well, especially older people who aren't up to preparing adequate meals. If your calorie count is too low or you eat too few nourishing foods, tell your physician before starting to take a newly prescribed medication. He

may need to adjust your dosage until your nutritional status improves.

To keep food/drug interactions at bay, follow these common sense tips:

- If you are taking a medication on a regular schedule with no problems, stick to that routine. If you always take your pill on an empty stomach—or a full stomach—try to avoid a sudden switch.

- If you experience unpleasant new symptoms while taking any medication—even a drug you have been using for a while—ask your doctor about the possibility of side effects or interactions.

- When your doctor prescribes a new medication, let him or her know what other medications you are taking, including nonprescription or herbal remedies and vitamin supplements. Also mention how much alcohol you drink.

- Let your doctor know if you follow a special or restricted diet—especially one that is unusually high or low in a particular kind of food—or if you plan to begin such a diet.

- Don't forget that water is a key nutrient as well, and necessary to the proper absorption of medicine. Make sure you drink the equivalent of eight glasses of water a day, particularly in hot weather when dehydration is more likely. □

Chapter 30

What Smokers Need To Do About Diet

f you're a smoker, you're probably painfully aware that the tide of public sentiment has turned overwhelmingly against you. No longer are you and your smoldering cigarette merely tolerated; you are now an outcast—banned, or at least discouraged, from lighting up almost everywhere.

Today, smokers are ostracized; even smoking in a smoking section can draw complaints. On any city street, see the smokers huddle in office-building doorways, because their workplaces are smoke-free. Smoking in the open air on a park bench is asking for trouble, and smoking in someone else's home—unless that someone is also a smoker—is totally out of the question.

Smokers, once perceived as sophisticates or mavericks, are seen these days to be either hopeless addicts or boorish pollution–spreaders.

However, though the movement to ban cigarette smoking is more vociferous and effective than ever, it is by no means new: Throughout history, there have been scores of public attempts to curb smoking by pun-

ishing or segregating smokers. For example, in Constantinople during the 1600's, those who smoked in public were executed—in public. But Turkish smokers continued to light up anyway.

Though the first Romanov czar, Mikhail Feodorovich, sentenced smokers to whippings, beatings, and nostril-slittings, Muscovites paid Europe's highest prices for tobacco. Russian smokers were known to sell their clothes to finance their habit.

King James I of England decreed tobacco to be immoral and unhealthy. But when he tried to tax tobacco into oblivion, he instead created a bustling black market for it.

In America, an aggressive anti-smoking campaign linking cigarettes with maladies from colorblindness to constipation was conducted in the years before and during Prohibition. Many states attempted to pass highly restrictive laws governing tobacco use. Typical was Illinois, where legislation was proposed to "disenfranchise and render

THE DANGERS

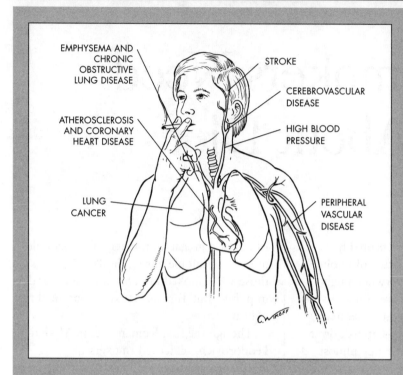

EMPHYSEMA AND
CHRONIC
OBSTRUCTIVE
LUNG DISEASE

STROKE

CEREBROVASCULAR
DISEASE

ATHEROSCLEROSIS
AND CORONARY
HEART DISEASE

HIGH BLOOD
PRESSURE

LUNG
CANCER

PERIPHERAL
VASCULAR
DISEASE

C. WIKOFF

Smoking does not inevitably lead to the diseases shown here; but it certainly increases the odds that you'll contract one or more of them. If you refuse to quit, you owe it to yourself to boost the protective elements in your diet to the highest levels considered safe by the experts.

[smokers] incapable of holding any office of trust or profit."

Once alcohol prohibition was achieved, it seemed that a similar fate was in store for tobacco. But by 1928 all anti-smoking regulations had been discredited or rescinded.

Today, the pendulum has swung again. We now know more than ever about the harmful effects of first- and second-hand smoke, and anti-smoking laws are beginning to reappear in response to a new round of attacks.
One thing remains clear, however: Despite extreme and punitive attempts to legislate the use of tobacco, people who are addicted to nicotine will continue to smoke. In light of this fact, according to the New York Academy of Sciences, any effort that reduces

the health risks associated with cigarette smoking is an "important health-care contribution to the peoples of the world."

The Risks a Smoker Must Combat

Although fewer people smoke now than ever before, more than one in six Americans—some 43 million people—still light up, according to the National Cancer Institute. These 43 million smokers place themselves at increased risk of cardiovascular and pulmonary diseases whose consequences can be painful, debilitating, or fatal. Such diseases include:

- Atherosclerosis (formation of fatty deposits in arteries) leading to conditions such as coronary heart disease
- Peripheral vascular disease (affects blood supply to the limbs)
- Cerebrovascular disease (affects blood supply to the brain)
- Emphysema and chronic obstructive lung disease

Additionally, smoking increases your risk of these and other cancers:

- Anogenital cancers
- Bladder cancer
- Cervical cancer
- Colon and rectal cancer
- Kidney cancer
- Acute leukemia
- Cancers of the larynx, pharynx, and mouth
- Lung cancer
- Pancreatic cancer
- Stomach cancer

Smokers are at a greater-than-average risk for scores of serious medical problems. In fact, in the words of a respected scientific journal, "it is difficult to find, in modern medical literature, a disease or abnormality which is not affected in some manner by cigarette smoking."

By now, you've surely heard the estimate that each cigarette you smoke shortens your life by eight minutes. You probably also recall former Surgeon General C. Everett Koop's warning that smoking is "the single most preventable cause of death, responsible for one out of every six deaths in the U.S." In addition, the American Cancer Society now states that 30 percent of all cancers are unequivocally caused by cigarette smoking.

Special Risks for Women

For women, smoking poses a number of additional dangers:

- Women smokers over the age of 35 have to stop taking birth control pills because of an increased risk of heart attacks and strokes.
- Smoking hastens development of osteoporosis, the "brittle bone" disease that affects many postmenopausal women. Studies indicate that women lose bone density in direct proportion to the number of cigarettes they smoke.
- Smoking when pregnant endangers your unborn baby, and can affect your new baby's health for years to come. Mothers who smoke have a higher risk of miscarriages. They more frequently give birth prematurely, more often to low birthweight babies.
- Maternal smoking has been associated with sudden infant death syndrome, impaired intellectual development of children, and other health and behavioral problems.
- Women smokers may have more difficulties associated with menopause; symptoms of menopause may arise earlier.

Cigarettes as Coffin Nails

Over 4,000 known toxic poisons—including formaldehyde, DDT and arsenic—are found in cigarettes. Here's an overview of just a few:

Nicotine. Defined by Dorland's Medical Dictionary as a "very poisonous alkaloid obtained from tobacco," nicotine appears to be unsafe at any level. One drop—the amount contained in 145 cigarettes—can be fatal. Nicotine causes blood vessels to constrict, which in turn raises your blood pressure. Nicotine causes an increase of blood fats, including cholesterol. Nicotine is highly addictive. Recovering alcoholics and drug addicts have reported that quitting smoking is harder than kicking drinking or drugs.

Tar. The tar in tobacco smoke contains chemicals called polynuclear aromatic hydrocarbons that scientists have implicated in some 40 to 80 percent of all human cancers.

Acetaldehyde. A disease-causing chemical found in cigarettes and smog, acetaldehyde acts as a free radical. Free radicals disrupt the body's normal molecular functions, and can cause damage which scientists have linked to accelerated aging and a variety of deadly diseases.

Heavy Metals. Lead, cadmium, radioactive polonium, and arsenic are just four of the poisonous heavy metals contained in cigarette smoke. These contribute to the suppression of the body's immune system and act as free radicals.

Carbon Monoxide and Nitrogen Oxide. These deadly gases destroy the ability of the blood to carry oxygen. They can oxidize blood fats and convert them into cancer-causing compounds.

The Best Advice For Smokers

If you're a smoker, try to quit. If you can't, make certain that you pay close attention to your diet and follow the recommendations in this chapter. Compelling evidence indicates that a diet rich in antioxidants (vitamins C, E, B-complex, and beta-carotene) may help protect your body against some of the ravages of smoking.

Ironically there is a solid body of evidence suggesting that smokers generally have *less* healthy diets than do nonsmokers. The studies vary, but nearly all bear out the fact that smokers eat fewer fruits, vegetables, whole grains, cereals and fiber than nonsmokers, while taking in significantly more meat, alcohol, coffee, fat, and cholesterol.

The research portrays smokers as a group who routinely fail to watch their health as closely as others. In 1987, the National Center for Health Statistics conducted a survey of 44,123 households to determine life-style differences among never, former, and current tobacco users. It found that, compared to nonsmokers, smokers:

- Take more risks
- Have more sexual partners
- Drink more alcohol
- Exercise and sleep less
- Don't take their vitamins as regularly as nonsmokers

And the more you smoke, the worse the picture looks: Poor health habits were found most often among the heaviest smokers. Despite all the grim statistics, however, it's obvious that most smokers fail to succumb to diseases directly attributable to their habit. What do the millions of smokers who never develop tobacco–related illnesses do differently? Quite possibly, these smokers may eat better and have healthier lifestyles. In fact, some studies show that the diets of former smokers more closely resemble those of never-smokers, suggesting that, at least in this group, there was a greater concern about general health.

Another clue: In Japan, where the per capita consumption of cigarettes is the world's highest, the incidence of lung cancer is nearly the world's lowest. Some experts credit the Japanese diet with the explanation: the Japanese eat less red meat and consume more fiber than do most Americans.

Supplements You Should Add to Your Diet

According to the New York Academy of Sciences, a variety of nutritional agents appear to reduce or inhibit the cancer–causing properties of cigarette smoke. These include antioxidant vitamins as well as other chemicals found in certain foods.

Elsewhere in this book, readers have been warned against taking vitamin supplements in excess of recommended daily allowances. They have been told that megadosing on vitamins—taking several times the recommended daily allowances of certain vitamins and nutrients—has not been shown to provide any health benefits.

However, smokers are in a nutritional class of their own. Their systems are continually bombarded with extraordinary levels of potent toxins. In view of this, smokers should weigh the probably minor risks of megadosing against the possible protective benefits that certain vitamins and minerals may provide.

Check with your doctor. If he agrees that the supplements are a safe bet for you, give them a try.

When considering which supplements to take, choose products from well-established, respected vitamin manufacturers. (See Chapter 2 for additional guidelines.) You should look for products that contain the following:

- Vitamin A (and its relatives, retinoids and retinoic acid);
- Vitamins C, E, and B-complex (especially B_{12})
- Beta-carotene
- Folic acid and folates
- Zinc
- Selenium

One approach to supplementation is typified in *Formula for Life,* by Eberhard and Phyllis Kronhausen. This is one of the better known books available about ways to protect yourself against the damage caused by environmental pollutants, stress, smoking, excess weight, and other threats to good health. The book notes that much—though not all—of the damage smoking does to your body is caused by free radicals, the highly reactive, unstable compounds that can oxidize (burn) molecules within the cells, including proteins, carbohydrates, fats, and even DNA. Conditions ranging from heart disease to cancer to cataracts have been blamed on the damage done by uncontrolled proliferation of free radicals in the body.

To keep free radicals at safe levels, the Kronhausens recommend the following "micronutrient menu" to their readers:

Vitamin C	2,000 milligrams
Vitamin E	100 international units (IU)
	(Others recommend 400 I.U.)
Glutathione	50–100 milligrams
	(an amino acid)
Beta-carotene	15 milligrams

B-complex Vitamins:

Thiamin (vitamin B_1)	80 milligrams
Riboflavin (B_2)	8 milligrams
Niacin (B_3)	40 milligrams
Calcium pantothenate (B_5)	240 milligrams
Pyridoxine	80 milligrams
hydrochloride (B_6)	
Cyanocobalamin (B_{12})	400 micrograms

Ergocalciferol (D_3)	125 I.U.
Calcium	250 milligrams
(as calcium carbonate)	

Some studies indicate that components of green tea (the kind served in many Asian restaurants) and red wine may be highly effective antioxidants.

In France, where consumption of both cigarettes and animal fats is high, the incidence of coronary heart disease is lower than would be expected. Some experts say red wine is the reason; studies have yet to find the ingredient responsible for this phenomenon.

Why Smokers Need Extra Fruits and Vegetables

Studies indicate that certain micronutrients found in fruits and vegetables may protect smokers against the toxic effects of tobacco smoke. Some of these nutrients are the same antioxidants provided by vitamin supplements, but others can be obtained only from the fruits and vegetables themselves.

The National Cancer Institute says that 5 to 9 daily servings of fruits and vegetables help protect against cancer. In the face of studies on the importance of antioxidant vitamins, smokers would be well-advised to eat at least nine servings, and even more, if possible. The National Cancer Institute defines a serving as 1 medium-sized fruit, 6 ounces of 100 percent fruit juice, a half cup of cooked vegetables, 1 cup of raw, leafy vegetables or a quarter cup of dried fruit.

Good choices include:

- Cruciferous vegetables—broccoli, cauliflower, cabbage, Brussels sprouts
- Green leafy vegetables—spinach, watercress, collard, turnip, and mustard greens, chard
- Citrus fruits
- Carrots, red peppers, winter squash, yams

More Fish, Less Meat for Smokers

Frequent consumption of the omega-3 polyunsaturated fatty acids found in fish may help protect smokers against chronic obstructive lung disease, according to one recent study. The researchers found that smokers who ate the most fish were less likely to have such respiratory problems as bronchitis, emphysema, or impaired lung function. They theorize that omega-3 acids inhibit the inflammatory processes triggered by tobacco smoke.

Since smoking raises your cholesterol level and promotes the development of fatty deposits in the arteries—just like the saturated fats in meat—a meat-eating smoker doubles his risk. So if you won't cut down on cigarettes, at least cut back on meat—and replace it with fish whenever you can.

TEN TIPS FOR QUITTING

(From Successful Programs and Successful Ex-smokers)

1. Pick a start date, not too far in the future. List all your reasons for quitting. Perhaps you want to see your children grow up, or be around to hold your first grandchild. Review your reasons daily before your quit date, then choose the one that's most important to you. Write it on several index cards and post them prominently around your home and office. Tuck one into your pocket. Tape one on your wallet. Stick one on the fridge. Put one wherever you keep cigarettes.

2. In the days leading up to "Quit Day," change your smoking habits. Switch to another brand. Use matches instead of a lighter, or vice versa. Keep track, and note on a piece of paper, when and why you smoke each cigarette. Delay smoking whenever you can. Start eliminating or delaying your "ritual" cigarettes—the morning-coffee cigarette or the after-dinner cigarette.

3. Decide whether you'll need support or will try "cold turkey." Join a smoke-ending program if you need the support of a group. Check with local heart and cancer groups to find a compatible class. Hypnosis is considered highly effective. See your doctor and get a prescription for a nicotine patch or nicotine gum. Get one of the video tapes on how to stop smoking. Read up!

4. Tell friends, co-workers, and family members that you're quitting and enlist their support. Tell them what day will be "Quit Day." Be specific about anything they can do to help—like calling you right after dinner, or taking a brisk walk with you at lunch time. You'll be amazed how supportive people are at a time like this! Consider asking a fellow smoker to join you in quitting.

5. When it's "Quit Day", quit. Make it a big production. Be extra kind to yourself. Reach for a carrot or a stick of gum instead of a smoke. Don't worry if you are short-tempered, nervous, or unable to concentrate. These withdrawal feelings will subside in a day or two. Think in terms of five minutes. Tell yourself, "I've gone five minutes without a smoke. I can go five more." Remember that each urge to smoke passes quickly. Visualize each urge as a big wave you're going to sail right over. Think positively. Physical activity is very helpful.

6. Remove all your smelly old ashtrays and smoking paraphernalia. Place flowers, potpourri, or framed pictures of loved ones where ashtrays and smoking areas used to be.

7. Have your teeth cleaned. Put your cigarette money in a jar and watch it grow every day. Then spend it on something special at the end of a week. Reward yourself by going to the movies or theater.

8. Drink lots of water—keep a glass handy to sip from at all times. A squeeze of lemon juice makes it more refreshing. You are likely to gain a couple of pounds, but if you watch what you eat and literally count calories, you probably won't go overboard.

9. For the first week or so, avoid situations where it's easy to cheat. Stay out of smoking sections and bars, and try to avoid your former smoking buddies—especially those who really don't want you to quit.

10. If you should slip and have a cigarette, don't think of it as a failure. Review your reasons for quitting, re-imprint them in your consciousness, and try again—maybe this time with a different support technique.

Are You Ready To Quit Yet?

Yes, it seems to be true: Smokers can, to some extent, curb at least some of tobacco smoke's damage—by taking special combinations of vitamins, eating at least nine servings of fruits and vegetables a day, increasing their consumption of fish, and lowering consumption of saturated fats.

But you have to ask yourself: Is it really worth it? Are the pleasures of smoking worth all the trouble and risk?

If you can unequivocally answer "yes," then dig into those vegetables, down those vitamins, tear into that halibut . . . and find an isolated place where you can light up. *And* keep your fingers crossed that you don't develop lung cancer, heart or respiratory disease, or any of the many other conditions that smoking may aggravate.

There are a Million Reasons for Not Quitting

If you are a truly addicted smoker, like most of those who smoke, deep down you really *do* want to quit. What prevents you from trying is your fear of the consequences.

You'll gain weight and get fat. Your job and life are already so stressful that you'll snap when you quit. You won't know what to do with your hands. You won't be able to concentrate. Quitting will hurt in awful ways you can't even imagine. Quitting might even be physically painful. And you know for sure that quitting will make you crazy, at least temporarily. There are even many smokers (the writer Kurt Vonnegut is one) who believe that quitting after a lifetime of smoking could wreak dangerous havoc on your body. Creative people fear losing their gifts. And statistics tell you that quitting smoking is difficult—even impossible for some people.

To make quitting successful, you must turn it into a challenge only you are smart and strong enough to overcome.

The Benefits of Quitting are Yours, Quickly

Those who quit smoking soon have much to celebrate. Within a day, your body's levels of toxic carbon monoxide and nicotine will rapidly decrease. Your sense of taste and smell may improve, as may your stamina. Though you may still cough, no longer will it be a smoker's cough; your cough is now one of recovery, as your lungs begin to detoxify themselves.

Your risk for pancreatic and esophageal cancer decreases almost immediately when you quit. By the end of your first nonsmoking year, your risk of a heart attack begins to decrease too. Eventually, your statistical risk of developing smoking-related diseases will mirror those of people who've never smoked at all: Sometime between your seventh and tenth nonsmoking anniversary, your statistical chance of having a heart attack, or developing bladder, lung, and other cancers approaches that of people who have never smoked. □

Keeping the Fun in Your Food

CHAPTER 31

Fitting Health into Your Everyday Meals

For most of us, switching to a healthier diet means changing some deep-seated habits: preparing dishes like mother never made them; spending more time in the fresh vegetable aisle of the supermarket; and keeping balance and nutrition in mind along with taste.

This change doesn't have to be a chore. It can be a pleasant, even exciting, process as long as we recognize that it *is* a big change—something that can only be accomplished gradually, not in an instant. Taking the time to examine your present eating patterns can help you decide which changes are most important right now, and which ones can be postponed until you've gotten comfortable with the first round of adjustments.

This chapter tells how to assess your current eating habits, zero in on healthy changes, and devise a plan that suits your own lifestyle and tastes. It then shows how to put that plan into practice through savvy shopping, healthier cooking, and balanced menu planning.

Step One:
Discover What You Really Eat

A food journal is a great way to evaluate your food habits. "Most people who have made successful lifestyle changes have used some form of record keeping," notes nutritionist Kathryn Parker, RD, of the Women's Diagnostic Center, Gainsville, Florida. "It's a great reality check." While keeping a food journal is the method recommended by many nutritionists, more abbreviated forms of record keeping can work just as well.

The results of a food journal analysis are likely to surprise you. People who fear that their eating habits are deplorable will probably discover they have pockets of healthy tastes and habits to build upon. And those who are sure they're on the nutrition honor roll may discover that their idea of a "portion" is two or even three times larger than what nutritionists have in mind. People often underestimate their daily intake by as much as 50 percent.

A food journal also helps you see how your eating habits fit into your everyday routine, allowing you to target mutually reinforcing habits for easier change. Research shows that this type of self-monitoring and daily record-keeping does help you modify in-grained behavior.

Any type of notebook, calendar, or computer file that is easy to consult frequently can serve as a food journal. Entries should include:

- What you ate
- How much you ate
- Where you ate
- What your motivation for eating was
- What else you were doing at the time

It's important to enter every meal and snack, including such "incidentals" as that bagel and coffee you had at the staff meeting, the two meatballs and chunk of cheese you ate while "test-tasting" the results of a dinner in progress, or even the box of cough drops you finished during the course of the day.

Once you've kept a journal for a week, put aside some time to analyze the results. Use the calorie and nutrient tables at the end of the book to calculate your calorie and fat intake for each meal and snack, and then add up your daily counts. This will give a realistic picture of what you currently eat.

Reading through the journal will raise your awareness of the specific foods you favor as well as your overall eating patterns. You will get to know your food cravings, and may find helpful patterns (such as a tendency not to snack in the evening if you've had a fruit desert with dinner). You can then incorporate this knowledge into your meal-planning. For example, if find you often crave sweets in the late afternoon, you can anticipate your desire and keep healthy substitutes like fruit on hand. Or, if you find that your motivation for eating is often not hunger but to reward yourself for a completed task, you can build this awareness into your plan by finding alternative ways to celebrate. Identifying your particular needs, desires and lifestyle will help you to create an individualized plan for improving your diet.

If the idea of keeping a complete food journal seems too bothersome, there are other ways to assess your daily intake of nutrients. Try focusing on one nutrient each week or month. For example, if you have a high cholesterol level you can record all the saturated fats you eat and then compare this figure with the recommended amount. When you have a good sense of your fat intake and how to adjust it, you can move on to another food group—for example, counting fruit and vegetable intake for a week. Another option is to consult a dietician for help in assessing your current nutritional status—a method particularly recommended for people with special medical needs and those with longstanding weight-control problems.

Reluctance to assess your current intake may itself signal an important attitude toward food. Many people think that nothing they now eat is nutritionally "good." They want to wipe the slate clean of all current habits and start over. It's a good idea to try to overcome this reaction, since virtually everyone has *some* good eating habits. It's easier to retain these patterns and plan improvements to be added, instead of totally rejecting all of your favorite meals. On the other hand, resistance may mean that now is not the right time in your life to change your eating habits. A dietetic makeover does involve some work and the food journal is merely the first step. People with serious health problems (such as binge eating) often avoid keeping track of food. If you find that you're afraid to keep a journal, you might want to consider consulting a professional.

Step Two: Compare the Real and Ideal

Issued by the U.S. Departments of Agriculture and Health and Human Services in 1992, the Food Pyramid provides the latest daily dietary guidelines for Americans. Use it as a guide to making healthy choices, ones that hopefully lead to a nutritionally balanced diet. The Pyramid is useful as a backdrop to any individualized nutrition plan. The overall recommendations are to:

- Eat a variety of foods
- Maintain a healthy weight
- Go easy on fat, saturated fat and cholesterol
- Eat plenty of vegetables, fruit, and grain products
- Use sugars, salt, sodium, and alcohol only in moderation

The Food Pyramid is divided into five food groups. At the bottom is the bread, cereal, rice and pasta group with a recommended six to eleven daily servings. The next level includes the vegetable group (3 to 5 daily servings) and the fruit group (2 to 4 daily servings). Next come 2 to 3 daily servings from the milk, yogurt, and cheese group, and another 2 to 3 servings from the meat, poultry, fish, dry beans, eggs and nut group.

On the top are fats, oils and sweets (to be used only sparingly).

When comparing your own diet to the Food Pyramid recommendations, first take a global view. Do you eat enough servings of fruit, vegetables, grains, and low fat dairy products every day? Do you overeat foods from certain groups such as beef, cheese, french fries, or chocolate? Keep in mind that while no foods need to be completely eliminated from a healthy diet, most Americans do need to adjust the amounts they eat from each of the food groups.

Individualizing the Food Pyramid

The paradox in today's nutrition research is that there are two opposing trends. The first is to search for common nutritional denominators for everyone—symbolized in the Food Pyramid. The second trend is to individualize nutritional needs. Your unique metabolism, health problems, tastes, lifestyle, and stress level may all affect the diet that's best for you.

The Food Pyramid is based on a 2,000 calorie a day diet that you may need to adjust according to your age, gender, and weight. Young children can eat smaller servings but should have the equivalent of 2 cups of milk per day. Optimal diets for teenagers and adults range between the following levels.

- 1,600 calories: This level is right for most inactive women and older adults.
- 2,200 calories: Most children, teenage girls, active women, and inactive men do well at this calorie level. Pregnant and breast-feeding women generally need more.
- 2,800 calories: For teenage boys, active men, and some very active women this caloric level is appropriate.

WHAT A CALORIE LEVEL ACTUALLY MEANS

	Lower: about 1,600	Moderate: about 2,200	Higher: about 2,800
Bread Group Servings	6	9	11
Vegetable Group Servings	3	4	5
Fruit Group Servings	2	3	4
Milk Group Servings	2-3[1]	2-3[1]	2-3[1]
Meat Group (ounces)	5	6	7

[1]Women who are pregnant or breastfeeding, teenagers, and young adults to age 24 need 3 servings.

The box on "What a Calorie Level Actually Means" shows what you typically should eat to maintain each level.

What's In a Serving? Serving size does count, and research shows that the average American portion is bigger than ever. A dinner-plate-size serving of pasta in restaurants and many homes equals 2 to 3 helpings of pasta on the Food Pyramid. A jumbo bagel equals 4 servings of bread. The box on "What Counts as a Serving" gives examples of serving sizes from the five food groups.

Adjusting for Activity Levels

Your current activity level profoundly affects your nutritional needs. Someone who cares for active youngsters, cleans house, works in the garden, and usually walks to do errands burns many more calories than one who drives to work and sits at a desk all day.

Likewise, someone who exercises for 30 to 60 minutes 3 to 4 times a week has different nutritional needs than a couch potato.

If you tend to lead a sedentary lifestyle, you need to be especially vigilant about your eating habits. Specifically, you need to limit your fat intake and be suspicious of your body's hunger signals. When a person is active, the body tends to give accurate messages about hunger levels. Sedentary people need to rely more on external guidelines for scheduling meals. An even better approach is to begin to move toward a more active lifestyle. A mild 20-minute walk or light workout will help you get in touch with your internal monitor, as well as increasing your metabolic rate, energy level, and stamina. Physical activity also allows you to eat more and is important in maintaining weight loss.

Active people who engage in physical workouts on a regular basis need to adjust their meal-plan accordingly. The most important recommendation is to eat carbohydrate-rich food within 1 to 2 hours of a vigorous workout. Stored energy in muscles, called glycogen, will be replenished by this food. Regular fluid intake before and during each workout is also important to maintain your energy level, since most energy loss during exercise is caused by mild dehydration. For more on exercise and energy, see Chapters 8 and 21.

Factoring in Your Specific Health Concerns
The Food Pyramid is a graphic representation of the basic dietary recommendations that most experts agree will keep your weight in control, provide needed vitamins and minerals, reduce cholesterol, and help you avoid heart disease, high blood pressure, and some cancers.

However, to reach specific health goals you need to modify the standard serving recommendations in the pyramid. If you want to lose weight, for example, you should reduce your intake of fat and sugars though you still need to eat at least the lowest number of recommended servings from each of the five major food groups. Those who seek to gain weight can increase the amounts of food they eat from each of the food groups.

If a high cholesterol level is your concern, cutting your intake of saturated fats is essential. Each of the five food groups should still be part of your daily menus, but substitute low-fat choices for such high-fat items as eggs, butter, salad dressings, oils and shortenings, cheese, ice cream, and other whole-milk byproducts. Eating the higher serving recommendation for grains, fruits, and vegetables, and the lower limit for lean meats and poultry is also good strategy.

WHAT COUNTS AS A SERVING

Breads, Cereals, Rice, and Pasta
1 slice of bread
1/2 cup of cooked rice or pasta
1/2 cup of cooked cereal
1 ounce of ready-to-eat cereal

Vegetables
1/2 cup of chopped raw or cooked vegetables
1 cup of leafy raw vegetables

Fruits
1 piece of fruit or melon wedge
3/4 cup of juice
1/2 cup of canned fruit
1/4 cup of dried fruit

Milk, Yogurt, and Cheese
1 cup of milk or yogurt
1-1/2 to 2 ounces of cheese

Meat, Poultry, Fish, Dry Beans, Eggs, and Nuts
2-1/2 to 3 ounces of cooked lean meat, poultry, or fish

Count 1/2 cup of cooked beans, or 1 egg, or 2 tablespoons of peanut butter as 1 ounce of lean meat (about 1/3 serving)

Source: *FDA Consumer*

Tailoring Your Menu to Your Lifestyle
Where you eat your food is an important factor when planning a weekly menu. Americans are eating out and ordering more take-out food than ever. In 1993, 43 percent of American food dollars were spent on food prepared outside the home, compared to 25 percent in 1955, according to the National Restaurant Association. If you are part of this trend, you need to factor that into your plan, rather than trying to change your lifestyle.

Home meals vs. restaurants. Record how many meals you actually prepare at home for a week or two. Afterwards, you can plan your shopping and meals based on a realistic picture of how often you cook. This helps to avoid frustration over spoiled food or the failure of a plan unsuited to your eating habits. Healthy strategies for dining out can be found in Chapter 38. It's usually easier, however, to improve your diet if you prepare food more often at home—where you control exactly what ingredients go into your meals. Gradual adjustments more often lead to success. If you find that you actually cook a meal once a week, for example, start by trying to cook twice a week. Or try a cooking class.

Singles and cooking for one. Single people usually have more flexible lifestyles and, therefore, need a flexible meal plan. They favor simple cooking strategies and quickie meals. If you take a few minutes to plan ahead, you can have nutrition at your fingertips. Cook a few meals at once and freeze them, and on those tired or rushed evenings, you'll have a dinner that just needs to be heated. Prepared microwave meals are also great for singles, but be aware that they should have no more than 10 to 15 grams of fat and no more than 1,000 milligrams of sodium. If you have the right food available, you are likely to save money and eat less fatty foods on the run.

A major issue for singles is the storage of fresh fruits and vegetables. One idea is to shop with a friend and share the vegetables or cook them together. If you're too busy to peel and chop, buy vegetables from the grocery store salad bar; you'll lose some vitamins due to previous chopping, but this is still a nutritious choice. If you buy fresh vegetables that don't last long, use them in the beginning of your week. Purchase others that will keep for a week or more, such as artichokes, beets, cabbage, carrots, and potatoes. Frozen vegetables are very useful for singles and have about the same nutritional value as fresh ones. Choose fruit that will keep well, such as apples, dried fruit, and citrus fruit. If you have a hard time remembering to eat fruit, keep some that doesn't need to be refrigerated on the table.

Working couples. Meal planning for working couples calls for both communication and independence. Many couples are on different schedules; if that's true in your case, flexibility is important. Eating with your partner is a good goal, but try to let go of the notion that all meals should be eaten together. If one of you gets home first, it may be better to eat a meal alone than to snack until the other arrives. If your schedules are exactly alike, meal-planning is simpler, but differences may still crop up over food preferences. It's usually best for everyone to make their own choices, rather than for one person to compromise and be left feeling unsatisfied and resentful.

Even with all these variables, meal-planning is still possible. Try sitting down on Sunday night and discussing what your week's schedule looks like, when you'll be able to eat together, and what you want to serve. Based on this, you can create a shopping list and a meal-plan for the week. A little preparation in the morning can go a long way for working couples. If you take out the ingredients or put the water in the pot when the sun rises, then you can come home at night and cook dinner with less thought and effort. Always have staples in the house for quickie meals on those evenings when cooking is out of the question.

Feeding a family. When you're cooking for a family, it's almost impossible to change your eating habits without affecting the entire group. Children are likely to provide the biggest challenge, but it's never too early to start a good nutrition plan for children. This doesn't mean putting them on the same plan as yourself. Instead, find where the two plans coincide and where flexibility is needed.

Research shows that the silent example is your most powerful tool for teaching children about healthy eating. Don't refer to "good" or "bad" foods, but rather show your children that there are *everyday* foods and *occasional* foods. High-fat foods can be "treats," whereas healthy foods can be eaten whenever hungry. Snacks are good for children and can be used as part of a regular daily diet. Fixed meal times, however, are the most reliable way to promote healthy eating habits. Nutritious foods are more appetizing when varied and colorful. Always include at least one of a child's favorite foods. Ask children to help you with the shopping and cooking. This gives you a teaching opportunity and encourages the kids to become involved in meal decisions. Dietitians advise parents to encourage children to develop their own food preferences and plan their own meals. Some suggestions to balance children's nutrition plans include: whole-grain crackers, fruits, low-fat cheese, mini-pizzas and vegetable sticks with low-fit dips.

Phases when the child wants the same food over and over are normal. If abnormal eating habits continue for long periods, consult a pediatrician. Teenagers may reject their parents' eating style; just continue to provide nutritious foods and set a good example. Many children and teens develop food idiosyncrasies which often change as fast as their shoe size if parents stay flexible and avoid criticism. Activity levels also affect children's dietary requirements. The main contributor to excess weight in childhood is inactivity. Encourage kids to participate in physical activities, games, or sports. When children are active, be sure to provide enough fluids and carbohydrates, including plenty of fruits, vegetables, starches, and grains.

Older People. Aging affects nutritional needs. Metabolism slows down in middle age, resulting in reduced calorie requirements and an increased need for these calories to be packed with nutrients. Food preferences may change, too. Dairy products become harder to digest. More fiber may be needed to promote digestion and relieve constipation. Calcium requirements rise in older women as hormonal changes deplete the body's supply. Aging also causes signals of thirst to weaken possibly leading to dehydration and making a regular routine of fluid intake very important.

A good meal plan for seniors must also take account of a potential increase in the need for vitamins and minerals. Heart problems may dictate a low-fat, low-cholesterol, low-salt diet. And some of the numerous medications prescribed for the elderly may conflict with even the best of meal plans. An in-depth look at the nutritional needs of the aged can be found in Chapter 20. For more on the conflict between food and drugs, turn to Chapter 29.

Step Three:
Design a Blueprint for Change

Without rules to serve as guideposts, it's almost impossible to reach a goal. However, inability to fit a set of arbitrary, unrealistic rules into your lifestyle is one of the most common reasons for a diet plan to fail. This failure often leads to conclusions such as, "If I can't measure all my portions, I'll never be healthy" or "since I hate cottage cheese, I'll never be able to lose weight." Overemphasis on rules also can lead you to categorize foods as "good" and "bad," promoting unnecessary feelings of denial and guilt if you cross the line. But while feeling rule-bound can defeat your plan, a complete lack of structure and an "anything goes" approach is also unlikely to work.

Which Rules Are Necessary?

Creating your own rules is the best way to build a strategy you can live by. After you've assessed your current eating habits and decided on your goals, you're ready to write your own rules. As you begin, learn to listen to your body. Cravings often reflect your body's real needs.

The key to good rule-making is to incorporate the foods you love into your plan. Your rules should fit your lifestyle, too. For example, if you often eat out make it a rule to dine in restaurants that provide a variety of healthy choices. If you've found that you consume too many calories while cooking, make it a rule to keep peeled carrots around for kitchen snacking. You might also ask your partner to "taste-test" your dishes. If being too careful during holiday meals dampens your good time, you can make a rule to be flexible on holidays but to return to your eating plan as soon as possible.

It also helps to formulate rules as steps toward a permanent change. For example, one man wanted to move toward low-fat dairy products, but hated the taste of skim milk in his morning coffee. He decided to keep a small container of Half and Half in the refrigerator to use with coffee, while switching to low-fat yogurt and cheeses to hold down his fat consumption. Months later, when his tastes had changed due to his first diet adjustments, he found he could enjoy his coffee with 2-percent milk.

Remember that it's not always necessary to sacrifice what you want for what you're told you need. For example, one woman strongly preferred toast to fruit in the morning. So she simply saved her fruit servings for mid-day and bedtime snacks.

To maintain a balanced diet try keeping a mental record of what you've eaten that day and what you plan to eat. Don't set yourself up for failure by making rules that are too ambitious, complex, or difficult to abide by. Remember: if one rule doesn't work out, you can always replace it with one that does!

Going Step by Step

Try to make the *process* of changing as rewarding as the results. Be patient. For this change to be real and long lasting, it's best to go slow. If the process feels unnatural and traumatic, it's unlikely to succeed. However, if it's easy and (relatively) pleasant then it may have a chance.

Approach change positively. Regard nutritious eating not as a punishment but as a liberation from all the side effects of unhealthy eating. Stop and appreciate the food you *are eating*, rather than focusing on what you *are not eating*. Focus on the benefits you hope to attain, and write them down to refer to in challenging situations. Talk about your accomplishments and allow yourself to feel good about changing.

Line up support. Research shows that supportive relationships are important in changing any habit. Tell others about the changes you're planning and the reasons you're making them, and enlist your friends' support. If possible, find a good role model who has succeeded in making nutritional changes or a support group of people who are facing similar situations.

Reinforce success. For long-term success you need positive reinforcement. A true improvement in health status will promote good feelings that feed on themselves as a constant reinforcement. Concrete rewards are a more tangible way to reinforce success. They can be anything that gives you pleasure, but should not involve food or drink.

A positive mind-set should be a constant reward. At the end of the day, don't waste time going over in your mind the goals you may not have met. Instead, savor what you *did* accomplish. Set small, tangible goals that you can reach with every meal—and remember to congratulate yourself for meeting them.

Step Four: Put Your Plan into Action

What's so important about breakfast? The evidence is quite conclusive that eating this first meal of the day is conducive to health. Breakfast provides the necessary nutrients for productive mornings, and also helps control eating throughout the day. Those who eat breakfast tend to have more nutritious diets, lower cholesterol and fat levels, and fewer excess pounds. Breakfast eaters also have stronger problem solving skills early in the day, are less tired, and eat less at lunch and dinner.

Best Strategies for Breakfast

Here's some help for those who "never eat breakfast." If you are one of those people who are never hungry in the morning, try eating a *small* breakfast every day for 2 weeks. This will give your body time to adjust to a new eating schedule. If you leave home early, try brown bagging your breakfast and eating it later in the morning.

The next best thing to eating breakfast is to compensate for the missed nourishment throughout the day. For example, have fruit as a mid-day snack. To replace calcium and grain loss, have a bowl of cereal as a nighttime snack.

Ingredients of a healthy breakfast. A balanced, filling, and energizing breakfast should include three major nutrients: carbohydrates, protein, and fiber. For most days of the week, high-fiber breads and cereals with fruit and low-fat milk deliver just the right mix.

Keep a variety of fresh fruit, dried fruit, and fruit juice to eat alone or add to dishes. Breads and cereals should be whole or mixed grains. Try to rotate different types of grain throughout the week. For bread toppings, try fat-free jams and jellies or low-fat cottage cheese. Dairy products should be low- or no-fat, including milk, cottage cheese, and yogurt.

Reserve eggs and breakfast meats for weekends or special occasions. For recipes, try mixing fresh eggs with frozen egg substitutes and egg whites to reduce the fat. Switch to lean ham, turkey bacon, lean ground turkey, and Canadian bacon. French toast and pancakes can make healthy breakfasts when cooked in non-stick pans, served without butter, and topped with jam, fruit or syrup, and powdered sugar.

Lunch: Never in the Same Place Twice

Here are ways of solving the lunch dilemma. Some working people who frequently eat lunch in restaurants choose to make it their main meal of the day, but most people eat more lightly at lunch because of habit and time constraints. Bringing food for lunch and snacks from home can save money and help you avoid temptations. If you work at home, constant access to the refrigerator can be a challenge. It's a good idea to schedule a lunch break, take the phone off the hook, and give yourself time to create and enjoy a satisfying meal.

Ingredients of a healthy lunch. The core of a healthy lunch usually includes soup, sandwich, and salad. You can create endless variations from basic lunch ingredients. Stock up on a wide range of vegetables for salads and sandwiches. Cut enough vegetables for a few days and store them in the refrigerator for easy use. Experiment with different flavored low-fat dips and dressings to liven them up.

Choose lean turkey or ham instead of bologna or salami for lunch meats. Use low-fat cheeses sparingly. Whole grain breads will be more satisfying and nutritious. Try creating different sandwich spreads and fillings made from beans, canned fish, cottage cheese, and tofu. Sardines and canned salmon or tuna (packed in water) are good choices. Broth-based soups are better than cheese- or cream-based soups. Eat low-fat corn chips

and pretzels with your sandwich if you wish. Fruit, frozen yogurt, or fig bars make a fine dessert. Use leftovers for easy lunches.

Dinner: Sorting Through the Options

Although dinner possibilities are countless, most Americans cook only 10 to 12 entrées, notes William Castelli, M.D., Director of the well-known Framingham Heart Study. Traditionally, these meals consist of large portions of meat, chicken, or fish, with smaller side dishes of vegetables and grains. Your challenge today is to reverse those ratios and use larger portions of vegetables and grains and smaller helpings of protein. Potatoes, rice, pasta and breads are becoming entrées, while meats and cheese are becoming side dishes.

For some people, experimenting with new recipes and adjusting old ones for healthier eating turns out to be fun—as long as there's some time set aside for learning new tricks. Alternating easy meals with more challenging dishes can keep the workload under control. When adjusting recipies, focus on reducing added fat and replacing it with herbs and spices. It may take some trial and error, but it's a worthwhile project to find a few new recipes for vegetarian meals or dishes that use small amounts of meat or fish that you really enjoy.

Ingredients of a healthy dinner. Planning a week's worth of dinner entrées will help you shape a varied, nutritious meal plan. A workable framework to create balance could be to base entrées on each of these groups once or twice a week:

- Beef or pork once
- Chicken or fish twice
- Pasta or other grain twice
- Vegetables and beans twice

Whatever your main dish, make two to three servings of vegetables part of almost every dinner. To increase the use of vegetables at dinner time try the following tricks:

- Grill vegetables while grilling your meat
- Add vegetables to sauce when making pasta
- Fill baked potatoes with steamed vegetables
- Stir-fry vegetables for quick meals
- Use leftover vegetables in salads or soups
- Use fresh or poached fruits in salads and for desert

Between-Meal Snacks

If you are hungry, eat something. Snacks have become such a common part of the American diet that recent studies show our three-meal-a-day lifestyle turning into five meals a day. Eating frequent small meals not only fits many of today's diverse lifestyles, it may even be healthier. Consequently, snacks take on a more central role in current meal-planning strategies.

Keep healthy choices in the foreground. If the first thing you see when you open the refrigerator is a large chocolate cake, it takes a lot of will power to look any further for a snack. But if your eye falls on an inviting plate of raw vegetables and dip, you're likely to go for it. Stocking up on healthy snacks is one of the best ways to ward off temptation. When you leave the house, consider packing healthy food to take along. If you're a person who likes to munch frequently, accept that fact and prepare for the inevitable. Here are some suggestions for healthy snacking:

- Prepare by making dips from fat-free yogurt, sour cream, mayonnaise, or cream cheese; try pureeing canned beans with herbs and spices for a tasty change of pace.
- Keep on hand a variety of raw vegetables such as carrots, celery sticks, zucchini, parsnip, cauliflower, or broccoli florets.
- Use fat-free tortilla chips, breadsticks, toasted pita bread, and cut-up vegetables for dips.
- For crunchy snacks, try pretzels, low-sodium crackers, unbuttered popcorn, graham crackers, and rice cakes.
- Satisfy your sweet tooth with fresh and dried fruit. Canned pineapple is particularly satisfying. Hard candies are high in calories but contain no fat and are useful if you can eat them sparingly.
- Breads, rolls, and bagels spread with jam or jelly can be healthy, filling snacks.

Stocking The Kitchen

Upgrading the nutritional value of the ingredients you stock in your pantry will automatically make for healthier home cooking. There is no need to restock all at once. As you experiment with different ingredients and run out of items, gradually replace them with healthier alternatives. Here are some suggestions.

- **Flour:** Substitute whole-grain flours (such as whole wheat, buckwheat, rye, and oat flour) for refined flours to provide more fiber as well as B vitamins. Soy flour is also a good source of protein.
- **Grains:** Brown rice is more nutritious than white rice because of its higher fiber content. Interesting quick-cooking grains include Texmati and pecan rice, bulgur, pre-cooked couscous, kasha, and instant polenta.

■ **Vegetable Oils:** Safflower, sunflower, and corn oils are high in polyunsaturated fat. Olive, canola, and peanut oils contain monounsaturated fat. Substituting either kind for saturated fats like butter will help to lower your cholesterol level. Avoid palm and coconut oils, which are full of saturated fat.

■ **Legumes:** Beans, peas, and lentils are an excellent source of protein and fiber. They also provide B vitamins, iron, and calcium. Legumes are a key element of any low-fat menu plan because they can be used as a meat substitute when combined with a grain.

■ **Condiments:** Get rid of high-sodium and high-fat condiments such as Worcestershire, soy, and cream sauces, and regular mayonnaise. Substitute flavored vinegar, tomato paste, lemon juice, and mustard. Stock up on herbs and spices and use them to replace salt.

Navigating the Supermarket

Some people prefer to plan and shop for one or two days at a time; others prefer a big supermarket shopping trip once every week or two. Whatever your approach, health-conscious shopping is the foundation of a healthy diet. A comprehensive shopping list can help you focus. To save time, some people create a master shopping list, make photocopies of it, and then simply check off needed items each week. If you work you may not have the energy to plan ahead, but you can keep a healthy paperback cookbook at work and, at the end of each day, pick out a recipe and get the ingredients on the way home.

Cruising the aisles of a supermarket, chock-full of new products and competing health claims, can be a bit overwhelming. To make shopping less of a chore, simplify and prioritize your goals. The first week you might want to focus on buying low-fat dairy products; the next week you can check for the sodium content in the foods you are purchasing and make low-salt substitutions. Another way to keep it simple is to look for whole foods with no added ingredients. For example, 100 percent fruit juice is a whole food, compared with a fruit drink that may have only 10 percent fruit juice. The closer you get to a whole food, the more nutrients you will consume. Here's a quick tour of the major departments, with an eye to your healthier choices.

Fresh produce aisle. Fruit is a good low-calorie source of carbohydrates, fiber, vitamins A and C, and potassium. Remember, however, that dried fruit is higher in calories and avocados are high in fat. Most fresh fruit will keep for a week, and some will need to ripen at home. When buying canned or frozen fruit, look for labels that say "unsweetened" or "packed in its own juices."

Vegetables provide fiber, vitamins A and C, potassium, calcium, and iron. They lose nutrients easily if not cooked properly, however. The fresher the vegetables, the more nutrients; precut and on-sale vegetables tend to be less nutritious. Always check vegetables for soft spots and bruises. Buy canned and frozen vegetables as substitutes for those out of season. Check labels for sodium content and for added cream or cheese sauces that are high in fat and calories.

As interest in healthy eating grows, many new varieties of vegetables and fruits reach the market. Experiment with them and you may find some new favorites.

WHAT THE HEALTH CLAIMS REALLY MEAN

Health claims are proliferating on supermarket packaging. For accurate information, rely on the new, government-mandated nutrition labels rather than manufacturers' claims. Here are the official definitions of common "health" catch-words.

■ **Low calorie:** These products have less than 40 calories a serving, but a "serving" may be tiny. Be sure to check the size.

■ **Reduced calorie:** This type of food has at least one-third less calories than comparable products. "Reduced calories" does not mean reduced fat, however.

■ **Light/lite:** Don't assume this means less calories; light/lite can refer to many variables such as color and taste. Read the nutrition label to check the validity of this claim.

■ **Sugar Free/sugarless:** These products have no table sugar, fructose, or corn syrup. Check for ingredients that sweeten the product.

■ **Diet/dietetic:** Such foods should meet the requirements of low- or reduced-calorie products. If not, look for a clear explanation of why the food is a diet product.

■ **Sodium free/low sodium/reduced sodium:** "Sodium free" means no more than 5 milligrams of sodium per serving. "Low sodium" food will not have more than 140 milligrams, and "reduced sodium" will have at least 75 percent less sodium than comparable products.

■ **Low/no cholesterol:** "No cholesterol" translates into no more than 2 milligrams of cholesterol per serving. "Low cholesterol" means 20 milligrams or less, and "reduced cholesterol" has 75 percent or less cholesterol than comparable products. Watch out for products that say "no cholesterol" but don't mention the saturated fat.

■ **Enriched:** When flour is processed it loses nutrients. "Enriched" means some have been put back. An enriched product may not be as nutritious as its unprocessed counterpart.

■ **Fortified:** To add vitamins and minerals not naturally contained in food is to fortify it. This may be beneficial, but only if you need to make up a deficiency.

The meat counter. Poultry and meat are excellent sources of protein, iron and B vitamins. Lean cuts of beef have reduced fat and, ounce for ounce, more nutrients. Eaten with the skin removed, poultry provides the protein with less fat. Since most Americans get too much fat and protein, cutting down on meat, choosing leaner cuts, and removing all visible fat is important for almost everyone. Ask the butcher to help you identify the leanest cuts.

■ "Prime cuts" usually have the most fat
■ "Choice" is moderately fat
■ "Select" is lean meat

Examine meat for visible fat, check the sell-by date, and inspect for damaged packaging. Look for labeling that gives fat-to-lean percentages.

Processed meats are not recommended for people watching calories, cholesterol, sodium, or fat content. If you want processed meats, look for low-fat varieties made from turkey or chicken.

The seafood counter. Fish is a prime source of protein, vitamins, and minerals. Fish is often low in fat; and even when it is fatty, it may contain omega-3 fatty acids that lower your triglyceride levels and reduce the danger of blood clots. Shellfish is being recommended again for its low calories and fat. Avoid dried, salted, and smoked fish if you are watching your sodium. Pickled fish is also high in sodium. Choose water-packed rather than oil-packed tuna to reduce calories and fat as much as possible. Rinsing canned tuna will wash away much of the excess sodium. When buying fish:

- Sniff before you buy
- Reject prewrapped fish with damaged packaging
- When possible, select fish stored unwrapped on ice in glass cases
- When buying whole fish make sure there is no yellowing along the cut line
- Make certain that fresh lobsters and crabs are alive when purchased
- Remember that precooked fresh fish is safe to eat only on the day prepared.

The dairy case. Eggs provide protein and vitamin A—but also a substantial amount of cholesterol. Check for cracks before buying eggs. When you open them, signs of freshness are that the yolk holds together and the white doesn't run. Cholesterol-free egg substitutes are available in the frozen-food section.

Milk gives you calcium, protein, B vitamins and vitamins A and D. However, whole milk and hard cheeses are high in saturated fats. In selecting products, look for low fat and skim milk that is fortified with vitamins A and D; cheese made from skim milk; and low fat cottage and farmer cheese. When buying milk, choose cartons on the bottom of the display case and get the milk just

before you are ready to pay. Substitute nonfat dry milk or 1 percent liquid skim milk for cream, rather than using nondairy substitutes that are high in fat. When buying yogurt, reduce calories by buying fat-free plain yogurt and adding your own fruit and flavorings.

Staples on the shelf. Beans, lentils, peas, peanuts, and soybeans (the legume family) provide protein, fiber, and many essential vitamins and minerals. Legumes may be used as meat substitutes when consumed with a balanced diet. However, some people have trouble digesting legumes. If they are not already part of your diet, introduce them gradually.

To make sure legumes are fresh, look for bright color; cracks or discolorations may mean they are old. Give tofu (bean curd) a try. It's a high-protein vegetable food that is very low in calories. Use it to supplement other foods; it will take on the flavor of any dish.

White bread, still the most common choice, loses 90% of its fiber during processing. Whole wheat, rye, and multigrain bread provide much more. Bread with 2 or more grams of fiber per slice is a good choice. Always check the sell-by date to ensure freshness.

Cereal, pasta, and rice are also grain products. Cereal is a source of fiber, vitamins, and minerals. When selecting cereals check for sugar, sodium, and calorie content. Granola cereals often are high in saturated fat. Read the nutrition label, rather than the packaging advertisements, for information. When reading labels check the serving sizes.

Pasta is a good source of complex carbohydrates, fiber, B vitamins, and iron. While pasta is a low-fat choice in itself, remember that adding a cream sauce can turn it into a high-fat meal. Stick with vegetable-based sauces instead. Rice also provides complex carbohydrates, protein, and sometimes fiber.

OUTFITTING A HIGH-HEALTH KITCHEN

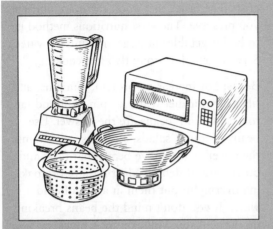

■ **Vegetable steamer:** This metal insert goes inside cooking pots. It holds vegetables above the water while cooking them with steam. This method preserves more of the nutrients than boiling in water.

■ **Non-stick pans:** These are used for sautéing meats and vegetables, frying eggs, and making omelettes with a minimum of butter or oil.

■ **Blender or food processor:** Both can mix, puree, chop, slice, and grate foods. Blenders can

be used to make nutritious drinks and soups. Food processors will chop and grate vegetables, making the preparation of healthy dishes less time-consuming.

■ **Microwave oven:** Because this speedy appliance uses moist heat, there is no need for butter or oil. The faster cooking preserves nutrients and leaves attractive color in fruits and vegetables.

■ **Wok:** Available in electric and stove-top models, this bowl-shaped pan is excellent for stir-frying meats and vegetables. Woks work well with little oil and cooks vegetables fast, preserving more nutrients.

■ **Skimmer/strainer:** Use this hand tool to remove congealed fat from the tops of casseroles, stews, and soups, thereby reducing fat and calories.

■ **Juicer:** This often cumbersome appliance converts fresh fruits and vegetables to juice. Use it to cut down on cost, sugar, and salt of commercial juices, while making fresh juice readily available.

■ **Hot-Air popcorn popper:** Popping corn without oil or butter keeps calories and fat low. It's great for late-night snacking.

White rice has little fiber left after processing; brown rice is a better source.

The current dietary rage is to replace saturated animal fats with unsaturated oils. This is a healthy move, but remember that vegetable oils are still 120 calories (per tablespoon) of pure fat, and that coconut, palm, and palm kernel oils do contain saturated fat. Try using small amounts of flavorful oils such as sesame, peanut, and olive oil. Remember that products advertising "100 percent vegetable oil" may still harbor highly saturated fats that can raise cholesterol levels

just as much as animal fat. Cholesterol itself never appears in vegetable oil, so don't be fooled by this manipulative advertising.

Nutrition-Wise Cooking

The latest cooking utensils make nutritious eating not only easy but quick. But remember that it takes a little time to learn how to use new equipment. Introduce new technology slowly. The box on "Outfitting a High-Health Kitchen" lists some of the best low- and high-tech items.

Often overlooked, food-preparation methods using high-health utensils can make a big difference in the quality of your diet. Use the following techniques to help preserve the nutrients in your food. These methods have the added benefit of reducing time spent in the kitchen.

Lean meats: The best methods for cooking meat and poultry are those that call for little or no addition of fat and, while draining off the fat already contained in the meat. These techniques include roasting, broiling, stir-frying, and microwaving.

Roasting and baking use dry heat. Broiling uses high, direct heat. Place the meat on a tray that allows fat to drip away.

Stir-frying is a very hot and fast method that requires little oil. If basting or marinating is necessary use non fat substances like lemon juice, vinegar, or wine. Always trim away obvious fat and whitish fat pads from under the skin. Steer away from high-fat cooking methods such as frying and batter frying.

Seafood: Eating fish is associated with a lower risk of heart disease. To preserve this health benefit, cook fish according to the amount of fat it contains. Grill or broil salmon, trout, and other fatty fish; use moist-cooking methods such as poaching to make flounder, haddock, and leaner fish taste better.

Vegetables: How you prepare and cook your vegetables will have dramatic results on their nutritional value. Wash them thoroughly but don't soak them; water will deplete nutrients. When vegetables are chopped, peeled, and cooked they lose vitamins. Try cooking them whole, or peel and chop just before cooking.

Cut the vegetables evenly so they cook for the same amount of time and, if you plan to freeze them, do it immediately after cooking. The goal is for vegetables to be tender and crisp. The faster they cook the more nutrients you preserve. The least nutritious method is to boil vegetables in large amounts of water. Serve vegetables promptly after cooking.

Beans: For increasing protein, vitamins, and fiber in your diet while keeping salt and fat to a minimum, beans are the answer. Use beans in soups, salads, and casseroles. Rinse them well and remove beans that float and other natural debris. Most require presoaking overnight; put them in a pot of cold water. If you don't mind the beans breaking up in the water, you can use a quicker method: Place the beans in a saucepan with 2 inches of water and bring to a boil over medium heat. Simmer for 2 to 3 minutes, turn off the heat, cover and let stand for 1 to 2 hours. Remove the residue from the top with a strainer. The skin will crack slightly when the beans are done. To reduce stomach upset and gas, after the beans have soaked drain the water and replace it with fresh water to simmer.

Pasta: Cook pasta until it is tender but still firm. Overcooking will drain it of nutrients. Don't rinse after cooking unless the recipe specifically calls for it—water washes away nutrients. Remember: cream-based, high-fat sauces counteract the benefits of this low-fat dish. □

CHAPTER 32

Keeping the Zest in Your Cooking: A Health-Conscious Guide

By now you have the mantra: low-fat; high-fiber; rich in fruits, vegetables, and grains. But how on earth can you put this into practice and still get anybody to the dinner table? Actually, the problem is not as insurmountable as it seems. The simple tips in this chapter and the next can help you turn shamelessly healthy food into truly exciting meals.

Don't worry about tracking down eye of newt, wing of bat, or other arcane ingredients, either. Common staple foods and equipment are all you need. You can then incorporate out-of-the-ordinary condiments, spices, or food combinations at your own pace. Begin by using healthy cooking techniques (baking instead of frying, for instance), substituting equivalent low-fat items in recipes (like using yogurt instead of mayonnaise), and seasoning foods in new ways (for example, topping vegetables with flavored vinegar or lemon juice rather than butter and salt). Gradually space your high-fat meals farther apart and fill in the gaps with intriguing, nutritious new dishes. Soon a new way of eating will become part of your lifestyle.

Nutritionally Correct Cooking Methods

Many Americans find fried foods and heavy cream sauces synonymous with "comfort." But this style of cooking is definitely on its way out. For healthy eating, throw away the deep-frier and roast, broil, bake, saute, poach, steam or microwave everything you cook. Or try baking in parchment paper; it's an easy, elegant way to cook meats, fish, vegetables, and even fruits.

Roasting. In this dry-heat method of cooking, food rests on a rack in a roasting pan, enabling fat to drip away during cooking. A chicken or turkey may require basting so it won't dry out; but be sure to use a low-fat broth or marinade, or separate the fat from the meat's own juices before using them. A measuring cup with a spout at the bottom is great for getting rid of fat. Simply pour the pan juices into the cup and let the fat rise to the top. The liquid at the bottom can then be poured back over the meat. Never roast at temperatures over 350 degrees Fahrenheit. Higher temperatures will sear the meat and lock fat inside.

Broiling. This method is similar to roasting, only the meat is placed directly under the heat.

Grilling. In this familiar outdoor barbecue cooking technique, meat is cooked over—rather than under—direct heat.

Baking. Unless you use some kind of breading, you will need a covered container for baking, the process requires a little more cooking liquid than roasting. Try low-fat broth, milk, water, or marinades like fruit juices, or wine. Non-stick cooking spray makes cleanup easier.

Sautéing. Ideal for foods that cook quickly, such as fish, thinly sliced meats, or vegetables, sautéing relies on constant movement to keep the food from sticking to the pan. Non-stick cooking spray works well with this method. The word *sauté* comes from the French *sauter* which means "to jump." Wok cooking and other stir-fry methods that keep food "jumping" in the pan borrow this concept.

Poaching. This easy technique simply calls for simmering the food in liquid.

Steaming. If you cannot eat your vegetables raw, steam them in a microwave oven or use a low-cost collapsible steamer basket that fits inside a pot. That way the vegetables scarcely touch the water. Use no more than about an inch of liquid to prevent the loss of vitamins and minerals. If you add herbs and spices to the water, the steam will impart a

delicate flavor to the vegetables. While the water is simmering, keep the lid tightly on the pot. Experiment to determine the time it takes for each of your favorite vegetables to reach the doneness you prefer. Broccoli will generally take three to four minutes; carrots, five minutes; green beans, four minutes; and small red potatoes, 10 minutes.

Microwaving. Microwave ovens cook efficiently because their energy heats the food, not the container or the appliance. Use only glass, plastic, or paper containers. Microwaves must be able to pass through the container to cook the food inside it; and metal containers reflect the waves, preventing the penetration of heat.

Here are a few tips for cooking by microwave:

- Be sure to stir or rotate foods halfway through cooking time to distribute moisture and heat evenly.
- Remember that sugar and fat attract energy, causing the food to cook faster.
- Reduce the liquid in your recipe by about one-quarter. Liquids do not evaporate during microwaving.
- To steam vegetables or facilitate the cooking of other foods, cover the dish with microwave-safe plastic wrap. To prevent explosions, make sure there is a small vent to let steam escape.
- Use the quick-cooking variety of rice or pasta.

MICROWAVING VEGETABLES: QUICK, EASY, HEALTHY

Here are some cooking tips from the United Fresh Fruit and Vegetable Association. Cooking times are approximate; exact time depends on oven and container. Microwave all vegetables on full power.

- Place whole vegetables at least one inch apart and turn them at least once.
- Pierce whole, unpeeled vegetables, such as squash or potatoes, before cooking to prevent their skins from bursting.
- Arrange vegetables so that the part that takes the longest to cook, like thick stalks, is toward the outside of the cooking dish.

Asparagus—Cut spears into 1/2-inch pieces. Microwave one pound in 2 tablespoons of water for 6 minutes.

Green beans—Cut beans in half. Microwave one pound in 1/4 cup water for 8 minutes.

Broccoli—Remove large leaves from one bunch of broccoli (about 1-1/2 pounds). Trim stalks; making a cut in the bottom of each. Microwave in 1/2 cup water for 11 minutes.

Cabbage—Wash, core and quarter a medium head (about 1-3/4 pounds). Microwave in 1/4 cup water for 11 minutes

Carrots—Slice into one-inch thick pieces. Microwave one pound in 1/4 cup water for 8 minutes.

Cauliflower—Microwave a whole head (one pound) in 1/4 cup water for 10 minutes. Or break into flowerets and microwave in 1/4 cup water for 8 minutes.

Corn-on-the-cob—Remove outer husks, carefully pull back inner husks, and remove silk. Replace husks and twist at the end to secure. Microwave, allowing 3–5 minutes per ear.

Mushrooms—Slice half a pound of washed, trimmed mushrooms. Microwave in 2 tablespoons of butter or margarine for 4 minutes.

Potatoes—To bake, prick clean potatoes several times to allow steam to escape. Arrange at least one inch apart on a paper towel. Microwave one potato 3 to 5 minutes; 2 potatoes 5 to 7-1/2 minutes; 3 potatoes 7 to 10 minutes; 4 potatoes 10-1/2 to 12 minutes.

Spinach—Remove stems from half a pound of spinach. Microwave in 1/4 cup water for 4 minutes.

Squash, acorn—Halve and scoop out seeds. Place cut side down in baking dish, microwave for 5-1/2 to 7-1/2 minutes per pound. Turn squash over. Place butter or margarine and brown sugar in each half, wrap in foil and let stand for 5 minutes.

Squash, summer and zucchini—Slice one pound. Microwave in 1/4 cup water for 8 minutes.

Tomatoes—Wash and halve tomatoes. Arrange in a circle on a dish and sprinkle with desired seasoning. Microwave 2 halves for 2–2 1/2 minutes; 4 halves, 3 to 4 minutes; 6 to 8 halves, 5 to 6 minutes.

Cooking with parchment paper. This method combines baking with steaming. Food is placed inside a packet made of folded parchment paper, then baked. As steam builds up inside, the food cooks gently without fat of any kind. Use this method when combining foods: for instance, cook fish in a packet with mushrooms and slivered carrots, or fruits with wine and raisins. You can find parchment paper in kitchenware stores. Aluminum foil and even brown packing paper will also work. Here's how it's done:

- Fold a 16-inch piece of parchment paper in half.
- Cut it as you would a valentine heart with the fold running down the center.
- Arrange the food in the center of one side of the heart, and fold the other side over it bringing the edges together.
- Crimp the edges together by making small, uniform folds, each one over the next, until the packet is completely sealed. Most foods will cook in 10 to 12 minutes at 400 degrees Fahrenheit.

The Trick to Healthy Substitutions

The simplest way to trim down a too-rich recipe is to use reduced-fat or reduced-calorie ingredients. Skim milk can easily replace whole milk in many recipes, and if skim milk is not robust enough—for example, in a cream soup—you can use evaporated skim milk or thicken with cornstarch or dry skim milk powder. Buttermilk is another option, depending on what you're making. It works quite well in waffles, as the editors of *Eating Well* discovered when they revamped a reader's recipe for their monthly "Rx for Recipes" feature. The original version called for three eggs, 1/2 cup of butter, and 1 cup of milk, and resulted in waffles with 343 calories and 19 grams of fat apiece. By replacing the three eggs with one whole egg plus two egg whites, and using 2 cups of skim-milk buttermilk instead of butter and whole milk, the editors created a "flavorful waffle" with only 220 calories and 4 grams of fat. Substituting 1 cup of whole wheat flour plus 1 cup of all purpose flour for the 2 cups of all-purpose flour specified in the original recipe provided additional fiber.

Eating Well's Waffles

1 cup	whole-wheat flour
1 cup	all-purpose white flour
1 1/2 tsp.	baking powder
1/2 tsp.	salt
1/4 tsp.	baking soda
2 cups	skim-milk buttermilk
1	large egg, separated, plus 2 egg whites
1 Tbs.	vanilla extract (optional)
1 Tbs.	vegetable oil plus extra for preparing the waffle iron
2 Tbs.	sugar

In a large bowl, stir together flours, baking powder, salt and baking soda. In a separate bowl, whisk together buttermilk, egg yolk, vanilla (if using) and oil. Add to the dry ingredients and stir with a wooden spoon just until moistened.

In a grease-free mixing bowl, beat the 3 egg whites with an electric mixer until soft peaks form. Add sugar and continue beating until stiff and glossy. Whisk one-quarter of the beaten egg whites into the batter. With a rubber spatula, fold in the remaining beaten egg whites.

Preheat waffle iron. Brush the surface lightly with oil. Fill the iron two-thirds full. Cook for 5 to 6 minutes, or until the waffles are crisp and golden. Repeat with the remaining batter, brushing the surface with oil before cooking each batch.

- Serves 6.
- Per serving: **Cal.** 220, **Pro.** 10 g, **Fat** 4 g, **Carb.** 38 g, **Sod.** 368 mg, **Chol.** 37 mg.

Reprinted with permission from Eating Well, *The Magazine of Food and Health.*

TRY THESE HEALTHY STAND-INS

Here are some substitutions that can help wring extra fat from your cooking.

Fats and Oils

Instead of:	Choose:
Marinating in oil	Marinades of vinegar, lemon juice, red or white wine, vermouth, yogurt, juice concentrate, tomato sauce, or well-seasoned broth
Creamy/oily salad dressing	Lemon juice, flavored vinegars, oil-free dressing
Cream/butter sauces	Tomato-based sauces
Regular mayonnaise	Low-fat yogurt; low-fat, reduced calorie mayonnaise
Butter or margarine as a topping for breads/rolls pancakes, waffles	Jam, jelly, fruit spread, marmalade, honey, fresh fruit, syrup (Use butter or margarine sparingly, if at all.)

Dairy

Instead of:	Choose:
Whole milk	Skim or low-fat (1 percent) milk (Add non-fat dry milk powder if necessary.)
Creamed cottage cheese	Dry curd or low-fat cottage cheese, farmer's cheese
Cream or whipped cream	Evaporated skim milk or whipped evaporated skim milk
Sour cream	Plain non-fat or low-fat yogurt or low-fat cottage cheese pureed in a blender
Cream cheese	Low-fat cottage cheese
Whole milk cheese	Part skim or low-fat cheeses
Whole eggs	Egg whites (two per whole egg) or egg substitute

Meat

Instead of:	Choose:
Bacon, sausage	Lean ham, Canadian bacon
Bologna, salami	Turkey breast
Marbled, fatty cuts such as rib roast, T-bone	Tenderloin, top or eye of round, round tip brisket, ground chuck

Adapted from: *Live Well The Low-Fat /High-Fiber Way.* New York, NY: The American Health Foundation Food Plan; 1990.

Another reader sent *Eating Well's* editors a recipe for the Greek dish *pastitsio*. The rich, creamy meat and pasta classic—with a whopping 723 calories and 45 grams of fat per serving!—called for 2 pounds of ground beef, 10 tablespoons of butter, 3 cups of cream, and three eggs. It's easy to see why the editors say this was the fattiest recipe to ever undergo a makeover. They began by using ground turkey instead of ground beef and reduced the total amount of meat by half a pound, replacing it with half a cup of bulghur. Bulghur is a fast-cooking type of wheat that results from precooking, drying, and cracking wheat berries. Like tofu, it takes on the flavor of foods with which it is cooked, and thus is a handy filler ingredient to reduce fat and calories from meats. The butter and cream were entirely eliminated, with evaporated skim milk used in their place. Low-fat cottage cheese enriched the sauce. Finally, the eggs and butter for the pasta layer, were omitted, resulting in a dish with only 467 calories and 12 grams of fat per serving.

Eating Well's Pastitsio

MEAT SAUCE

1 tsp.	olive or vegetable oil
1	large onion, finely chopped
1 1/2 lbs.	lean ground beef or ground turkey
3/4 cup	dry white wine
1 6-oz. can	tomato paste
1/2 cup	bulgur
3/4 tsp.	cinnamon
3/4 tsp.	nutmeg
3/4 tsp.	allspice
1 tsp.	salt
1/2 tsp.	freshly ground black pepper

CREAM SAUCE

2 cups	1% cottage cheese (1 lb.)
1 1/2	cups evaporated skim milk (12-oz. can)
1 cup	defatted reduced-sodium chicken stock
2 Tbs.	all-purpose white flour
1/2 cup	freshly grated Kefalotýri, Asiago, or Parmesan cheese (1 oz.) salt & freshly ground black pepper to taste

PASTA

1 lb.	elbow macaroni or ziti
6 Tbs.	freshly grated Kefalot´yri, Asiago, or Parmesan cheese (3/4 oz.)
1 tsp.	vegetable oil
1/2 tsp	salt
2 Tbs.	chopped fresh parsley (optional)

To make meat sauce: In a large nonstick skillet, heat oil over medium heat; add onions and saute until softened, about 5 minutes. Add ground meat and cook, breaking it up with a wooden spoon, until no longer pink, about 5 minutes. Drain off fat. Add 1 cup water, wine, tomato paste, bulgur, spices, salt and pepper. Simmer, uncovered, over low heat, stirring occasionally, until the bulgur is tender, about 20 minutes. Taste and adjust seasonings.

To make cream sauce: In a food processor or blender, puree cottage cheese until completely smooth. Set aside. In a medium-sized heavy saucepan, combine evaporated skim milk and 3/4 cup chicken stock. Heat over medium heat until scalding. In a small bowl, stir together flour and the remaining 1/4 cup cold chicken stock until smooth. Stir into the hot milk mixture and cook, stirring constantly, until thickened, about 2 minutes. Remove from the heat and whisk in the pureed cottage cheese and grated cheese. Season with salt and a generous grinding of pepper. To prevent a skin from forming, place wax paper or plastic wrap directly over the surface and set aside.

To make pasta: In a large pot of boiling salted water, cook macaroni or ziti until *al dente*, 8 to 10 minutes. Drain and return to the pot. Toss with 1/4 cup grated cheese, oil and salt.

To assemble and bake *pastitsio*: Preheat oven to 350 degrees F. Spray a 9-by-13-inch baking dish with nonstick cooking spray. Spread half of the pasta mixture over the bottom of the prepared dish. Top with one third of the cream sauce. Spoon all of the meat sauce over, spreading evenly. Cover with another third of the cream sauce. Top with the remaining pasta mixture and cover with the remaining cream sauce. Sprinkle with the remaining 2 Tbs. grated cheese. (*Pastitsio* can be assembled ahead and stored, covered, in the refrigerator for up to 2 days or in the freezer for up to 3 months. If frozen, thaw in the refrigerator before proceeding.) Bake for 40 to 50 minutes, or until bubbling and golden. Sprinkle with parsley, if using, and serve.

■ Serves 10.
■ Per serving: **Cal.** 467, **Pro.** 33 g, **Fat** 12 g, **Carb.** 52 g, **Sod.** 929 mg, **Chol.** 55 mg.

Reprinted with permission from Eating Well, The Magazine of Food and Health.

Other grains can also substitute for meats in a recipe. Rice, barley, quinoa (pronounced "KEEN-wa"), and kasha all work well either to lend fullness to a dish with less meat than usual or to make a meatless dish more filling. Barley, probably the world's oldest grain crop, is a low-starch staple. The seeds of quinoa, an annual wild-growing herb are rich in protein and high in fiber. Their saponin coating has a bitter taste; so you'll need to rinse them with water before using. Kasha is cracked, roasted buckwheat groats. You don't have to rely on these exotic grains, however. Ordinary rice will often do just as well.

Get Maximum Leverage from Seasonings

Since our taste buds recognize only four basic flavors—sweet, salty, sour and bitter—there is no real substitute for salt; but by over-stimulating the other areas of the tongue with extremely flavorful foods it is possible to actually "fool" the taste buds. Flavored vinegars, oil, chutneys, mustards, and herb blends are just right for the job because they pack a tantalizing punch in small amounts.

Flavored Vinegars

Add zest to salads, sauces, and marinades with this new culinary craze. Several varieties are available in most supermarkets, or you can create your own by combining various herbs or edible flower blossoms with vinegars made from cider, red or white wine, or rice wine. Although there are no rules about combinations, you might want to try cider vinegar with basil, mint and dill or full-bodied red wine vinegar with pungent herbs such as oregano and rosemary. White wine vinegar is the most versatile kind, blending well with almost any single herb or combination of herbs; and sweet, mild rice wine vinegar blends nicely with delicate herbs such as mint or lavender.

To make your own flavored vinegar:

- Make sure the jar or bottle is completely sterile and dry.
- Place herbs in the container and pour vinegar over them. A good ratio is one cup of fresh herbs (or 1/3 cup dried herbs) to one quart of vinegar.
- If you place the container in a sunny location, it will steep more quickly and will be ready to use in about two weeks. It will take about a month in a shadier spot.
- When it's ready, strain the vinegar through a coffee filter into the bottle you'll use for storage. Add a sprig of the herb that flavors the vinegar, if you like.

If you're not feeling adventurous enough to experiment on your own, here are a couple of the many combinations you can try.

Vivid Vinaigrette

Use this delightful vinegar the next time you make a vinaigrette dressing.

2 sprigs chervil
2 sprigs basil
2 sprigs tarragon
1 sprig thyme
6 chive blades
1 quart white wine vinegar

Mediterranean Blend

This hearty mixture works as well in meat marinades as it does on a salad.

2 sprigs oregano
1 sprig rosemary
1 sprig thyme
2 garlic cloves
1 small hot red pepper
1 quart white wine vinegar

Flavored Oils

Use flavored oils as you do flavored vinegars—but don't go overboard. Even mono- or polyunsaturated oils such as olive oil contain relatively high amounts of calories and fat. For instance, one tablespoon of olive oil has 14 grams of fat and 120 calories.

Add flavored oils to salads, sauces, and marinades and use them when you grill or sauté meats and vegetables. They are as easy to make as vinegar; however, they can't be stored indefinitely (as vinegars can) since they tend to become rancid. Keeping them in the refrigerator will extend their life to about three months.

Here are some suggestions for adding your favorite flavors to an oil:

- Start with a dry, sterile container.
- Place the herbs in the jar or bottle and pour oil over them. You will need one cup of fresh herbs—or 1/3 cup dried—for every quart of oil.
- If you use garlic, remove it after the oil is finished steeping (about 2 weeks) or the taste will become overpowering.
- Since mold can develop if the ingredients aren't completely covered with oil, it's a good idea to strain the flavored oil into another bottle and discard the herbs. Don't add a sprig of the dominant herb (as you would with vinegar) unless you plan to continue adding oil to cover it.
- Store in a cool place out of direct sunlight, or in the refrigerator.

Here's one combination that goes especially well with seafood. Experiment with any other ingredients that catch your fancy.

Maritime Marinade

3 sprigs dill
3 sprigs parsley
3 sprigs tarragon
3 sprigs thyme
1 clove garlic
1 tsp. coriander
1 tsp. black peppercorns
Grated peel of 1 lemon
1 quart olive oil

Chutneys

If ever a seasoning could overwhelm the taste buds, it would be chutney. This condiment is a combination of fruit, hot spices, sweet vegetables, and tart flavorings. The word chutney actually comes from the Hindustani word *chatni*, which means "strong spices."

To make chutney, cut fruits or vegetables into small pieces—or puree them—and add vinegar, sugar, herbs, and spices. Cook the mixture until it has the consistency of jam. Chutney can usually be stored in the refrigerator for up to two months.

Here's a recipe for one of the classic chutnies. Use it as you would other condiments, such as mustard or horseradish.

Major Jones Chutney

3/4 pound	tart green apples, unpeeled and finely chopped (2 apples or about 2 cups)
1 cup	finely chopped raisins
1 tsp.	corn oil
1 tsp.	ground mustard seed or crushed whole mustard seeds
1 tsp.	ground coriander
3/4 tsp.	ground ginger
3/4 tsp.	chili powder
1/4 tsp.	ground turmeric
1/4 tsp.	ground cumin
1/4 tsp.	garlic powder
1/8 tsp.	cayenne pepper
2-1/2 Tbs.	red wine vinegar
1-1/2 cups	water

Combine the chopped apples and raisins in a large mixing bowl. Mix thoroughly and set aside. Heat the oil in a heavy saucepan and add all of the spices, mixing well. Combine the vinegar and the water, add to the spice mixture and bring to a boil. Then add the apple-raisin mixture and cook, uncovered, over low heat, stirring occasionally, for about 1 hour and 15 minutes, or until the liquid is absorbed and the apples are completely tender. Cool to room temperature and store in a covered container in the refrigerator.

■ Makes 2 cups
■ 2 tablespoons contain approximately: 30 calories, 5 mg. sodium

From: Secrets of Salt-Free Cooking, the 101 Productions series. Copyright 1991 by Jeanne Jones Inc. Reprinted with permission.

QUICK TIP FOR REDUCING SALT

Not only can you cut down on salt by replacing it with herbs and spices in recipes, but you can also remove much of the naturally occurring salt in foods such as feta cheese, capers, pickled vegetables, sauerkraut, ham, and other smoked meats. Simply soak the foods in cold water from 15 to 30 minutes. If the food is really salty, you may need to drain the water after 15 minutes, refill the container, and soak for another 15 to 30 minutes.

Mustard

The pungent flavor of mustard makes it a great condiment for everything from fish to chicken and beef. It's also great with vegetables. If you want to whip up a quick batch of homemade mustard, it's easiest to start with a prepared mustard, such as Dijon; but if you feel more adventurous, you can use powdered mustard or grind various kinds of mustard seeds. You can vary the sharpness of your mustard by steeping it in various liquids. Use vinegar for a mild flavor, white wine for a Dijon-type flavor, flat beer for a fiery taste, or plain water for the hottest mustard of all. You can also add whichever herbs you like—for example, dill or fennel for fish, or tarragon for chicken. Put all the ingredients you choose in an air-tight jar. Mustard will usually last up to 3 months if you store it in a cool, dark place.

Here's a recipe for Thyme Mustard from *Herbs in the Kitchen* that you can vary by using chives, oregano, savory, or tarragon in place of thyme. To make it sweeter, add more honey. You can also divide it in two batches and flavor each with a different herb. Whatever you decide, plan on mellowing the mustard for 3 to 4 weeks; it will be very hot when first prepared. The texture will depend on how finely you grind the seeds. It's best to use a mortar and pestle or spice mill, but if you plan to use a food processor, soak the mustard seeds in water for 2 or 3 hours beforehand.

Thyme Mustard

1 1/2 cups	mustard seed, freshly ground
1/2 cup	water
1/4 cup	white wine vinegar
1/4 tsp.	salt
1/4 tsp.	freshly ground white pepper
1 1/2 tsp.	honey
1 Tbs.	minced thyme

Blend the ground mustard seed with the water and vinegar in a bowl. The mustard will absorb the liquid as it stands. Add the salt, pepper, honey, and thyme and blend well. Add a little water if necessary to bring the mustard to a spreading consistency.

Pack into jars and keep refrigerated until ready to use.

■ Makes about 2 1/2 cups

From: Herbs in the Kitchen *by Carolyn Dille and Susan Belsinger. Loveland, CO: Interweave Press, Inc.; 1992.*

Herb blends instead of salt

Instead of a salt shaker, why not combine your favorite spices in a shaker and put it on the table to use at mealtime. You can easily combine basil, rosemary, tarragon, and marjoram to serve with chicken or turkey; and a blend of savory, sage, cumin, coriander, ginger, and thyme goes well with pork. For Italian meals, shake on parsley, oregano, and basil, mixed with a little cayenne pepper and fennel. Classic herbs for fish are dill, chives, lemon thyme, tarragon, and chervil. Here are a few all-purpose mixtures you might want to try. See which one you want to make part of your daily diet.

Four-Spice Blend

This mixture is practically a staple in France, where it's used for meats, vegetables, soups, and sauces. It's especially good on carrots, turnips, and parsnips.

5 Tbs.	ground cloves
3 Tbs.	ground ginger
3 Tbs.	ground nutmeg
3 Tbs.	ground white pepper

Piquant Blend

1 Tbs.	ground black pepper
1 Tbs.	ground cloves
2 Tbs.	sweet paprika
1 tsp.	ground coriander
1/2 tsp.	garlic powder
1/2 tsp.	grated dried orange rind

Eastern Blend

2 Tbs.	cardamom seeds
1 4-inch	cinnamon stick
2 tsp.	cumin seeds
2 tsp.	whole cloves
2 tsp.	black peppercorns
1/2	whole nutmeg

Place all ingredients in an electric blender or coffee grinder and process until finely ground. In India and Pakistan, where this mixture is used as a table seasoning, it is known as "garam masala."

Herb blends not only work well in shakers on the dinner table, but make a quick dip when combined with non-fat or low-fat sour cream, cream cheese, or plain yogurt. And that's just the beginning. For more ideas on delicious ways to use herbs, turn to Chapter 35.

A Few Ideas to Start With

The new style of healthy cooking has an important bonus: It's frequently easier than old-fashioned cuisine, with its complicated sauces and elaborate desserts. The fresh imaginative recipes you'll find reprinted below show how much can be accomplished with simple combinations of unexpected ingredients. After you've tried a few, you may find yourself experimenting with some new ideas of your own. The key point is to make the food fun. Healthy eating definitely does not have to be dreary.

BOUNTIFUL BREAKFASTS

Fruity Amaranth Muffins

A delicious breakfast treat or anytime snack.

1 1/2 cups	low-fat milk or calcium-fortified soy milk
1/4 cup	safflower oil
2 Tbs.	honey or brown rice syrup
1/2 tsp.	vanilla
2 Tbs.	lemon juice
1 cup	diced mixed dried fruit
1 1/2 cups	amaranth flour
1/2 cup	whole wheat flour
1/2 cup	sunflower seeds
1 Tbs.	baking powder
1/4 tsp.	cinnamon

Preheat oven to 375° Fahrenheit.
Oil muffin tins.

HOW TO PICK A HEALTHY BREAKFAST CEREAL

Faced with such a huge selection, how can you zero-in on cereals healthy enough to eat on a regular basis? Here are a few clues to look for.

1. Choose whole grains: Ingredients listed on the box should mention whole grains (such as rolled oats or whole wheat) or whole grain flour. Watch for the words "flour," "milled flour," or "meal," since this usually means "refined," and hence less nutritious.

2. Each serving should have three or four grams of fiber: You'll get the most fiber from one ounce (about 1/2 cup) of Kellogg's All-Bran with Extra Fiber (14 grams) or from General Mills Fiber One (13 grams), but you don't have to aim that high if these cereals fail to appeal.

3. Watch the sugar: If you're counting calories, remember that sugary cereals can cost you.

4. Don't be fooled by vitamin content: Don't choose "fortified" cereal based solely on vitamin content. You could just as easily take a vitamin pill.

5. Hold the salt: If you like salt but need to cut down, don't unnecessarily waste your daily sodium allotment on breakfast. If you stick with lightweight cereals such as flakes, you can usually keep sodium below 250 to 300 milligrams per ounce. But watch out for the heavier, denser cereals: They can contain up to 600 milligrams of sodium per ounce.

6. Watch granola and mueslis: Granola can be high in fat, although some companies (Health Valley, Alpen, Breadshop, and Kellogg) now make low-fat varieties. Muesli, the European version of granola, is often lower in fat; but contrary to their reputation, neither granola nor muesli is high in fiber.

Combine first 5 ingredients in a small mixing bowl. Stir in dried fruit. Set aside. Combine remaining ingredients in a large mixing bowl. Add liquid ingredients to dry ones. Stir just until moistened. Spoon batter into muffin tins, filling 2/3 full. Bake until tops are brown and a toothpick inserted in the center comes out clean, about 35 minutes. Remove from oven and cool in tins for 5 minutes. Remove muffins from tins and place onto a wire rack to finish cooling completely.

- Makes 12 muffins
- Per muffin: **Cal.** 244 **Pro.** 7 g **Fat** 10 g **Sod.** 140 mg **Carb.** 35 g **Chol.** 1 mg

From: Vegetarian Gourmet *Magazine. 1994;3:11.*

Orange-Fig Muffins

1 1/2 cups	all-purpose flour
3 Tbs.	sugar
4 tsp.	baking powder
3 cups	Common Sense™ Oat Bran cereal, any variety
1/2 tsp.	grated orange peel
1 3/4 cups	orange juice
3 Tbs.	vegetable oil
4	egg whites
1/2 cup	chopped, dried figs

Stir together flour, sugar and baking powder; set aside. In a large mixing bowl, combine Common Sense Oat Bran cereal, orange peel, orange juice, oil, egg whites, and figs; beat well. Add dry ingredients to cereal mixture, stirring only until combined. Portion batter evenly into 12 lightly greased 2 1/2-inch muffin-pan cups. Bake in 400°F oven about 28 minutes or until golden brown. Serve hot.

- Yield: 12 muffins
- Per Serving (1 muffin): **Cal. 200**
  Dietary fiber 3 g **Fat** 4 g
  Sat. Fat less than 1 g **Chol.** 0 mg

From: Live Well The Low-Fat/High-Fiber Way. *The American Health Foundation Food Plan. New York, NY: 1990.*

Banana-Raisin French Toast

With a nutritious surprise filling, this low-fat French toast is sure to please children.

1	ripe banana, peeled
2 tsp.	frozen orange-juice concentrate
4 slices	cinnamon-raisin bread
2 large	egg whites
1/4 cup	skim milk
1/4 cup	nonfat or low-fat yogurt
1 1/2 Tbs.	maple syrup or honey
1 tsp.	butter

In a small, shallow bowl, mash banana coarsely with a fork. Stir in orange-juice concentrate. Spread the banana mixture over 2 slices of bread and top with the remaining 2 slices of bread, forming 2 sandwiches. In a pie plate, whisk together egg whites and milk; add sandwiches and soak for about 20 seconds. Turn sandwiches over and soak for 20 seconds longer. Transfer the sandwiches to a plate. In a small bowl, stir together yogurt and maple syrup or honey. Set aside. In a nonstick skillet, melt 1/2 tsp. butter over low heat. Tilt the pan to swirl the butter

around the skillet. With a metal spatula, place the sandwiches in the pan, and cook until the underside is browned, 5 to 7 minutes. Lift the sandwiches and add the remaining 1/2 tsp. butter. Turn over and cook for 5 to 7 minutes longer, or until browned. Serve with the sweetened yogurt.

- Serves 2.
- Per serving: **Cal.** 302 **Pro.** 11 g **Fat** 4 g
  Sod. 317 mg **Carb.** 57 g **Chol.** 7 mg

Reprinted with permission from Eating Well, *The Magazine of Food and Health.*

Turkey & Apple Sausage Patties

To ensure a moist sausage, be sure to use breadcrumbs made by whirling fresh or day-old bread in a food processor.

2 tsp.	vegetable oil
1	onion, finely chopped
2	tart apples, such as Granny Smith, peeled and grated
1 lb.	ground turkey
1 cup	fresh breadcrumbs (4 slices bread)
2	large egg whites
2 tsp.	rubbed dried sage
1 1/2 tsp.	salt
1/2 tsp.	freshly ground black pepper
1/4 tsp.	freshly grated nutmeg
1/4 tsp.	allspice

Preheat oven to 450 degrees F. Spray a baking sheet with nonstick cooking spray or line it with parchment paper.

In a nonstick skillet, heat oil over medium heat. Add onions and sauté until softened, about 3 minutes. Add apples and sauté for 3 to 5 minutes longer, or until the apples are very tender. Transfer to a large bowl and let cool completely. Add turkey, breadcrumbs, egg whites, sage, salt, pepper, nutmeg and allspice; mix well. Divide the sausage mixture into 16 portions and form into 3/4-inch-thick patties. (The patties can be prepared ahead and stored, well wrapped, in the freezer for up to 3 months.) Place the patties on the prepared baking sheet and bake until the outside is golden brown and the interior is no longer pink, about 10 minutes for fresh patties or 20 minutes for frozen patties.

■ Makes 16 patties, serves 8.
■ Per serving: **Cal.** 92 **Pro.** 12 g **Fat** 5 g
  Sod. 552 mg **Carb.** 16 g **Chol.** 36 mg

Reprinted with permission from Eating Well, *The Magazine of Food and Health.*

Eating Well's Cinnamon Rolls

DOUGH

3 1/2–4 cups	all-purpose white flour
1 cup	whole-wheat flour
1 pkg.	active dry yeast (1 Tbs.)
1/2 cup	nonfat cottage cheese
1 cup	plus 1 Tbs. skim milk
1/3	cup sugar
2 Tbs.	vegetable oil
1/2 tsp.	salt
2	large eggs, lightly beaten
1	large egg white

FILLING

1/2 cup	packed light brown sugar
1/4 cup	dark corn syrup
1 Tbs.	ground cinnamon
1/2 cup	golden raisins
1/4 cup	chopped toasted pecans

GLAZE

1 1/4 cups	confectioners' sugar
1–2 Tbs.	skim milk
1 tsp.	corn syrup
1/2 tsp.	pure vanilla extract

To make dough: In a large mixing bowl, combine 1 1/2 cups white flour, whole-wheat flour and yeast. Place cottage cheese in a cheesecloth-lined sieve over a bowl. Gather cheesecloth into a ball and squeeze out moisture from cottage cheese. (You should have about 1/4 cup cottage-cheese solids remaining.) Transfer the cottage-cheese solids to the sieve and press them through the sieve into a small saucepan. Stir in 1 cup milk, sugar, oil and salt; heat, stirring, until warm (120–130 degrees F). Stir into the flour mixture. Add eggs and egg white; beat with an electric mixer on low speed for 30 seconds, scraping the sides of the bowl. Beat on high speed for 3 minutes. Using a wooden spoon (or dough hook of mixer), stir in 2 cups white flour. Turn the dough onto a lightly floured surface and knead for about 5 minutes, adding enough of the remaining flour to make a soft, smooth dough. (It will be slightly sticky.) Place the dough in a lightly oiled bowl and turn once. Cover with plastic wrap and let rise in a warm place until doubled in bulk, about 1 hour.

To make filling and bake rolls: In a small saucepan, combine brown sugar, corn syrup and cinnamon; heat gently, stirring, until smooth. Set aside to cool. Punch dough down. Turn out onto a lightly floured surface. Cover and let rest for 10 minutes. Roll or pat into a 12-by-18-inch rectangle. Spread the brown sugar mixture over the dough. Sprinkle with raisins and pecans. Starting at the long edge, roll up jelly-roll fashion. Pinch the edges of dough together along the length of the roll. With a sharp knife, slice the roll into 12 pieces. Spray a 9-by-13-inch baking dish with nonstick cooking spray, and place the cinnamon rolls, cut-side up and slightly apart, in the dish. Cover with plastic wrap and let rise in a warm place until nearly doubled, about 45 minutes. (Alternatively, refrigerate for 2 to 24 hours, then let stand in a warm place for 30 minutes.)

Meanwhile, preheat oven to 375 degrees F. Brush rolls with 1 Tbs. milk. Bake for 25 to 30 minutes, or until light brown. Transfer to a rack and let cool slightly in the pan.

To make glaze: In a small bowl, stir together confectioners' sugar, 1 Tbs. milk, corn syrup and vanilla. Add more milk, if necessary, to make a drizzling consistency. Drizzle the glaze over the rolls and serve them warm.

■ Makes 12 cinnamon rolls.
■ Per serving: **Cal.** 367 **Pro.** 9 g **Fat** 73 g **Sod.** 127 mg **Carb.** 73 g **Chol.** 36 mg.

Reprinted with permission from Eating Well, *The Magazine of Food and Health.*

Frozen Fruit Slush

This healthful treat makes a versatile snack for you and your children. For an unusual twist, try this for breakfast.

3	bananas, ripe
1/2 cup	lemon juice
1 cup	orange juice
4 cup	pineapple juice

Blend all ingredients in a blender until smooth. Combine crushed ice and water to the desired consistency ending up with a total of 5 cups. Add the blended fruits and serve. Or freeze the blended fruit juices in a wide unbreakable bowl or pan. Scrape frozen fruit mixture out with an ice cream scoop or spoon and put into a glass. Pour clear diet pop over the top to achieve the desired consistency and serve. Or freeze into popsicles.

■ Serves 12
■ Per Serving: **Cal.** 82 **Pro.** trace **Fat** trace **Sod.** 1 mg **Carb.** 20 g **Chol.** ?

From: Recipes to Lower Your Fat Thermostat *by LaRene Gaunt. Provo, UT: Copyright 1992, 1884 by Vitality House International, Inc. All rights reserved. Used by permission.*

Norwegian Pancakes

These delicate pancakes are delicious and almost fat-free. Contrary to the impression created by its name, buttermilk is a low-fat (1 or 1 1/2 percent butterfat) liquid. It is so named because it is the liquid left behind when the cream is skimmed from the milk to make butter.

DRY INGREDIENTS

1 cup	whole-wheat flour
1 cup	all-purpose flour
1 Tbs.	sugar
2 tsp.	baking soda
1/8 tsp.	salt (optional)

WET INGREDIENTS

1	egg
3 cups	buttermilk
1/4 tsp.	vanilla extract

POSSIBLE TOPPINGS

1/2 cup	fruit butter (e.g., apple, pear, peach)
2 cups	plain nonfat or low-fat yogurt
3 cups	berries, sliced if large

In a large bowl, combine the dry ingredients, mixing them well. In a medium-sized bowl, beat the egg lightly, and add the buttermilk and vanilla, mixing the ingredients well. When you are ready to cook the pancakes, lightly oil a nonstick griddle (for example, spray it with vegetable oil), and heat it over medium heat. Make a well in the dry ingredients, and pour in the wet ingredients, mixing the two just enough to moisten the dry ingredients. On the heated griddle, pour sufficient batter to make 4-inch pancakes—4 of them at a time on an 11-inch square griddle. Cook the pancakes until they begin to bubble on the surface, then flip them over, and lightly brown them on the other side. Repeat the procedure until all the batter is used up, re-oiling the griddle only to prevent the pancakes from sticking to it. Serve the pancakes with the desired toppings.

Reprinted from JANE BRODY'S GOOD FOOD GOURMET: Recipes and Menus for Delicious and Healthful Eating, *with the permission of W.W. Norton & Company, Inc. Copyright © 1990 by Jane E. Brody.*

NOVEL LOW-FAT SNACKS

Mexican Tabbouleh

Preparation tip: For the best consistency, prepare the bulgur, the cut-up vegetables, and the dressing separately in advance, and combine them about 1 hour before serving the tabbouleh.

Serving suggestion: Instead of (or in addition to) tortilla chips, you could serve this with scoops made out of firm fresh vegetables: wedges of red, green, and yellow peppers, chunks of celery, leaves of Belgian endive, or diagonally cut slices of a large carrot.
For maximum flavor, bring the tabbouleh to room temperature before serving it.

SALAD

1 cup	bulgur, medium- or fine-grind
1 6-oz. can	spicy hot V8 juice or Snappy Tom or tomato juice spiked with Worcestershire sauce and hot pepper sauce
10 oz.	beef broth (1 1/8 cups)
1	medium cucumber, peeled, seeded, and diced (1 cup)
2 to 3	firm plum tomatoes or 1 large firm tomato, chopped
1/2 cup	diced sweet green pepper
1/2 cup	chopped fresh parsley
1/4 cup	sliced scallions (including the green tops)
1 to 2 Tbs.	chopped cilantro
1	minced jalapeño (1 tablespoon), or to taste

DRESSING

1/4 cup	fresh lime juice
1 Tbs.	olive oil
1 tsp.	thyme, crumbled
1 tsp.	minced garlic (1 large clove)
	Cayenne or freshly ground
	black pepper to taste

Place the bulgur in a medium-sized heat-proof bowl. In a small saucepan, heat the juice and the broth just to boiling, and pour the liquid over the bulgur, stirring the mixture once. Let the bulgur stand for about 1 hour. Then drain off any remaining liquid, pressing lightly on the bulgur to extract any excess moisture. Let the bulgur cool, then chill it until 1 hour before serving time. In another bowl, combine the remaining salad ingredients. Cover the bowl, and refrigerate it until 1 hour before serving time. In a small jar or bowl, combine the dressing ingredients. One hour before serving the salad, add the vegetable mixture to the bulgur, pour on the dressing, and toss the ingredients to combine them well. Let the tabbouleh come to room temperature.

■ 6 to 8 salad servings or 10 to 12 hors-d'oeuvre servings

Reprinted from JANE BRODY'S GOOD FOOD GOURMET: Recipes and Menus for Delicious and Healthful Eating, *with the permission of W.W. Norton & Company, Inc. Copyright © 1990 by Jane E. Brody.*

Spinach Dip

This very low-fat dip has a mild Roquefort flavor that really enhances fresh vegetables that have been steamed tender-crisp and then chilled.

Serving suggestion: Serve this dip with carrots, green beans, cauliflower, or broccoli that have been steamed tender-crisp.

1 large clove garlic, peeled and minced
1 Tbs. olive oil
1 10-oz. package frozen chopped spinach, thawed and squeezed to remove excess liquid
1/2 cup plain nonfat or low-fat yogurt
1/3 cup grated Parmesan
1/4 tsp. salt
1/4 tsp. pepper

In a small skillet over low heat, sauté the garlic in the oil for 1 minute or until the garlic is tender (be careful not to burn the garlic). Combine the garlic and oil with the remaining ingredients in a blender or food processor, processing the ingredients until they are smooth. Cover the dip, and chill it until serving time.

Reprinted from JANE BRODY'S GOOD FOOD GOURMET: Recipes and Menus for Delicious and Healthful Eating, *with the permission of W.W. Norton & Company, Inc. Copyright © 1990 by Jane E. Brody.*

BL's Beans

From the kitchen of nutrition director [of the Center for Science in the Public Interest] Bonnie Liebman. Spoon it over toasted tortillas and it's a main dish. Scoop it up with fat-free tortilla chips or green pepper slices and it's a dip.

4 medium onions, chopped
2 green peppers, chopped
4 cloves garlic, crushed
2 Tbs. olive oil
3 16-oz. cans pinto beans, drained
   and rinsed
1 16-oz. can tomatoes, no salt added,
   chopped
1 8-oz. can tomato sauce, no salt added
1/2 tsp. cayenne or more, to taste
1 Tbs. each oregano and basil (optional)
1 tsp. cumin or more, to taste
Juice from 1/2 lemon

Saute the chopped onions, green peppers, and garlic in the oil in a large skillet. Mash about half of the beans in a bowl. Add the mashed beans plus the whole beans, tomatoes, tomato sauce, spices, and lemon juice to the skillet. Cook about 20 minutes, uncovered, until the excess liquid cooks out.

■ Serves 8
■ Per serving: **Cal.** 243 **Pro.** 10 g **Fat** 5 g
  Sod. 297 mg **Carb.** 42 g

Copyright 1994, CSPI. Reprinted from Nutrition Action Healthletter *(1875 Connecticut Ave., N.W., Suite 300, Washington, D.C. 20009. $24.00 for 10 issues.)*

NEW APPROACHES TO LUNCH

Smoked Turkey & Celery Root on Pumpernickel

Seasoned with a mustard dressing, peppery celery root is a good match for the smoked turkey.

4 tsp.	nonfat yogurt
4 tsp.	Dijon mustard
2 tsp.	reduced-calorie mayonnaise
1 1/3 cups	grated peeled celery root freshly ground black pepper to taste
1/2 lb.	smoked turkey breast, sliced
4 large	lettuce leaves, rinsed and dried
8 slices	pumpernickel bread

In a medium bowl, whisk together yogurt, mustard and mayonnaise. Stir in celery root and season with pepper.

To assemble sandwiches, layer smoked turkey, celery root mixture and lettuce between slices of pumpernickel.

■ Serves 4.
■ Per serving: **Cal.** 285 **Pro.** 17 g **Fat** 39 g
  Sod. 454 mg **Carb.** 35 g **Chol.** 1mg.

Reprinted with permission from Eating Well, *The Magazine of Food and Health.*

Crab Salad in Pita Pockets

A fresh, lively dressing of ginger, jalapeño and lime juice replaces mayonnaise in this luxurious sandwich filling.

1 Tbs.	red-wine vinegar
4 tsp.	olive or vegetable oil
2 tsp.	fresh lime juice
3/4 lb.	lump crabmeat, excess liquid squeezed out
3/4 cup	finely chopped celery heart with leaves

1/4 cup   minced red onion
2 tsp.   minced jalapeño pepper
                or to taste
1 tsp.   minced peeled gingerroot
salt & freshly ground black pepper to taste
2 8-inch pita breads, cut in half crosswise
4 large lettuce leaves, rinsed and dried

In a medium-sized bowl, whisk together vinegar, oil, and lime juice. Add crabmeat, celery, red onion, jalapeño and ginger; toss well. Season with salt and pepper. To assemble sandwiches, line pita halves with lettuce and fill with crab salad.

■ Serves 4.
■ Per serving: **Cal.** 189 **Pro.** 18 g **Fat** 7 g
  Sod. 554 g **Carb.** 14 g **Chol.** 85 mg

Reprinted with permission from Eating Well, *The Magazine of Food and Health.*

Black Bean Soup

2 cans   (15 oz. each) black beans,
                undrained
2 cups   chicken broth
1 cup   chopped onions
1/2 cup   chopped carrots
1/2 cup   chopped celery
2   bay leaves
1/4 cup   sliced green onions
1/4 cup   chopped red bell pepper

Place 1 can beans and 1 cup of the chicken broth in an electric blender container. Process until smooth except for small pieces of skin. In 2-quart saucepan, combine processed beans, remaining broth, the 1 cup onions, carrots, celery and bay leaves. Cook over medium heat, stirring occasionally, until bean mixture starts to boil. Reduce heat and simmer 15 minutes or until vegetables are tender. Add remaining can of beans and bring mixture to boil. Remove bay leaves and serve garnished with green onions and red bell pepper.

■ Yield: 5 cups
■ Per Serving: (1 1/4 cups) **Cal.** 264
  Dietary fiber 13 g **Fat** 2 g **Sat. fat** 0.2 g
  Chol. 0.5 mg

From: Live Well The Low-Fat/High-Fiber Way. *The American Health Foundation Food Plan. New York, NY: 1990.*

SUMPTUOUS MAIN DISHES

Basmati Rice and Beef Salad

This salad can be adapted to taste and ingredient availability.

Preparation tips: The "hotness" of the dish can be adjusted to taste by using more or less hot curry powder (or none at all). The salad can be served warm or at room temperature.

5 quarts   boiling water
1 Tbs.   salt (optional)
2 cups   basmati long-grain brown rice
                 or an alternative
                 (see "Preparation tips," above)
1 lb.   lean boneless beefsteak, 1/2-inch
                 thick, well trimmed, and sliced
                 into 1/4-inch strips
Salt to taste (optional)
Freshly ground black pepper to taste
1 1/2 Tbs. vegetable oil (preferably canola),
                 divided
1 Tbs.   cornstarch

1 tsp.	sugar
1 1/2 cups	water
3 Tbs	reduced-sodium soy sauce
4 tsp.	white-wine vinegar
1 lb.	carrots, scraped and thinly sliced on the diagonal
1 1/2 cups	chopped onion
1 Tbs.	minced gingerroot
2 tsp.	minced garlic (2 large cloves)
1 1/2 tsp.	hot curry powder
1 1/2 to 2 cups	frozen peas
1 bunch	scallions (including the green tops), thinly sliced

In a large kettle, combine the 5 quarts of boiling water with the 1 tablespoon of salt (if you are using it) and the rice. Stir the ingredients, bring the water back to a boil, stir the ingredients again, and boil the rice for 15 minutes (10 minutes if you are using white rice). Drain the rice in a large strainer, rinse the rice, and drain it again. Bring about 2 inches of water to a boil in a large sauce pan. Place the strainer of rice over the boiling water, cover the rice with a dishtowel (be sure to fold the towel in so that it will not burn), and tightly cover the pan with a lid. Steam the rice for 20 minutes, or until it is dry and fluffy. Transfer the rice to a large bowl. While the rice cooks, sprinkle the beef with the salt (if desired) and pepper. Heat 1/2 tablespoon of the oil in a large nonstick skillet, and brown the beef quickly. Transfer the beef and any juices to a medium-sized bowl, and set the bowl aside. Prepare the sauce in a small bowl by mixing the cornstarch with

the sugar, the 1 1/2 cups of water, soy sauce, vinegar, and any juices from the cooled beef. Stir the ingredients to combine them thoroughly. Set the sauce aside. Heat the remaining 1 tablespoon oil in the skillet, add the carrots and onion, and cook the vegetables, tossing them often, until they are tender crisp. Stir in the gingerroot, garlic, and curry powder, and stir-fry the ingredients for 30 seconds. Add the peas. Stir the sauce mixture once again, and add it to the pan. Bring the mixture to a boil, and cook the ingredients, tossing them occasionally, over medium heat for 2 minutes or until the sauce is slightly thickened. Stir in the reserved beef. Add the vegetable-and-beef mixture to the reserved rice. Add the scallions. Toss the mixture to combine the ingredients well, and serve the salad warm or at room temperature.

■ Serves 6

Reprinted from JANE BRODY'S GOOD FOOD GOURMET: Recipes and Menus for Delicious and Healthful Eating, *with the permission of W.W. Norton & Company, Inc. Copyright © 1990 by Jane E. Brody.*

Pineapple Ham Stir-Fry

Sweet and succulent! Your family will love this dish.

1 16-oz. can	pineapple chunks, juice packed
1/2 cup	orange juice
1 Tbs.	soy sauce
1/4 tsp.	chicken bouillon granules
1 clove	garlic, minced
1/8 tsp.	black pepper
4 tsp.	cornstarch
1/4 cup	cold water
1 cup	chicken stock
6 oz.	lean ham, diced
1 med.	green pepper, cut into 1" squares
3 cups	brown rice cooked

Drain pineapple, reserving juice. Combine orange juice, soy sauce, bouillon granules, garlic, black pepper and reserved pineapple juice. Set aside. Whisk cornstarch into 1/4 cup cold water. Set aside. Heat Wok or heavy non-stick skillet until very hot. Add chicken stock, ham and green pepper. Cook until ham is just browned, about 4 minutes. Remove from Wok. Combine orange juice mixture and pineapple chunks in Wok. Cover and cook 2 minutes. Remove pineapple with slotted spoon. Return ham to juice in Wok. Add cornstarch mixture. Cook and stir until thickened. Adjust thickness with chicken stock or water. Return pineapple to Wok. Serve over brown rice.

■ Serves 6

■ Per serving: **Cal.** 204 **Pro.** 8 g **Fat** 4 g **Sod.** 323 mg **Carb.** 33 g

From: Recipes to Lower Your Fat Thermostat *by LaRene Gaunt. Provo, UT: Copyright 1992, 1984 by Vitality House International, Inc. All rights reserved. Used by permission.*

Spicy Hawaiian Stir-Fry

Pineapple and chile peppers create a fragrant and exotic blend of flavors.

SPICY RICE VINEGAR MARINADE:

1/2 cup	vegetable broth
2 Tbs.	low-sodium tamari or soy sauce
2 Tbs.	rice vinegar
2 tsp.	arrowroot or cornstarch
1 tsp.	sugar
1/4 tsp.	crushed red pepper flakes
1 lb.	firm tofu, drained and cubed (about 2 cups)

1 (10 oz.) can unsweetened pineapple chunks	
1 large	green bell pepper, cut into 1" chunks
1 Tbs.	canola oil
4	scallions, chopped
1/2 cup	snow peas, trimmed and halved on the diagonal
1 tsp.	toasted sesame oil

Combine marinade ingredients in a deep dish. Marinate tofu for 10 minutes. Drain, reserving marinade. Set aside. Drain pineapple, adding juice to reserved marinade. Saute pepper in 2 teaspoons canola oil for 5 minutes. Add scallions, snow peas and pineapple and stir-fry for 2 minutes. Remove from skillet and set aside. Add sesame oil and remaining one teaspoon canola oil to skillet and stir-fry tofu until browned, about 8 minutes. Add pineapple mixture and reserved marinade to tofu. Cook and stir until thickened and bubbly, about 8 minutes. Serve immediately over brown rice or crisp chow mein noodles.

■ Serves 4

■ Per serving: **Cal.** 228 **Pro.** 20 g **Fat** 15 g **Sod.** 320 mg **Carb.** 23 g **Chol.** 0 mg **Calcium** 251 mg.

From: Vegetarian Gourmet. *1994; Vol. 3.*

Seafood Pasta Supreme

PASTA
1 pound lobster spacarelli or plain macaroni as long as they are not too dense.
Large pot boiling water
2 tsp. salt (optional)
1 Tbs. oil

SAUCE

1 Tbs.	olive oil
1/2 lb.	shrimp, shelled and deveined
1/2 lb.	sea scallops, sliced into 1/4-inch rounds

1 Tbs.	minced garlic (3 large cloves)
1/2 cup	sliced scallions
2 cups	peas, cooked if raw, thawed if frozen
2 cups	fresh tomatoes, peeled (if desired) and cut into 1/2-inch dice
1/2 cup	pasta cooking liquid
1 Tbs.	minced fresh basil or 1 tsp. dried basil
1/2 tsp.	oregano, crumbled

Salt to taste (optional)
Freshly ground black pepper to taste
1/4 cup minced fresh parsley
Grated Parmesan or
Romano for garnish (optional)

To make the pasta, place the pasta in the boiling water with the salt (if desired) and oil. Return the water quickly to a boil, and cook the pasta for 15 minutes or until it is *al dente*. Drain the pasta, and transfer it to a heated serving bowl or large platter. While the pasta cooks, prepare the sauce. Heat the oil in a large skillet. Add the shrimp, and saute them for 1 minute. Add the scallops, garlic, and scallions, and cook them for 2 minutes. Add the remaining ingredients except for the cheese, and heat the sauce, stirring it gently. Pour the sauce over the pasta, toss the ingredients together, and serve the pasta immediately with the grated cheese (if desired).

■ Serves 6

Reprinted from JANE BRODY'S GOOD FOOD GOURMET: Recipes and Menus for Delicious and Healthful Eating, *with the permission of W.W. Norton & Company, Inc. Copyright © 1990 by Jane E. Brody.*

Chicken Spinach Manicotti

FILLING:

1/4 pound fresh mushrooms	
2 cups	cooked chicken meat
1/2 cup	well drained, cooked spinach
1/3 cup	freshly grated parmesan cheese
1 egg	(or 2 egg whites or egg substitute equivalent to 1 egg)

Freshly ground black pepper

Sauté the mushrooms in a little oil. Chop together with the chicken and spinach until fine. Stir in the Parmesan cheese, the egg, and pepper.

PASTA:

12 manicotti tubes, cooked according to package instructions

Fill manicotti tubes and place in an oiled 11 X 7-inch shallow baking dish.

SAUCE:

2 Tbs. melted margarine
1 1/2 Tbs. flour
1 13-oz. can evaporated skim milk
Freshly ground black pepper and nutmeg
2 Tbs. parmesan cheese, grated

Blend margarine and flour. Cook one minute over moderate heat. Gradually add the evaporated skim milk, stirring constantly with a whisk. Heat till sauce bubbles, then season with pepper and nutmeg. Remove from the heat and add the grated Parmesan cheese. Pour sauce over manicotti. Sprinkle with 1/3 cup of grated Parmesan cheese and bake at 375°F. for 10 minutes or until cheese browns.

■ Yield: 6 servings
■ Approx. Cal/Serv.: 460

From The American Heart Association Cookbook, Fourth Edition *by Ruth Eshleman and Mary Winston. Copyright © 1984 by The American Heart Association. Reprinted by permission of David McKay Co., a division of Random House, Inc.*

Charcoal Grilled Shiitakes with Rosemary and Garlic

Mushrooms take on a woodsy flavor when grilled over charcoal.

8 oz.	shiitake mushrooms (about 3 cups)
1 Tbs.	extra-virgin olive oil
1 Tbs.	low-sodium tamari or soy sauce
1 Tbs.	crushed fresh garlic
1 tsp.	minced fresh rosemary or 1/2 tsp. dried
1 tsp.	pure maple syrup (optional)
1 tsp.	toasted sesame oil (optional)

Salt and black pepper to taste

Rinse mushrooms. Remove and discard stems. Toss mushrooms with remaining ingredients in a large bowl and marinate for at least 5 minutes. Grill mushroom caps over coals until slightly charred, about 3 minutes per side. Serve hot.

Hints: Use any large, firm exotic mushroom, such as portabello, in place of shiitakes. Broil mushrooms 4" from heat in your broiler.

■ Serves 4
■ Per serving: **Cal.** 218 **Pro.** 6 g **Fat** 5 g **Sod.** 158 mg **Carb.** 45 g **Chol.** 0 mg

From: Vegetarian Gourmet *Magazine. Vol. 3, Issue 3, 1994 (No. 11).*

SIDE DISHES WITH SNAP

Quinoa (The Basic Recipe)

Before cooking, always rinse the grain well to remove a slightly bitter coating.

1 3/4 cups water
1 cup Quinoa

Rinse Quinoa thoroughly, either by using a strainer or by running fresh water over the Quinoa in a pot. Drain excess water. Place Quinoa and water in a 1 1/2 quart sauce pan and bring to a boil. Reduce to a simmer, cover and cook until all of the water is absorbed (about 15 minutes). You will know that the Quinoa is done when all the grains have turned from white to transparent, and the spiral-like germ has separated. Makes 3 cups.

Nutty Broccoli

SAUCE:

2 cups	yogurt
1	egg
1/4 cup	Parmesan cheese

Dash of cayenne (optional)

NUT LAYER:

1	large onion, sliced
1 cup	mushrooms, sliced
1	green pepper, sliced thinly
2–3	cloves garlic, minced
1/2 cup	minced parsley
1/4 cup	sunflower seeds
1 Tbs.	fresh dill
1 Tbs.	tamari
1/2 lb.	fresh broccoli
2 cups	cooked Quinoa (see recipe above.)

Saute onion, pepper, mushrooms, and garlic until peppers are soft and mushroom liquid is gone. Stir in rest of nut layer ingredients. Steam broccoli till just tender. In an 8″ sq.

buttered pan arrange Quinoa, nut layer mix, broccoli, and sauce. Sprinkle with sesame seeds and dash of cayenne. Bake at 350 degrees for 30 minutes.

Reprinted with permission from White Mountain Farm, Inc., Mosca, CO.

Twice Baked Potatoes, Cottage Style

4	medium potatoes, baked
1 cup	low-fat cottage cheese
1/2 cup	low-fat milk
1 Tbs.	onion, minced

Freshly ground black pepper
Paprika
Dried parsley flakes

Cut hot potatoes in half lengthwise. Scoop out potatoes, leaving skins intact for restuffing. With wire whisk beat potatoes with cottage cheese, milk, and onion. Spoon mixture back into skins. Sprinkle with paprika and parsley flakes. Bake 10 minutes or until just golden.

■ Yield: 8 servings
■ Approx. Cal per serv.: 90

From The American Heart Association Cookbook, Fourth Edition *by Ruth Eshleman and Mary Winston. Copyright © 1984 by The American Heart Association. Reprinted by permission of David McKay Co., a division of Random House, Inc.*

Brussels Sprouts and Pecans

2 10-ounce	packages frozen brussels sprouts, thawed
3 Tbs.	margarine
4 Tbs.	flour
3/4 cup	nonfat dry milk
1 3/4 cups	boiling chicken broth
1/4 tsp.	nutmeg
1/4 cup	chopped pecans
1 cup	packaged stuffing mix

Cook the Brussels sprouts, uncovered to preserve the color, in a small amount of boiling salt water until tender. Prepare the sauce. Melt 3 tablespoons of margarine over low heat and blend in the flour. Cook 1 minute, stirring. Add dry milk, then boiling chicken broth all at once, beating with a wire whisk to blend. Cook and stir until sauce comes to a boil and thickens. Remove from heat and stir in nutmeg and pecans. Place cooked sprouts in an oiled 1 1/2-quart casserole. Pour in the cream sauce, and top with the stuffing mix. Bake at 400° F. in oven till topping is lightly browned, about 10 minutes.

■ Yield: 8 servings
■ Approx. cal/serv.: 160

From The American Heart Association Cookbook, Fourth Edition *by Ruth Eshleman and Mary Winston. Copyright © 1984 by The American Heart Association. Reprinted by permission of David McKay Co., a division of Random House, Inc.*

Arugula and Fennel Salad

Arugula is also known as roquette and rugola. But by any name, it is a now-popular nippy green that, if not carried locally, could be grown in a window box from early spring until the first frost. It's worth the effort. And once you try this salad, you'll know why.

DRESSING

2 Tbs.	red-wine vinegar
2 Tbs.	olive oil
1 tsp.	Dijon-style mustard
1/2 tsp.	salt (optional)
1/4 tsp.	freshly ground black pepper

SALAD

2 bunches arugula, tough stems removed
  and leaves torn in half
1 bulb fennel, cored and cut crosswise
  into 1/8-inch slices
1/3 cup lightly toasted pine nuts

In a salad bowl, whisk together the dressing
ingredients. Add the arugula, fennel, and
pine nuts. Toss the salad lightly, and serve it
immediately.

■ Serves 4

Reprinted from JANE BRODY'S GOOD FOOD
GOURMET: Recipes and Menus for Delicious and
Healthful Eating, *with the permission of W.W.
Norton & Company, Inc. Copyright © 1990 by
Jane E. Brody.*

Lentil Salad with Sorrel

The small green French lentils are delicious
in salads and retain their shape better than
most. The common brown lentils will work;
be sure they are cooked until just tender.
With a loaf of crusty bread and a simple,
fruity red wine, this is a good main course
salad for lunch, supper, or a picnic.

1 1/2 cups lentils
about 1/3 cup olive oil
1 small onion, diced fine
2 or 3 medium-sized ripe tomatoes, diced
2 garlic cloves, minced
2 or 3 cooked new potatoes, diced
Juice of 1/2 lemon, or to taste
Salt and freshly ground pepper
1 cup shredded sorrel leaves
3 ounces (85 g) fresh mild goat cheese
  or feta cheese

Rinse and pick over the lentils. Put them in a
pan with water to cover by 1/2 inch. Bring to
a boil, then reduce heat and simmer, covered,
until they are just tender, from 20 to 30 min-

FROZEN DESERTS 101

Don't be fooled by a label that says "non-fat" or "low-fat" on a frozen dessert container, because the claim may refer only to the dairy ingredients and not to any added nuts, oils or butter. And never assume that frozen yogurt automatically means healthier eating. While the fat content of some frozen yogurt products can be zero, others may have as much as regular ice cream! Here are a few more facts about frozen desserts:

■ Ice milk often has half the fat of regular ice cream—but read the label. While most companies base their figures on a half-cup serving, most people eat a full cup.

■ A dairy dessert can be fat-free and still have loads of sugar.

■ Frozen yogurt may claim to have active cultures, but none of the available brands have as much as regular yogurt.

■ To appear healthier than ice cream, frozen yogurt products usually measure a serving as three ounces, while most ice cream and ice milk companies use a four-ounce measure.

Copyright 1994, CSPI. Adapted from Nutrition Action Healthletter (1875 Connecticut Ave., N.W., Suite 300, Washington, D.C. 20009. $24.00 for 10 issues.)

utes. When the lentils are done, spread them
on a baking sheet and toss with the olive oil.
Let them cool slightly, then stir in the onion,
tomatoes, garlic, and potatoes. Season with
lemon juice, salt, and pepper. When the
lentils are at room temperature, stir in the
sorrel leaves and crumble in the goat cheese.

The flavor improves if the salad is refrigerated for 3 to 4 hours, then brought to cool room temperature before serving.

■ Serves 6 to 8

From: Herbs in the Kitchen *by Carolyn Dille and Susan Belsinger. Loveland, CO: Interweave Press, Inc.; 1992.*

Ratatouille

1/4 cup	oil
2 cloves	garlic, chopped
4	onions, thinly sliced
3	green peppers, cut in strips
1	eggplant, diced
4	zucchini squash, cubed
4 or 5	fresh tomatoes, peeled; or
	1 large can, drained
1-2 Tbs.	fennel seed
Freshly ground black pepper	
1/2 tsp.	oregano
1/2 tsp.	dill
1/4 cup	lemon juice

Heat oil until a haze forms. Sauté onions and garlic until golden brown, then add green pepper strips, eggplant and squash; continue cooking for about 5 minutes, stirring occasionally.

Put in the tomatoes, pepper, oregano, fennel and dill. Cover and cook at a low temperature for about 15 minutes, stirring occasionally. Uncover and continue cooking for 15 minutes to allow excess liquid to evaporate. Sprinkle on lemon juice.

Serve hot or cold.

■ Yield: 2 quarts
■ Approx. cal/serv.: 1/2 cup = 150

From The American Heart Association Cookbook, Fourth Edition *by Ruth Eshleman and Mary Winston. Copyright © 1984 by The American Heart Association. Reprinted by permission of David McKay Co., a division of Random House, Inc.*

Sweet Potato Special

Preparation tips: This can be prepared two days ahead for baking. Cover the dish and refrigerate it, but bring it to room temperature before baking it. Although canned pineapple can be used, the flavor is not as good as when fresh fruit is used.

5 pounds	sweet potatoes
Water to cover	
1 12-ounce package pitted prunes	
1 cup water	
2 cups (1/2 large) fresh pineapple, slivered	
1/4 cup dark brown sugar (optional)	
1 Tbs. butter or margarine (optional)	

Cook the potatoes, whole and unpeeled, in water to cover until they are very soft. Drain the potatoes, pierce them one at a time with a fork, peel them, place them in a large bowl, and mash them. Preheat the oven to 350°F. In a small saucepan, cook the prunes in the 1 cup of water for 5 minutes. Add the prunes, their cooking liquid, and the pineapple to the potatoes, mixing the ingredients to combine them well. Place the potato mixture in a large ovenproof casserole. Sprinkle the potatoes with brown sugar (if desired), and dot the top with the butter or margarine (if you wish). Place the uncovered casserole in the hot oven, and bake the potatoes for 20 minutes or until the potatoes are heated through.

■ Serves 10

Reprinted from JANE BRODY'S GOOD FOOD GOURMET: Recipes and Menus for Delicious and Healthful Eating, *with the permission of W.W. Norton & Company, Inc. Copyright © 1990 by Jane E. Brody.*

UNBELIEVABLY HEALTHY DESSERTS

Strawberry Cheesecake

A fabulous low-fat variation of this all time favorite dessert.

2 cups	fresh strawberries
2	bananas
2 cups	low-fat yogurt
1 tsp.	vanilla
2	egg whites
1 env.	unflavored gelatin
2 Tbs.	boiling water
1	unbaked Grape-Nuts Pie Crust (Below)

Combine 1 cup strawberries, bananas, yogurt, vanilla, egg whites, gelatin and boiling water in blender on high speed for 2 minutes. Pour into Grape-Nuts Pie Crust. Bake at 350°F for 1 hour. Refrigerate for 3 hours. Top with remaining 1 cup fresh strawberries before serving.

■ Serves 6

Grape-Nuts Pie Crust

Isn't this a great idea? Only a trace of fat and a terrific taste.

1 6 oz. can apple juice concentrate
1 1/2 cups Grape-Nuts cereal

Mix juice with Grape-Nuts and let stand for a few minutes until moisture is absorbed. Press into a 9" non-stick pie pan. Bake at 350°F for 12 minutes. Cool. Fill with fruit and yogurt pudding. Serve.

■ Serves 6
■ Per serving: **Cal.** 164 **Pro.** 4 g **Fat** trace **Sod.** 148 mg **Carb.** 36 g.

From: Recipes to Lower Your Fat Thermostat *by LaRene Gaunt. Provo, UT: Copyright 1992, 1984 by Vitality House International, Inc. All rights reserved. Used by permission.*

Quinoa Pudding

3 cups	cooked Quinoa
1 cup	milk grated rind of lemon and orange
1/4 cup	sugar
1 tsp	vanilla
2 eggs	
1/2 cup	raisins & almonds (optional)

pinch of nutmeg, cinnamon and cloves

Heat Quinoa in milk until it is soft and milk is absorbed. Add other ingredients, stirring after each addition. This is a variation of the old rice pudding, use your favorite recipe.

Reprinted with permission from White Mountain Farm Inc.,

Simple Soft Ice Cream

1 cup nonfat dry milk
3 cups water
2 Tbs sugar
Vanilla extract to taste

Blend all ingredients in a blender until smooth. For a variety of flavors, replace vanilla extract with banana, cherry or maple extract. Freeze in shallow pan. Just before serving, thaw slightly and break into small chunks. Whip until soft. Spoon into 4 dishes, top with fresh fruit and enjoy.

From: Recipes to Lower Your Fat Thermostat *by LaRene Gaunt. Provo, UT: Copyright 1992, 1884 by Vitality House International, Inc. All rights reserved. Used by permission.* □

FOR MORE RECIPE IDEAS

Each of the books from which these recipes were drawn contains a wealth of other inventive, healthy dishes. Check your local bookstore or order directly from the publishers at the addresses listed below.

Eating Well, The Magazine of Food and Health
Contact:
Eating Well
Ferry Road
Charlotte, VT 05445
Phone orders: 800-678-0541
Fax: 802-425-3307

Herbs in the Kitchen
by Carolyn Dille and Susan Belsinger, 1992
$26.95
Contact:
Interweave Press Inc.
201 East Fourth Street
Loveland, CO 80537
Phone orders: 800-645-3675
Fax orders: 970-667-8317
Other inquiries: 970-669-7672

The International Menu Diabetic Cookbook
by Betty Marks, 1985
Contact:
Contemporary Books, Inc.
Two Prudential Plaza, Suite 1200
Chicago, IL 60601
Phone: 312-540-4500
Fax: 312-540-4657

Jane Brody's Good Food Gourmet
by Jane Brody, 1990
Contact:
W. W. Norton & Company
500 Fifth Avenue
New York, NY 10110
Phone: 212-354-5500
Fax: 212-869-0856

Nutrition Action Healthletter
$24.00 (10 issues)
Contact:
Center for Science in the Public Interest
1875 Connecticut Avenue, N.W., Suite 300
Washington, D.C. 20009
Phone: 202-332-9110
Fax: 202-265-4954

Recipes to Lower Your Fat Thermostat
by LaRene Gaunt, 1992
Contact:
Vitality House International, Inc.
1675 North Freedom Boulevard, #11C
Provo, UT 84604
Phone: 800-748-5100
Fax: 801-373-5370

Vegetarian Gourmet Magazine
$15.95 (5 issues)
Contact:
Chariot Publishing, Inc.
P.O. Box 7641
Riverton, NJ 08077
Phone: 800-628-8244
Fax: 717-278-2233

The World in Your Kitchen
by Troth Wells, 1993
$16.95
Contact:
The Crossing Press
P.O. Box 1048
Freedom, CA 95019
Phone orders: 408-777-1048
Fax orders: 408-722-2749

CHAPTER 33

Improving Your Diet with International Flair

If your low-fat, high-fiber diet is beginning to seem . . . well . . . just a little bit *dull,* it's probably time for a bit of adventure. International cuisine, at home or away, can lend zest to your diet without adding fat. You just need to know which dishes to choose.

Some foreign cuisines have gained well-deserved reputations for being healthier than our own. Chinese, Japanese, and Greek menus, for example, are all studded with delicious dishes that meet the most stringent of requirements for healthy dining. Other cuisines—particularly Mexican and French—are noted for the opposite.

Still, it's quite possible to cook a healthy French meal, and equally easy to order a fat-soaked, salt-laden disaster at your local Chinese restaurant. This chapter sorts out which items to order and which to reject from nearly a dozen ethnic cuisines. You'll find a surprising range of healthy options in even the worst of these diets. But first, a few general guidelines.

Strategies for Healthy International Dining

It's a good rule of thumb to keep your international adventure to less than 800 calories, with no more than 30% coming from fat. Code words for high-fat (high-calorie) menu selections are listed in the box on the next page, together with warning signs of sodium. These signals are not foolproof—not every dish prepared in broth, for example, is high in salt. Nor should you forego every breaded entree. The words are merely a reminder to think twice about what may go into the dish.

■ **Ask questions; make requests.** Never be afraid to ask your server how a meal is prepared, or to request changes in cooking methods. Most restaurants will use less butter or oil, for example, if you ask. For a list of restaurants that serve low-fat meals, try calling your local chapter of the American Heart Association.

■ **Have an extra side dish of grains or vegetables**—or both—unless these foods are already the basis of your entree. Then mix

WARNING SIGNS OF FAT AND SODIUM

High fat	High sodium
Battered	Smoked
Fried	Pickled
Breaded	Barbecued
Creamed	Marinated
Au gratin	Parmesan
Scalloped	In broth
Hollandaise	Teriyaki
Escalloped	Creole

your entrée with the extra food. This reduces the fat and sodium quotient of the meal—provided you . . .

- **Don't clean your plate.** There's nothing wrong with left-overs—or doggy bags.
- **Don't start with fat-laden munchies.** At restaurants, ask that complimentary chips and hors d'oeuvres be removed. If you know you'll keep nibbling, why tempt yourself?
- **Trim fat from meat**—or ask the server to have it done. This is an easy saving that costs nothing in diminished enjoyment.
- **Go in for variety.** No single ethnic cuisine holds the key to longer life. The Japanese have a low rate of heart disease—but a high rate of stomach cancer. The secret lies in choosing the best of each nationality's diet, and rejecting the heart-stoppers.

French

In the 1960s and 70s, French food was filled with cream and butter. Now, the trend is toward lighter cooking, with a focus on fresh garden ingredients and fewer flavors to confuse the palate. Light-minded chefs choose top-quality foods at the peak of their flavor, in season, and cook them as simply as possible.

The French currently eat about as much saturated fat as the Americans and British, and have similar levels of total cholesterol, according to the World Health Organization. However, their fatality rate from coronary heart disease isn't much higher than that of the Japanese and Chinese, who eat much less saturated fat and have lower cholesterol levels. In fact, France's rate of heart disease is the world's second lowest—after Japan's. The French also match the U.S. and the United Kingdom in terms of high blood pressure and—at least in men—cigarette smoking. Why, then, are French hearts apparently healthier?

One proposed explanation is wine. The people in the nations with the longest life expectancies in the world—Crete and Japan—both drink moderate amounts of alcohol. It's thought that this may help the heart by impeding the development of blood clots which, by blocking the supply of blood to the heart muscle, can cause a heart attack. Despite this theory, however, health officials hesitate to recommend alcohol, lest people become carried away with it. Officials also note that drinking can increase your risk of certain cancers and other diseases.

Whether you take wine or not, avoid haute cuisine or cuisine bourgeois. Both terms

WHAT'S OKAY AND WHAT TO WATCH WHEN EATING. . .

 French

Go ahead and enjoy

- Salade nicoise, spinach salad (without bacon), endive and watercress salad
- Consommé and other stock–based soups
- Stews like bouillabaisse or ratatouille
- Poached or steamed seafood
- Seared or oven–roasted scallops or salmon
- Sauces labeled coulis, vegetable puree, or reduction
- Roast chicken or chicken in wine sauce
- French bread
- Fresh or poached fruit

But hold back on

- Cassoulet, gratins, quiches (they're made with a lot of egg and cheese)
- Soufflés (heavy with eggs)
- Sweetbreads (fatty meat)
- Duck or goose (tend to be fatty)
- Paté (also fatty)
- béarnaise, beurre blanc, and other dairy–based sauces
- Fondue or crepes
- Brioches, croissants, eclairs, and other pastry

indicate that butter, cream, pork lard, goose fat, and eggs are used liberally. Nouvelle cuisine tends to be healthier. Choose simple meals, with few if any sauces, which tend to be high in sodium. When you do opt for an entree with sauce, try to select one that's wine-based rather than one filled with cream or butter. When dining out, remember that sauces are not always mentioned on the menu. Ask your server if your meal has a sauce and, if so, how it's prepared.

To turn your kitchen into a haven of light French food, keep these staple ingredients handy:

- Olive oil
- Red wine vinegar
- Dijon mustard
- Defatted chicken stock
- Shallots, garlic, chervil, chives, parsley, and tarragon

Italian

It's important to distinguish between northern and southern Italian cuisine. Southern Italy traditionally follows a Mediterranean diet, with lots of grains, fruits and vegetables, olive oil instead of butter, and little meat. This is thought to be one of the healthiest ethnic cuisines in the world, and some authorities even recommend it over the

U.S. Food Guide Pyramid. (See Chapter 1 for more information.) Northern Italian meals, in contrast, are full of beef, veal, butter, and cream—and have a totally different effect on your fat and calorie count. Not surprisingly, northern Italians have much higher rates of heart disease than their southern countrymen.

Unfortunately, Italian restaurants in this country tend to mirror the fat content of northern cuisine. An analysis of 15 popular dishes as served in 21 mid-priced restaurants in three major cities revealed that one order of fettuccini Alfredo includes nearly 435 calories from saturated fat—as much as 3 pints of Breyer's Butter Almond ice cream. The analysis, commissioned by the Center for Science in the Public Interest, a research group in Washington, DC, also found that eggplant parmigiana with spaghetti has the fat and calories of five egg rolls (1,208 calories, 62 grams of fat, 46 percent of calories from fat), and that an appetizer of fried cala-

WHAT'S OKAY AND WHAT TO WATCH WHEN EATING. . .

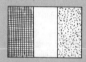 Italian

Go ahead and enjoy

- Vegetable antipasto (roasted peppers and zucchini, grilled mushrooms, caponata)
- Salads such as panzanella (with tomatoes tomatoes and bread)
- Pasta with tomato- or wine-based sauce without meat. Marinara is a good tomato-based sauce. Red or white clam sauce is okay, too
- Pasta e fagioli (pasta and bean soup) Minestrone soup (if no meat)
- Ribollito (a thick vegetarian stew)
- Cioppino (seafood stew)
- Grilled game, veal, and fish
- Chicken cacciatore
- Snapper in cartoccio (baked in parchment)
- Marinated calamari
- Pasta primavera (pasta with vegetables). Make sure there is no cream or butter sauce
- Eggplant pomodoro style
- Italian ice

But hold back on

- Meat or cheese antipasti
- Cannelloni, ravioli, lasagna, and other cheese-filled pastas
- Pasta with pesto or cream sauces, such as carbonara and Alfredo
- Risotto (a rice dish cooked with butter and cheese)
- Eggplant with cheese or veal parmigiana
- Veal or chicken piccata, marsala, and saltimbocca
- Garlic bread made with butter
- Cannoli or other cream pastries
- Pancetta, prosciutto, pecorino cheese

mari delivers 924 milligrams of cholesterol—more than a four-egg omelet.

Nevertheless, it's easy to have a delicious Italian meal without wallowing in fat. Virtually all pasta dishes except those with cream or cheese sauces derive less than 30 percent of their calories from fat, and less than 10 percent from saturated fat. The sauce can be tomato, clam, even meat or meatballs—just avoid Alfredo, carbonara, and other cream or cheese variations. If you prefer not to have pasta as your main meal, add some on the side. This can stretch your food to make a second meal—spreading the main-dish fat and calories over a couple of sittings. When eating with friends in a restaurant, try ordering a pasta dish for every meat- or cheese-based entree, sharing the food, and taking home the leftovers. You'll get to sample a variety of dishes without breaking your calorie and fat budget.

Also make a side dish of vegetables or a salad with endive, radicchio, or other greens a part of your meal. When dining out, this can help make up for the restaurants' frequent failure to serve vegetables with pasta entrées. Be choosy with the vegetables, though: they are often soaked with butter or oil. And order the salad dressing on the side. Remember too, that a tablespoon of grated parmesan cheese adds 2 grams of fat to your meal, one of

which is saturated. If you're watching sodium, you should be aware that most Italian restaurant entrées supply 1,500 milligrams, making it hard to stay within the Recommended Daily Allowance of 2,400 milligrams.

Preparing healthy Italian food is almost as easy as "a loaf of bread, a jug of wine, and thou." Pasta with a jar of sauce (check the label for fat and sodium) enlivened by chopped onion, pepper, tomato, garlic, and herbs makes a quick, tasty, healthy meal. If you must add meat to the sauce, use ground turkey or lean beef. Squeeze garlic into soups, vegetables, sauces, and salads for extra flavor and its heart-healthy dividends. Use herbs such as basil, parsley, rosemary, and oregano to add flavor and variety in place of salt.

Freshness is a key to Italian foods' tastiness. But you also need to keep these staples on hand:

- Balsamic and red wine vinegars
- Cannelini beans and chick-peas, dried
- Extra virgin olive oil
- Dried pasta in a variety of shapes
- Coarse cornmeal (for polenta)
- Porcini mushrooms, dried
- Italian plum tomatoes, canned
- Parmigiano-Reggiano cheese, in chunks for grating
- Part-skim ricotta cheese (low in fat, tastes like real Italian ricotta cheese)
- Garlic, basil, oregano, rosemary, sage

WHAT'S OKAY AND WHAT TO WATCH WHEN EATING. . .

 Greek

Go ahead and enjoy

- Torato (cold soup with eggplant, peppers, and yogurt)
- Grilled fish or octopus
- Skewered and grilled vegetable and meat dishes, such as souvlaki and shish kebab
- Grilled lamb chops, roast leg of lamb, braised lamb shanks
- Fish baked with plaki sauce
- Grilled fish with parsley or lemon sauces
- Garlic dips from giant white beans

But hold back on

- Taramasalata (creamy fish-roe dip)
- Meats in avgolemono (egg-based lemon sauce)
- Moussaka and pastitsio (casseroles made with eggs and cheese)
- Skordalia (almond-garlic sauce)
- Gyros

Greek

Greek cuisine is another example of the Mediterranean diet. In fact, it was the observation that people on the Greek island of Crete had only one-twentieth the American death rate from heart disease that helped spur interest in the Mediterranean diet.

Breads are the center of Greek meals; other foods are considered accompaniments. Milk is seldom used as a beverage. Meat traditionally is reserved for special occasions, vegetables are often main courses, and pasta is almost as popular as in Italy. Rice is also featured in many dishes. Sauces are built on wine, stocks, tomato, and yogurt rather than cream. As in southern Italy, olive oil is popular. Lentils and beans are commonly used in appetizers and main courses. Greek feta cheese (white cheese made from sheep's milk and preserved in brine), is lighter than average—but to keep salt content as low as possible, be sure to rinse before serving. Lamb is a favorite meat. Trim it carefully and cook on the grill to keep fat to a minimum. Seafood dishes also are common. Fruit is an every-day dessert. Baklava, a rich pastry, is reserved for special occasions.

If you're interested in trying some light Greek cooking, stock up on the following:

- Olive oil ("pure" is fine)
- Red and white wine vinegars
- Lemon juice
- Orzo (rice-shaped pasta), short macaroni, and rice
- Dried cannelini beans, lentils, yellow split peas

- Plain low-fat or non-fat yogurt for sauces
- Tomatoes, canned
- Garlic, oregano, rosemary, parsley

Chinese

With its reliance on rice and vegetables, and sparing use of meat, Chinese food is a model of healthy dining. At least, that's true in China. A study of eating habits in rural China found that the average diet includes 77 percent carbohydrates and 15 percent fat, compared to the 35 to 40 percent fat in the American diet. Perhaps it's no surprise that the Chinese develop heart disease at a far lower rate than Americans.

Chinese restaurants in the U.S. tend to use more meat and sauce than found in China, but still serve a relatively high-vegetable cuisine. Stir-frying, a method of cooking quickly in a lightly oiled hot wok, retains more vitamins than the traditional American methods of cooking. According to a University of Nebraska study, beef prepared this way retains more vitamin B_6 and thiamin than it does when broiled or microwaved.

One of the organizations that developed the Mediterranean Diet Pyramid is now working on an Asian diet formula. Its work is based on studies by T. Colin Campbell, PhD, a researcher at Cornell University, who has been examining the nutritional benefits of the Asian diet since 1984. He and his colleagues are investigating the theory that eating more plant foods (grains, fruits, vegetables, and beans) can help prevent chronic degenerative diseases. Evidence so far indicates that even

small amounts of animal food (both meat and dairy products) significantly increase cholesterol levels.

Among Dr. Campbell's findings:

- People in rural China get 20 to 30 percent more calories than Americans but are 25 percent thinner.
- The Chinese eat a third less protein than we do, and only a tenth as much animal protein.
- Men in China have much lower cholesterol levels than American men.
- The Chinese are only half to one-third as likely to develop colon cancers as are Americans.
- The Chinese diet is high in antioxidant nu-

TOFU TIPS

Although tofu, a major source of soy and protein in Chinese food, derives a little more than half its calories from fat, most of the fat is unsaturated. To use tofu, slice it into chunks and use it in place of meat in recipes. It has little flavor of its own, but picks up the taste of whatever surrounds it. Cover unused tofu with water and refrigerate it. Change the water at least every other day.

- Make eggless egg salad or mock chicken salad using firm tofu as a base.
- Marinate and grill tofu just as you would chicken or beef. Serve in fajitas or on top of salads.
- Stir-fry chunks of tofu with vegetables and serve over rice.
- Prepare chili, substituting crumbled tofu for ground meat.
- Simmer soup made with soy milk, then add tofu to create a robust low-fat meal.

Source: *Environmental Nutrition*, May 1994, p 4,.

trients that, according to some researchers, may help inhibit growth of cancer.

Other research also demonstrates the health value of Asian food. Green tea, the type usually served without charge in Chinese and Japanese restaurants, has been linked to a lower risk of esophageal cancer. Other studies have suggested that this kind of tea may also block the growth of other kinds of tumors. Researchers attribute the tea's effects to its antioxidant chemicals.

Asians tend to rely on soy rather than meat for much of their protein; and this may give a double boost to their health. The soy not only replaces animal fat, but may also confer benefits of its own. An ingredient in soy is thought to reduce or prevent formation of artery-clogging fat deposits on blood vessels' walls. According to some reports, individuals whose cholesterol levels exceed 250 can reduce them by as much as 25 percent simply by substituting soy for animal protein.

Soy also appears to have some cancer-fighting properties. More than 30 studies confirm the ability of one ingredient of soy, a substance called an isoflavone, to prevent growth of cancer cells—at least in a test tube. Isoflavones in soy may mimic estrogen, a female sex hormone. This could trick the body into producing less of the real thing. Since growth of some cancers in women is promoted by estrogen, the benefits of reduced levels seem obvious. Asian women, who eat lots of soy, have lower estrogen levels than American women, as well as half the breast-cancer rate and fewer symptoms at menopause. Japanese women do not have a term for hot flashes and do not experience premenstrual syndrome.

Some evidence suggests that soy may help prevent cancer in men, too. Japanese men who eat lots of rice and the soy-based product called tofu have lower rates of prostate cancer. Those raised on the American diet (high saturated fat) are more likely to develop prostate cancer. There is no definite proof that it's the Japanese diet that lowers cancer rates, however.

Chinese culinary style varies by region. The names you usually see on menus, such as Cantonese and Szechuan, refer to areas known for a particular style of cooking. Cantonese food, from southern China, emphasizes pork, chicken, and dumplings. Szechuan cuisine, from inland China, is noted for its hot, spicy seasonings, with many high-fat meat dishes fried in oil. Northern menus characteristic of Beijing feature sweet-and-sour dishes, duck, noodles, and steamed breads. Coastal dishes from Shanghai naturally include more seafood.

The base of all Chinese meals is rice; the Chinese eat three to four mouthfuls of unseasoned rice for each mouthful of highly seasoned toppings. The yin-yang rule for a big Chinese meal is one salty, one sweet; one stir-fried, one steamed; one bland, one hot; one stewed, one pickled.

Although traditional Chinese food is healthy, you need to be choosy when dining out. Americanized Chinese restaurant food often is fried or otherwise prepared in oil. A fried egg roll, for instance, usually derives more than half of its 200 calories from fat. And a highly publicized analysis commissioned by the Center for Science in the Public Interest (CSPI), found that a typical serving

WHAT'S OKAY AND WHAT TO WATCH WHEN EATING. . .

 Chinese

Go ahead and enjoy

- Hot–and–sour soup
- Wonton soup
- Steamed vegetable dumplings
- Chinese greens
- Steamed or braised whole fish or scallops with black–bean sauce (avoid black–bean sauce if you are watching sodium intake)
- Chicken or eggplant steamed or braised
- Steamed beef with pea pods
- Stir-fry dishes (go easy on the oil or use broth instead)
- Dishes made with sliced rather than diced meat (dicing can be used to hide a fatty cut of meat)
- Rice—preferably brown, but steamed white is fine
- Chicken and broccoli
- Vegetable dishes with mushrooms, broccoli, water chestnuts, bamboo shoots, bok choy, squash, snow peas, lotus root.

But hold back on

- Fried egg rolls
- Fried dumplings, pork or beef dumplings
- Sweet–and–sour pork
- Seafood with lobster sauce
- Egg Fu Yung
- Spare ribs
- Pressed duck, Peking duck
- Anything "crispy" or "batter coated" (usually deep fried)
- Fried rice
- Kung Pao chicken (heavy on nuts, high in fat)

---

of Kung Pao chicken, with more than 40 percent of its calories from fat, is loaded with a total 76 grams—more fat than the 66 grams the government says we should eat all day.

Nevertheless, the analysis gave Chinese cooking in general a clean bill of health. Based on an examination of 15 popular dishes from 20 mid-priced Chinese restaurants in Washington, DC, Chicago, and San Francisco, it found that saturated fat overall was lower than in most American food. Almost all entrées derived much less than 10 percent of calories from saturated fat—the target recommended by the Food and Drug Administration. Another study of main courses in Chinese restaurants, this time in

Dallas-Fort Worth, found that fat, at 8 to 32 grams, was well within accepted guidelines.

On the other hand, Chinese food is often high in sodium—something to be aware of if you have high blood pressure. Oyster- and black-bean sauces are major culprits, but the CSPI analysis found that most dishes included at least 2,000 milligrams—nearly the entire recommended daily intake of 2,400 milligrams.

Chinese cooking is notorious for its use of monosodium glutamate (MSG), which can be unpleasant for anyone sensitive to it. However, MSG is a completely optional ingredient, and many Chinese restaurants will omit it on request. Even so, be wary when dining out: Pre-made sauces and stocks used in restaurants usually contain it, so keeping it out of the rest of the entrée may not make the food MSG-free.

To get the peak health benefits offered by Chinese cuisine, try these tactics whenever cooking at home, ordering take-out, or going out to eat:

■ Add rice to your entrée. "One cup rice, one cup entrée" is a good rule. Split an entree with a friend or save the leftovers. This distributes the sodium and fat in the main course between the two of you or over more than one meal.

■ Choose vegetables, dumplings, dim sum, and other dishes that are steamed rather than fried or sautéed.

■ Share a dish of steamed vegetables. If you are eating alone and want a non-vegetarian entree, have one vegetable dish and another with meat or fish. This dilutes the meal's total fat content—provided you have leftovers.

■ Peel any batter-fried skin off of chicken or fish.

■ Get more vegetables and less meat in meat dishes.

■ Use fewer nuts—they raise fat content.

■ Avoid fried rice—many versions contain egg, which raises fat and cholesterol. Fried rice also has 1 to 2 tablespoons more oil than other rice. If you must have it, ask for vegetable fried rice and mix it with steamed rice.

■ Ask for brown rice at the restaurant or make your own at home—it has more fiber and nutrients than white rice.

■ If you must eat crispy beef or other oily, fried dishes, share a single portion with your group.

■ Avoid breaded meat or shrimp dishes. They're almost always fried.

■ Use reduced-sodium soy sauce if sodium is a concern.

■ Don't add soy sauce to stir-fry dishes.

■ To reduce sodium, season food at the table with Chinese hot mustard or rice vinegar rather than soy sauce.

■ Don't add butter, margarine, or salt to rice while cooking. Don't use packaged rice mixes—they're high in sodium and fat.

■ Use no more than an ounce or so of meat per serving—or none at all.

■ When stir frying, blanch vegetables first. This can cut the oil needed by half, according to Barbara Tropp of China Moon Cafe in San Francisco.

■ In restaurants, look for "heart-healthy," "low-fat," or "Buddha's delight" (vegetarian) sections on the menu.

WHAT'S OKAY AND WHAT TO WATCH WHEN EATING. . .

Japanese

Go ahead and enjoy

- Miso soup (unless you're on a low-sodium diet)
- Sushi (except surimi and salmon caviar), sashimi
- Sunomono (cucumber salad)
- Yakitori (grilled or broiled chicken)
- Chiri nabe (fish stew)
- Yosenabe (a seafood-and-vegetable stew)
- Shabu-shabu (a variety of vegetables and meats boiled in broth)
- Teriyaki
- Tofu and other soybean dishes
- Rice and noodles
- Rice crackers

But hold back on

- Tempura or agemono (food is deep fried)
- Egg dishes such as oyako-donburi
- Salted, smoked, or pickled fish
- Pan-fried pork
- Tonkatsu (fried pork)
- Breaded meat, fish, or chicken
- Sukiyaki
- Fried tofu

For cooking Chinese at home, lay in a supply of these basics—readily available in most supermarkets—then branch out as your recipes dictate:

- Short- or medium-grain rice
- Egg noodles
- Reduced-sodium soy sauce
- Corn or peanut oil
- Sesame oil
- Fermented black beans
- Fresh ginger, scallions, garlic, red pepper flakes

Japanese

The fat content of Japanese cuisine is among the lowest in the world—many dishes contain less than 20 percent. Like Chinese cooking, Japanese food traditionally uses plenty of grains and vegetables, accented with meat or fish as well as tofu and other soybean products. This may be one reason why Japan enjoys a relatively low rate of many cancers—and the world's lowest rate of heart disease. The seaweed used in sushi and Japanese stews is high in calcium, magnesium, and iodine. But beware of smoked, salted, and pickled Japanese specialties. They are suspected culprits in the high rates of stroke and stomach cancer in Japan.

Here are some tips for making your Japanese meal as healthy as it can be, at home or in a restaurant:

■ Keep sauces on the side; they are usually served that way in restaurants.

■ Watch out for soups—they can be salty.

■ Look for the word yakimono on menus or in cookbooks—it means broiled, a healthier mode of cooking.

■ Buy or eat sushi (or sashimi) only at a clean restaurant with a good reputation. Unclean raw fish can make you sick. Do consider trying sushi, as it has no added fat and contains omega-3 fatty acids, which may be heart-healthy.

■ Minimize use of soy and teriyaki sauce.

■ Go easy on tempura (deep-fried food) and tonkatsu (deep-fried pork).

■ Consider trying nebemono—one-pot meals with names like yosenabe and shabu-shabu.

■ If you're concerned about sodium, avoid dishes using miso (fermented soybean paste) and smoked or pickled fish.

■ Opt for fresh fruit over sweet bean-cake (yokan) as your dessert.

Mexican

Americans now spend more on salsa than they do on ketchup—a startling demonstration of Mexican foods' soaring popularity. The new craze for Mexican dining is not, however, all that compatible with our new-found interest in light cuisine. If you order grilled fish or chicken in a tomatillo sauce, or a jicama salad with a light vinaigrette, your Mexican food is probably healthy. But, many of the most popular meals at large, mid-priced, non-fast-food chains are loaded with salt and fat.

A 1994 evaluation commissioned by the Center for Science in the Public Interest found that rice at mid-priced Mexican chains and some independent restaurants in four major cities had more than 800 milligrams of sodium, about a third of what we should eat all day. Beans contained almost as much. Worse yet, an order of beef-and-cheese nachos packed 59 percent of its calories in fat (versus the recommended target of 30 percent), a chicken burrito dinner included a day-and-a-half's worth of sodium, and a chile relleno dinner derived 79 percent of its 487 calories from fat. According to CSPI, making a meal of just the side dishes of rice and beans, guacamole, and sour cream at mid-price chains gives you nearly two thirds of the fat and three fourths of the saturated fat and sodium that the government says you should eat all day.

It's not hard to see why so many Mexican dishes are loaded with fat. Remember that enchiladas are tortillas softened in oil. Tacos are deep-fried tortillas. In chimichangas, both the filling and shell are prepared in boiling oil. Favorite Americanized dishes such as beef burritos with cheese and sour cream are also high in both fat and calories, often thanks to the toppings. A plain tostado (a corn tortilla with refried beans) has only 140 calories. Add on sour cream, guacamole, and cheese, and, voila—300 calories. How can this happen? Consider the numbers:

Sour cream (1 tablespoon) = 26 calories and 2.5 grams fat

Guacamole (1 tablespoon) = 23 calories and 1.5 grams fat

At least guacamole (mashed avocado and tomato) contains mostly monounsaturated

WHAT'S OKAY AND WHAT TO WATCH WHEN EATING. . .

 # Mexican or Southwest

Go ahead and enjoy

- Gazpacho soup (cold soup)
- Albondigo soup (vegetables and meatballs)
- Black bean and vegetable soup
- Fajitas or tacos al carbon, especially with seafood (hold the sour cream)
- Burrito with vegetables, whole beans (not refried), or chicken
- Soft taco with chicken
- Tostado, bean or chicken
- Steamed tortilla
- Enchilada, bean
- Mesquite-grilled chicken, seafood, or lean cuts of beef or pork, especially with fresh salsa
- Fish or chicken marinated in lime juice (called seviche when made with fish)
- Rice and whole beans
- Shredded lettuce and tomato
- Salsa

But hold back on

- Tortilla chips and nachos
- Guacamole
- Chimichangas (fried)
- Burritos with beef or cheese
- Hard-shell tacos (fried)
- Flautas (deep-fried tacos and burritos), taquitos (fried)
- Fried tortillas
- Enchiladas, cheese and/or beef
- Quesadillas
- Dishes with poblano aioli (chile mayonnaise) or cilantro pesto (nuts and oil)
- Refried beans, also called frijoles
- Chilies rellanos
- Chile con queso
- Anything with sour cream
- Tamales
- Chorizo (sausages)
- Frozen margaritas and pina coladas

fat—which can increase "good" (HDL) cholesterol. Still, try substituting lettuce, tomato, and onion as your flavor enhancers. Feel free to use salsa, which has less than 5 calories and little fat per tablespoon.

Unlike Old El Paso and other supermarket refried beans, most restaurant-cooked refried beans are prepared in lard with bacon or cheese. Don't forget either, that salads, a safe option in most other types of restaurants, can consist of fried foods in an oily tortilla shell when you dine out Mexican-style.

Indeed, of all the main dishes tested by CSPI, only chicken fajitas registered fewer than 30% calories from fat—and just 5% from saturated fat. Fajitas consist of marinated chicken breast sautéed with onions and green peppers—a relatively healthy combination. Also in their favor: You assemble the final product at the table and therefore control what goes into the tortilla. (Skip the sour cream and guacamole.)

With the introduction of reduced-fat menu options such as Taco Bell's line of "Border Lights," it's becoming a bit easier to go out for a healthy Mexican meal. There are numerous health-saving tactics to be tried as well—both at the restaurant and at home:

- Choose steamed or baked tortillas rather than fried; use whole wheat tortillas at home.
- Ask for nonrefried beans when dining out; use no-fat black beans for home cooking.
- Avoid combination plates, they're likely to be fattier.
- Don't get side dishes, or choose marinated vegetables.
- Use salsa on your main course instead of sour cream and cheese. Do the same with the tomatoes and onions and hot peppers (pico de gallo) that come with many restaurant dishes—ask for some if it's not offered.
- At home or away, use low-fat or nonfat sour cream.

In many ways, Southwest cooking is Mexican food with these principles at work. It uses little or no sour cream and less cheese and butter. Rice and beans are still the core of the meal, but supporting roles are played by grilled or raw fresh vegetables. There's lots of fresh salsa and pure chile puree. Salads are green, not fried. Watch out, though, for Tex-Mex. It's heavy in barbecued or fried meats. Cal-Mex is a lighter choice, with more fresh vegetables.

When stocking up on Mexican ingredients, read labels and avoid products containing coconut oil, palm oil, and lard, all high in saturated fat. Look for brands saying "no salt added." Supermarket salsa generally has 40 to 180 milligrams of sodium per tablespoon, so look for brands with a "no salt added" label if you're watching your sodium. Here are some of the staples to keep on hand:

- Dried pinto and black beans
- Corn and whole–wheat tortillas
- Rice (preferably brown)
- White cornmeal
- Chilies, dried (cascabels, guajillos) and fresh (Anaheims, jalapenos, poblanos, serranos)

When shopping for groceries, focus on:

- Tomatoes
- Avocados
- Corn on the cob
- Squashes, especially zucchini and pumpkin
- Jicama
- Limes, apples, mangoes, papayas, pineapples
- Cilantro (Chinese parsley, coriander greens)

Indian

Indian cuisine is rich in healthy ingredients: plenty of grains, vegetables, beans, and yogurt accented with meat or fish. Typical dishes contain lentils, chickpeas, rice, beans, and spices such as cardamom, cinnamon, and cloves. Popular meat recipes include lamb and chicken marinated in a healthy, yogurt-and-spice sauce.

However, there can be plenty of fat hidden in preparation. Many dishes are soaked in clarified butter (ghee), which can raise the proportion of calories from fat to 50 percent. Others are swimming in coconut oil, one of the few vegetable oils that is almost entirely saturated fat. Check on the curry sauce, for instance. Most curries are made with coconut milk, though healthier yogurt-based sauces are sometimes available. Saffron rice may sound healthy, but some versions are cooked with ghee. Always ask restaurants how the food is prepared; some will use lighter oils on request.

Among your healthier choices: tandoori chicken and fish dishes, made in a clay oven and marinated in Indian spices, entrées with yogurt marinades; vegetarian dishes made with lentils, spices, and grains. You might want to try some of the chutneys, too; but these thick condiments made from spices, sugar, vinegar, and fruits are sometimes too sweet or spicy for many people.

Make liberal use of Indian breads (baked, not fried) such as chaputi. Wrap a bit of the entrée in a tortilla-like piece of chapati and garnish with chutney. A couple of entrées with a variety of breads can easily make a filling meal for 4.

WHAT'S OKAY AND WHAT TO WATCH WHEN EATING. . .

 # Indian

Go ahead and enjoy

- Karhi (chick-pea soup)
- Mulligatawny or dal rasam (lentil soups)
- Dry pulkas (unleavened wheat bread)
- Nann (a bread, without butter, baked)
- Chapati (tortilla-like bread, baked)
- Kulcha (baked bread)
- Salad or vegetables with yogurt dressing
- Dal (lentils)
- Tandoori, masala, tikka, or vindaloo-style dishes
- Dishes marinated in yogurt
- Yogurt-based curries
- Khur (a milk-and-rice dessert)

But hold back on

- Samosa (fried meat or vegetables wrapped in dough—very high in fat)
- Bhatura, paratha, poori (fried breads)
- Pakori (deep-fried breads and vegetables)
- Ghee, or clarified butter (ask if this is used in preparing your meal; it may not appear on the menu, and it raises fat content dramatically)
- Coconut milk (again, ask if this is used in preparing your meal—it raises fat content dramatically)
- Dishes with the words kandhari, malai, or korma (indicate lots of cream or coconut)
- Most rice or cheese puddings, honeyed pastries

WHAT'S OKAY AND WHAT TO WATCH WHEN EATING. . .

Middle Eastern

Go ahead and enjoy	But hold back on
■ Hummus (mashed chick peas) without the traditional drizzle of oil on top	■ Saganaki (contains fried cheese and butter)
■ Baba ghanoush (mashed eggplant)	■ Falafel (deep fried)
■ Pita bread	■ Fried lamb patties
■ Ful medames (fava beans and chick peas)	■ Lamb stews
■ Any salad, including tabouleh, tabouli, or fattoush	■ Kasseri (cheese and butter casserole)
■ Lentil soup	■ Arat (a strong, alcoholic, chalk-white drink)
■ Rice pilaf	
■ Shish kebab	
■ Kibbe (baked meat with wheat, onions, and pine nuts)	
■ Kofta (ground beef with parsley and onions) grilled, not fried	

Middle Eastern

Prepared Middle Eastern dishes sold at supermarkets or restaurants may be high in fat, as they contain a fair amount of oil, tahini (sesame seed paste, somewhat like peanut butter), and whole-milk yogurt. When making them at home, substitute low-fat or non-fat yogurt, and use it to stretch dishes made with oil or tahini.

(On the brighter side, tahini and olive oil are mostly healthier unsaturated fat.)

Many of the healthiest Middle Eastern dishes are based on grains and legumes. Most are usually served with pita bread, which is nearly fat-free. Here are some examples:

■ Hummus—a dip made from mashed chickpeas seasoned with garlic, lemon juice, olive oil, and sometimes tahini.
■ Tabouli—a salad of bulgur (parboiled cracked wheat) combined with chopped vegetables and herbs.

A subset of Middle Eastern cooking is the Lebanese cuisine, considered by some to be among the world's healthiest. It features fresh vegetables, legumes, rice, bulgur wheat, seafood, and lamb. Common herbs and seasonings are mint, parsley, onions, garlic, oregano, cumin, and olive oil. A typical meal consists of grape leaves stuffed with rice, chickpeas served as a dip, parsley and bulgur-wheat salad, eggplant, seafood, and lamb. Beware, however, if you're on a reduced-sodium diet: Lebanese food can be extremely salty.

Cajun

When French colonists from Acadia, an area now known as Nova Scotia, moved to the Louisiana coast, they came to be known as Cajuns. They are noted for their red-hot spicy cooking, a blend of French and Creole cuisine. Cajun dishes tend to use lots of seafood, cooked as a stew and served over rice. They often start with a roux made from heated oil and flour mixed with liquid to form a sauce base. Vegetables and meat or seafood and seasonings are then added. Gumbo and jambalaya (rice, chicken, ham, pork, sausage, broth, vegetables, and seasonings) are familiar specialties. Watch out for lard in cooking, and remember that Cajun seasonings are typically high in sodium.

WHAT'S OKAY AND WHAT TO WATCH WHEN EATING. . .

 Cajun

Go ahead and enjoy

- Seafood gumbo
- Red beans, pinto beans, and rice (without sausage)
- Greens (kale, mustard greens, okra)
- Corn bread (if not fried)
- Shrimp creole (in a tomato sauce over rice)
- Blackened fish or chicken (heavily seasoned and cooked quickly with very little oil)
- Boiled seafood dishes, such as shrimp or crab boil
- Jambalaya (omit fatty ingredients)

But hold back on

- Bisques (cream-broth soups) or étouffé (soup or stew with lots of butter); corn or fish chowder
- Dirty rice (fried rice with fatty meats)
- Sausage dishes such as boudin or andouille
- Hush puppies (fried corn bread)
- Jambalaya
- Crab cakes, (if fried. Grilled or broiled cakes are okay.)
- Batter-fried seafood
- Gravy, honeyed dressings
- "Mud pies" and other rich desserts

WHAT'S OKAY AND WHAT TO WATCH WHEN EATING. . .

 Thai

Go ahead and enjoy

- Lemon-grass soups like tom yum koong (shrimp and chili paste)
- Po tak (seafood soup)
- Pad Thai (stir-fried noodles and sprouts)
- Forest salad
- Larb (minty chicken salad)
- Yum neua (broiled beef with onions)
- Sauteed ginger beef or chicken (request minimal oil)

But hold back on

- Coconut-milk-based soups and curries
- Royal tofu (fried)
- Hot Thai catfish (fried)
- Hae Kuen (deep-fried prawn cake—try requesting a stir-fried variation)
- Pla sam rod (a deep-fried fish—try requesting a stir-fried variation)
- Peanut sauce
- Yum koon chaing (sausage with peppers

Thai

With its unusual herbs and spices—lemon grass, lime leaves, and Thai basil—Thai cuisine offers a fascinating change of pace. But be selective. While Thai stir-fry has the same vitamin-packed benefits as Chinese and Japanese dishes prepared this way, many dishes are laced with fat-laden coconut milk. Curried dishes, in particular, often contain coconut milk, which can raise their fat content to more than 40 percent. Many other entrées are prepared with cream. When dining out ask how foods are prepared—the use of coconut milk or cream may not be obvious. If cream is involved, ask that milk be substituted. As always, avoid deep-fried foods, go easy on dishes with nuts, and load up on rice and vegetables. Remember, too, when first trying Thai food that it can be *very* hot. □

Chapter 34

Adding Global Savoir-Faire to Your Regular Meals

Perking up your new, healthier diet with a hint of the exotic doesn't have to be a chore. In fact, you'll find that many exciting foreign recipes take no more effort than the fat-laden "comfort food" of the past. You'll be surprised, too, at how easy it is to find the ingredients. Though international dishes often call for spices, vegetables, and grains not often used in American cooking, you're still likely to find virtually all of them in today's jumbo supermarkets. If you can't, in most metropolitan areas, specialty stores and farmers' markets will usually fill the gaps.

As the sampler of recipes in this chapter shows, healthy, highly nutritious cooking definitely does not have to be boring and ordinary. On the contrary, it can open up an intriguing new world of enjoyment.

Cuisine Fusion

Experiments with dishes that you don't normally cook and ingredients you've never thought to try not only adds instant variety to your menus, but also gives you a chance to judge which new spices, vegetables, and cooking techniques to add to regular kitchen repertoire. Such culinary hybridization has become a popular trend among chefs at top restaurants around the country. Called "cuisine fusion," the blending of two or more diverse cooking techniques or ingredients from other countries can result in such dishes as chicken fajita pitas, pizza-filled egg rolls, and croissant sandwiches. To get your creative juices flowing, here is a recipe for Oriental Stir-Fry Pizza that won first place at the 1994 Pizza Expo in Las Vegas. It is reprinted with the permission of its creator, Phillip Koenig of *The Silver Spoon* in Louisville, KY:

Oriental Stir-Fry Pizza

STIR-FRY MEDLEY

1 Tbs.	olive oil
1 tsp.	grated fresh gingerroot
1/2 cup	grilled chicken
1/2 cup	chopped red bell peppers
1/2 cup	snow peas
1/4 cup	sliced celery
3	scallions, sliced
1	eight oz. jar baby corn ear, drained

PIZZA:

2 Tbs.	sesame seeds
1	commercially prepared prebaked pizza crust
1/4 cup	commercially prepared peanut satay sauce (or see recipe below)
1/2 cup	shredded cheese
1 Tbs.	chopped honey-roasted peanuts
2 Tbs.	rice noodles (or chow mein noodles)

To make medley: Heat oil over medium-high heat in a wok. Add gingerroot and stir-fry for 30 seconds. Add remaining ingredients and stir-fry until vegetables are tender-crisp, about 4 minutes. Remove from heat and set aside.

To assemble: Preheat oven to 450° F. Place sesame seeds in a skillet and dry-roast over medium-low heat, stirring constantly, until uniformly golden brown, about 5 minutes. Remove from heat and set aside. Place crust on pizza pan and brush with peanut satay sauce to within 1″ of the edge. Sprinkle with toasted sesame seeds and top evenly with stir-fry medley. Sprinkle with cheese and peanuts. Bake until cheese is melted and topping is hot, about 8 minutes. Remove from oven, let cool for 5 minutes. Sprinkle with rice or chow mein noodles, slice into wedges and serve.

Peanut Satay Sauce

Peanut satay sauce is a great topping for pork loin, chicken, or even pasta. It packs a lot of flavor—but also significant amounts of fat— so don't overdo. The following recipe, also from Phillip Koenig, is more than you will need for one Oriental Stir-Fry Pizza, but it will keep in the refrigerator for several months.

6 cloves of garlic, pounded
3 shallots or small white onions
2 Tbs. cayenne pepper
1/2 lemon peel
1 Tbs. olive oil
1 Tbs. lemon juice
1 12 oz. jar of crunchy peanut butter
15 oz. water
1/3 cup sugar
1–2 tsp. salt, or to taste

Stir-fry garlic, shallots, cayenne, and lemon peel in oil. Remove lemon peel, add lemon juice and simmer for 1 minute. Add peanut butter and water. Bring to a boil, add sugar and salt. Boil until thickened.

Dining Out in Your Own Home

No matter how dreadful a cuisine's reputation for healthiness may be, there's always something worthwhile to be drawn from it. (See Chapter 33, "Improving Your Diet With International Flair," for tips on what to adopt and what to avoid in the leading foreign cuisines.) The meal plans that follow show how, with a little judicious selection, you can bring the excitement of international dining to your own table without the calories and fat.

France

What cook could ignore the world's most famous cuisine? To keep French cooking healthy, simply avoid heavy cream sauces, rich patés, and fat-laced casseroles, and stick with the ingredients the region is known for: fresh vegetables, herbs and olive oil. Although dishes vary from province to province, most reflect the French obsession with fresh produce. Gardens abound in almost every backyard, window box, and terrace.

The French consider vegetables and herbs

essential to every meal; and they pride themselves on their ability to use herbs and other seasonings to enhance a dish, rather than to overwhelm it. Meals usually consist of a light appetizer such as a salad, a soup, an entree, a vegetable dish, and a fruity dessert. And there is almost always wine and bread.

French menu: *Artichauts Vinaigrette* (artichokes with vinaigrette dressing), *Soup au Pistou* (vegetable soup), *Bar Provencal* (sea bass with tomatoes), *Carottes Persillees Avec Champignon* (parsley carrots with mushrooms), *Brioche* (French rolls), and *Mousse de Myrtilles* (blueberry mousse).

Artichauts Vinaigrette

(Artichokes with Vinaigrette Dressing)

VINAIGRETTE DRESSING
1 tsp. capers, rinsed and chopped
1 Tbs. minced chives
1 Tbs. minced parsley
4 artichokes
Juice of 1/2 lemon
1 Tbs. vinegar
Salt

Combine vinaigrette dressing with capers, chives, and parsley and blend thoroughly. Refrigerate until ready to use.

Snap stems off the artichokes and break off any small leaves at the base. Trim the bottoms so that artichokes will stand upright. With a sharp knife, cut an inch off tops and also trim points of remaining leaves using scissors. Rinse well in cold water. Rub cut leaves with lemon juice and immerse artichokes in bath of vinegar and water until ready to cook. Bring 4–5 quarts of water to a boil in a large saucepan with a little salt. Drop in artichokes, cover with 2 layers of cheesecloth, and boil, uncovered, for 40–50 minutes, until leaves pull off easily. Drain upside down in colander. Searve each, warm or cold, with 1–2 Tbs. vinaigrette.

- Serves 4
- Per serving: **Cal.** 112 **Pro.** 4 g **Fat** 4 g **Sod.** 86 mg **Carb.** 15 g.

From: The International Menu Diabetic Cookbook *by Betty Marks. Copyright © 1985. Used with permission of Contemporary Books, Chicago.*

Soup au Pistou

SOUP

1 1/4 oz.	sorted uncooked red kidney beans, rinsed
1 oz.	sorted uncooked great northern beans, rinsed
2 quarts	water
1/2 cup	each, diced onion and sliced celery
6 oz.	pared potato, cut into 1/4-inch cubes
4	small plum tomatoes, blanched, peeled, seeded, and diced
3/4 cup	each, sliced carrots and zucchini
1/2 cup	diagonally sliced green beans
2 Tbs.	tomato paste
2	bay leaves
3 oz.	uncooked small macaroni (e.g., ditalini, elbows)

Dash pepper

PISTOU

1 cup fresh basil leaves
2 Tbs. hot water
1 Tbs. plus 1 tsp. olive oil
2 garlic cloves, minced
1 oz. grated Parmesan cheese

To prepare soup: In a 4-quart saucepan combine beans; add water and bring to a boil. Reduce heat to low, add onion and celery, and simmer for 30 minutes. Add remaining ingredients for soup except macaroni and simmer until vegetables and beans are tender, 45 minutes to 1 hour. Add macaroni, stir, and cook for about 5 minutes.

To prepare pistou: While macaroni is cooking, in blender container combine all ingredients for pistou except cheese; process until smooth, scraping down sides of container as necessary. Transfer to small bowl and stir in cheese.

To serve: Remove and discard bay leaves from soup. Into each of 8 soup bowls, spoon 1/8 of the pistou, then ladle 1/8 of the soup over pistou; serve immediately.

- Serves 8, about 1 cup each
- Per serving: **Cal.** 148 **Pro.** 6 g **Fat** 4 g **Sod.** 116 mg **Carb.** 23 g **Chol.** 3 mg

From: Weight Watchers New International Cookbook. *New York, NY: NAL Penguin Inc; 1985*

Bar Provencal

(Sea Bass with Tomatoes)

Juice of 1 lemon
2 Tbs. plus 1 tsp. safflower oil
Dash cayenne
1 1/2 lbs. sea bass fillets or fillets of other
  firm white fish
1 cup chopped onions
2 green peppers, cored, seeded, and
  cut into strips
2 cloves garlic, minced
1 lb. tomatoes, peeled, seeded, and chopped
Pinch fennel seeds
Pinch dried thyme
4 peppercorns
1 Tbs. fresh oregano or 1/4 Tbs. dried
1/4 cup chopped parsley
1 lemon, sliced

Mix lemon juice and 2 Tbs. safflower oil with cayenne. Wash fish and pat fry. Place fish in oil/lemon mixture, cover, and refrigerate several hours. Drain, but reserve liquid. Heat 1 tsp. oil in nonstick saucepan and saute onions until soft. Then add peppers and garlic and cook 5–10 minutes. Add tomatoes, fennel seeds, thyme, peppercorns, oregano, and half the parsley and cook until all vegetables are tender. Broil fish about 4 inches from heat source, brushing with marinade and turning. Cooking time depends on thickness of fish, but fish is ready when it flakes when pierced with fork. Remove fish from broiler and place in center of a warm serving platter. Spoon vegetables alongside fish on the platter. Top with lemon. Sprinkle fish with remaining parsley.

From: The International Menu Diabetic Cookbook *by Betty Marks. Copyright © 1985. Used with permission of Contemporary Books, Chicago.*

Carottes Persillees Avec Champignons

(Parsley Carrots with Mushrooms)

1 lb.	carrots, scraped, trimmed, and julienned
1 tsp.	fructose
1/2 cup	seltzer
1 Tbs	butter divided
Few grinds	black pepper
1 cup	sliced mushrooms
2 Tbs.	minced parsley

Place carrots in enamel or nonstick saucepan with fructose, seltzer, 1/2 Tbs. butter, and pepper. Bring carrots to boil, cover, and simmer 30 minutes, until tender. Add mushrooms and cook a few minutes longer. Drain off any remaining liquid. When ready to serve, add remaining butter and parsley. Heat, toss, and serve.

■ Serves 4

■ Per serving: **Cal.** 89 **Pro.** 2 g **Fat** 3 g **Sod.** 84 mg **Carb.** 13.5 g

From: The International Menu Diabetic Cookbook by Betty Marks. *Copyright © 1985. Used with permission of Contemporary Books, Chicago.*

Brioche

Enjoy a continental breakfast of Brioche spread with marmalade and served with coffee or tea. These delicious French rolls can be frozen, individually wrapped; just reheat when ready to use.

1 packet fast-rising active dry yeast
2 Tbs. each warm water (see yeast
    package directions for temperature)
    and granulated sugar
6 large eggs
1/3 cup plus 2 tsp. margarine, softened
Dash salt
2 1/4 cups plus 2 Tbs. all-purpose
    flour, divided
1 cup cake flour

Spray twelve 2 1/2-inch-diameter muffin pan cups or 12 individual brioche pans with nonstick cooking spray; set aside. In mixing bowl sprinkle yeast over water; add sugar and stir to dissolve. Let stand until mixture becomes foamy, about 5 minutes. Using electric mixer at medium speed, beat in 5 eggs, 1 at a time; add margarine and salt and beat until well combined. Beat in 2 1/4 cups all-purpose flour and the cake flour, beating until dough becomes smooth and sticky, about 3 minutes. Scrape down sides of bowl; cover bowl with a clean damp towel or plastic wrap and let stand in warm draft-free area until dough doubles in volume, about 45 minutes. Sprinkle work surface with remaining 2 Tbs. flour and turn dough out onto floured surface; gently shape into 12-inch-long loaf. Cut off 1/4 of dough and set aside; cut remaining loaf into 12 equal portions and shape each into a smooth ball, tucking all ends under. Place dough balls, seam-side down, in sprayed pan. Cut remaining dough into 12 equal portions and shape each into a small ball. Using finger, press down center of each large dough ball, making an indentation; dip bottom of each small ball into water, then, pressing gently but firmly, press a small ball into each indentation. Lightly beat remaining egg and, using pastry brush, brush an equal amount over surface of each roll; let stand in warm draft-free area until rolls double in volume.

■ Serves 12, 1 Roll Each

From: Weight Watchers New International Cookbook. *New York, NY: NAL Penguin Inc.; 1985.*

Mousse de Myrtilles

(Blueberry Mousse)

1 1/2 cups	fresh blueberries
1/4 cup	concentrated frozen apple juice
1 package	unflavored gelatin
1/4 cup	cold water
2 Tbs.	plain low-fat yogurt
1/2 tsp.	ground cinnamon
2	egg whites, beaten stiff

Combine blueberries and apple juice in saucepan and bring to boil. Reduce heat and boil down to 1 cup, mashing berries against side of pan. Remove from heat and chill. Sprinkle gelatin over cold water in a cup, then place in bowl of hot water to dissolve. Stir gelatin into blueberries, setting the bowl over ice. Stir until berries thicken. Fold in yogurt and cinnamon and beat in egg whites. Pour into serving dish and place in freezer for about 1–2 hours, until firm.

■ Serves 6

■ Per serving: **Cal.** 50 **Pro.** 2.5 g **Fat** 0 g **Sod.** 21 mg **Carb.** 10 g

From: The International Menu Diabetic Cookbook *by Betty Marks. Copyright © 1985. Used with permission of Contemporary Books, Chicago.*

China

Chinese cuisine has been in existence for at least 5,000 years. As in France, the dishes vary from province to province, and there is a focus on fresh vegetables. Semi-tropical south China, with its abundance of seafood and agricultural products, is the home of the "haute cuisine" with which most Americans are familiar: Cantonese cooking. Vegetarian dishes and rice dishes come mainly from eastern China. In the north, where wheat is grown instead of rice, you'll find noodles, crepes, dumplings, and pancakes. Finally, Western China, a humid region where chiles were traditionally used as a means to preserve food, gave birth to fiery Szechuan and Hunan cooking.

With over a billion people to feed, Chinese farmers concentrate on growing efficient food crops such as rice, wheat, soybeans (hence, tofu), and legumes on the available land. Seasonings such as ginger, garlic and scallions are often used for taste as well as fragrance, with no one flavor predominating. Soy sauce is to the Chinese what salt is to the West. Steaming and stir-frying, the most common cooking techniques, help vegetables retain both their crunch and their nutrients.

Meals often have a message in China. Bamboo shoots are served to wish guests good health and rice symbolizes fertility. Noodles, which represent longevity, are served whole, because it is considered bad luck to break them. As you sit down to enjoy a Chinese meal, such as this one, wish your fellow diners "ho yum ho sic" (good drinking, good eating).

Chinese menu: *Chinese Cold Noodles in Sesame Sauce, Stir-Fried Vegetables, Lemon Chicken,* and *Yang Tao* (kiwifruit).

Chinese Cold Noodles in Sesame Sauce

3 Tbs.	canned chicken broth
2 Tbs.	smooth peanut butter
1 Tbs.	soy sauce
1/4 tsp.	minced pared gingerroot
1/8 tsp.	minced fresh garlic
1/2 tsp.	Chinese sesame oil
1 cup	chopped thin spaghetti, chilled
1/4 cup	chopped scallions (green onions)
1/2 oz.	shelled roasted peanuts, chopped
Dash ground red pepper, or to taste	

In small saucepan combine broth, peanut butter, soy sauce, ginger, and garlic and cook over medium heat, stirring frequently, until mixture comes to a boil; remove from heat and stir in oil and pepper. Transfer to small bowl, cover with plastic wrap, and refrigerate for at least 30 minutes. In serving bowl combine spaghetti with sauce and toss to combine; sprinkle with scallions and peanuts.

- Serves 2
- Per serving: **Cal.** 222 **Pro.** 9 g **Fat** 12 g **Sod.** 863 mg **Carb.** 22 g **Chol.** 0 mg

From: Weight Watchers New International Cookbook. *New York, NY: NAL Penguin Inc.; 1985.*

Stir-Fried Vegetables

1 Tbs.	sesame oil
1 Tbs.	low-sodium soy sauce
1 tsp	finely chopped fresh gingerroot
3 cups	assorted vegetables (green beans, red or green peppers, broccoli, mushrooms, zucchini, yellow squash, bamboo shoots, water chestnuts, etc.), cut into 1/2-inch pieces

Mix oil, soy, and ginger in wok or large non-stick skillet. Add vegetables and cook quickly, stirring with chopsticks. Vegetables should be crisp. Cook softest vegetables last. Remove from heat and serve.

- Serves 4
- Per serving: **Cal.** 76 **Pro.** 4 g **Fat** 4 g **Sod.** 141 mg **Carb.** 6 g

From: The International Menu Diabetic Cookbook *by Betty Marks. Copyright © 1985. Used with permission of Contemporary Books, Chicago.*

Lemon Chicken

1/2 cup	fresh lemon juice
1 Tbs.	lime juice
1 1/2 Tbs.	walnut oil
1/1/2 Tbs.	low-sodium soy sauce
2 tsp.	Dijon mustard
1 pound	skinless, boneless chicken breasts
4	lemon wedges
Dash cayenne	

Combine lemon and lime juice, oil, soy, mustard, and cayenne. Marinate chicken breasts in this for 4 hours or more in a cool place. Cut chicken breasts into 4 pieces and poach in the marinade in a saucepan until tender, about 10 minutes. Transfer chicken to warm platter and reduce marinade until thick. Then spoon over chicken and serve with lemon wedges.

- Serves 4
- Per serving: **Cal.** 200 **Pro.** 27.5 g **Fat** 8 g **Sod.** 284 mg **Carb.** 45 g

From: The International Menu Diabetic Cookbook *by Betty Marks. Copyright © 1985. Used with permission of Contemporary Books, Chicago.*

Yang Tao

(Kiwifruit)
4 kiwifruits, peeled and sliced
1 tangerine, peeled and sectioned
1/2 teaspoon peeled and
    finely chopped fresh gingerroot
Fresh mint (optional)

Arrange kiwifruit slices on dessert dishes. Place a few tangerine sections next to them or in center. Garnish with touch of ginger and mint sprig, if desired.

- Serves 4
- Per serving: **Cal.** 44 **Pro.** 1 g **Fat.** 0 **Sod.** 0 **Carb.** 10 g

From: The International Menu Diabetic Cookbook *by Betty Marks. Copyright © 1985. Used with permission of Contemporary Books, Chicago.*

Italy

While the Chinese blend all flavors together in harmony, the Italians insist that each ingredient retain its own unmistakable identity. For this reason, Italian cooking is less complicated than most other types of cuisines.

Although Italy is smaller than California, it has more regional cuisines than the entire United States. Olive oil, cheese, tomatoes and pasta predominate in each section of the country, but Italian cooks insist there are distinct regional differences. In the cosmopolitan north, for instance, the cuisine reflects the prosperous economy: with fresh egg pastas and rice, meats, cheeses and mushrooms, all often heavily buttered. In the less populated areas of the south, where cheeses are most often made from sheep's milk, and fish often replaces meat, the food is more heavily seasoned. Garlic, fresh herbs and hot peppers are used with abandon.

Traditionally, the main midday meal brings the entire family together, often for several hours. The *pranzo di mezzogiorno*, as it is known, sets the pace for the rest of the day. Why not serve a traditional Italian meal on a weekend or another day when all your loved ones gather? You will need several courses of equal size (Italian meals don't build up to a main entree). Our menu plan outline provides recipes for each course except the cheese; that is up to you. Start your meal with a hearty *Mangia!* It means "Eat!" in Italian.

Italian menu: *Primo Piatto (first course):* Zuppa di Broccoli (broccoli soup with tubettini); *Secondo Piatto (second course):* Conchiglie con Pettine (conchiglie with scallops); *Contorno (contour):* Insalata di Barbabietola e Radicchio (beet and radicchio salad); *Fromaggio* (cheese); *Dolce (dessert):* Mele Infornate (stuffed baked apples).

Broccoli Soup with Tubettini

1 large	bunch broccoli (about 1 1/2 lbs.)
1 Tbs.	olive oil
1/2 cup	minced red onion
1/2 cup	minced celery, strings removed before mincing
5 1/2 cups	Chicken Broth, preferably homemade, or defatted low-sodium canned
1 Tbs.	minced fresh sage or 1 tsp. crumbled dried sage
1/2 tsp.	coarse salt
1/4 tsp.	crushed red pepper flakes
1/2 cup	tubettini (tiny tubular pasta)
2 Tbs.	freshly grated imported Parmesan cheese, for serving

Remove florets from broccoli, leaving about 1/2 inch of their stems. Cut florets into 1/2-inch pieces. Wash in cold water, drain, and set aside. Remove and discard the large coarse leaves from stems and cut off about 1/2 inch of the tough lower part of stalks. Wash thoroughly and peel stalks with vegetable peeler. Cut stalks in half lengthwise and then into 1/2-inch pieces. In a heavy 5-quart pot, heat olive oil over medium-low heat. Add onion and celery and cook, stirring frequently, until vegetables are limp, about 3 minutes. (If vegetables start to stick to bottom of pan, stir in 2 tablespoons broth to prevent scorching.) Add broccoli stems, broth, sage, salt, and pepper flakes. Bring to a boil and add tubettini. Cook, uncovered, over medium-high heat until the pasta is barely al dente, about 7 minutes. Add florets

OLIVE OILS ARE NOT ALL CREATED EQUAL

Italians judge olive oils the way the French weigh the merits of wines, and there is actually good reason to do so. Soil quality, weather conditions, the type of olive, and the preparation technique combine to create vast differences in the oils:

Extra-virgin, cold pressed or first pressed olive oil

This designation means the finest olives were hand picked and then pressed—only once!—by hand or with a small machine. The low-acid oil has a strong, fruity flavor and aroma, and it may appear cloudy or slightly greenish in color. Use it raw, in salad dressings or bread toppings for example. Because it has a low smoking point, it does not make a good cooking oil.

Virgin olive oil

Better for cooking because it stands up to heat, but higher in acid content, Virgin olive oil comes from riper and lower grade olives than extra-virgin. Although it is pressed the same way, it usually tastes blander and has a yellowish color.

Pure olive oil

To make this oil, the residual pulp of the olives used for virgin olive oil is re-pressed using heat. Hydraulic machines do this work in large factories. Pure olive oil is ideal for cooking because it is the least expensive, but it tastes blander than virgin oil and has a paler color.

Switching to olive oil from butter is a definite plus for your health; but you still need to use a little moderation. Although the fat in olive oil is not the harmful saturated variety, it still amounts to 14 grams per tablespoon. Each tablespoon also contributes 120 calories to your diet.

---

and continue cooking until pasta and florets are cooked, about 5 minutes. Transfer to bowls, sprinkle each with 1 teaspoon Parmesan cheese, and serve.

■ Makes 9 cups, serves 6
■ Per serving: **Cal.** 142 **Fat** 4 gm **Sod.** 228 mg **Chol.** 2 mg

From: Lean Italian Cooking, *by Anne Casale. Copyright © 1994 by Anne Casale. Reprinted by permission of Ballantine Books, a division of Random House, Inc.*

Conchiglie with Scallops

1 lb.	sea or bay scallops
2 Tbs.	plus 2 tsp. extra virgin olive oil
1/2 cup	fresh bread crumbs made from cubed Italian or French bread, including crust, coarsely ground in food processor or blender
2 Tbs.	minced Italian parsley leaves
1 Tbs.	minced garlic
6	large ripe plum tomatoes (1 lb.), blanched, peeled, cored, seeded, and coarsely chopped
1/2 tsp.	coarse salt
1/2 tsp.	crushed red pepper flakes
12 oz.	conchiglie (medium-size shell pasta)

Wash scallops several times in cold water to remove sand. Blot dry with paper towel. If using bay scallops, leave whole, if using sea scallops, cut horizontally into 1/2-inch slices; set aside. In a small nonstick skillet, heat 2 tsp. oil over medium heat. Add bread crumbs and toast until golden, stirring frequently to prevent scorching. Remove from heat and stir in minced parsley. In a 12-inch skillet, heat remaining 2 Tbs. oil over medium heat. Add garlic, turn heat to low, and cook until very lightly golden. Add the tomatoes and simmer, mashing down the tomato pulp with a wooden spoon. Cook until sauce comes to a slow boil, about 1 minute. Stir in scallops and cook, stirring frequently, for 3 minutes. Season with salt and pepper flakes. Remove from heat. Cook pasta in 6 quarts boiling water with 2 teaspoons coarse salt until *al dente*. Drain pasta and transfer to 4 serving bowls. Spoon sauce over each portion. Sprinkle each serving with toasted bread crumbs and serve.

■ Serves 4

■ Per serving: **Cal.** 538 **Fat** 11 gm **Sod.** 708 mg **Chol.** 37 mg

From: Lean Italian Cooking, *by Anne Casale. Copyright © 1994 by Anne Casale. Reprinted by permission of Ballantine Books, a division of Random House, Inc.*

Beet and Radicchio Salad

1	small red onion (2 oz.), peeled and sliced paper-thin
1 1/4 lbs.	(5 or 6) medium-size beets
1	medium head radicchio (about 6 oz.), halved, cored, leaves separated, washed, spun dry, and cut into thin julienne strips
1 1/2 Tbs.	minced fresh mint leaves
1/2 tsp.	coarse salt
1/2 tsp.	freshly milled black pepper
1 Tbs.	red wine vinegar
2 1/2 Tbs.	extra virgin olive oil

Place sliced onions in a small bowl with 3 ice cubes and cover with cold water. Refrigerate for at least 1 hour. (Soaking the onion will ensure crispness.) Wash and trim beets, leaving 2 inches of the stems and the root ends intact to prevent color from oozing out during boiling. Place in a medium-size pot and cover with water; cover pot and bring to a boil. Cook beets, partially covered, over high heat until tender when pierced with a metal cake tester, about 20 to 40 minutes. Drain in colander and let cool until you can slip off the skins; slice off the stems. Quarter beets and cut into 1/2-inch wedges. Drain onion, blot dry with paper towel, and combine with beets. Arrange in center of serving platter and surround with julienned strips of radicchio. In a small bowl, combine mint, salt, pepper, and vinegar; stir with fork or small whisk to combine. Add oil, a little at a time, whisking until dressing is well combined. Spoon dressing over salad and serve.

■ Serves 4

■ Per serving: **Cal.** 129 **Fat** 9 gm **Sod.** 256 mg **Chol.** 0 mg

From: Lean Italian Cooking, *by Anne Casale. Copyright © 1994 by Anne Casale. Reprinted by permission of Ballantine Books, a division of Random House, Inc.*

Stuffed Baked Apples

6	medium-size baking apples, preferably Rome (about 2 1/2 lbs.)
1/2 cup	dark raisins
1/3 cup	lightly packed light brown sugar
1 tsp.	ground cinnamon
2 Tbs.	dark rum or brandy
1/2 cup	dark corn syrup
1 tsp.	pure vanilla extract
1 tsp.	freshly ground nutmeg
1 1/2	cup unsweetened apple juice

Adjust oven rack to center of oven and pre-heat to 350° F. Using a melon baller, core apples from stem end without cutting through to bottom. Using a vegetable peeler, peel off skin about halfway down each apple. In a small bowl, combine raisins, brown sugar, cinnamon, and rum. Fill cavity of each apple with raisin mixture. Place apples in a 9 × 13 × 2-inch baking dish. In a small bowl, combine dark corn syrup with vanilla. Spoon mixture over apples; sprinkle each with nutmeg. Pour apple juice into bottom of baking dish. Place in oven and bake apples for 20 minutes. Using a bulb-type baster, baste apples with pan juices. Continue baking and basting every 10 minutes until apples are extremely tender when tested with a cake tester, about 45 minutes. Remove from oven and keep basting with pan juices every 5 minutes until apples are well coated with glaze. Serve warm or at room temperature with a little glaze over each.

- Serves 6
- Per serving: **Cal.** 218 **Fat** 64 gm **Sod.** 31 mg **Chol.** 0 mg

From: Lean Italian Cooking, *by Anne Casale.*
Copyright © 1994 by Anne Casale. Reprinted by
permission of Ballantine Books, a division of
Random House, Inc.

India

The subcontinent of India stretches some 2,000 miles from east to west and north to south, accounting for the rich diversity of its cuisine. In the south and east, heavy rainfall encourages cultivation of rice; but in the dry north, wheat and barley are staples and the people eat bread with their meals. Many kinds of fruits are grown in the mountainous inland regions, and seafood is popular along the coasts.

More important than any type of food in India, though, are the spices. Most renowned is curry, typically a blend of cardamom, coriander, turmeric, cumin, and ginger, but subject to variation from one household to the next. Curry dishes are usually served with chutney or a cooling *raita*, a salad-like combination of ingredients with a yogurt base.

Vegetarian meals are also popular in India. The concept of *ahimsa*—nonviolence toward, and reverence for all life — is widespread. Some Indians refuse to eat eggs, for fear of disturbing embryonic life; and some would rather forego root vegetables than disturb the worms around them. On the other hand, many Indians eat fish, which they refer to as "fruit of the sea."

Our menu offers you the choice of a meal with chicken and *Naan* (a type of bread), or a vegetarian meal with rice. You may want to serve all the courses in small bowls on individual trays, or *thalis*, as they do in India. Place a thali—with the rice or bread in the center, the main dishes on the right, and supporting dishes (like chutneys and raitas) on the left—on the floor beside each diner. Food is eaten with the fingers, and instead of napkins, water bowls are used to clean the hands.

Indian menu: *Tandoori Chicken* with *Naan* (buns) or *Mixed Vegetable Curry* with *Radish Raita.*

Tandoori Chicken

1 cup	chopped onions
1/2 cup	plain low-fat yogurt
1/4 cup	fresh lemon or lime juice
1 Tbs.	seeded chopped mild or hot green chili pepper
3 to 6	small garlic cloves
1 tsp.	minced pared gingerroot
1/8 tsp.	each ground turmeric, ground cinnamon, ground cardamom, ground cloves, and ground allspice
1	chicken (3 pounds), cut into 8 pieces and skinned
2 tsp.	olive or vegetable oil
Dash salt	

Garnish: 1 Tbs. chopped fresh cilantro (Chinese parsley)

In blender container combine onions, yogurt, juice, chili pepper, garlic, and seasonings; process until smooth, scraping down sides of container as necessary. Using sharp knife, cut slits in chicken but do not pierce to the bone; transfer chicken to 1-quart stainless-steel or glass bowl and add yogurt mixture, rubbing mixture into chicken parts to coat. Cover bowl with plastic wrap and refrigerate for at least 8 hours. Preheat oven to 475° F. Transfer chicken to rack in roasting pan and brush with any remaining marinade; roast for 15 to 20 minutes. Brush chicken pieces with oil and continue roasting until, when chicken is pierced with a knife, juices run clear, about 10 minutes longer. Transfer chicken to serving platter and pour pan juices over chicken; serve sprinkled with cilantro leaves.

- Serves 4
- Per serving: **Cal.** 278 **Pro.** 35 g **Fat** 11 g **Sod.** 155 mg **Carb.** 8 g **Chol.** 103 mg

From: Weight Watchers New International Cookbook. *New York, NY: NAL Penguin Inc.; 1985.*

Naan

1 packet	fast-rising active dry yeast
3/4 cup	warm water (see yeast package directions for temperature), divided
2 tsp.	granulated sugar
1/4 cup	margarine, melted, divided
1/4 cup	plain low-fat yogurt
1	egg
2 1/4 cups plus 1 Tbs.	all-purpose flour, divided
1 tsp.	salt
2 tsp.	poppy seed or sesame seed

In a cup sprinkle yeast over 1/4 cup water; stir in sugar and let stand until foamy, about 5 minutes. In mixing bowl, using electric mixer at medium speed, combine remaining 1/2 cup water with 3 tablespoons margarine and the yogurt and egg, beating until blended; add 2 1/4 cups flour and the salt and yeast mixture and mix to form a soft sticky dough. Spray a bowl with nonstick cooking spray and transfer dough to sprayed bowl; cover with clean damp towel or plastic wrap and let stand in warm draft-free area until dough is doubled in volume, about 30 minutes. Preheat oven to 450° F. Sprinkle work surface with remaining tablespoon flour; turn dough out onto floured surface, cut into 12 equal pieces, and shape each into a ball. Working on floured surface to prevent sticking, pat each ball into an oval, about 4 inches in diameter and 1/4 inch thick. On each of 2 baking sheets arrange 6 ovals; brush each with an equal amount of remaining margarine and sprinkle with poppy (or sesame) seed. Bake until puffed and browned, 10 to 12 minutes. Serve hot.

■ Serves 12, 1 bun each
■ Per serving: **Cal.** 138 **Pro.** 4 g **Fat** 5 g **Sod.** 238 mg **Carb.** 20 g **Chol.** 23 mg

From: Weight Watchers New International Cookbook. *New York, NY: NAL Penguin Inc.; 1985.*

Mixed Vegetable Curry

2 small hot green chili peppers,
   seeded and minced
2 small garlic cloves, minced
1/8 tsp. each ground cumin,
   ground coriander and ground turmeric
1 Tbs. plus 1 tsp. olive or vegetable oil
6 oz. diced pared potatoes
1 cup each diced onions, carrots,
   red bell peppers, and green bell peppers
3 medium tomatoes, blanched,
   peeled, and chopped
1 tsp. salt
3/4 to 1 cup water
1 cup cooked long-grain rice (hot)
Garnish: chopped fresh cilantro
   (Chinese parsley) or Italian (flat-leaf)
   parsley leaves

Using a mortar and pestle, crush together chili peppers, garlic, cumin, coriander, and turmeric to form a paste. In 12- or 14-inch skillet heat oil; add chili pepper mixture and

cook, stirring constantly, for 2 to 3 minutes. Add potatoes, onions, carrots, bell peppers, tomatoes, and salt, stirring to combine; add enough water to just cover the vegetables and, stirring constantly, bring to a boil. Reduce heat and let simmer until vegetables are tender, 15 to 20 minutes. To serve, mound vegetable mixture on serving platter, mound rice alongside vegetables, and sprinkle rice and vegetables with cilantro or parsley.

■ Serves 4
■ Per serving: **Cal.** 207 **Pro.** 5 g **Fat** 5 g **Sod.** 578 mg **Carb.** 37 g **Chol.** 0 mg

From: Weight Watchers New International Cookbook. *New York, NY: NAL Penguin Inc.; 1985.*

Radish Raita

1 cup   grated radishes
1/2 tsp.   salt
1/4 cup   plain low-fat yogurt
Dash each ground cumin and
           ground red pepper
Garnish: mint sprig

In colander sprinkle radishes with salt; let drain for 30 minutes. Squeeze out any excess water and transfer radishes to bowl; stir in yogurt and cumin. Serve sprinkled with red pepper and garnished with mint.

■ Makes 2 servings
■ Per serving: **Cal.** 28 **Pro.** 2 g **Fat** 0.5 g **Sod.** 577 mg **Carb.** 4 g **Chol.** 2 mg

From: Weight Watchers New International Cookbook. *New York, NY: NAL Penguin Inc.; 1985.*

Middle East

At the crossroads of Europe, Asia and Africa lies what Westerners refer to as "the Middle East." Technically, the region consists of only Iraq, Syria, Jordon, Lebanon, and Israel; but for many people the term encompasses all the countries of south-west Asia and northern Africa.

Known as "the cradle of civilization," this region is thought to be the birthplace of agriculture. Three of the world's great religions—Judaism, Christianity, and Islam—all spread outward from this central cultural pressure-cooker. Today, as through the centuries, it is an area characterized by intense political and social conflict.

Middle Eastern meat eaters usually stick to lamb; religious restrictions make pork a rarity. Indeed the cuisine of the region focuses on vegetables, (eggplant, squash and tomato), that are generally stuffed or wrapped in grape leaves; dried fruits (raisins and dates); nuts and seeds (almonds, walnuts, and sesame—often made into a paste called tahina); and legumes (fava beans, lentils and chickpeas). Middle Easterners sometimes serve meats as a *mezza*, in which a wide array of dishes served like appetizers replace a single main entree. Guests may sample as many dishes as they like. But, in contrast to a buffet, all the dishes are placed on trays or spread on a large cloth on the floor and remain within arm's reach of all guests throughout the meal. Diners lounge on low cushions or stools and clean their hands in water bowls. The diners linger for hours, talking, eating, and drinking strong coffee or mint tea.

Use the recipes in this chapter for your own *mezza*, or choose one or two for a main entree.

Middle Eastern Mezza: *Hummus bi tahina* (chickpea dip) with pita bread, *Iman bayaldi* (stuffed eggplant), *Mahasha* (stuffed tomatoes), *Morroccan lentils, Tabbouli* (bulghur wheat salad), *Roz bil tamar* (Rice with dates and almonds), *Borani esfanaj* (spinach and yogurt salad), *Ma'mounia* (semolina halva dessert). Additions could include cold fish, hard-boiled eggs, a bowl of raisins and nuts, and a platter of herb sprigs such as mint, tarragon, chives, dill, and parsley.

Hummus bi Tahini

(Garbanzo/chickpea dip)

1 1/4 cups garbanzos/chickpeas,
   cooked (keep the water)
3 cloves   garlic, crushed
A little milk or retained cooking water
1 Tbs. tahini*
Juice of 2 lemons
Salt and pepper
Olive oil
1/4 tsp. paprika
1/2 Tbs. fresh parsley, chopped

*Paste made from ground sesame seeds, available from whole-food stores.

Put the cooked garbanzos/chickpeas into a blender with the garlic, and some of the retained cooking water or milk. You may need to do this in two or three lots as the garbanzos/chickpeas are quite stiff. Add the milk or retained cooking water as necessary to make a smooth, creamy consistency. Now spoon in the tahini, add the lemon juice and salt and pepper. Whizz the mixture once more and check the flavors, adding more salt, tahini or lemon juice as desired. Turn the hummus into a shallow bowl and pour on a little olive oil to cover the surface with a thin film, scatter the parsley over and sprinkle on the paprika. Serve with hot pita bread and chopped cucumber, carrots, fennel root, bell pepper or celery sticks.

■ Serves 4–6

From: The World in Your Kitchen, by Troth Wells. Freedom, CA: The Crossing Press; 1993

Imam Bayaldi

(Stuffed Eggplant)

4 eggplants
Oil
1 onion, finely sliced
4 cloves garlic, crushed
1 green bell pepper, chopped
6 tomatoes, chopped
Squeeze of lemon juice
1 cup monterey jack or cheddar cheese,
    grated or 1 cup yogurt
Salt and pepper
1 Tbs. fresh parsley, chopped

Heat oven to 325° F. First of all, put the egg-plants into the oven to cook for 10 minutes or so. While they are baking, heat the oil in a pan and cook the onion until it turns soft and transparent. Now add the garlic and stir this round for a few moments but do not let it brown. The green bell pepper goes in next, and when it has softened put in the

tomatoes. Continue to cook gently for a few minutes. Meanwhile, remove the eggplants from the oven and when they are cool enough to handle, cut off the stalk end and slice them in halves, lengthwise. Remove as much of the pulp as you can, using a tea-spoon or sharp knife, without damaging the skins. Chop up the pulp and add it to the pan with the onion and other vegetables. Squeeze in some lemon juice and season. Arrange the eggplant halves in an ovenproof dish and pile the cooked mixture into them, and around them if there is some left over. Put the dish into the oven for 10 minutes, with the cheese on top if using, and cook for a few minutes or until the cheese has melted and turned golden. Remove from the oven, scatter the parsley over and serve either hot or cold, with yogurt if using.

■ Serves 4

From: The World in Your Kitchen, by Troth Wells. Freedom, CA: The Crossing Press; 1993

Mahasha

(Stuffed tomatoes)

4 large tomatoes
Oil
2 Tbs. fresh cilantro/coriander leaves,
    chopped
1 tsp. curry powder
1/2–1 tsp. chili powder
2 tsp. cumin seeds
1 tsp. mustard seeds
1 clove garlic, crushed
Salt
1/2 lbs. potatoes, mashed
1/3 cup peas

Heat oven to 325° F. To begin, slice the tomatoes in half and carefully scoop out the pulp and seeds; keep these for later use. Then heat up some oil in a pan and when it is very hot, toss in the cilantro/coriander leaves and let them crisp up. Now add the curry powder, chili, cumin seeds, mustard seeds and garlic to the fried cilantro/coriander leaves. Mix well and sprinkle on salt as required. Cook for a minute or two before adding the mashed potato, the peas and the tomato pulp. Stir all the ingredients well to distribute the spices. Fill the tomatoes with the mixture and place them in a shallow ovenproof dish. Bake for 15–20 minutes and serve hot or cold.

■ Serves 4

From: The World in Your Kitchen, *by Troth Wells. Freedom, CA: The Crossing Press; 1993*

Moroccan Lentils

2 cups	brown lentils
1	large onion, chopped
4 cups	water
1 tsp.	salt
3 Tbs.	olive oil
2 cups	chopped tomatoes
1/4 cup	olive oil
1	large bay leaf
4	garlic cloves, minced
1/2 cup	chopped parsley
1 tsp.	cayenne pepper, or to taste

Wash and pick over the lentils and put them in a heavy 3-quart saucepan with a tight fitting lid. Add the onion to the saucepan with the water, salt, and 3 tablespoons olive oil. Bring to a boil, reduce heat and simmer for 30 minutes or until most of the liquid has been absorbed. Add the tomatoes, olive oil, bay leaf, garlic, parsley, and cayenne pepper.

Simmer for 20 minutes, stirring occasionally. Transfer to a heated serving dish and serve hot.

■ Serves 6

From: Herbs in the Kitchen *by Carolyn Dille and Susan Belsinger. Loveland, CO: Interweave Press, Inc.; 1992.*

Tabbouleh

(Bulgur wheat salad)

1/2 cup bulgur
A few lettuce leaves
4 Tbs. fresh parsley, chopped
2 Tbs. fresh mint, chopped
1 onion, finely sliced
4 tomatoes, chopped
4 Tbs. lemon juice
4 Tbs. olive oil
Salt and pepper

First, soak the bulgur for 20 minutes or so in enough cold water to cover. Then drain well. Line a salad bowl with the lettuce leaves and then spoon in the bulgur. Scatter in 3 tablespoons of the parsley together with the mint, onion and tomatoes and mix them in. Now combine the lemon juice with the oil, season with salt and pepper and mix well. Pour this over and toss the salad to coat the ingredients evenly. Sprinkle the remaining spoonful of parsley on top.

■ Serves 4–6

From: The World in Your Kitchen *by Troth Wells. Freedom, CA: The Crossing Press; 1993*

Roz bil Tamar

(Rice with dates and almonds)

2 Tbs.	margarine
1 cup	almonds
1 cup	dates, pitted
1 cup	raisins
1 tsp.	rose water or a little grated orange rind
1 cup	rice, cooked
Salt	

Melt the margarine in a large pan and when it is gently bubbling, add the almonds. Fry them, stirring often, for one or two minutes. Next put in the dates and raisins, adding more margarine if necessary. Keep stirring so that nothing sticks or burns, and cook for a few minutes until the dried fruit begins to plump up. Now heap the rice on top of the fruit and nut mixture: cover. Cook over a very gentle heat, or place in a low oven, for 10–20 minutes to let everything heat through. Just before serving, sprinkle on the rose water and garnish with additional almonds and orange peel.

■ Serves 4

From: The World in Your Kitchen, *by Troth Wells. Freedom, CA: The Crossing Press; 1993*

Borani Esfanaj

(Spinach and yogurt salad)

2 Tbs. oil
1 onion, finely chopped
2 cloves garlic, crushed
1 pound spinach, chopped
Salt and pepper
1 cup yogurt

Heat the oil and sauté the onion for several minutes until it is golden. Then add the garlic and after a minute or two, put in the spinach and seasoning. Cook the spinach, turning from time to time, until it has settled and softened. Transfer it to a serving dish and let it cool. When ready to serve, blend in the yogurt and mix well.

■ Serves 4

From: The World in Your Kitchen, *by Troth Wells. Freedom, CA: The Crossing Press; 1993*

Ma'mounia

(Semolina halva dessert)

1 Tbs.	margarine
1 cup	semolina
2 1/2 cups	milk (or half milk, half water)
1/2 cup	sugar
1 tsp.	ground cinnamon
1 Tbs.	pignoles/pine nuts (optional)

Heat the margarine in a saucepan and add the semolina. Cook it gently and stir it round for about 5 minutes until it deepens in color. In a separate pan, bring the milk or milk and water to the boil with the sugar and then pour this gradually over the semolina. Stir over a low heat and cook until the mixture thickens. When it is ready, set the pan aside, covered, for 15 minutes. And then serve it, cool, with cinnamon and the pignoles/pine nuts on top.

■ Serves 4

From: The World in Your Kitchen, *by Troth Wells. Freedom, CA: The Crossing Press; 1993*

Working Those Odd New Vegetables into Your Cooking

Gone are the days when turnips were the most exotic option in the produce section. Now we're confronted by a growing assortment of weird vegetables with unpronounceable names. Browse through any large array of produce and you'll find an odd assortment of dry, tuberous bulbs; vaguely familiar-looking spiky globes with leafy tops; and stringy sprouts that must surely have grown in a cellar. These peculiar specimens certainly look "interesting," but what on earth do you do with them?

If you find yourself shying away from the vegetable shelves these days, stop and think again. Those pallid, misshapen roots and sprouts can actually be quite delicious. All you need to overcome "veggie-phobia" is a bit of information on what to choose and how to prepare. Once you've made a few experiments, you'll find that cooking with exotic vegetables, such as jicama, kohlrabi, enoki mushrooms, and sunchokes, can add a pleasing new dimension to everyday dining.

Here are some tips from the United Fresh Fruit and Vegetable Association on the best ways to approach these unfamiliar foreign plants. The sample recipes we've included only hint at the many possibilities they offer.

Alfalfa Sprouts. Delicate and thread-like alfalfa sprouts have a nutty, mild taste and are high in vitamins and minerals.

■ *Selection and Storage:* Keep refrigerated.
■ *Preparation:* Alfalfa sprouts are a great addition to sandwiches, tacos and salads.

Artichokes. Artichokes have a subtle, sweet and somewhat nutty flavor.

■ *Selection and Storage:* Look for compact globes that feel heavy and are plump and fresh-looking. Avoid any with loose or spreading leaves. During the spring, artichokes should be bright green; during the winter they will appear bronzed. Keep them cold and somewhat damp until you're ready to cook them; try to use them within a few days of purchase.
■ *Preparation:* Rinse each artichoke in cold water and cut off the stem close to the base. Remove any small, loose, or discolored leaves at the bottom. Cut off about 1 inch from the top; snip the thorny tips off the remaining leaves using kitchen shears. Simmer uncovered in 2 inches of water 25 to 30 minutes. Drain upside down.

If you are unacquainted with the art of eating an artichoke, you're not alone. Simply pull off the outer leaves, dip them into any favorite sauce, and draw the leaf end through your teeth to scrape off the edible portion. After you've worked your way around the artichoke, you'll come to light-colored leaves tipped with purple. Pull these away and scrape out the prickly, fuzzy "choke." Underneath lies the succulent heart.

Artichokes with Fresh Tomato Sauce

1 lemon, sliced
1 1/2 tsp. salt, divided
4 medium-size artichokes
2 Tbs. olive oil
1/2 cup chopped onion
2 cloves garlic, minced
4 medium tomatoes, peeled,
   chopped (3 cups)
1/4 cup chopped parsley
2 Tbs. freshly squeezed lemon juice
1/2 tsp. dried leaf basil, crushed
1/4 tsp. dried rosemary, crushed

In large saucepan, bring 299 water to boiling; add lemon slices, 1 teaspoon salt and prepared artichokes. Cover. Simmer 25–30 minutes, until stem ends of artichokes are tender when pierced with a fork and leaves pull easily from the base. Remove from pan, drain upside down. In large skillet, heat oil; saute onion and garlic until soft. Stir in remaining ingredients. Simmer over low heat 15 minutes, stirring occasionally. Place artichokes on serving platter. Spoon tomato sauce around artichokes.

■ Serves 4.

Recipe courtesy of: United Fresh Fruit and Vegetable Association, Alexandria, Virginia

Bean Sprouts. These low-calorie sprouts are crispy and nutty.

■ *Selection and Storage:* Select fresh, crisp sprouts with moist tips. Shorter sprouts will be the most tender. Store in a plastic bag in the refrigerator and use as soon as possible.
■ *Preparation:* Raw bean sprouts add flavor to salads and can be stir-fried with other vegetables.

Bok Choy. Also called Chinese chard, this vegetable has broad white or greenish-white stalks with loose, dark green leaves. It is sweet and mild tasting.

■ *Selection and Storage:* Select firm, crisp heads. Store unwashed in a plastic bag in the refrigerator and use within a few days.
■ *Preparation:* Cut off the root end, separate stalks and remove any tough or wilted leaves. Cut leaves from stems and slice in one inch pieces. Slice stems diagonally in thick chunks. Bok choy can be stir-fried or served raw in salads.

Celeriac. Also known as celery root, celeriac is a celery-like plant with a thick edible root. The crunchy root tastes like celery with walnut overtones.

■ *Selection and Storage:* Select roots that are small; larger roots tend to be woody. Discard tops and keep the roots cold and humid.
■ *Preparation:* Scrub and peel off brown skin. Cube or shred and dip into lemon juice to preserve the color. Add raw, shredded or julienned strips of celery root to salads and vegetable trays, or sauté or stir-fry them.

Chayote (shy-o-tay). This squash-like vegetable is also known as the vegetable pear. It is round to pear-shaped with smooth or ribbed skin and a delicate flavor.

■ *Selection and Storage:* Choose dark green, hard chayote. Store in the refrigerator.
■ *Preparation:* You can steam, stuff, or bake chayote. Use it in any recipe calling for summer or winter squash.

Daikon. This large, white, high-calcium Japanese radish, tastes hotter than the American variety.

■ *Selection and Storage:* Select daikons that are clean and free of cuts or bruises. Store in the refrigerator.
■ *Preparation:* Serve raw in salads, pickled as a relish, or simmered in soup.

Enoki Mushrooms. Exotic and creamy white, enoki mushrooms have long slender stems and very small round caps.

■ *Selection and Storage:* Select fresh-looking mushrooms and keep them in the refrigerator.
■ *Preparation:* Remove about one inch from the bottom of the stems, rinse and separate. Use raw in salads or add to stir-fry recipes at the last minute.

Fennel. This feathery-topped vegetable has a celery-like appearance and an enlarged bulb-like base. A native of the Mediterranean, fennel is often called *finocchio,* or *anise.* It has a licorice flavor.

■ *Selection and Storage:* Choose fennel with a firm, light green or white bulb. Avoid discolored or cracked bulbs. Refrigerate in plastic wrap or bags and use within a few days.
■ *Preparation:* Wash and remove tough outer stalks. Trim the stalks to the point where they join the bulb, removing any wilted or bruised layers. To serve raw, slice lengthwise into strips; for braising, halve or quarter the bulbs; for sautés or stir-frys, cut the bulb diagonally.

Jícama (HEE-ka-ma). Jícama is a brown root with the delicate flavor and texture of a water chestnut.

■ *Selection and Storage:* Choose well formed jicama free of bruises. Smaller ones are less woody. Refrigerate, unwashed, wrapped in plastic.
■ *Preparation:* Serve raw, cut in strips to use with dip, or slice into salads. Because it stays crisp when cooked, jicama is great for sautéing or stir-frying.

Orange-Jícama Salad

SALAD

2 cups	fresh orange sections (from about 4 oranges)
1 lb.	jícama, peeled and thinly sliced into 2 3 1/4-inch pieces
1	medium red onion, peeled, thinly sliced crosswise, and separated into rings
8 cups	torn lettuce leaves (preferably romaine and red-leaf)
1/3 cup	pine nuts, toasted (optional)

DRESSING

1/3 cup	orange juice (preferably fresh)
1/4 cup	fresh lime juice
2 Tbs.	red-wine vinegar
1 Tbs.	olive oil
1/2 tsp.	salt (optional)
1/4 tsp.	freshly ground black pepper

In a large bowl, combine the orange sections, jícama, and onion. In a small bowl, whisk together the dressing ingredients. Add the dressing to the orange mixture, toss the in gredients gently, cover the bowl, and chill the salad until serving time.

At serving time, add the lettuce and the pine nuts (if desired), and toss the salad once more.

■ Serves 8

Reprinted from JANE BRODY'S GOOD FOOD GOURMET: Recipes and Menus for Delicious and Healthful Eating, *with the permission of W. W. Norton & Company, Inc. Copyright © 1990 by Jane E. Brody.*

Kohlrabi. A cross between cabbage ("kohl") and turnip ("rabi"), kohlrabi has tasty leaves, stems and roots. The leaves have an earthy, cabbage flavor, while the stems taste something like radishes.

■ *Selection and Storage:* Buy globes about 2 inches in diameter; if they are larger, they can taste tough and bitter. Store in the refrigerator.
■ *Preparation:* Trim stems just before using, then wash, peel, and cut in strips for dipping or to add to stir-fry combinations. To cook the bulb, trim but don't peel, cover in lightly salted water and bring to a boil. Cook until tender, about 30 minutes. Steam kohlrabi the same way; it may take 5 to 10 minutes longer than boiling. Peel after cooking.

Nopales. Also called cactus leaves, nopales taste like crisp green beans.

■ *Selection and Storage:* Choose firm, fresh-looking leaves (the smaller ones are more tender). Store in the refrigerator.
■ *Preparation:* Carefully remove thorn eyes with a vegetable peeler. Cut de-spined leaves in small pieces and boil in salted water until tender, about 10 minutes. Serve with freshly chopped tomatoes and onions.

Rutabaga. Although often placed in the same category as turnips, rutabagas are very different botanically. They are orange-yellow, with a smooth, dense texture and mellow flavor.

■ *Selection and Storage:* Look for firm, smooth-skinned globes that feel heavy for their size. Store in the refrigerator up to 4 weeks.
■ *Preparation:* Remove skin with a paring knife or vegetable peeler. Dice or slice, then cook until tender by steaming, baking, sautéing, or microwaving. They can also be added to soups or stews.

Parsnips. Cream-colored parsnips are similar to carrots and have a sweet, nutty flavor.

■ *Selection and Storage:* Look for firm, well-formed roots. Very large ones may be fibrous and taste bitter. Parsnips can be kept refrigerated in a plastic bag up to 1 month.
■ *Preparation:* Remove skin with a peeler. Serve them raw or cooked, as you would carrots.

Salsify. Sometimes called "oyster plant" because it tastes a bit like oysters, this vegetable resembles parsnips, with heavy, grassy tops. Roots are grey-white in color, with firm, juicy flesh.

■ *Selection and Storage:* Buy medium-size, firm, clean roots. Refrigerate in a crisper for 3 to 4 days.
■ *Preparation:* Trim, peel, and cut in 2 inch pieces. Place in boiling salted water; add one teaspoon of vinegar for each inch of water. Cook 5 to 10 minutes, drain, and season.

Spaghetti Squash. A novel vegetable prized for its golden yellow, crisp flesh, which breaks into strands after cooking. Its slightly sweet flavor and unique appearance add a distinctive accent to any meal.

■ *Selection and Storage:* Look for yellow evenly colored squash; avoid any that have a greenish tinge. Stored in a cool, dry place; they will keep for several weeks.

■ *Preparation:* Bake, boil, steam, or microwave spaghetti squash. Be sure not to overcook it, or it will become watery and taste bland. To microwave, pierce the skin in several places. A 3 pound squash, which will serve 6 to 8 people, will cook in 12 to 15 minutes on high power. Boiling will take about 20 to 30 minutes, depending on size. The squash is done when a fork can easily pierce the skin. When it is cool enough to handle, split the squash lengthwise and remove the seeds and fibrous portion. To loosen the strands, gently run a fork over the flesh. Serve in place of pasta, tossed with flavored oils or cheese; or top the strands with a zesty vinaigrette dressing and serve cold.

Sunchokes. Also known as Jerusalem artichokes, sunchokes have a flavor similar to globe artichokes. They have a gnarled, knobby appearance and a nutty taste.

■ *Selection and Storage:* Look for firm, clean tubers with no soft spots. Store in the refrigerator.

■ *Preparation:* Remove skin and serve raw in salads; they can also be broiled, sautéed or mashed.

Jerusalem Artichokes and Peas

1/2 pound Jerusalem artichokes (sunchokes)
2 Tbs. extra virgin olive oil
1/2 cup thinly sliced scallions
One 9-ounce package tiny frozen peas, defrosted and well drained
1/2 tsp. crushed fennel seed
1/2 tsp. coarse salt
1/2 tsp. freshly milled black pepper

With a vegetable peeler, remove thin outer skin from each artichoke. Thoroughly wash several times in cold water, drain, and blot dry. (Chokes will turn a light beige color after cleaning.) Slice each in half crosswise and then lengthwise into 1/4-inch strips. In a deep 3 1/2-quart saucepan, heat oil over medium heat. Add scallions, turn heat to low, and cook until softened but not brown, about 2 minutes. Stir in artichokes, cover pan, and cook just until tender-crisp, about 5 to 8 minutes. Stir in peas and fennel. Cook for an additional 3 minutes. Season with salt and pepper. Transfer to bowl and serve.

■ Serves 4
■ Per serving: **Cal.** 138 **Fat** 7 gm
  Sod. 271 mg **Chol.** 0 mg

From: Lean Italian Cooking, by Anne Casale. Copyright © 1994 by Anne Casale. Reprinted by permission of Ballantine Books, a division of Random House, Inc.

Tomatillos. Appropriately called Mexican sauce tomatoes, tomatillos add spicy flavor to sauces. They are yellowish-green, bright green, or purplish-green in color and are covered with a papery husk. The flavor is tart and similar to a green apple.

■ *Selection and Storage:* Keep in a cool, well-ventilated, dry place. Do not remove the husks.

FOR MORE RECIPES...

You can many of the cookbooks cited in this chapter directly from the publishers. For more information, check the box at the end of Chapter 32.

■ *Preparation:* Slice raw tomatillos in salads or tacos; steam in a small amount of water for 5 minutes for a sauce-like consistency; or combine chopped tomatillos, onions, peppers, and spices with low-fat or non-fat sour cream for a spicy dip to serve with tortilla chips.

Turnips. This snappy-flavored vegetable has white skin and flesh, topped with edible leaves. It is a member of the mustard family.

■ *Selection and Storage:* Find turnips that are heavy and smooth with fresh, green leaves. Store in the refrigerator. Although you can keep the root for up to a week, you should eat the greens in 2 to 4 days.

■ *Preparation:* Remove skin with a peeler. Dice or slice and cook until tender by steaming, baking, sautéing, or microwaving. Turnips also taste delicious in soups or stews.

Warm Potato and Turnip Salad with Sorrel

1 1/2 lbs. new potatoes
1 pound small turnips with tops,
   about 2 bunches
3 oz. pancetta or salt pork
1 garlic clove, finely minced
3 Tbs. olive oil
About 1 tsp. white wine vinegar
Salt and freshly ground pepper
       1 cup shredded sorrel leaves

Scrub the potatoes and turnips and cook them in water to cover by 1 inch until they are just tender. Drain them and let them stand until they are just cool enough to peel. Cut the pancetta into 1/2-inch dice. Cook it over medium-low heat until it is golden brown and there are about 2 tablespoons of rendered fat in the pan. Peel and cut the vegetables into 1-inch (2-cm) dice. Put them in the pan with the oil and sprinkle the vinegar, salt, and pepper over them. Heat the vegetables over medium heat, shaking the pan frequently. When they are heated through, transfer them to a bowl and toss with the sorrel leaves and pancetta. Serve the salad immediately.

■ Serves 6

From: Herbs in the Kitchen *by Carolyn Dille and Susan Belsinger. Loveland, CO: Interweave Press, Inc.; 1992.* □

CHAPTER 35

Herbs and Spices: Your Allies for Healthier Meals

You've probably never stopped to add it up, but the typical American now uses nearly two *pounds* of spices annually. The per capita consumption of chili peppers has surpassed that of green peas; and chili pepper farm acreage is greater than that devoted to celery and honeydew melons.

According to the American Spice Trade Association, spice consumption in the U.S. has increased 50 percent in the last 10 years. As a nation, we consume 821 million pounds annually. At the present rate of growth, the figure should rise to a billion pounds by the year 2000.

The reasons for this phenomenon range from what retailers refer to as the "pizza boom" to a growth in our interest in ethnic cuisines and an increase in the number of immigrants from regions known for their hot and spicy foods. As people became aware of the delights of Mexican and Thai cuisines, for example, supermarkets saw the wisdom of stocking cilantro and lemongrass. But one of the most critical factors in the booming sales of both the spicier spices and the milder herbs is Americans' growing awareness of and commitment to healthier eating.

Spicing Up a Healthful Diet

Reducing the fat in food is the number-one food-related concern in the United States, according to a 1993 survey conducted by the Food Marketing Institute in Chicago. Home cooks are also anxious to keep levels of salt to a minimum. But as you remove fat and salt, you begin to create a flavor gap. High in flavor and low in fat, sodium, and calories, herbs and spices can bridge the gulf in taste-appeal, making bland, good-for-you foods like beans, whole grains, and vegetables surprisingly exciting.

Moreover, as our forefathers always knew, spices and herbs have healthful properties of their own. Ginger ale worked for a tummy upset in your mother's era, and it still works today. But scientists are now beginning to confirm that some spices can also help stave off life-threatening diseases ranging from heart disease to cancer.

The Healing Herbs and Spices

Eastern countries, such as China and India, have appreciated the dual function of herbs and spices for millennia. Now, Western medicine is attempting to identify and isolate the beneficial compounds in a variety of familiar substances that pack a powerful biological punch.

Bay Leaves

Bay leaves—like cinnamon, turmeric, and cloves—help to regulate the body's level of insulin, the hormone that carries blood sugar into the cells. All four of these spices are under study as possible treatments for Type II (adult onset) diabetes, a disease that occurs when the body produces insulin, but not in sufficient quantities to meet its needs. Right now, however, dried bay leaves aren't a help. The sharp leaves can puncture the wall of the digestive tract, and should never be eaten.

Chili Peppers

Capsaicin, the active ingredient in hot chilies (and the cause of that burning, fiery sensation on the tongue), is so biologically active that it is now being sold by prescription, in ointment form, for pain relief. In lower doses, it is also available over the counter. In at least one study, researchers also found that capsaicin may fend off migraine headaches.

Cinnamon

In laboratory studies, cinnamon—together with turmeric, cloves, and bay leaves—tripled the ability of insulin to metabolize glucose, the blood sugar that supplies us with energy.

While some diabetics who are taking a quarter teaspoon or so of cinnamon with their morning oatmeal have reported better blood sugar control, there are no major studies to back up its therapeutic effect and it can't be used as a replacement for regular medication. Since cinnamon can be toxic in high doses (see the section on risks later in this chapter), diabetics and others should be careful about overdoing it in their diets.

Cloves

Cloves—like cinnamon, turmeric, and bay leaves—triple the ability of insulin to metabolize glucose in the lab, thus helping our bodies burn the sugar we need for energy.

Cumin

Israeli scientists have identified cumin, an ancient spice known in Biblical times and widely enjoyed today (especially in bean and lentil dishes) as one of several spices with anti-cancer properties. When urologists at Western Galilee Regional Hospital analyzed the eating habits of patients with some kind of urological cancer (such as bladder or prostate cancer) and patients free of disease, they concluded that dietary differences were a significant factor.

Among the spices examined, cumin appeared to be the most potent cancer-preventive. While only 12 percent of patients with cancer said they seasoned their foods with cumin, 40 percent of those *without* cancer reporting using the spice.

Similarly, researchers in India who tested the effectiveness of 20 different spices and leafy vegetables in preventing cancer identified cumin as a heavyweight in the battle to combat this serious disease. The spice greatly increased the activity of a chemical called GST, a detoxification enzyme known to protect against certain kinds of cancer. Cumin

THE LORE AND LURE OF SPICES

The discovery of spices and herbs may have taken place before the dawn of civilization. These important plant products not only enhanced the flavor of food, but kept it from spoiling. They also were among the world's first medicinal remedies. Indeed, in ancient times, people prized spices more highly than gold or jewels, and spice merchants jealously guarded their sources of the precious stuff.

Most spices come from tropical and subtropical trees, shrubs, and vines, and are typically processed from the part of the plant that contains flavorful oils. Ginseng and horseradish come from the roots of their plants, for example; saffron and cloves from the flowers; caraway and sesame from the seed; cinnamon from the bark; and pepper and vanilla from the fruit. Herbs, on the other hand, are usually the leaves of plants that grow in temperate regions.

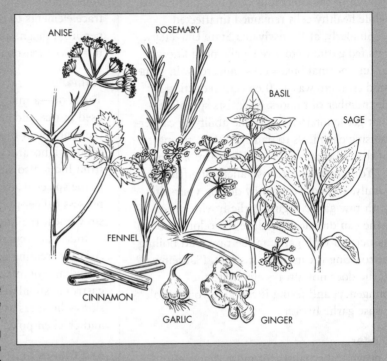

Most of the spices and many of the herbs we use today came originally from plants native to the Far East, India, and the Mediterranean. Among the few spices native to the New World is one of today's most popular seasonings: the red pepper from which chili and cayenne are made.

Nowadays, many of the spices that once grew only in the Far East are being cultivated in other tropical countries, and a wide range of formerly exotic spices are commonly available at a reasonable cost. It's a good thing, too, given Americans insatiable demands for new ways to liven their diets.

was also found to block 83 percent of the chromosome damage normally caused by a powerful cancer-causing chemical, while poppy seeds prevented 80 percent, and turmeric, 54 percent.

Garlic

This remarkable and odoriferous condiment not only wards off vampires, it also appears to protect against elevated levels of serum cholesterol, high blood pressure, and perhaps even cancer. And substances found in garlic have even been found to have antibiotic properties.

At the UCLA School of Medicine, researchers added aged garlic extract to test tubes containing cancer cells from humans and mice. A week later, they found that the growth of the cancerous cells had diminished, while healthy cells remained unaffected.

Similarly, at Pennsylvania State University, rats fed garlic were given a chemical known to turn normal breast cells cancerous. In some studies, there was a 70 percent reduction in the number of tumors. Scientists speculate that garlic interferes with the ability of cancer-causing chemicals to damage DNA, the part of the cell that carries hereditary information.

You don't have to risk alienating friends, family, and co-workers by dosing yourself with raw garlic. Aging garlic in vinegar or wine can drastically reduce the odor problem associated with garlic in the raw; and boiling or roasting it can make it sweet. (Sautéing garlic does not always eliminate the pungency; and frying it can give your whole house garlic breath.)

Ginger

Known to herbalists for more than a thousand years, ginger is particularly valued as a preventive for nausea. Not long ago, a group of Danish physicians tested ginger as a remedy for a type of pregnancy nausea so severe that it can require hospitalization. Clearly, the doctors were reluctant to prescribe drugs because of possible dangers to the developing baby, so they compared powdered ginger capsules (4 pills, or 1 gram, per day—about the same amount of ginger that you would get in a portion of ginger cake) with a dummy pill. All the women took each treatment for 4 days—not knowing which they were getting. At the end, some 70 percent said they felt better on the ginger regimen, and reported no side effects.

Parsley

When sprinkled liberally over food, parsley adds small but significant amounts of several trace elements to the diet; for example, copper, iron, magnesium, molybdenum, and zinc. It is also a reasonably good source of calcium.

Turmeric

Turmeric—a mild, slightly bitter, golden spice used in rice and curry mixtures—is one of the four spices that triple the activity of insulin in laboratory tests. Preliminary studies from India also suggest that two compounds in the spice—Curcumin I and II—may possess cancer-preventing properties and possibly boost the immune system.

Indeed, curcumin is used in many parts of Asia for treating a wide variety of ailments, including eye infections, blood diseases, gastrointestinal ailments, and—applied to the skin—the sores associated with smallpox and chicken pox.

And Others . . .

Decades of research link a diet rich in beta-carotene with a reduced risk of cancer and heart disease. This nutrient works as an antioxidant, possibly preventing the growth of cancer cells and protecting delicate arteries that feed the heart. Beta-carotene can be found in a variety of fruits and vegetables, but herbs, too, are a rich and often overlooked source. Among the highest in beta-carotene are basil, coriander, dill, fennel leaves, mint, parsley, and rosemary.

MAKING SPICES DO THE WORK OF SALT

When reducing the salt in your diet, you should:

- Check your spices and herbs regularly, replacing them as soon as they lose their aroma and color
- Increase the amount of spices and herbs in recipes by about 25 percent while decreasing salt by half or more
- Finely crush all herbs
- Reserve about 25 percent of the seasonings to add in the last 10 minutes of a long-cooking dish
- Double the marinating time to ensure that the flavors completely penetrate the meat or poultry

Vibrant Combinations for Every Kind of Meal

Poultry   Rosemary and thyme
Tarragon, marjoram, garlic [and onion]
Cumin, bay leaf, and saffron (or turmeric)
Ginger, cinnamon, and allspice
Curry powder, thyme [and onion]

Fish and Seafood
Cumin and oregano
Tarragon, thyme, parsley, and garlic
Thyme, fennel, saffron, and red pepper
Ginger, sesame, and white pepper
Cilantro, parsley, cumin, and garlic

Beef   Thyme, bay leaf [and onion]
Ginger, dry mustard, and garlic
Dill, nutmeg, and allspice
Black pepper, bay leaf, and cloves
Chili powder, cinnamon, and oregano

Pork   Caraway, red pepper, and paprika
Thyme, dry mustard, and sage
Oregano and bay leaf
Anise, ginger, and sesame
Tarragon, bay leaf, and garlic

Vegetables

Beans   Marjoram and rosemary
Caraway and dry mustard
Broccoli   Ginger and garlic
Sesame and nutmeg
Cabbage   Celery seeds and dill
Curry powder and nutmeg
Carrots   Cinnamon and nutmeg
Ginger [and onion]
Corn   Chili powder and cumin
Dill [and onion]
Peas   Anise [and onion]
Rosemary and marjoram
Spinach   Curry powder and ginger
Nutmeg and garlic

Summer Squash
Mint and parsley
Tarragon and garlic
Winter Squash
Cinnamon and nutmeg
Allspice and red pepper
Tomatoes   Basil and rosemary
Cinnamon and ginger

Potatoes, Rice, and Pasta

Potatoes   Dill, parsley [and onion]
Caraway [and onion]
Nutmeg and chives
Rice   Chili powder and cumin
Curry powder, ginger and coriander
Cinnamon, cardamom, and cloves
Pasta   Basil, rosemary, and parsley
Cumin, turmeric, and red pepper
Oregano and thyme

Fruits

Apples   Cinnamon, allspice and nutmeg
Ginger and curry powder
Bananas   Allspice and cinnamon
Nutmeg and ginger
Peaches   Coriander and mint
Cinnamon and ginger
Oranges   Cinnamon and cloves
Poppy [and onion]
Pears   Ginger and cardamom
Black (or red) pepper and cinnamon
Cranberries
Allspice and coriander
Cinnamon and dry mustard
Strawberries or kiwi fruit
Cinnamon and ginger
Black pepper and nutmeg

Source: American Spice Trade Association

The Risks of Overdoing It

The ancient Greeks advised moderation in all things. This is especially true when it comes to using herbs and spices, which may be irritating or even hazardous to your health—particularly in large doses.

Cinnamon

In large quantities, cinnamon can irritate mucous membranes; bring on severe digestive problems (such as nausea, vomiting, diarrhea, gassiness, bloating, and rectal burning), cause depression; and interfere with concentration. In some people, it prompts a strong allergic reaction.

Cinnamon oil has also been known to cause contact dermatitis in bakers who hand-knead dough. Cinnamic aldehyde, used as a flavoring in toothpaste, can cause stomatitis (inflammation of the lining of the mouth) and cheilitis (cracks and scaling in the corners of the lips).

Once affected by cinnamon, some individuals may find themselves more sensitive to other substances, including the flavoring agents in chewing gum, fragrances, and sunscreens. Cinnamates, present in some colas, ice creams, pastries, chocolates, and other candies, may produce hives and skin eruptions in sensitive individuals.

Licorice

People who eat large amounts of licorice may develop shortness of breath, swelling of the abdomen and ankles and weight gain due to fluid retention, headaches, muscle weakness, and heart palpitations. For those who are particularly sensitive, even a small amount can be troublesome. The culprit is glycyrrhizic acid, the active component in licorice, which is related chemically to several hormones. Glycyrrhizic acid can produce a whole host of biological effects, such as steroidal and estrogenic activity, potassium depletion, and muscle weakness. It can also diminish the effect of certain medications, particularly those used to control blood pressure and treat heart conditions.

Mustard

Surprisingly, mustard contains a powerful poison: allyl isothiocyanate. When mustard seeds are crushed, this potent irritant is released. Typically, it affects the stomach and bowel. In laboratory experiments, allyl isothiocyanate has caused high blood pressure in animals. Humans report severe skin and respiratory problems, coronary thrombosis (a blood clot in a coronary artery), and heart attacks from long-term, high-volume consumption of prepared mustard or other contact with the seeds. Some scientists have suggested that mustard can actually create ulcers in the walls of an artery. Allyl isothiocyanate can also be found in horseradish, broccoli, and cabbage.

Nutmeg and Mace

Like cinnamon, nutmeg is best used judiciously: a little bit is infinitely preferable to a large quantity. Nutmeg (and mace, which comes from the same plant) contains myristicin, a kind of narcotic. In excess, it can cause hallucinations. Searching for an "organic" high, some people have consumed large quantities of nutmeg, which is cheaper and more readily available than other mind-altering drugs. However, those who use it are not apt to repeat the experience. After-effects of excessive doses of nutmeg include severe and extremely unpleasant headaches, cramps, and nausea. Extremely high doses can lead to liver damage and even death.

Red peppers

Capsaicin, the substance responsible for the pungency of hot peppers, is a highly irritating substance, so concentrated that the tongue can detect it in a solution of one part capsaicin to a million parts of water. We are all familiar with the "chili effect," the sweating and salivation that comes after eating foods high in capsaicin. These reactions may be reflexes resulting from the direct effects of this irritating substance on the pain fibers in the mucous membranes of the mouth.

People once thought that all highly spiced foods created gastric problems (one of the reasons why physicians used to treat all stomach ulcers with bland diets). Although we now know that a bacteria is responsible for most ulcers, experts still believe that capsaicin can cause mucosal damage in the stomach, including increased shedding of surface cells and bleeding. It may also—in large doses—trigger cancer.

Twenty Popular Herbs and Spices and How to Use Them

For those who want a blast of flavor without paying the price in terms of a larger waistline or a boost in their blood pressure, herbs and spices are the answer. Here is one case where it pays to experiment.

Anise. Similar in flavor to cumin, caraway, dill, and fennel, anise is native to the Middle East and Mediterranean. Usually sold in the form of seeds, this licorice-flavored spice is particularly good in soups, stews, and baked goods, and with fish, chicken, or pork.

PURCHASE, HANDLING, AND STORAGE TIPS

■ The best way to learn about spices and herbs is to actually try them. Crush a little in the palm of your hand, smell it, and taste it.

■ Dried herbs tend to have a stronger flavor than fresh ones, so use a third to a quarter less in your recipes.

■ Whole spices offer the best value and keep the longest. Black peppercorns for example, could last for years with proper care. The flavor of ground pepper, however, begins to degrade immediately after grinding. In general, you should consider replacing your spices whenever the color begins to pale or the aroma fades or at least every six months.

■ Buy in small quantities or share the contents of more economical, larger packages with friends. If you patronize stores that sell in bulk, ask about the age of the spice. Don't buy if the spices are exposed to light or stored in open bins.

■ Never keep spices and herbs on a shelf over the stove. The heat will leach away all the aromatic oils. Be sure your spices are in air-tight sealed containers and store them in a cool, dark, dry place, such as the refrigerator.

Basil. Often paired with tomatoes, this aromatic herb has a slight licorice taste. It's delicious in Italian-style tomato sauces, on pizza, and in salads. It also tastes good in soups and vegetable dishes and with eggs, fish, lamb, and chicken.

Bay leaves. The ancient symbol of victory and honor, bay leaves—which grow on the laurel tree—originated in the Mediterranean.

TAKING ON AN INTERNATIONAL FLAVOR

Each ethnic cuisine has its own unique set of flavors. This table pinpoints the spices that can transform a mundane meal into an exotic culinary experience.

Italian	French	Chinese	Spanish	Indian	Greek	Russian
Garlic	Tarragon	Ginger	Saffron	Red pepper	Oregano	Dill weed
Basil	Chervil	Anise seeds	Paprika	Chilies	Mint	Coriander
Oregano	Parsley	Garlic	Garlic	Saffron	Garlic	leaves
Parsley	Thyme	Red pepper	Parsley	Mint	Cinnamon	(Cilantro)
Rosemary	Rosemary	Sesame seeds	Cumin seeds	Cumin seeds	Dill weed	Parsley
Bay Leaves	Nutmeg	Star anise		Coriander	Nutmeg	Mint
Nutmeg	Saffron			seeds &		
Fennel seeds	Bay leaves			leaves		
Red pepper	Garlic			(cilantro)		
Marjoram	Green &			Garlic		
Sage	pink			Turmeric		
	peppercorns			Nutmeg		
				Cinnamon		
				Ginger		
				Anise seeds		
				Dill weed		
				Cloves		
				Mace		
				Cardamom seeds		
				Mustard seeds		
				Sesame seeds		
				Fenugreek		

Mexican	German	Middle Eastern	North African	Hungarian	Indonesian	Scandinavian
Chilies	Caraway	Allspice	Red pepper	Paprika	Chillies	Cardamom seeds
Oregano	seeds	Oregano	Cumin seeds	Poppy seeds	Garlic	Nutmeg
Cumin seeds	Dill seeds	Marjoram	Coriander	Caraway	Red pepper	Dill seeds & weed
Sesame seeds	& weed	Mint	seeds	seeds	Bay leaves	White pepper
Cinnamon	Cinnamon	Sesame seeds	& leaves	Garlic	Ginger	Mustard seeds
Coriander	Ginger	Garlic	(cilantro)	White pepper	Coriander	
leaves	Nutmeg	Dill weed	Mint		seeds	
(cilantro)	White	Cinnamon	Saffron		Turmeric	
	pepper	Cumin seeds	Garlic		Curry powder	
	Juniper	Coriander	Cinnamon			
	berries	seeds	Ginger			
	Allspice	& leaves	Turmeric			
	Mustard	(cilantro)				
	seeds &	Anise seeds				
	powder					

Source: American Spice Trade Association

They add a subtle, yet distinctive flavor to soups and stews, marinades, and roasts. The stiff, sharp leaf doesn't soften with cooking however; so always remove it from the dish before serving.

Black pepper. America's favorite spice is great with everything, but especially good on meat, fish, vegetable dishes, and salads.

Caraway. These dark brown seeds have a pungent aroma and taste a bit like licorice. They add a distinctive flavor to breads and other baked goods, pork dishes, and cabbage.

Cinnamon. One of the oldest known spices, cinnamon comes from the bark of a tree in the laurel family. Whole sticks enhance hot beverages and add flavor to pickles; ground cinnamon adds savor to pork, squash, and baked goods.

Cloves. Cloves are the unopened buds of an evergreen tree native to Indonesia. Their warm aroma and sharp taste enhance baked goods, cereals, and autumn vegetables such as parsnips, squash, and pumpkin.

Cumin. This ancient spice is the chief ingredient in chili powder. It is particularly savory in casseroles, salads, stews, and vegetable dishes.

Dill. The dill plant, related to parsley, produces flavorful seeds and leaves. The seeds, with their hint of caraway, are used in pickled foods, stews, coleslaw, and savory bread. The leaves are good in salads and sprinkled on fish.

Ginger. Ginger root is available fresh, dried, powdered, preserved, and crystallized. It is particularly well-suited to baked goods, and blends well with other spices as a seasoning for meat and chicken. Ginger also adds zip to sauces, stir fries, salads, and marinades.

Marjoram. Related to oregano, marjoram is particularly delicious in tomato dishes and with fish, vegetables, lamb, veal, chicken, and eggs.

Mint. Peppermint and spearmint are the most commonly available varieties of mint. This herb makes a tasty addition to beverages, fruit, yogurt, lamb, and vegetables.

Mustard Seed. Mustard, a spice with a distinctive, hot, musty flavor, comes in two forms: whole seeds and powder. The seeds are good in pickles and salad dressings. Dry mustard powder goes well with meat, chicken, fish, cheese, and eggs. It also adds zest to a sauce.

Nutmeg and Mace. Nutmeg is the seed and mace, the covering of the seed of a species of evergreen tree. Nutmeg is the sweeter and more delicate of the two. Both are excellent in baked goods, sauces, and casseroles.

Oregano. Similar to, but more pungent than marjoram, oregano is an important ingredient in Greek and Italian cooking. It is especially good with tomato dishes and on pizza, vegetables, pork and chicken.

Paprika. Orangy-red paprika is made from the fruit of the capsicum pepper and ranges in taste from mild to slightly hot. Cooks often add paprika to soups and stews, and sprinkle it on beef, pork, and beans; usually regarded as just garnish, when used generously it can add an intriguing new flavor to your meals.

Poppy Seeds. The rich, sweet, nutty taste of poppy seeds enhances salads, pasta, and baked goods.

Red Pepper. Pungent red pepper, also known as cayenne, should be used with discretion. It heats up soups, stews, curries, salad dressings, sauces, and of course, chili; and is especially flavorful when blended with other spices.

Sesame Seeds. Believed to be the oldest plant grown for its oil, sesame is also one of the oldest spices. Its mild, sweet, slightly nutty flavor can be enhanced by toasting. It is outstanding in baked goods and sprinkled over salads, vegetables, casseroles, rice, and pasta.

Thyme. A member of the mint family, thyme is a favorite in savory baked goods, vegetable casseroles, soups, stews, lamb, poultry, and fish dishes. □

Chapter 36

How the Most Popular Cookbooks Measure Up on Health

Until a few years ago, it was sufficient for a cookbook to be clear, simple, and crammed with tasty recipes. But now that we're learning of food's true impact on health, there's another factor in the equation: A really good cookbook must not only please the palate, but do it in a way that optimizes good health.

Take a careful look at the cookbooks you turn to most frequently. Do they keep calling for butter, cream, eggs, and whole milk? If so, they're part of the great American love affair with saturated fat and cholesterol—and they're becoming out of date. There is a whole new generation of cookbooks available now that emphasizes lower fat, lower cholesterol, lower salt, lower sugar, and higher fiber—along with good taste. In fact, even many of the standard cookbooks we all grew up with have been revised to fit into our new, more health-conscious way of dining. And many modern cookbooks now offer nutritional analysis of each dish—a great help to anyone trying to maintain health at its peak.

Fortunately, as long as your aim is a generally balanced diet, there's no need to toss out all of your favorite traditional recipes. Even the most outrageously rich concoction can do no harm if you reserve it for special occasions or a once-in-a-while change of pace. Your old stand-bys and your special occasion cookbooks may also be full of useful food preparation tips, and their recipes can inspire you to create your own healthy, culinary masterpieces. Rather than replace your collection, you merely need to refresh it. Adding a couple of the more imaginative new health-conscious cookbooks—and using them regularly—may well be enough to bring your overall diet up to par.

CORE COOKBOOKS FOR TODAY'S HEALTH-CONSCIOUS KITCHEN

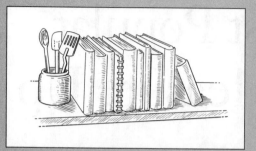

Your library should include at least one easy-to-follow "how-to" cookbook, one vegetarian cookbook, both a basic and a gourmet low-fat cookbook, and a dessert cookbook that offers low-fat choices. Our panel of experts recommends you consider the following books when building a library:

Basic Traditional

- Betty Crocker's New Choices Cookbook
- The Good Housekeeping Illustrated Cookbook
- Joy of Cooking

Vegetarian

- Life's Simple Pleasures: Fine Vegetarian Cooking for Sharing and Celebration
- Moosewood Cookbook
- New Vegetarian Cuisine

Basic Low-Fat

- The American Heart Association Cookbook
- The Healthy Heart Cookbook
- The Wellness Low-Fat Cookbook

Gourmet Low-Fat

- Cooking Light Cookbook, 1994
- The Light Touch Cookbook: All-Time Favorite Recipes Made Healthful and Delicious
- Jane Brody's Good Food Gourmet

Low-fat Dessert

- Have Your Cake and Eat It, Too
- The dessert sections of Cooking Light, 1994, or Jane Brody's Good Food Gourmet

To get extra mileage from an older cookbook, check into the *What's In It?* series of guides to cookbooks, published by Nutrinfo. The series provides per-serving nutrition information for many popular cookbooks, including *The Fannie Farmer Cookbook*, *The Silver Palate Cookbook*, *The Way to Cook*, and others. Write Nutrinfo at 40 Spring Street, Watertown, MA 02272, or phone them at 800-676-6686. Each guide is $4.95 plus $1.00 shipping and handling.

What to Look For in a Cookbook

Some cookbooks seem better than others even before you try the recipes. Here's a quick checklist to use at the bookstore.

- Is the book easy to read? Is the type large enough; are the steps clearly indicated?
- Is nutritional analysis part of the actual recipe? Experts say to watch for this. A table elsewhere in the book isn't convenient—and isn't enough.
- Do the recipes include preparation time? This information is especially helpful when you're cooking a dish for the first time.
- Does the book call for special ingredients or equipment that you don't have? If so, don't buy the book unless you plan to make those purchases, too.
- Do the recipes seem familiar; do they duplicate many you already have? A better choice might be a cookbook that offers new ideas or combinations of foods that you've never tried, or describes new techniques.

- Does the book fit your cooking style? Are there so many steps it seems impossible to follow, or are the recipes so simple they threaten to bore you?
- Is the book explicitly health conscious?
- Does it offer alternatives or ways to adapt the recipes to special diets?

If a book meets most of these requirements, you don't have to reject it because the recipes have more fat, salt, sugar or less fiber than you want. However, you will have to put some thought into making substitutions to improve the nutritional content. Frequently, you can succeed at this without losing flavor. For instance,

To Reduce Fat:
- Substitute skim milk for whole milk.
- Replace sour cream with non-fat yogurt.
- Use evaporated skim milk instead of cream.
- Switch to low- or non-fat cheese from whole-milk cheese.
- Use egg whites or egg substitute instead of whole eggs.
- Replace fat with applesauce or fruit puree in baking.
- Substitute oil for butter, and decrease the amount by half.
- Use cooking sprays in nonstick cookware rather than greasing the pan.

To Reduce Sugar:
- Decrease sugar by up to half the amount specified.

To Reduce Salt:
- Replace salt with herbs and spices. (See Chapter 35 for ideas.)

To Increase Fiber:
- Replace half the white flour with whole wheat flour.

How Experts Rate Today's Favorites

To help you zero in on some of the healthier cookbooks available today, we asked a panel of expert nutritionists to rate some of the most popular basic traditional and specialty cookbooks. Their standard of judgment was the diet currently considered generally healthiest: low in fat and cholesterol, high in complex carbohydrates. The panel also considered the taste appeal of the dishes and ease of preparation.

Rating scale:

🍎🍎🍎 = Healthy recipes with few or no modifications needed

🍎🍎 = Many recipes need modifications for inclusion in a healthy diet

🍎 = For special occasions or reference only

General Cookbooks

🍎🍎🍎

Better Homes and Gardens Family Favorites Made Lighter
Meredith, 1992. ($14.95)

A traditional cookbook goes low-fat, with one recipe per page, color photos and menu ideas. This book lowers the fat, cholesterol, and sodium in such traditional favorites as scalloped corn, sweet and sour pork, and barbecued ribs.

Nutrient analysis: yes
Modifications needed: none

🍎🍎

Better Homes and Gardens New Cookbook
Bantam, 1984. ($7.99)

Lots of reliable recipes and good general information. Clearly written, with good pictures. Includes food safety and preparation tips, but offers no guidelines for healthy recipes. Many recipes are high in fat and calories and call for more fat than is really needed.

Nutrient analysis: yes, but not with recipes
Modifications needed: make low-fat substitutions

🍎🍎

Betty Crocker's Cookbook
Prentice Hall, 1993. ($14)

Always a classic, with good basic techniques, plenty of pictures, and basic recipes. Attractive photos and presentation, but little information on healthy eating. Recipes use more fat than really needed.

Nutrient analysis: yes, but not with recipes
Modifications needed: make low-fat substitutions

🍎🍎🍎

Betty Crocker's New Choices Cookbook
Prentice Hall, 1993. ($23)

A traditional name in cookbooks takes a new healthy approach to the basics. Practical and useful. Most recipes are low in fat, sodium, cholesterol, and calories; includes advice on how to revise favorite traditional recipes.

Nutrient analysis: yes
Modifications needed: none

🍎🍎

Fannie Farmer Cookbook
By Marion Cunningham
Bantam, 1983. ($7.99)

An excellent—though not especially healthy—all-purpose cooking reference, that ranges from basic to gourmet. Includes microwave information. Covers kitchen design, meal planning, and food composition. No guidelines for healthy diet. Some recipes have been modified to reduce fat somewhat, but most are traditional, high-fat, high-calorie.

Nutrient analysis: yes, but not with recipes
Modifications needed: make low-fat substitutions

🍎

James Beard's American Cookery
By James Beard
Little, Brown, 1980. ($18.95)

A classic roundup of American recipes. Also provides interesting information on evolution of cooking in America. Beard's opinionated writing is fun to read, but there is a lot of cream in his cooking. You'll need to make significant changes to most recipes before including them in your diet.

Nutrient analysis: no
Modifications needed: make low-fat substitutions

🍎🍎🍎

Jane Brody's Good Food Gourmet
By Jane Brody
Bantam, 1992. ($15)

A bounty of healthy, delicious dishes. Health-oriented, but balanced: not all vegetarian or extremely low fat. These informative, basic recipes use common ingredients—and for the most part—yield good results. Some portions contain more protein than often recommended, but you can cut the amount without sacrificing taste.

Nutrient analysis: no
Modifications needed: reduce the amount of protein per portion

The Good Housekeeping Illustrated Cookbook
Hearst Books, 1988. ($27)

A great basic cookbook: full of useful, easy-to-follow, reliable recipes with good illustrations that are particularly helpful for the beginner. Provides menus with different themes, seasonal menus and recipes, hints for using herbs and spices, summary of vitamins and minerals. The recipes, however, are traditional, not low-fat, high-fiber or low-salt.

Nutrient analysis: no, only calories and an overview
Modifications needed: make low-fat substitutions, reduce salt, increase fiber

Joy of Cooking
By Irma Rombauer
NAL-Dutton, 1989. ($4.50)

A comprehensive guide on how to cook nearly everything. Many food professionals and amateur cooks consider it a must for every kitchen. Includes basic cooking techniques and traditional recipes as well as background on seasonal food, food storage, and food handling. Recipes cover the spectrum from healthful to high-fat, so select and combine them with care. Last revised in 1964,

the book makes no attempt to favor low-fat, low-salt, low-calorie, or low-sugar dishes.

Nutrient analysis: no
Modifications needed: make low-fat substitutions, reduce salt, increase fiber

The New Basics Cookbook
By Julee Rosso and Sheila Lukens
Workman, 1989. ($19.95)

Excellent recipes well-written and presented, but full of fat. The recipe for basic mashed potatoes, for example, calls for 4 tablespoons butter, 1/2 cup milk, and 1/4 cup sour cream—a high fat approach to what can be a non-fat dish. But the chapter introductions are descriptive and inviting, and there is excellent information on cooking equipment, a conversion chart, and a glossary of cooking terms. Some complicated techniques, some hard-to-find foods, no preparation time included, and no discussion of modifying for fat content. Many of the recipes would still be good with much less fat.

Nutrient analysis: no
Modifications needed: make low-fat substitutions, lower salt

The New York Times Cookbook
By Craig Claiborne
HarperCollins, 1990. ($30.)

This encyclopedic reference book has reliable and varied recipes, but may be difficult for the beginner. Probably not the cookbook you would browse through looking for something to make for dinner tonight. The recipes are high in fat.

Nutrient analysis: no
Modifications needed: make low-fat substitutions

🍎
The New York Times 60-Minute Gourmet
By Pierre Franey
Fawcett, 1982. ($6.95)

Quick, tasty recipes that are easy to cook and high in fat. Cut the fat, and it's a winner.

Nutrient analysis: no
Modifications needed: make low-fat substitutions

🍎
The Silver Palate Cookbook
By Julee Rosso and Sheila Lukens
Workman, 1982. ($12.95)

Creative, delicious recipes that are fun for entertaining but very high in fat. Good if you want to make something different and special. Information on cooking techniques, sections on brunch and drinks, metric conversion charts. Complex recipes, not quick or easy to prepare. No preparation time or low-calorie modifications included. Some hard-to-find and expensive ingredients.

Nutrient analysis: no
Modifications needed: make low-fat substitutions, reduce salt, increase fiber

🍎
The Way to Cook
By Julia Child
Knopf, 1993. ($30)

Excellent recipes with clear, step-by-step instructions and photo illustrations. Focuses on classic cooking, with a French slant, the book presents complicated recipes for good tasting, very high-fat dishes.

Nutrient analysis: no
Modifications needed: make low-fat substitutions

Specialty Cookbooks

🍎🍎🍎
American Heart Association Cookbook
Ballantine, 1994.($6.99)

More than a cookbook, this is a guide to low-fat food shopping, menu planning, dining out, and cooking. Also explains how to adapt recipes and prepare quick and easy low-fat meals. There are 600 simple, easy-to-follow recipes here for basic foods. All use common ingredients and are heart-healthy. Some recipes, however, may lack taste appeal.

Nutrient analysis: yes
Modifications needed: none

🍎🍎🍎
American Heart Association Low-Fat, Low-Cholesterol Cookbook
By Scott M. Grundy and Mary Winston
Times Books, 1991. ($13)

Practical and exciting recipes from expert authors. Simple, easy-to-follow recipes for basic foods. But you may need to add a little spice.

Nutrient analysis: yes
Modifications needed: none

🍎🍎
A Thousand Recipes Chinese Cookbook
By Gloria B. Miller
S&S Trade, 1984. ($20)

Although not specifically written to fit into a healthy diet, the recipes tend to reduce fat consumption by using minimal amounts of meat and dairy products. The mixed vegetable and grain dishes are high fiber. The introduction describes philosophy and basics of Chinese cuisine and includes excellent tips on how to select quality ingredients. No preparation time included.

Nutrient analysis: no
Modifications needed: keep oil to a minimum in preparation

🍎🍎🍎

Butter Busters

By Pam Mycoskie
Warner, 1994. ($16.99)

Many, many easy-to-prepare, low-fat recipes that rely on artificial substitutes to lower fat and calories. Unfortunately, not all recipes succeed in preserving taste appeal.

Nutrient analysis: yes
Modifications needed: none

🍎🍎🍎

Cooking for a New Earth: A New Approach to Home Cooking that Promotes Wholesome Eating and Healthy Living

By Carl Jerome
Henry Holt, 1993. ($12.95)

Creative, simple, nutritious recipes with good guidelines for healthful eating.

Nutrient analysis: no
Modifications needed: none

🍎🍎🍎

Cooking Light Cookbook, 1994

Oxmoor House, 1993. ($24.95)

A wonderful series (1991-1995) with good advice on exercise, beautiful color photographs, and over 400 low-fat, low-sodium recipes that taste great.

Nutrient analysis: yes
Modifications needed: none

🍎🍎🍎

Eat More, Weigh Less: Dr. Dean Ornish's Life Choice Program for Losing Weight Safely While Eating Abundantly

By Dean Ornish
HarperCollins, 1994. ($13)

Guidelines and 250 recipes for those ready to adopt a diet with less than 10 percent fat. Informative, scientific approach with no calorie counting and no measuring of portion sizes.

Good selection of main-course vegetarian recipes. Uses herbs and spices to add flavor without salt. Includes whole grains in many dishes and gives numerous tips for improving taste without using fat. These creative recipes can be time-consuming to prepare, however, and may call for hard-to-find ingredients.

Nutrient analysis: yes
Modifications needed: none

🍎

Essentials of Classic Italian Cooking

by Marcella Hazan
Knopf, 1992. ($30)

This easy-to-use cookbook covers everything you need to know to cook Italian food. But you do need to be selective and make plenty of substitutions: The recipes are high in fat.

Nutrient analysis: no
Modifications needed: make low-fat substitutions

BEST BETS FOR BETTER BAKING

Casual substitution of ingredients in baking often leads to poor results. Because most baked products are high in fat, you'll probably need to practice portion control to include them in a healthy diet. Here are three popular baking books, one with special modifications for low-fat diets.

Fanny Farmer Baking Book

By Marion Cunningham
Knopf, 1984. $25

A wide selection of recipes that produce great baked goods. Not low in fat. Make low-fat modifications where possible and partake sparingly. No nutritional analysis.

Have Your Cake and Eat It, Too

By Susan Purdy
Morrow, 1993. $25

An excellent book that offers scores of techniques for reducing fat when baking. The creative recipes are tasty and reliable. Nutritional analysis with the recipes.

The King Arthur Flour 200th Anniversary Cookbook

By Brinna Sands
The Countryman Press, 1992. $21

A good baking manual with wonderful recipes. Although not necessarily low-fat, it is health conscious and includes a nutrition section. Another section is devoted to whole-wheat baking.

There's also a good newsletter for bakers, *The Baking Sheet,* published by Sands, Taylor & Wood Co., distributors of King Arthur Flour. P.O. Box 876, Norwich, Vermont 05055. Eight issues are $18. Nutritional analysis is included with each recipe.

Graham Kerr's Minimax Cookbook

By Graham Kerr
Doubleday, 1992. ($25)

Good philosophy on dietary change and how to make it happen in the kitchen. The book includes 150 easy-to-follow low-fat recipes; but its overall organization is confusing and results are not always reliable. Augmented with attractive photos and a helpful discussion of equipment and techniques. Provides time and cost estimates for each recipe.

Nutrient analysis: yes
Modifications needed: none

Great Good Food: Luscious Lower Fat Cooking

By Julee Rosso
Crown, 1993. ($19)

Lots of interesting recipes, but results are not always predictable. Some recipes have flavor problems, others don't yield the amount indicated, so the calorie count is inaccurate. Still, the book includes some useful techniques, an emphasis on fresh ingredients, basic nutrition information, and a host of new ideas for modifying basic recipes.

Nutrient analysis: yes
Modifications needed: make low-fat substitutions, increase fiber

🍎🍎🍎

The Healthy Heart Cookbook
Oxmoor House, 1992. ($24.99)

Uses the same beautiful format as the *Cooking Light* series. Features over 350 heart healthy recipes, menu plans, and tips for reducing fat and modifying favorite recipes.

Nutrient analysis: yes
Modifications needed: none

🍎🍎🍎

In the Kitchen with Rosie
By Rosie Daly
Knopf, 1994. ($14.95)

A choice selection of tasty, low-fat recipes—and an excellent way to see if a spa-style menu suits you. Well-presented recipes give good results, taste delicious, and use common foods in uncommon ways. But the recipes are few in number, have lots of steps, and sometimes call for hard-to-find ingredients. The best-selling cookbook of all time.

Nutrient analysis: yes
Modifications needed: none

🍎🍎🍎

Life's Simple Pleasures: Fine Vegetarian Cooking for Sharing and Celebration
By Karen Mangum
Pacific Press, 1990. ($24.95)

Six complete menus for each of the four seasons, featuring 140 low-fat recipes. The more than 60 beautiful photographs illustrating the recipes inspire you to try the dishes. The food pleases the palate and the book pleases the eye.

Nutrient analysis: yes
Modifications needed: none

🍎🍎🍎

The Light Touch Cookbook: All-Time Favorite Recipes Made Healthful and Delicious
By Marie Simmons
Chapters, 1992. ($19.95)

A beautiful and useful cookbook with great photographs. Simmons, who is known for creating excellent recipes, focuses here on low-fat dishes. Many are lightened-up classics. Wonderful use of spices to pick up the flavor when the fat is missing. Well written and clear: a fancy cookbook that is really very practical.

Nutrient analysis: yes
Modifications needed: none

🍎

Mastering the Art of French Cooking, Volume 1
By Julia Child, Louisette Bertholie and Simone Beck
Knopf, 1970. ($25)

An undisputed classic for anyone interested in cooking in general and French cooking in particular, but not a cookbook to use every day. The recipes taste wonderful, but they're complex and generally very high in fat.

Nutrient analysis: no
Modifications needed: make low-fat substitutions

🍎🍎

The Mediterranean Diet Cookbook

By Nancy Harmon Jenkins
Bantam, 1994. $27.95

Tempting, easy-to-follow recipes, useful information on healthful eating habits, and a helpful section on structuring mealtimes—all tucked into a somewhat confusing format. The flavors may take some getting used to, and even though olive oil is a "good" oil, there's too much of it here. You can reduce the oil called for in most recipes by at least half. A steady diet of this cooking also might leave you short of calcium.

Nutrient analysis: yes
Modifications needed: decrease oil

🍎🍎

Moosewood Cookbook

By Mollie Katzen
Ten Speed Press, 1992. ($19.95)

A classic vegetarian cookbook, this revised 1992 edition is significantly more healthful than the original 1979 volume, but it still offers great recipes presented in a friendly manner. Unfortunately, some recipes still have more fat than recommended.

Nutrient analysis: no
Modifications needed: make low-fat substitutions

🍎🍎🍎

New Vegetarian Cuisine

By Linda Rosensweig and Prevention Magazine Editors
Rodale Press, 1993. ($26.95)

Low-fat vegetarian food that tastes good. Over 250 recipes for pasta, grains, beans, soups, and salads.

Nutrient analysis: yes
Modifications needed: none

🍎🍎🍎

Quick and Healthy:
For People Who Say They Don't Have Time
To Cook Healthy Meals

By Brenda J. Ponichtera
ScaleDown, 1991. ($16.95)

Designed for the busy family. More than 180 quick and tasty low-fat recipes and time-saving tips. Provides grocery lists and menus.

Nutrient analysis: yes
Modifications needed: none

🍎🍎

365 Ways to Cook Chicken

By Cheryl Sedaker
HarperCollins, 1986. ($16.95)

An abundance of easy ways to serve chicken, that versatile, low-fat favorite. Recipes are reliable and varied, but sometimes too high in extra fat. Includes preparation times. The "Chicken Lite" section, an introduction to the low-fat benefits of cooking with chicken, is good but needs a nutrient analysis.

Nutrient analysis: no
Modifications needed: make low-fat substitutions

🍎🍎

365 Ways to Cook Pasta

By Marie Simmons
HarperCollins, 1988. ($17.95)

Plenty of recipes for everybody's favorite food. Many are quick and easy: all are clearly presented. But there are only 10 pages of light and easy recipes: and many dishes

FOR MORE HEALTHY NEW RECIPES:

If you want to add to your repertoire of healthy recipes, consider these newsletters and magazines.

Magazines

Eating Well, the Magazine of Food & Health. Ferry Road, P.O. Box 1001, Charlotte, Vermont 05445-1001. Six issues for $18.

Cooking Light, the Magazine of Food and Fitness. P.O. Box 830549, Birmingham, AL 35283-0549. Nine issues for $18.

Newsletters

The Cookbook Review, 60 Kinnaird Street, Cambridge MA 02139. Six issues for $24.

Nutrition Action Health Letter, The Center for Science in the Public Interest, 1875 Connecticut Avenue, N.W., Suite 300, Washington, DC 20009-5728. 10 issues for $24.

call for more butter, oil, and cream than experts consider wise today. High carbohydrate cooking can be lower in fat than this. Cut the fat and it's great.

Nutrient analysis: no
Modifications needed: make low-fat substitutions

🍎🍎

The Vegetarian Epicure Volume 1
By Anna Thomas
Knopf, 1972. ($16.95)

A classic vegetarian cookbook—one of the first and most enduring—with interesting, simple recipes for tasty vegetarian food. The book is easy to read but there's no attempt at low-fat, low-cholesterol cooking.

Nutritional analysis: no
Modifications needed: make low-fat substitutions

🍎🍎🍎

The Weight Watchers Complete Cookbook & Program Basics
Macmillan, 1994. ($25)

Good low-fat recipes with sound nutritional information and tips for weight reduction. Provides sample meal plans, holiday menus, basic recipes, and techniques. Tracking amounts/exchanges (part of the Weight Watchers approach) may be burdensome for some people.

Nutrient analysis: yes
Modifications needed: none

🍎🍎🍎

The Wellness Low-Fat Cookbook
University of California at Berkeley Wellness Letter Staff
Rebus, 1994. ($24.95)

An excellent low-fat cookbook. Highly rated for its solid nutritional advice and its collection of tasty, clearly written recipes. Includes good photographs.

Nutrient analysis: yes
Modifications needed: none ◻

Chapter 37

Junk Food: How Much Can You Get Away With?

When the snack products and convenience foods now popularly termed "junk food" began to crackle and crunch their way off production lines in the 1950s, it seemed like a liberating trend, a response to the nation's increasing affluence and decreasing time for food preparation. The appeal of junk food can be summarized in four words: cheap, quick, easy, and fun. Unfortunately, the rapid increase of fun foods in the American diet has also had a depressing effect on our nutritional health.

What Is Junk Food?

Junk food is now defined as any food packed with "empty calories"—an abundance of fat, sugar, sodium, and chemicals—and little nutritional value. Fast food items, such as hamburgers, fries, tacos, and fried chicken, are considered junk food when the amount of fat, calories, sodium, and chemicals they harbor is disproportionate to their total nutritional value. Satisfying your appetite with this kind of food may lead to

nutritional deficiencies, high cholesterol levels, and eventually heart problems. Although many health authorities insist that there is no such thing as junk food, consumers find it a useful term for distinguishing nourishing food from products whose chief appeal is fun, convenience, and addictive taste ("bet you can't eat just one").

Cash registers across the country ring up an astounding amount in sales of fast foods and snacks (candy, sweets, chips, cookies, ice cream and cakes). Americans today spend about $9 billion a year on candy and gum and $1.8 billion on potato chips. Among the 66 million Americans eating at least one meal a day out, 33 percent choose fast food.

While this national orgy of snacking may pose a threat to our collective health, junk food is not inherently "poison" and it's not necessary to completely avoid it to live a healthy life. Nutritionists have retreated from advising a complete denial of any food, realizing that the forbidden fruit can become an obsession. Eating a candy bar once in a while isn't going to ruin your health, and, depending on your choices, a meal at a fast food restaurant doesn't have to be a diet disaster.

In the pages ahead, you'll find some strategies for navigating the junk food maze, including insights into its appeal, guidelines on how much you can eat guilt-free, and tips for staying under that limit through moderation, compensation, and substitution. Victor Herbert, MD, JD, Professor of Medicine at Mount Sinai and Bronx Veteran Affairs Medical Centers makes the case in a nutshell: "All food is health food in moderation, all food is junk food in excess."

Junk Food's Appeal

The dazzling spread of both fast food outlets and snack products keeps them constantly "in your face." Fast food outlets have become an international symbol of American culture, and the industry is growing at an overwhelming rate both abroad and at home. In 1994 alone, McDonald's added 1,000 outlets worldwide; Subway, the submarine sandwich specialty shop, set up 25 new restaurants a week; and Pizza Hut opened a restaurant somewhere on the globe every four hours. The industry is also invading new territories such as hospitals, schools, and mass merchandise stores like WalMart. The National Restaurant Association believes that when the 1994 numbers are totaled, they will show that consumers for the first time have spent more on fast food than on restaurant meals. With increased spending on take-out meals, fast food is also invading the home, as well as turning our cars and desks into dining rooms.

If you feel that junk food is constantly being pushed on you, you're right. As any parent of young children knows, candy and gum are displayed conveniently close to the supermarket cash register. Fast food chains spend an average of nearly $1 billion a year in television advertising. Junk food is advertised as "fun food" and "cool" food, with the majority of the advertising directed at children and teens. The fast food industry openly competes for children's attention with offers of toys, special cups, kid clubs, playgrounds, and Disney videotapes. Surveys have told the industry's chieftains that parents often let children make restaurant choices, and 83 percent of the time, kids under 17 choose fast food.

But all this marketing effort would not work if junk food did not fundamentally appeal to American needs and lifestyles. There are probably some people who have never raced out to buy a candy bar or a burger and fries after dealing with a stalled car, angry boss, or irritable loved one. But most of us have found solace in junk food in times of stress. If this happens only occasionally, little harm is done. But if binging on high fat, high sodium products is a common coping tool for you, it is likely to become a source of physical stress itself.

Along with stress, time-pressure heightens the appeal of junk food, known for its speed and convenience. The snack and fast food industries thrive on impulse eating. Many people today eat when they have a free moment, not at pre-set meal times. Junk food allows you to eat without planning, without dressing up, without making a lot of decisions, sometimes without even getting out of your car. The menus at fast food restaurants and products in convenience stores are consistent, predictable, familiar, comfortable. They fit well into our hurried, pressured lifestyles.

These trends are not likely to reverse themselves. The results of the national low-fat eating campaign are telling. According to a recent *New York Times* article, Americans are choosing to adjust, rather than funda-mentally change their eating habits. Few peo-ple are rushing out to stock up on vegetables and grains. "Instead," says the *Times*, "there has been a stampede to buy packaged foods emblazoned with a 'no fat' or 'low fat' label." Indeed, for many this is now the only seal of approval needed, regardless of the product's other ingredients—or lack of them.

We have become dependent on the conve-nience, and even nutritionists now accept the fact that snacking, or "grazing" (eating five

THREE SQUARES A DAY (FAST FOOD STYLE)

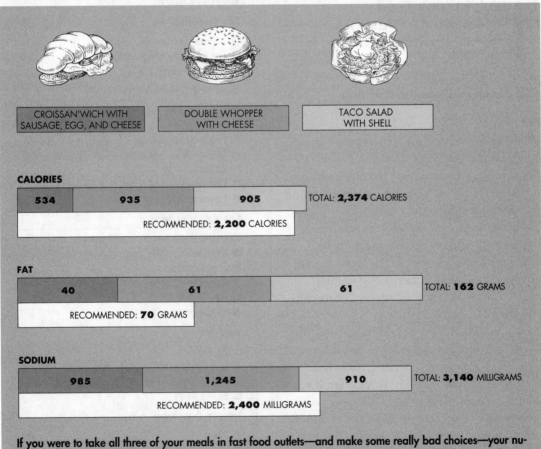

| CROISSAN'WICH WITH SAUSAGE, EGG, AND CHEESE | DOUBLE WHOPPER WITH CHEESE | TACO SALAD WITH SHELL |

CALORIES

| 534 | 935 | 905 | TOTAL: **2,374** CALORIES |

RECOMMENDED: **2,200** CALORIES

FAT

| 40 | 61 | 61 | TOTAL: **162** GRAMS |

RECOMMENDED: **70** GRAMS

SODIUM

| 985 | 1,245 | 910 | TOTAL: **3,140** MILLIGRAMS |

RECOMMENDED: **2,400** MILLIGRAMS

If you were to take all three of your meals in fast food outlets—and make some really bad choices—your nu-tritional profile for the day would look like the graph above. Although your calories would be more or less in line, you would have eaten more than double the recommended amount of fat and nearly 750 excess mil-ligrams of sodium. And that's not counting fries and dessert! The moral: While you don't have to completely give up those fat-laden burgers and breakfast sandwiches, you don't want to make a habit of them either.

or six small meals, rather than three square ones a day) can be a healthy eating pattern. Snacks are necessary for growing children, who receive 25 percent of their daily caloric intake from snacking. But what you eat, and how much, does make a difference. Low-fat snacking is associated with lower weight, lower serum cholesterol, and better blood glucose control. But Americans tend to reach for high-fat snacks: we now get 40 percent of our daily fat intake from snacks.

The Junk in Junk Food

The new nutrition labels mandated by the federal government allow us to take a closer look at what we are eating. And what we are eating is too much fat, salt, and protein, and too little fiber.

Fat

What we find is that fat is by far the biggest component of most junk food. A Nestle Crunch Bar gets 72 of its 150 calories from fat; a bag of potato chips has 10-11 grams of fat per ounce. Palm and coconut oil, which are highly saturated vegetable fats, are used in making a wide variety of snack foods. And so-called "healthy" snack foods are not always that healthy either; a bag of "natural" potato chips gets 60 percent of its calories from fat.

Red meat is still the biggest contributor of fat to the American diet, with butter, dressing, and frying oil coming in second. Most fast food items contain 40 to 50 percent fat. If you choose a Burger King Double Whopper with Cheese, you've ordered up 935 calories and 61 grams of fat. Compare that with the Burger King Broiler Chicken Sandwich at a more reasonable 320 calories and 10 grams of fat.

HEALTHIER SNACKS

Supermarkets and health food stores are stocked with an increasing variety of low-fat, low-calorie junk food. Here are some you might like as much as the old-fashioned kind.

New Crunchies:
- Low fat baked cheese puffs
- Low sodium, low-fat chips (Cape Cod, Louise's, Old El Paso)
- Whole wheat pretzels
- Sesame sticks

For Chocoholics:
- Instant diet hot chocolate
- Fat free chocolate cookies
- Chocolate syrup

Dips and Condiments:
- Dip mixes by Hain
- Fresh salsas
- Lite mayonnaise (tofu-based) and ketchup
- Low-sodium mustard and Worcestershire sauce
- Chutney (fruit or vegetable based relishes)
- Horseradish

For a Sweet tooth:
- Low-calorie candies or lifesavers
- Hard candy, jelly beans
- Marshmallows
- Angel food cake
- Apple crisps
- Whipped toppings

Cookies:
- Fig bars
- Gingersnaps
- R.W Frookie Cookies & Apple Fruit Cookie
- Snackwell's

Frozen Desserts:
- Sherbet
- Frozen yogurt
- Ice milk
- Frozen tofu
- Frozen fruit juice bars

Salt

Along with fat, most junk food is high in sodium, which can aggravate high blood pressure, leading ultimately to strokes and congestive heart failure. Some canned foods and frozen dinners are also known for their high sodium content. The National Academy of Science recommends no more than 2,400 milligrams of sodium a day, or just over one teaspoon. Yet a Burger King Chicken Sandwich has 1,417 milligrams of sodium and Hardee's Big Country Breakfast with Sausage has 1,980 milligrams. Remember that most of the sodium we eat is added when foods are manufactured and cooked. French fries are one of the lowest sodium foods you can find—until you pick up the salt shaker.

Too Much Protein, Too Little Fiber

Our bodies need protein, and fast food chains often advertise this fact to appear healthy. However, all we need to function normally is less than 2 ounces a day. The average American diet provides this much and more without our having to give it a thought. A large hamburger provides more than half the protein we need in a day; combine it with a shake and fries and you'll have met all your protein needs. You will also have consumed 1,779 calories—enough for a whole day for most people. Fast food provides protein, yes—but only with the extra fat and calories that most of us definitely do not need.

While junk food gives us too much of many food elements, it provides too little fiber. A high-fiber diet helps reduce your odds of many major disorders, such as heart disease, diabetes, and colon cancer.

Americans eat an average of 10 grams of fiber daily while the National Cancer Institute recommends eating two to three times this amount. More fiber-enriched foods are beginning to reach the market, which is a start; but beware of high-fiber candy bars. These products often get 35 percent of their calories from fat, compared with the 21 percent fat in regular candy bars. They also contain less than 7 percent of the Recommended Daily Allowance of all vitamins and minerals. Reading labels can really help!

The Fun Food Industry Reforms

Twenty years ago you couldn't find any low-fat or low-sodium products in the supermarket. Increasing public awareness of the relationship between health and nutrition has changed all that. Consumer groups have demanded that companies disclose ingredients and cooking methods used in their products. The Center for Science in the Public Interest (CSPI) started looking at fast food in 1983, and the work of this group and others has led to introduction of bills for ingredient labeling and orders from state attorneys general enjoining companies from deceptive advertising.

Many magazine articles and TV shows have picked up on the topic and the fast food industry has begun to take nutrition into account when designing new menus. Some packaged and canned food manufacturers have also adjusted basic recipes and cooking methods, and new healthier product versions are appearing in confusing proliferation. With reduced-fat versions of such classic health offenders as Ruffles potato chips and Doritos corn chips now reaching the market, the low-fat/low-salt revolution is almost complete.

Still, while these products greatly expand your choices, it's important to remember that many of them are merely "healthier" junk food, not truly nutritious eating. You should use them to satisfy occasional cravings, not as diet staples. If a product contains fat and a disproportionate amount of calories in relation to its nutritional value, it is still considered "junky" food.

Be aware, too, that reading labels is even more important with convenience and snack foods than with regular items. Do not take "health" labels at face value. Many "low-fat" or "no fat" products are still very high in calories, and foods that sound healthy may not be!

Carrot cake for instance, sounds nice and healthy. But 40 to 50 percent of the calories in carrot cake are from fat. In fast food restaurants, remember that so-called healthier versions may actually just be smaller portions. KFC Lite'n Crispy skin-free chicken has the same amount of fat per ounce (50 percent fat calories) as Extra Crispy; the only difference between the two is their weight: 3 ounces instead of 5 ounces.

Studying labels is a good habit, but you don't have to spend your life doing it. Once you've found new products that satisfy your appetite, decide how often you ought to eat them, then relax and enjoy!

Fast Food Chains Discover Health

Fast food chains hopped aboard the low-fat/low-salt bandwagon several years ago. They've changed some of their cooking techniques and added some new, healthier choices. All the major hamburger chains have switched from beef fat to vegetable shortening for all frying (definitely an improvement, but still a source of extra calories and fat). Sodium content has also started downward. Taco Bell cut 750 milligrams of sodium from its Taco Salad with

shell; Wendy's reduced the sodium in its chili by 30 percent; and Jack in the Box stopped salting burgers during the grilling process.

Many chains now offer grilled and broiled foods alongside their fried dishes. Arby's added a Grilled Chicken Barbecue Sandwich; Burger King removed half the fat from its BK Broiler Chicken Sandwich; and Wendy's added a Grilled Chicken Sandwich.

Muffins, low-fat milk, and salads have been added to many chain menus. Dairy Queen and Baskin-Robbins have introduced low-fat frozen yogurt and nonfat yogurt. Even Dunkin' Donuts eliminated egg yolks from doughnuts, switched to low-calorie mayonnaise, and introduced bagels.

A 1994 Consumer Report study shows, however, that although fast food companies are offering lower-fat items, most people still order those foods that are heavy in fat, saturated fat and other nutrients that should be limited in a prudent diet. Remember the "Best Bet" in the nearby box the next time you roll into a fast food outlet.

Where (and How) to Draw the Line

"Everyone, including those with dietary health issues, can get away with 500 empty calories a week," says Andrea Weiss, RD, MS, Metabolic Support Specialist at Maimonides Medical Center in New York. Does that sound like too little? Not if you remember that all food has some nutritional value and that those calories are not considered "empty." A fast food meal of 1,000 calories, for example, is likely to contain 500 empty calories. "Therefore, most of us can

BEST BETS IN THE FAST FOOD CHAINS

	Calories	Fat (grams)	Sodium (milligrams)
Burger King			
BK Broiler Chicken Sandwich	267	8	412
Chef Salad (easy on dressing)	178	9	568
Chunky Chicken Salad (easy on dressing)	142	4	443
Chicken Tenders, 6 pieces	236	13	541
Hamburger	272	11	505
McDonald's			
Fat-free Apple Bran Muffin	180	0	200
McLean Deluxe	320	10	670
Chunky Chicken Salad	150	4	230
Chicken McNuggets, 6 pieces	270	15	580
Small Hamburger	255	9	490
Wendy's			
Baked Potato, plain	270	0	20
Grilled Chicken Sandwich	320	9	715
Junior Hamburger	260	9	570
Chili, 9 oz.	220	7	750
Hardee's			
Pancakes, 3	280	2	890
Chicken Stix, 6 pieces	210	9	680
Grilled Chicken Sandwich	310	9	890
Hamburger	270	10	490
Side Salad	20	0	15
Pizza Hut			
Pan Pizza, Cheese, medium 2 slices	492	18	940
Thin 'n Crispy Pizza, Cheese, medium, 2 slices	398	17	867
L. J. Silver			
Seafood Salad	230	5	580
Rice Pilaf	210	2	570
Light Portion Baked Fish with lemon, 2 pieces, with rice pilaf and small salad	320	6	650
Jack-in-the-Box			
Hamburger	267	11	556
Chicken Fajita Pita	292	8	703
Baskin-Robbins			
Fat Free Just Chocolate Vanilla Twist (frozen dairy dessert) 1/2 cup	100	0	0
Coconut, small (5 oz.)	100	0	50

CHOOSING THE LESSER EVIL

Six Best and Worst Snacks at the Supermarket

Best: Popcorn with chili or onion powder	55 calories
Worst: Potato chips	155 calories
Best: Ice Milk	95-140 calories
Worst: Ice Cream	250-375 calories
Best: Chocolate syrup	50-60 calories
Worst: Candy bar	270 calories
Best: Slice of angel food cake with strawberries	150 calories
Worst: Strawberry shortcake	400 calories
Best: Apple crisp with cereal topping	180 calories
Worst: Apple pie	400 calories
Best: Popsicle	65 calories
Worst: Ice cream bar	162 calories

Best and Worst Choices at Six Fast Food Chains

	Calories	Fat (grams)	Sodium (milligrams)
Burger King			
Best: Hamburger	272	11	505
Worst: Double Whopper with Cheese	935	61	1245
Best: BK Broiler Chicken Sandwich	267	8	728
Worst: Chicken Sandwich (fried)	686	40	1417
Best: Croissan'wich with Egg and Cheese	315	20	607
Worst: Croissan'wich with Sausage, Egg and Cheese	534	40	985
Arby's			
Best: Light Roast Beef Deluxe	296	10	826
Worst: Roast Beef, Super	529	28	798
Best: Baked Potato, Plain	240	2	58
Worst: Baked Potato, Deluxe	621	36	605
Best: Chicken Fajita Pita	256	9	787
Worst: Chicken Cordon Bleu	658	37	1824

afford one junk food splurge a week," says Ms. Weiss. Your 500 weekly calories can translate into almost anything: a lunch of burger and fries, a hefty candy bar, or a large bag of potato chips.

How can you keep your junk food consumption down to these relatively modest levels? The solution is to find an approach that works well with your own lifestyle and eating patterns. The following strategies can be combined to fit your individual needs.

Best and Worst Choices at Six Fast Food Chains	Calories	Fat (grams)	Sodium (milligrams)
McDonald's			
Best: Hamburger	255	9	490
Worst: McRib Sandwich	445	22	972
Best: Grilled Chicken Sandwich	252	4	740
Worst: McChicken	415	20	770
Best: Muffin, Fat-free Apple Bran	180	0	200
Worst: Danish, Cinnamon Raisin	440	21	430
Wendy's			
Best: Jr. Hamburger	260	9	570
Worst: Big Classic, Double with Cheese	820	51	1555
Best: Grilled Chicken Sandwich	320	9	715
Worst: Fish Filet Sandwich	460	25	780
Best: Chili (9 oz.)	220	7	750
Worst: Biggie French Fries (6 oz.)	449	22	271
Taco Bell			
Best: Chicken Burrito, no Red Sauce	334	12	880
Worst: Burrito Supreme, with Red Sauce	503	22	1181
Best: Chicken Salad	125	8	252
Worst: Taco Salad with shell	905	61	910
Best: Pintos 'n Cheese with Red Sauce	190	9	642
Worst: Nachos Bellgrande	649	35	997
KFC			
Best: Lite'n Crispy Drumstick	242	14	—
Worst: Colonel's Chicken Sandwich	482	27	—
Best: Original Recipe Thigh	294	20	619
Worst: Extra Tasty Crispy Thigh	406	30	688
Best: Mashed Potatoes and Gravy	71	2	339
Worst: French Fries	244	12	139

Moderation

Let's say your lifestyle demands eating whatever is immediately available, rather than planning a weekly indulgence. In cases like this, consistent moderation is a good technique. Nutritionist Victor Herbert notes that "a Big Mac contains all the vitamins, minerals, and nutrients we need for health; but it also contains too much fat. Two Big Macs a week is health food, a Big Mac every day is junk food."

There are two ways of moderating your junk food intake: You can limit the number of times a week you indulge; or you can clean

ORDER IT YOUR WAY

As you can see from the best/worst lists, what you choose to eat can greatly affect the nutritional quality of your meal. Fast food chains are not required to disclose nutrition information, creating a problem for the health-conscious consumer. However, if you remember a few basic guidelines (fried foods are fat-filled; adding cheese adds extra fat) you'll be ready to make some healthy choices. Because selections change so often, don't hesitate to ask your favorite chain for nutritional information. Most fast food chains will provide it on request. Your overall objectives are to reduce fat, calories, and sodium, and add fiber. Here are some specific tactics to employ:

■ Avoid or cut back on condiments:
—mayonnaise (2 tablespoons = 194 calories, 21 grams fat)
—tartar sauce (134 calories, 14 grams fat, per serving)
—cheese (Processed American, 92 calories, 7 grams fat, per serving)
—salad dressing (2 ounces Olive Oil and Vinegar = 310 calories, 33 grams fat)

■ Choose grilled or broiled versions of foods, rather than fried alternatives (see "Choosing the Lesser Evil" box for comparisons).

■ Order plain burgers or cheeseburgers, rather than the "deluxe" versions.

■ To reduce sodium, cut down on pickles, mustard and ketchup.

■ When ordering pizza, get vegetable toppings and a thin crust.

■ Visit the salad bar for fiber; fill up on vegetables, fruit, and beans.

■ Go easy on processed meats like bacon, pepperoni, and sausage, which are high in fat and sodium.

■ Choose muffins, pancakes, and low-fat milk for breakfast foods, while avoiding biscuits (235 calories, 12 grams fat) and croissants (180 calories, 10 grams fat.).

■ Supplement kids meals with milk.

■ Try the leaner beef versions of your favorite sandwich.

■ Choose smaller portions of food or reduce servings by one-third.

■ Remove skin from fried chicken (a major reservoir of fat) and fill out your meal with corn on the cob, mashed potato, and salad.

■ Order grain versions of bread whenever available.

■ Use baked potatoes as a side dish without elaborate toppings.

■ Reduce calories by choosing juice or low-fat milk instead of soft drinks (8-10 teaspoons of sugar per 12 ounce can) or milk shakes (10 ounces = 300-400 calories).

up your choice of foods. For some, a small amount of real chocolate is more satisfying than a lot of low-fat chocolate. For others, more frequent—but healthier—junk proves an easier way to change. If you adjust the salt and fat content of your fast food meals, you can eat them more often. When you order fast food, get a hamburger a la carte rather than as a complete dinner and ask for it without mayonnaise. Try ordering smaller portions, skipping the fried items, and avoiding the extras. Steer clear of Quarter-Pounders and Double Whoppers. (For more tips, see the "Order It Your Way" box.)

The same principles apply to supermarket snacks. Either splurge and eat a fistful of cookies once a week or eat one cookie a day. Choose the approach that works best for you; either is better than no change at all. Listen to your appetite and use adjusted portions and ingredients—rather than denial—to moderate your diet.

Compensation

If you are not the moderating type and can't imagine limiting yourself to only 500 empty calories a week, try compensating. The 500 calorie limit is meant for those who don't get regular exercise. If you're physically active, you can afford more calories. If you really, really love these empty calories, adopt an exercise program that will burn them up, make sure the rest of your diet is extra healthy, and go to it!

Overall healthy eating in itself can serve to compensate for empty calories. According to dietician Weiss, "If you are eating a healthy diet, you can probably afford to eat 1,000 empty calories a week." Some nutritionists suggest 80 percent healthy food, 20 percent empty calories as a formula for compensation.

Try picking up an order of fries at McDonald's and eating it at home with a low-fat meal. People who are conscious of their diet and eat nutritionally rich foods, can feel secure with an occasional indulgence. These "safety valves" may help you stick with an overall low-fat diet without feeling unfairly denied.

Substitution

It is amazing how many empty calories you can save with simple substitutions. For example, a piece of angel food cake with strawberries is a healthy 150 calories, compared to a slice of strawberry shortcake (with whipped cream), which weighs in at 400 calories.

For some people, favorite snacks are a problem that even 1,000 empty calories a week can't satisfy. In such situations, substitution can be an important dietary aide. Everyday more products are being created to satisfy common cravings with less calories, fat, and sodium. If you live for ice cream, find a low-fat variety that your taste buds enjoy. If salty snacks are your downfall, switch from high-fat nuts to low-fat pretzels. Check the "Healthier Snacks" list shown earlier. Read nutrition labels, choose well, and always be prepared with a satisfactory substitute. Keep in mind though, that switching to these products only cuts down on dietary offenders; it doesn't necessarily increase your intake of valuable nutrients and fiber.

Junk and the Kids

Kids like junk food; and they do require extra calories between meals. Nutritionists feel that because children and teenagers expend a tremendous amount of energy, they often can safely in-

---

FINDING FIBER IN FAST FOOD

■ Try beans. Fried-chicken chains may serve baked beans; Wendy's serves chili with beans, and Mexican chains serve refried beans. Salad bars often offer kidney and garbanzo beans.

■ Eat the skin of your baked potato. (It's high in vitamins, too.)

■ Look for whole-grain breads. Subway and Wendy's offer wheat products. Although a small percentage is actually whole-grain, this is still a better choice.

■ Fill up with fruits and vegetables from the salad bar.

dulge in some junk food, as long as it doesn't push nutritious food out of their diets.

On the other hand, a steady intake of fatty foods from childhood to adulthood greatly increases the risk of serious diseases. The key to dealing with this dilemma is to return to the notion that some foods should be reserved as "treats" and to teach children that these foods are to be eaten only occasionally, along with a large variety of choices from five basic food groups. When teaching children about food decisions, explain your reasoning, and try to set a good example. If older children rebel against parental eating habits, don't fret; eventually most will return to the patterns they acquired at home.

Set standards for kids that allow them the extra calories they need without turning treat foods into staples. Some parents keep only healthful foods in the house, but allow sweets at restaurants, birthday parties, or movies. Nutritionists say that growing children shouldn't eat more than one fast food meal a week. And one night a week will satisfy most children's demands while reinforcing the idea that this type of food is a treat.

At the community level, you can request that schools and recreation centers upgrade their menus and change the snacks offered in vending machines. A 1993 American Academy of Pediatrics study offered a low-fat meal as one of two daily lunch choices in 16 elementary schools and found, "With this intervention the fat content of the average lunch selected by students dropped from 36 percent to 30 percent calories from fat." This strategy is especially effective because it simply changes the kids' available choices instead of attempting to change their attitudes about low-fat foods." Changes like these in the outside world can encourage better eating without increasing tension between parents and children.

Coming Soon to a Restaurant Near You: Vegetarian Fast Food

Keep your eye out for more alternative fast food; the vegetarian fast food industry is quickly expanding. Machessmo Mouse is a fast food chain on the west coast known for its healthy burritos, tacos, and salads. Dharma serves vegetarian fast food in California, with double-decker vegetarian sandwiches, beans, and frozen yogurt. (Be on the alert for added cheese in vegetarian food; it significantly raises the fat content. Watch out for fat-laden avocado, too.)

The invention of the Gardenburger made vegetarian fast food a reality. Gardenburgers are made of mushrooms, onions, rolled oats. They're shaped like hamburgers, but pack one-third the calories. Ingredients vary according to brand name. Now health food stores carry Gardentaco, Gardensausage and Gardensteak, all with less than half the fat of the real thing. □

Chapter 38

The Secret to Healthy Restaurant Dining

Is dining out your great escape? Do you seize those precious hours, throw your fat counter to the wind, and indulge in a thoroughly delicious, luxuriously incorrect meal? If your restaurant excursions are limited to an occasional night on the town, there's absolutely no reason for you to do otherwise. Any reasonable nutrition program allows for a little variety. And at restaurant prices, you really should get something you enjoy.

But today, eating out is a way of life for many people. More than 66 million Americans eat at least one meal a day outside the home, getting about one-third of their daily calories from restaurant food. In fact, 42 percent of American food dollars are now spent on eating out, according to the National Restaurant Association.

For working people, eating out is more than just convenient to their on-the-go lifestyle. It has become an integral part of the work routine: Power breakfasts, business luncheons, and dinners with clients have become keys to networking and success in professional circles.

Busy parents and single people are also buying an increasing amount of take-out foods and eating restaurant-prepared dishes at home. As a result, restaurant meals now comprise a significant portion of many Americans' total nutritional intake. If you're part of this group, treating every restaurant meal as a special occasion, with all nutritional rules suspended, can seriously affect your health.

Most people find it much more difficult to manage their diets when eating out, according to the American Institute for Cancer Research. At home it's possible to select healthy ingredients and cooking methods and control portion sizes. In restaurants, however, the abundance of tantalizing choices on the menu may make equally delicious lower-fat foods seem mundane. And the social and festive setting tends to put us in a mood for indulgence.

Recognizing this problem is the first step in overcoming it. The principles of good nutrition that guide your food choices at home are still applicable to the meals you eat out.

The good news is that restaurant menu planners are beginning to recognize the growing demand for healthier cuisine. An overwhelming majority of Americans now understand that good diet plays a role in the prevention of such serious illness as heart disease and cancer, according to a 1993 survey conducted by the Restaurant Association. So, more and more restaurants, including fast food outlets, are responding with an expanded selection of healthier foods. About 40 percent of restaurant owners now offer special dishes that are lower in fat, cholesterol, sodium, and calories, often marked with a heart symbol or similar graphic. And inventing healthy dishes that also thrill the taste buds has become a hallmark of many young talented chefs. (Ever try whole wheat, spinach, or artichoke pasta?) Dining out sensibly is becoming easier than ever before.

Strategies for Restaurant Dining

With the right coping strategies, you can eat out as often as you wish—and still maintain a healthy diet. Start by developing a personal list of convenient restaurants that offer a selection of appetizing, healthy dishes that you enjoy. Restaurants that serve a wide variety of fish, poultry, and lean meat, excellent salads, or interesting pasta give you the best chance to make nutritionally sound choices. If you're on a stringent diet for medical or weight-loss purposes, you may want to call a restaurant beforehand to see if they will accommodate your requests for low-fat food preparation.

On the way to a new (or old favorite) dining spot, it's helpful to mentally review the healthy dishes you like and seldom prepare at home. For example, if you rarely cook fish or shellfish at home you may want to concentrate on this category when eating out.

Or if you don't usually eat fruit desserts at home, you could decide to order sorbet whenever it's on the restaurant menu. A general idea of what you're going to order is the first line of defense against an intriguing but too rich menu.

When you know you'll be eating dinner in an enticing restaurant, you can limit yourself to lean, low-calorie foods for breakfast and lunch. But don't skip morning or afternoon meals in order to "save up" calories for a large restaurant dinner. This can leave you ravenous and lead to over ordering and overeating.

A few minutes before entering the restaurant, try visualizing the scenario and menu. Focus on how you can achieve a balanced, enjoyable meal. If you've already eaten liberally during the day, you may decide to focus on low-fat and low-calorie dishes. If you've been more careful, it's possible to order a more indulgent entree (while limiting the amount of fat in the appetizer, salad, and dessert).

Be prepared, too, for another distraction: the suggestions of the waiter and the food choices of your dining companions. You may be exhorted to go along with the crowd, or be bombarded with exclamations like, "No cheese, what's a baked potato without cheese?" Don't feel you have to offer a full explanation. A simple "I prefer it that way," or "I enjoy healthy eating" will do. If asked if you're on a diet, you might reply, "No, this is just the way I like to eat." If you dine out often with co-workers or family, ask for support. You can explain the motivation for your choice: "I've resolved to eat low-fat meals in restaurants."

Certainly, it's not necessary to order a "nutritionally correct" meal every time you step

QUESTIONS TO ASK THE WAITER

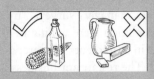

What type of fat do you use during preparation? Foods prepared with unsaturated oils, such as corn, safflower and sesame, are preferred over those made with saturated fats like butter, cream, and beef suet. Saturated fats can increase your blood cholesterol levels.

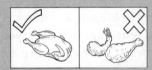

What cooking methods do you use? Broiled, steamed, poached, boiled, baked or stir-fried dishes are preferable to oilier pan-fried and deep-fried dishes. A fried chicken or fish fillet can soak up as much as three to four times the fat found in prime steak.

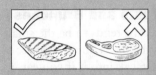

Which cuts of meat do you use? Some fatty red meat will have from 20 to 30 grams of fat per 3.5-ounce cooked serving. However, lean roasts and steaks, with visible fat trimmed, will run between 6 and 9 grams of fat for a 3.5-ounce cooked serving. Lean steaks include choice or select grades or flank, club, tenderloin, sirloin and London broil; lean roasts include eye of round, top and bottom round, and sirloin tip. Fatty steaks include ribeye, T-bone, New York strip, skirt steak, and porterhouse; fatty roasts include blade, chuck, rib, and brisket.

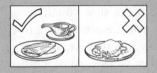

Is the dish served with sauce or added butter? If so, ask that butter be left off and that sauce be served on the side so you can use just a little to moisten the dish.

into a restaurant. Dining out is meant to be a joy. If once in awhile you crave a steak or piece of pie, enjoy. It's possible to include some high-fat and high-calorie dishes a couple of times a week and still be eating a healthful, low-fat diet overall. A little forethought about your restaurant eating patterns can go a long way in establishing better nutrition, however.

Making the Menu Work for You

The standard dinner menu is set up to encourage ordering an appetizer, soup or salad, main course, and desert. Often the "prix fixe" or "early bird special" menus are a good buy and therefore a temptation. But if they en-

courage you to eat much more food than you feel comfortable with, they're no bargain. Such a lineup is great for a special occasion, but an extravagance for everyday dining.

Many diners would prefer that restaurants offer special pricing on smaller portions. Serving different amounts for different appetites was endorsed by 74 percent of respondents to a 1993 Restaurant Association survey as the number one step that restaurants should take to address nutrition concerns. However, while some restaurants do offer "appetizer" and "entree" sizes of pasta dishes, the idea of different sizes across the board has yet to catch on.

Meanwhile, feel free to break the habit of ordering something from each menu category. Try sharing a main course with your dining companions to keep portions small. And remember that you don't have to order an entree when dining out. Some people prefer to start with a light soup or salad, then have an appetizer served when the other diners receive their entree. Add a side dish of a baked potato or vegetable to make a more filling meal (but watch the toppings!).

Doubling up on appetizers and skipping a main dish is a particularly good strategy with some ethnic cuisines, such as Indian, Thai, Middle-Eastern, or Chinese. That gives you the opportunity to sample many exotic tastes at one sitting. Spanish restaurants often offer *tapas:* snack-sized portions of main course selections. But be aware that nibbling, too, needs to be limited. Many small portions of different foods can easily add up to much more fat and calories than one hefty entree!

If you see nothing on the menu that pleases both your palate and your health consciousness, ask the waiter if you can design your own dish. Pasta and tomato sauce, broiled chicken or fish without sauce, or plain rice and vegetables are examples of dishes that most any restaurant can provide. Too often, dishes that sound healthy are served with sauces or added butter that can bring the calorie count for a piece of fish, for example, up to that of a broiled steak. Don't hesitate to ask the waiter about how the dish is prepared and presented.

If you have food allergies or dietary restrictions you can mold menu selections to fit your special needs. There's no reason why the restaurant staff can't cater to your need for healthy food. Don't hesitate to ask for substitutions or special preparation. Three out of five restaurant managers surveyed by the Restaurant Association were willing to make substitutions in ingredients and preparation when asked. The restaurant business is highly competitive; managers have learned that flexibility is key to keeping a steady clientele. Any good restaurant will allow you to order what you want. After all, you're the paying customer.

Better Breakfasts and Brunches

Though breakfast tends to be the smallest meal of the day, a lot of calories and fat can sneak into it if you eat in a restaurant. The traditional breakfast of eggs, hash browns, and sausage is fine on occasion; but don't make it the way you greet every new morning. Loading up on heavy food early in the day can slow you down at work or school. If you are accustomed to big breakfasts, you may find that you feel surprisingly better when you switch to meals that depend more on fiber to fill you up.

If you can't make time for a leisurely, sit-down breakfast at home, you'll probably pick something up on the way to work. This makes convenience the number one characteristic you're looking for. Even so, convenient foods don't have to be unhealthy ones. Most delis, breakfast stands, coffee shops, and convenience stores stock good food: fresh fruit, juices, low-fat muffins, single-serving packages of cereal, and low-fat milk, cottage cheese, and yogurt. These choices are just as handy as a sticky doughnut or a gooey Danish, and healthier too—especially if grabbing breakfast on the run is part of your daily routine.

Consumer demand has led many fast food restaurants to add health-oriented items to the menu. Opt for the bran or low-fat muffins over biscuits, croissants, and breakfast-meat sandwiches, which are typically loaded with fat. Most chain restaurants also have a selection of cereals; get a high-fiber, unsweetened variety and be sure to ask if low-fat milk is available.

Here are some ways to improve your breakfast order:

Fresh fruit—a grapefruit half, melon, or fruit salad—is a better choice than juice. Whole fruit is more filling and gives you extra fiber.

Pancakes and waffles, while tough to prepare at home, are fun to order in restaurants. Whole-wheat selections are best. Skip or minimize the butter and syrup, and instead top them with jam, unsweetened fruit, or low-fat yogurt.

Cereal is an excellent choice when eaten with skim milk and fruit. Choose whole-grain cereals, such as shredded wheat, oatmeal, or bran; stay away from the sugar-coated variety. Ask that hot cereals like oatmeal or grits be prepared without butter. Order butter on the side if you really must have some. Limit the amount of granola you eat. Despite its healthy reputation, it is often prepared with coconut or other artery-clogging saturated oils and lots of sugar.

Poached or soft-boiled eggs are a better selection than oily scrambled or fried eggs. Poached eggs over whole wheat toast can be a tasty substitution for buttered toast. But remember: If your cholesterol level is high, you're better off skipping eggs entirely for most of the time.

Meat at breakfast is best reserved for a treat at Sunday brunch. If you do order meat, choose Canadian bacon or lean ham instead of bacon or sausage.

Hash browns and french fried potatoes should also be viewed as a treat, not a breakfast staple. Ask if they come with your dish. If so, either request that they be left off the plate or ask if you can substitute a vegetable or a fruit salad.

Muffins, like salad bars, have mistakenly become synonymous with healthy eating. However, many muffins (even the celebrated oat bran variety) can be high in fat, calories, and sugar if baked with oil, nuts, and raisins. Many places now offer fat- or sugar-free muffins. If not, a plain bran or corn muffin is your best bet. If your muffin leaves grease stains on the take-out bag, you need to try a different variety.

Toast, an English muffin, or a bagel are good choices. But they may arrive at your table smothered in butter or cream cheese. Ask for spreads to be served on the side. Better yet, use jam or preserves instead.

All pastries such as **doughnuts**, croissants, coffee cake, biscuits, sweet rolls, and Danishes are best avoided. If you do order a pastry, make it a plain doughnut instead of one that is glazed, iced, or filled with cream, cheese, or chocolate.

Low-fat cottage cheese or low-fat ricotta make for healthier spreads than cream cheese or butter.

Skim milk is better in your coffee or tea than whole milk or dairy creamers. Avoid powdered milk substitutes; they are often high in saturated fat. Real powdered nonfat milk, however, is a good alternative.

Breakfast bars demand special care, for they may offer the temptation of high-fat food at a bargain price. Stick with muffins, bread, or fruit rather than pastries, eggs, hash browns, or meats.

Your Tactics at Lunch

Make lunch the flex point in your meal plan for the day, adjusting it to compensate for what you'll eat that evening.

If you foresee a big dinner, then a light, balanced lunch is the way to go. Even if you are having a business meal, keeping it light makes sense; the company and conversation, not the food, are likely to be the focus. Why "waste" calories on dishes you'll barely notice you're eating? If business companions ask why you chose soup and a large salad over prime rib, explain that you need to feel energetic when you get back to work; heavier foods and a full stomach can leave you feeling sluggish. Fortunately, now that the three-martini lunch is a thing of the past, many business lunch spots are catering to the demand for lighter fare.

"Light" doesn't mean "nothing," however. Under-eating at lunch can be a problem too. People who find themselves too busy to remember to eat during the work day wind up feeling dizzy and tired late in the afternoon— a situation that makes them prone to grab the nearest apple turnover or chocolate bar.

If you have little time to cook in the evening, eating a bigger meal at lunch can be a health booster. In fact, many nutritionists wish they could revise the American style of eating to make the mid-day meal the largest of the day. "Because we usually burn more calories during the day, it may make more sense to eat our largest meal at lunchtime," says Kathryn A. Parker, a registered dietitian in Gainseville, Florida. "Otherwise we end up filling up the tank at night, just when the engine is turned off."

Sandwich Bites

Whether you decide to make lunch a big meal or small one, be sure to balance your food choices with those you make at morning and night. In addition to the guidelines in the dinner section of this chapter, follow these sandwich tips:

- Choose sandwiches on whole-grain breads, bagels, English muffins, or rolls, which generally have only 1 to 2 grams of fat. A croissant can contain 12 to 20 grams of fat.
- Be aware that seafood salads, like tuna or shrimp, often come loaded with cholesterol-rich mayonnaise; order them without the dressing.
- Order sandwiches made without butter, mayonnaise, or other fatty spreads; or ask that the spread be served on the side. Mustard or salsa makes a great sandwich spread.
- Choose turkey or lean ham as sandwich meats; they contain only 1 to 2 grams of fat per ounce. Bologna or salami are high-fat cold cuts with 6 to 8 grams of fat per ounce.

SALAD BAR SAMPLER

Item	Serving	Calories	Fat
Bacon bits	2 teaspoons	54	3 grams
Olives	5	25	2 grams
Parmesan cheese	1/4 cup	111	7 grams
Eggs, chopped	2 tablespoons	27	2 grams
Cheddar cheese	2 tablespoons	57	4.5 grams
Feta cheese	1/4 cup	75	6 grams
Italian dressing	1 tablespoon	69	7 grams
Typical low-fat Italian dressing	1 tablespoon	16	0.5 grams

- Have the urge for something crunchy? To accompany your sandwich, choose pretzels or breadsticks (1 gram of fat per ounce) rather than potato or nacho chips (10 grams of fat per ounce.)
- Skip the cheese on sandwiches or use the low-fat variety.

Reconnoitering The Salad Bar

Health concerns gave birth to the salad bar, but this simple spread of cut, raw vegetables was soon invaded by lots of little temptations. Today it takes a bit of care to create a healthy plate from a salad bar that may offer a variety of cheeses, meats, breads, soups, pasta and potato salads, and even desserts. In fact, you can easily leave the salad bar without any of the vegetables you so health-consciously sought! Here are some things to keep in mind:

Dressings provide from 50 to 80 percent of the calories in tossed, Greek, Caesar, and spinach salad. For example, a Greek salad (3 cups lettuce, 1/2 ounce anchovies, 1/8 cucumber, 1/4 tomato, 1 ounce feta cheese, and 1 olive) with 2 tablespoons of dressing has 300 calories; without dressing it has only 135. A tossed salad with 2 tablespoons of dressing has about 174 calories; without dressing it only has 36. Use low-fat dressing or try a no-fat solution—opt for a vinegar, lemon, mustard, and herb combination.

French, Russian, blue cheese, creamy Italian, mayonnaise or oil dressings, should be limited to 1 tablespoon. Experiment with substituting grated cheese for creamy dressings on salads.

Cottage or feta cheese is a healthier choice than fattier Swiss, cheddar, or American. Stay away from salad ingredients like avocados, anchovies, eggs and bacon.

Tuna, lean beef, or chicken make better additions to your salad rather than bologna, ham, and salami.

Croutons and bacon bits are best skipped or limited. You can add a crunchy texture by crowning your salad with bean sprouts.

ALCOHOL CALORIE SAMPLER

Item	Serving	Calories
Beer	12 ounces	146 calories
Gin (90 proof)	1.5 ounces	110
Whiskey (86 proof)	1.5 ounces	105
Rum (80 proof)	1.5 ounces	97
Vodka (80 proof)	1.5 ounces	97
Wine, red	4 ounces	85
Wine, white	4 ounces	80
Champagne	4 ounces	79
Cordials/liqueur	1.5 ounces	146-186

A look at mixed drinks

Cocktails and mixed drinks can be even higher in calories when they include creamy, sweet ingredients. If you prefer mixed drinks, choose lower-calorie, lower-fat mixers such as orange, lime, lemon, cranberry, vegetable, or tomato juice. Club soda and sparkling water are great no-calorie mixers.

Cocktail calories

- Eggnog (4 ounces with rum): 309 calories, 14.5 grams fat
- Brandy Alexander (3.5 ounces brandy, creme de cacao, and heavy cream): 305 calories, 11 grams fat
- White Russian (2.75 ounces vodka, coffee liqueurs, and heavy cream): 236 calories, 5.5 grams fat
- Pina colada (4.5 ounces rum, coconut cream, sugar, and pineapple juice): 262 calories, 2.5 grams fat

Kidney beans or chick peas demand moderation. Steer clear of the three-bean salad, which often has a dressing high in fat and sodium.

A roll with your salad will fill you up. Whole-wheat rolls are a good choice, with only 72 calories and less than 1 gram of fat. If the bread is good, fresh and warm, you won't miss the butter.

If you want "just a taste" of the higher fat items, save it for your second trip to the salad bar. This way your stomach will be full of healthy greens, minimizing your risk of turning a dollop of potato salad into a plateful.

Passing the Cocktail Hour

Restaurant profits depend heavily on the sale of alcohol, so it's no accident that dinner ordering rituals encourage drinking. After a cocktail, many people who seldom drink at home drift into ordering a second or third in the restaurant. Unless health problems forbid, there's little harm in having a drink or two. But there's also little sense in allowing eager waiters to pressure you into ordering more than you really want.

The bar or cocktail lounge is often where we end up meeting dinner companions or waiting for our table. But you don't have to drink alcohol just because it's handy. Most bars will serve coffee and soft drinks. Often that's a good way to start the evening, even if you plan on alcoholic beverages later on.

Drinks in the cocktail lounge can make you prone to carelessness when you finally order the meal. Cocktail bars tend to offer peanuts, mini hot dogs, fried chicken wings, and chips—salty foods that increase your thirst and make it more likely that you'll order another drink. Eating such bar fare not only adds calories, but, with healthy eating already thrown out the window, can give you an excuse to go all out at dinner.

The calories of the drinks themselves are not to be overlooked either. They can add up, especially since many restaurants serve oversized drinks. Remember that each beer can "cost" you the equivalent of three bread sticks or eight large clams on the half shell. Here are a few guidelines to help you navigate the cocktail lounge:

- Try to go straight to the dining room, not first to the bar. Make sure to have a reservation so you don't have to wait for a table; or dine earlier, during the less crowded times.
- Cut down on the number and size of your drinks as well as their alcohol content. Drinking just one beer a day can add 54,000 calories (or 16 pounds) to your diet over a year.
- Order non-alcoholic beer, wine, and mixed drinks. This will cut calories by more than half.
- Buy wine by the glass, rather than by the bottle, to help limit consumption.
- Have your drink with your meal, not before.
- Always ask for water along with your drink so that you're not sipping alcohol simply to quench your thirst.
- Extend the drink itself with water, club soda, juice, or other mixers.

Making the Most of Dinner

Dinner is generally the largest meal of the day, particularly if you're eating out. Even so, a key strategy is to keep portions modest. Unfortunately, restaurant owners know that many diners feel cheated by small portions. Oversized dinner plates, filled to the rim, are therefore all too often the norm.

"A serving of meat should be about the size of the palm of your hand," says Kathryn A. Parker, R.D. "This amounts to about a 3- to 4-ounce serving. But restaurants almost always give you a bigger piece of meat—

typically a 6-ounce serving." If you go to a restaurant that prides itself on huge portions, plan to save part of the meal and have it for lunch the next day. If you are still a member of the "clean plate club" from childhood, you can ask the waiter to serve only half of the entree and bring you the rest in a doggie bag at the end of the meal. And if you feel a 3-ounce steak won't fill you up, Ms. Parker suggests ordering a second baked potato or other vegetable to satisfy your appetite.

How long you take to eat can affect how much you eat. The key to monitoring your true appetite is to eat slowly, with awareness. Eat a moderate portion of your entree, then put down your fork and enjoy the conversation. Set a mental timer for 10 minutes, recommends registered dietitian Mary Lee Chin. If you are still hungry after that time, then eat more of your entree or order something else.

Here are some tips for dealing with the dinner menu:

Savvy Starts
- Choose a light, satisfying appetizer: Shrimp cocktail (5 jumbo shrimp with 2 tablespoons of cocktail sauce) has only 124 calories and less than 1 gram of fat. A half cup of fresh fruit cup with orange sherbet has 130 calories and less than 1 gram of fat.
- Order clear rather than cream soups. The latter have lots of fat and calories. Consomme, wonton, and Manhattan clam chowder are better choices. If you do order a cream soup, make it a cup, not a bowl.

- Ask for salad dressing on the side, and use it sparingly. Basalmic vinegar makes a great substitute for salad dressing (it doesn't need to be cut with oil because of it's sweet flavor). Salsa, soy sauce, or a spritz of lemon or lime can also dress your greens.
- Remember that fried foods have astronomical amounts of calories and fat. For example:
- Fried clams (18 small): 342 calories and 19 grams of fat
- Ten potato skins sprinkled with cheddar cheese: 1,034 calories and 60.5 grams of fat
- A 7-ounce platter of nachos (approximately 48 chips) with 12 ounces of cheddar cheese and one cup of salsa: 2,498 calories and 174.5 grams of fat!

Excellent Entrées

- Seafood is a healthy choice if prepared with a minimum of oil. Even the fattiest fish tends to have no more fat than the leanest of meat. Light and flaky fish—such as flounder, pike, haddock, red snapper, and grouper—have about 1 to 2 grams of fat per 3.5-ounce serving. Fattier varieties, such as salmon and tuna, may run about 7 grams per 3.5-ounce serving. Ask for fish to be broiled in lemon juice or white wine.

- Order skinless white-meat poultry. More than half the fat in poultry is in and around the skin, and dark meat has about twice the fat of white. Avoid frying, which can double the overall fat content of the dish; and don't even think about batter-dipping and frying. It can increase the fat content five or six fold! Stuffed poultry dishes also tend to be high in fat.

- Pasta- and rice-based dishes are an excellent choice if you're careful about the sauce. Fettuccine Alfredo can have more than 1,000 calories in a 3-cup serving, with 60 grams of fat. Pasta made with a tomato sauce provides 72 percent less fat and half the calories.

- Don't mistake quiches and omelets for lighter fare, even if the menu bills them that way. Food prepared with cheese or a pastry crust is probably going to be high in fat.

- Eat red meat sparingly. Nutritionists recommend switching a good part of your red meat intake over to vegetables, grains, poultry, and fish. When eating beef, veal or pork, choose lean cuts and keep the fat content down in other portions of your meal. Avoid organ meats such as liver, which are lower in fat, but high in cholesterol.

- The sauce counts. Cream sauces such as, hollandaise, bearnaise, and newburg are loaded with fat. The hollandaise sauce in eggs Benedict accounts for more than 50 percent of the calories and close to 70 percent of the fat in the dish.

- Accompany your entree with vegetables that have been minimally cooked and prepared with little oil, butter, or cheese. Overcooking drains veggies of vitamins. Roasted vegetables are a delicious new alternative now gaining in popularity. Ask for baked, roasted, or mashed potatoes instead of fries or chips. Be sparing with butter and sour cream on baked potatoes. Try accenting your spuds with Worcestershire, Tabasco sauce, or mustard.

DESSERT COUNTDOWN

Dessert	Amount	Calories	Fat (grams)
Peach sorbet	1/2 cup	110	0
Marble cheesecake	2-inch piece	442	30
Carrot cake	1/12 cake	676	37
Hot fudge sundae	1 cup vanilla 1/4 cup fudge 4 tablespoons whipped cream 1 cherry	642	37

A Just Dessert

If your whole reason for going out is the view of that dessert cart rolling slowly to your table, then plan an occasional indulgence! You can compensate with a lean appetizer and entree.

Do save rich desserts for an occasional treat, however, especially if you eat out regularly. Most of the time you can enjoy fresh fruit after the meal. Restaurants often offer more exotic varieties of fruit than you would buy for yourself at home. If fruit isn't offered in the dessert section of the menu, check the appetizers or ask the waiter. Fruit-based desserts like sorbet are also a good choice.

If you do order a rich dessert, keep the serving small by sharing with someone or requesting that the waiter only serve a half portion. Remember that desserts made with cream cheese—like cheese cake and carrot cake—are high in fat. If you *must* have ice cream and the only offering on the menu is a hot fudge sundae, you can still request a small bowl of your favorite flavor without the sauce or whipped cream.

Savoring Ethnic Cuisine

Part of the adventure of dining out is sampling exotic tastes and enjoying unusual aromas that rarely fill our own kitchens. But, unfamiliarity with the language, ingredients, and preparation of dishes offered at an ethnic restaurant may leave you wondering what, exactly, you are ordering. Take heart. Healthy meals can be found in any type of cuisine if you know what to look for. Here are some points to keep in mind when visiting some of the more popular types of ethnic restaurants. For additional tips (and some other nationalities) see Chapter 33, "Improving Your Diet with International Flair."

Italian

Italian cuisine offers a rich variety of vegetable, bean, and pasta dishes. Try to steer clear of dishes labeled "Crema" or "fritto" style, indicating a heavy preparation; "pomodora" (tomato) suggests a lighter preparation. When ordering meat dishes, choose poultry or veal over sausage and beef specialties. Order seafood sauteed in wine rather than oil. Be aware that breading and cheese coatings ring up the calories in these dishes. Opt for meatless, tomato-based sauces, such as marinara or pizzaola, rather than cream sauces. Clam or calamari sauces are another tasty, lower-fat alternative to meat or cream sauces.

Healthy Picks
- Minestrone or consomme
- Cioppino (seafood soup)
- A salad of Italian greens, fava beans, drained Italian tuna, plum tomatoes, and slices of skim-milk mozzarella, with oil and vinegar on the side
- Chicken piccata or cacciatore
- Eggplant pomodora
- Polenta and grilled mushrooms
- Roasted peppers and sun-dried tomatoes over pasta
- Shrimp sauteed in wine sauce
- Italian ice

Avoid
- Antipasto salad (usually oil-soaked)
- Garlic bread
- Dishes made with large amounts of cheese, meats, or oils: for example, rich meat lasagna, manicotti, cannelloni, pesto, and anything cooked "Parmigiana" style
- Cream pastries

Mexican

Salsa is the great gift of Mexican cuisine; it adds an abundance of flavor to everything, and has almost no calories. Use salsa, or taco sauce as a topping or dip instead of sour cream, cheese, or guacamole (avocados are one of the few fruits very high in fat). Opt for plain black or pinto rather than refried beans. Avoid fried dishes and those prepared

with lots of cheese. Seafood or chicken in tomato-based or vegetable sauces are good choices. Order a la carte; combination dinners are often served with refried beans, sour cream, guacamole, cheese, and fried foods. It's fine to have one or two of these selections, but not all of them.

Healthy Picks
- Black bean soup or gazpacho
- Tortillas or soft tacos (unfried) filled with chicken, seafood, or vegetables
- Seafood burritos or enchiladas (with a minimum of cheese)
- Soft flour tortillas with chili con carne, black beans, or Mexican rice
- Camarones de hacha (shrimp in tomato coriander sauce)
- Arroz con pollo (boneless chicken with rice)
- Baked bananas, fresh jicama, or pineapple

Avoid
- Nacho chips
- Fried foods such as chimichangas and taquitos

Chinese

The typical Chinese restaurant menu is filled with vegetables, rice and noodles, making healthy eating an easy task. It also gives you the opportunity to eat a variety of vegetables you probably don't get very often, such as snow peas, water chestnuts, bamboo shoots, bok choy, lotus root, and mushrooms. Preparation is key: stir-fried or steamed dishes are better than those that are deep fried.

Chinese restaurants often make menu items to order: Ask that oils be used sparingly and that the flavor enhancer monosodium glutamate (MSG) be left out if it bothers you. You can also request that shrimp, scallops, or chicken be substituted for beef in menu entrées. The red meat preferred in Chinese cooking tends to be very lean, however. Use soy sauce sparingly—it contains 800 milligrams of sodium in each tablespoon.

Healthy Picks
- Wonton soup
- Steamed rice
- Steamed dumplings
- Fish steamed with ginger and scallions
- Steamed vegetables, lean meats, chicken, tofu, and seafood dishes in a light wine sauce; when ordering stir fried, ask for as little oil as possible
- Moo shu vegetables
- Moo goo gai pan chicken
- Shrimp with snow peas
- Fortune cookie

Avoid
- Dishes in heavy sauces, such as lobster sauce, garlic sauce, or sweet and sour sauce
- Egg rolls
- Pressed duck
- Fried rice
- "Crispy" or batter-dipped dishes
- Spareribs
- Egg foo yung
- Chow mein noodles

Japanese

Japanese cuisine is an especially healthy dining option, stressing soybean-based foods, small quantities of fish and meat, and rice and noodles. If you don't like to eat raw fish, order sushi made with just vegetables. Try the cooked crab or shrimp. Substitute shrimp, scallops, or chicken for beef in entrées. Augment your meal with steamed or stir-fried vegetables. Eat pickled, smoked, and salted dishes sparingly. Limit the amount of rice you eat—it's served in an abundance.

Healthy Picks
- Miso soup
- Gyoza (meat or seafood dumplings)
- Sashimi
- Sushi
- Hibachi chicken or lean beef
- Teriyaki-style meats, chicken, or fish, preferably steamed, grilled, or broiled
- Mandarin orange sections, sherbet, and fresh fruit

Avoid
- Fried bean curd
- Tempura, or other foods battered and fried
- Agemono
- Katsu dishes

French

French food varies in style: Provencal and Riviera-style cooking favor olive oil rather than butter or lard, and feature fish and vegetable dishes. Haute cuisine and cuisine bourgeoise both include heavy use of butter, cream, pork lard, goose fat, and eggs. Those looking to eat extra light should look for cuisine minceur, which means the "cuisine of slenderness," and dishes served "en papillote," or steamed in a paper envelope. If you can't resist a dish with a heavy French cream sauce, ask for a half- or appetizer-size portion.

Healthy Picks
- Consomme or seviche
- Salad nicoise (ask for dressing on the side)
- Herbed vegetables
- Coq au vin (chicken in wine)
- Pot-au-feu (stewed chicken)
- Bouillabaisse (fish stew)
- Poached quenelles (steamed fish dumplings)
- Ratatouille (eggplant, zucchini, and tomato casserole)
- Sorbet
- Fresh pears or other fruit in wine sauce

Avoid
- Puff-pastry appetizers
- Terrines or patés
- Hollandaise, bearnaise, bechamel, beurre blanc, veloute, and Mornay sauces
- "Au gratin" or "en casserole" dishes
- Pork or goose dishes
- Croissants
- Quiche
- Fondue
- Crepes
- Heavy pastries

Indian-Pakistani

The essence of Indian cuisine is its careful balance of unique spices and seasonings that create exciting flavors. Nonfried foods and vegetable and bean dishes come to life with spices (without much fat). Ask that dishes be prepared with a minimum of ghee (clarified butter). Look for Tandoori dishes, which are baked in a clay oven.

Healthy Picks
- Mulligatawny or lentil (Dahl rasam) soup
- Chapati (unleavened bread) and nan (leavened bread)
- Items prepared without frying or added ghee
- Curry dishes made with chicken, lobster, shrimp, lentils, or vegetables
- Chicken or fish tandoori
- Mango or papaya slices

Avoid
- Fried breads
- Coconut soup
- Fried entrées or rices
- Dishes prepared with coconut cream □

Nutrition, A to Z

ALPHA-TOCOPHEROL

See Vitamin E

ARGININE

See Nonessential Amino Acids

ASCORBIC ACID

See Vitamin C

ASPARTIC ACID

See Nonessential Amino Acids

BETA-CAROTENE

See Vitamin A

BETA-TOCOPHEROL

See Vitamin E

BIOTIN

What it is
Biotin, sometimes called vitamin H is produced naturally within the body by normal intestinal bacteria. This supply is all that a normal, healthy adult needs. Biotin is one of the water-soluble vitamins. There is no synthetic form available.

What it does
Biotin helps the body form fatty acids and process amino acids, starches, and sugars.

Why you need it
Biotin helps maintain the health of the body's sweat glands, nerve tissue, blood cells, bone marrow, skin, hair, and male sex glands.

Can you take too much?
Scientists currently consider natural biotin supplements to be non-toxic. Doses of 50 to 100 times the recommended intake have caused no ill effects.

Recommended daily allowances
The government has not yet established an official recommended dietary allowance (RDA) for biotin.

ADULTS

The estimated adequate intake for everyone 11 years of age and older is 100 to 200 micrograms per day.

CHILDREN

The following daily amounts are estimated to be adequate for children.

Infants up to 6 months:	35 micrograms
Ages 6 to 12 months:	50 micrograms
Ages 1 to 3 years:	65 micrograms
Ages 4 to 6 years:	85 micrograms
Ages 7 to 10 years:	120 micrograms

Best dietary sources
Biotin is found in dairy products, including butter, cheese, and milk; nuts, including cashews, peanuts, and walnuts; vegetables, including green peas, lentils, soybeans, and split peas; meats; organ meats, especially calves liver; chicken; eggs; fish, including mackerel and tuna; whole grain foods, including brown rice, bulgur, wheat, and oats; sunflower seeds; and brewer's yeast.

BRANCHED-CHAIN AMINO ACIDS

What they are
Three essential amino acids—leucine, isoleucine, and valine—form the so-called branched chain. Amino acids are the building blocks of protein. These three are among those considered "essential" because

they cannot be manufactured in the body and must be obtained through diet.

What they do
Along with the other amino acids, the branched-chain acids are the raw material used by the body to manufacture human proteins. These proteins are a vital component of all the body's cells.

Why you need them
Scientific evidence shows that branched-chain amino acids may help restore muscle mass following surgery, an injury, or trauma. They also help in people who have liver disease. There currently is no evidence that extra branched-chain amino acids are beneficial for healthy individuals. However, a general deficiency of protein in the diet can cause a loss of stamina, lowered resistance to infection, slow healing of wounds, weakness, and depression.

Can you take too much?
Amino acids are rarely toxic, even in large amounts.

Recommended daily allowances
There is no official recommended dietary allowance for the branched-chain amino acids, either separately or as a group.

The estimated adult daily requirement for leucine is nearly 9 milligrams per pound of body weight. Infants require almost 5 times that amount; children need approximately twice the adult requirement.

For isoleusine, the estimated adult daily requirement is about 6 milligrams per pound of body weight. Infants require more than 3 times that amount; the requirement for children is about twice the adult amount.

The estimated adult daily requirement for valine is also about 6 milligrams per pound of body weight. Infants require more than 4 times that amount, while children need about twice the adult requirement.

Your total daily requirement for protein in general is the number of grams equal to half your body weight. For instance, if you weigh 160 pounds, you need 80 grams of protein daily.

Best dietary sources
These and other amino acids are available in most meat and dairy products.

CALCIFIDOL

See Vitamin D

CALCITROL

See Vitamin D

CALCIUM

What it is
Calcium and phosphorus — the two most abundant minerals in our bodies — work together to keep our bones and teeth healthy. Calcium is found in many foods — most notably dairy products — and is also available as natural and synthetic supplements. You will need a prescription for certain forms of calcium; others can be purchased over the counter.

What it does
Fully 99 percent of our calcium deposits are stored in the bones. In response to the body's needs, calcium moves out of the bones into the bloodstream and then back into the bones for continued storage. Most of the remaining 1 percent of our calcium supply is located in body fluids, where it helps transmit nerve impulses. Calcium also promotes blood coagulation and plays an

essential role in enabling muscles, such as the heart, to relax and contract.

Why you need it

Calcium is essential to a child's normal growth and development, and everyone needs an adequate supply to keep bones and teeth strong and healthy. Because of the part it plays in muscle activity, some people take it to prevent muscle cramps; others use it to alleviate their severe muscle spasms that accompany a disorder called tetany.

One of calcium's more recently — and widely — publicized benefits is its ability to stave off the brittle-bone disease osteoporosis when used in combination with estrogen.

Can you take too much?

Doses above 2,000 milligrams per day can lead to potentially serious problems, including development of kidney stones. A loss of appetite, constipation, drowsiness, dry mouth or a metallic taste in the mouth, headache, and a feeling of fatigue or weakness could be early warning signs that there is too much calcium in your system. Later signs may include confusion, depression, nausea, vomiting, pain in bones or muscles, high blood pressure, increased thirst or urination, increased sensitivity of the eyes or skin to light, itchy skin or rash, and a slow or irregular heartbeat. If you notice any of these symptoms and you think the amount of calcium you have been taking could be the source of the problem, stop using the supplements and call your doctor. If you think your heartbeat is either irregular or slow, seek medical attention immediately.

Recommended daily allowances

ADULTS

The basic allowance for everyone 18 years of age and older is 800 milligrams.

Women need an additional 400 milligrams of calcium each day during pregnancy and as long as they breastfeed. Do not take megadoses of calcium during pregnancy or while breastfeeding. Calcium does pass into the breast milk.

Many experts believe that we need more calcium than the official recommendation and suggest the following amounts: 1,000 milligrams of calcium per day for premenopausal women and, due to the risk of osteoporosis, 1,500 milligrams for postmenopausal women and for both elderly men and women past the age of 65.

CHILDREN

Infants up to 6 months:	400 milligrams
Ages 6 to 12 months:	600 milligrams
Ages 1 to 10 years:	800 milligrams
Ages 11 to 24 years:	1,200 milligrams

All calcium supplements are not created equal. The body only absorbs part of the calcium it takes in, and different forms of calcium provide varying amounts of this mineral. Calcium citrate may provide a bit more usable calcium than other forms, and is less likely to have side effects. Calcium carbonate is often recommended because it contains the highest percentage of absorbable calcium. It is also the cheapest and has the added advantage of acting as an antacid. Two 1,250- or 1,500-milligram tablets of calcium carbonate per day will provide 1,000 milligrams of what is called "available" calcium to the body.

To get the same 1,000 milligrams from other forms of calcium, you need to take up to 12 tablets a day. Divide the following amounts into more than one dose and take them after meals: two 1,600-milligram tablets of calcium phosphate, five 950-milligram tablets of calcium citrate, eleven 1,000-milligram tablets of calcium gluconate, twelve 650-milligram tablets of calcium lactate, and 12 teaspoons of calcium glubionate. Chelated calcium tablets and combinations of calcium and other vitamins and minerals such as vitamin D and magnesium offer no special advantage. Also avoid bone meal and dolomite—they may contain toxic lead, mercury, and arsenic.

Whichever supplement you choose, check the information supplied with it to determine the dosage that will supply the amount of calcium you need. Remember too, that smoking and drinking alcohol, coffee, or tea increases the amount of calcium that your body will lose.

Best dietary sources
Calcium is found in dairy products, shrimp, canned salmon and sardines, green leafy vegetables, Brazil nuts and almonds, molasses, soybeans, and tofu.

One cup of yogurt contains up to 415 milligrams of calcium. There are 300 milligrams in 1 cup of skim milk, and 290 milligrams in 1 cup of whole milk. One slice of Swiss cheese provides 270 milligrams; 1 cup of cottage cheese, 230 milligrams; 1 ounce of cheddar cheese, 200 milligrams; 1 stalk of broccoli, cooked, 160 milligrams; and one 4-ounce piece of tofu, 150 milligrams.

CAROTENE

See Vitamin A

CHLORIDE

What it is
Chloride is a component of hydrochloric (stomach) acid. This mineral is also found in various salt products. Natural and synthetic supplements are available.

What it does
Chloride helps maintain the acid balance in the body's cells and fluids.

Why you need it
Chloride is essential to good health. Without it, the delicate chemical balance in the body will go awry.

Can you take too much?
Too much — or too little — chloride in your system can lead to weakness or confusion. At the extreme, you could go into a coma.

Recommended daily allowances
ADULTS

The RDA for everyone 18 years of age and older is 1.75 to 5.1 grams.

CHILDREN

Infants up to 6 months	0.275 to 0.7 grams
Ages 6 to 12 months	0.4 to 1.2 grams
Ages 1 to 3 years	0.5 to 1.5 grams
Ages 4 to 6 years:	0.7 to 2.1 grams
Ages 7 to 10 years:	0.925 to 2.775 grams
Ages 11 to 17 years:	1.4 to 4.2 grams

Best dietary sources:
Most of our chloride intake comes from table salt, which contains sodium chloride; salt substitutes, which contain potassium chloride and sea salt.

CHOLECALCIFEROL

See Vitamin D

CHOLINE

What it is
Choline, present to some degree in all our food, plays an important role in the nervous system. Natural and synthetic supplements are available. Choline is also a component

of lecithin, another nutrient available in supplement form. It is part of the B complex of vitamins.

What it does

The body uses choline to make acetylcholine, a substance essential for transmission of signals in many parts of the nervous system. Choline also aids in the transport of fats into the body's cells, and is vital to the health of the liver and kidneys.

Why you need it

Although choline deficiency is rare, it can lead to internal bleeding in the kidneys, excessively high blood pressure, heart disease, and degeneration of the liver.

If you have high cholesterol and triglyceride levels and are taking nicotinic acid (a form of niacin) as a treatment, you may need choline supplements, since high levels of niacin can deplete the choline in your system.

Can you take too much?

Sustained megadosing (above 6,000 milligrams) can cause dizziness, nausea, and vomiting. If you develop any of these symptoms, stop taking the choline supplement and call your physician.

Recommended daily allowances

The government has not yet established a recommended dietary allowance (RDA) for choline. A typical diet provides 500 to 900 milligrams daily. Taking more than 1 gram of supplementary choline per day is not generally recommended; and healthy women should not take choline supplements at all during pregnancy or while breastfeeding.

Best dietary sources

Foods richest in choline include cabbage, cauliflower, chickpeas, green beans, lentils, soybeans, split peas, calves' liver, eggs, rice, and soy lecithin.

CHROMIUM

What it is

Chromium is one of the minerals that the body needs in only trace amounts. It is found in a variety of meats, seafood, dairy products, eggs, and whole-grain foods.

What it does

Chromium helps the body to convert blood sugar (glucose) into energy. It also makes insulin work more efficiently and effectively.

Why you need it

Because chromium makes it easier for the body to burn glucose, chromium supplements have recently been touted as energy-boosters. In addition, chromium's alliance with insulin makes it especially important for diabetics. It can help some people who develop diabetes as older adults better tolerate glucose, thereby reducing the amount of insulin they need to control their sugar levels.

Can you take too much?

The chromium in food and vitamin/mineral supplements poses no danger. Indeed, Americans are thought to not get enough. However, long-term exposure on the job has reportedly led to skin problems, perforation of the nasal septum, liver or kidney impairment, and lung cancer in some people.

Recommended daily allowances

The government has not yet established the recommended daily amount (RDA) of chromium. The estimated safe and adequate daily intake is as follows:

ADULTS

All adults:	50 to 200 micrograms.

CHILDREN

Infants up to six
months: 1 to 40 micrograms
Ages 6 to 12 months: 20 to 60 micrograms
Ages 1 to 3 years: 20 to 80 micrograms
Ages 4 to 6 years: 30 to 120 micrograms
Age 7 and older: 50 to 200 micrograms

Women should avoid chromium supplements during pregnancy and while they are breastfeeding an infant.

Best dietary sources
You can obtain chromium from meats, including beef, chicken, and calves' liver; fish, oysters, and other seafood; cheese and other dairy products; eggs; fresh fruit; potatoes (with skin); whole grain products; brewer's yeast; and condiments such as black pepper and thyme.

COBALAMIN

See Vitamin B₁₂

COBALT

What it is
Cobalt, one of the minerals we need in just trace amounts, is stored in the liver. This mineral is readily available in a well-balanced diet, and deficiencies are rare.

What it does
Cobalt is closely related to vitamin B_{12}, and is therefore essential to the production of the red blood cells that carry oxygen throughout the body.

Why you need it
An inadequate supply of cobalt can lead to the condition called pernicious anemia. Symptoms include digestive problems, weight loss, and a burning feeling in the tongue.

What's too much?
Megadoses of cobalt—in the range of 20 to 30 milligrams per day — can lead to serious problems. Cobalt toxicity can cause the thyroid gland to grow too large in infants or to become enlarged in adults. The heart may also grow too large and, and congestive heart failure could result. In addition, excessive cobalt exposure can lead to an abnormally high level of red blood cells.

Recommended daily allowances
Cobalt deficiencies are extremely rare, and the government has yet to establish a recommended dietary allowance.

Best dietary sources
The small amounts of cobalt in a well-balanced diet will satisfy the cobalt requirements of most people. The richest sources are meats, particularly kidney and liver; clams and oysters; milk; figs; and buckwheat. There is some cobalt available in vegetables such as cabbage, lettuce, and spinach; but strict vegetarians are at greater risk of a deficiency than others.

COPPER

What it is
Copper is one of the minerals used by the body in only trace amount. It is an essential ingredient of proteins and enzymes.

What it does
Copper plays a major role in the body's ability to store and use iron. This important mineral triggers the release of iron, which then forms the hemoglobin in red blood cells. The body also uses this mineral to produce various enzymes it needs to maintain its tissues.

Why you need it

Because of its role in the production of hemoglobin, copper helps to prevent anemia. A deficiency of copper, though rare, can lead to weakness, poor respiration, and skin sores.

Can you take too much?

Nausea, vomiting, stomach pain, and muscle aches may be signs that you have too much copper in your system. Excessive amounts of copper can lead to anemia in some people.

Recommended daily allowances

The government has not yet established a recommended dietary allowance (RDA) for copper. Estimated safe and adequate daily intake is as follows:

ADULTS

All adults:	2 to 3 milligrams

Women should not take megadoses of copper during pregnancy or while they are breastfeeding.

CHILDREN

Infants up to 6 months:	0.5 to 0.7 milligrams
Ages 6 to 12 months:	0.7 to 1 milligrams
Ages 1 to 3 years:	1 to 1.5 milligrams
Ages 4 to 6 years:	1.5 to 2 milligrams
Ages 7 to 10 years:	2 to 2.5 milligrams
Age 11 and older:	2 to 3 milligrams

Best dietary sources

You can obtain copper from nuts, including Brazil nuts, cashews, hazelnuts, peanuts and walnuts; barley and lentils; honey and blackstrap molasses; mussels, oysters, and salmon; mushrooms; oats; and wheat germ.

CYANOCOBALAMIN

See Vitamin B12

CYSTEINE

See Nonessential Amino Acids

DELTA-TOCOPHEROL

See Vitamin E

DHA

See Omega-3 Fatty Acids

DIBASIC CALCIUM PHOSPHATE

See Calcium

DIHYDROTACHYSTEROL

See Vitamin D

DOCOSAHEXAENOIC ACID

See Omega-3 Fatty Acids

EICOSOPENTAENOIC ACID

See Omega-3 Fatty Acids

EPA

See Omega-3 Fatty Acids

ERGOCALCIFEROL

See Vitamin D

EVENING PRIMROSE OIL

See Gamma-Linolenic Acid

FERROUS FUMARATE

See Iron

FERROUS GLUCONATE

See Iron

FERROUS SULFATE

See Iron

FIBER

What it is
Fiber is the material that gives plants their stability and structure. There are two types: soluble fiber, which dissolves within the digestive system, and insoluble fiber, which is unaffected by digestion. Both pass through the body without being absorbed.

Fiber is found to some degree in all vegetables, fruits, nuts, and grains, and is also available as a supplement.

What it does
Fiber acts much like a sponge, and is able to absorb many times its weight in water. Soluble fiber absorbs cholesterol-containing bile from the digestive system and clears it from the body.

Why you need it
Insoluble fiber adds bulk to bowel movements, helping to prevent constipation, hemorrhoids, diverticulosis, and—over the long-term—colorectal cancer. Soluble fiber helps reduce the levels of cholesterol and triglycerides in the blood and works to moderate blood sugar levels as well.

Can you take too much?
A sudden increase in fiber intake can cause bloating and gas. Tremendous amounts could cause a blockage in the large intestine, although this is a rare occurrence. A diet with 25 grams of fiber for each 1,000 calories eaten is considered high in fiber.

Recommended daily allowances
There is no official recommended dietary allowance (RDA) for fiber. Nutrition experts advise intake of at least 20 to 30 grams a day.

Although no problems have surfaced, women who are pregnant or breastfeeding should not use fiber supplements unless prescribed by a physician. Fiber supplements are hazardous to children younger than two years of age.

Best dietary sources
Good sources of fiber include: fruits and vegetables, nuts, seeds, and whole-grain products. Beans and lentils are excellent sources of soluble fiber.

FISH OILS

See Omega-3 Fatty Acids

FLUORIDE

What it is
Fluoride, one of the minerals we require in only trace amounts, is best known as sodium fluoride, an ingredient in many toothpastes. Fluoride occurs naturally in some foods, and supplements are also available, with a physician's prescription.

What it does
Fluoride helps the body retain the calcium it needs for strong bones and teeth.

Why you need it
Fluoride supplements are prescribed to prevent dental cavities in children living where the fluoride level in the drinking water is inadequate. Children who need extra fluoride generally keep taking supplements until they are 16 years old. Physicians also use fluoride, along with

calcium and vitamin D to treat osteoporosis. It is important to note that this treatment must be supervised by a doctor.

Can you take too much?

A dose of fluoride 2,500 times the standard recommendation can be fatal. Smaller overdoses can eventually lead to stomach cramps or pain, diarrhea, black stools, and vomiting, which could be bloody. A feeling of faintness, shallow breathing, increased saliva, tremors, and an unusual feeling of excitement are also potential warning signs of fluoride toxicity. Stop taking fluoride and call your doctor if you develop any of these symptoms.

Recommended daily allowances

The government has not yet established a recommended dietary allowance (RDA) for fluoride. The estimated safe and adequate daily intake is as follows:

ADULTS

All adults:	1.5 to 4 milligrams

The experts disagree about whether it is safe — or beneficial — to take fluoride supplements during pregnancy. At this time experts feel that breastfeeding mothers who take additional fluoride need not anticipate problems with their infants. However, it is best to discuss your specific needs with your physician and to avoid taking megadoses of fluoride while pregnant or breastfeeding.

CHILDREN

Infants up to 6 months:	0.1 to 0.5 milligrams
Ages 6 to 12 months:	0.2 to 1 milligrams
Ages 1 to 3 years:	0.5 to 1.5 milligrams
Ages 4 to 6 years:	1 to 2.5 milligrams
Ages 7 to 10 years:	1.5 to 2.5 milligrams
Age 11 and older:	1.5 to 4 milligrams

Best dietary sources

Fluoride can be found in organ meats, including calves' liver and kidneys; fish and seafood, including cod, canned salmon, and canned sardines; apples; eggs; and tea. Note, however, that the amount of fluoride in these foods can vary greatly. It is much higher in areas where the soil is rich, and the water is fluoridated.

FOLACIN

See Folic Acid

FOLATE

See Folic Acid

FOLIC ACID

What it is

Folic acid is a water-soluble vitamin known by many other names—vitamin B9, folate, folacin, and tetrahydrofolic acid. It is available in fresh leafy green vegetables and liver. Folic acid is also manufactured synthetically and is included in most multivitamin supplements. An injectable form is available by prescription.

What it does

Folic acid is essential for the formation of the DNA that makes up our genes and the RNA that transmits their instructions. It is particularly important in the body's production of red blood cells. Folic acid deficiency results in megaloblastic anemia, an anemia similar to that caused by vitamin B12 deficiency. Symptoms include weight loss, digestive problems, and a burning feeling in the tongue.

Why you need it

Folic acid helps us grow and develop normally. It also regulates nerve cell development in the embryo and the developing baby. Folic acid supplements are used to treat the anemia that may occur with alcoholism, liver disease, pregnancy, breastfeeding, or the use of oral contraceptives.

Can you take too much?

Very high amounts of folic acid have been taken over long periods of time without any adverse effects. However, there is a chance that prolonged use of large amounts might lead to the formation of folacin crystals in the kidneys or cause severe neurologic problems. Symptoms such as loss of appetite, nausea, gas, and abdominal bloating may occur if you take more than 1,500 micrograms of folic acid per day.

Recommended daily allowances

ADULTS

For everyone 11 years and older the official recommended dietary allowance is 400 micrograms.

Women need an additional 400 micrograms of folic acid each day during pregnancy. (It is believed that folic acid supplementation during pregnancy may prevent the development of neural tube defects that can lead to mental retardation.) Breastfeeding mothers need an extra 100 micrograms of folic acid per day.

Many others may also require additional folic acid. People who do not eat a well-balanced diet, those over the age of 55, people who abuse alcohol or other drugs, and women who take oral contraceptives should discuss the need for folic acid supplementation with their physicians.

CHILDREN

Infants up to 6 months:	30 micrograms
Ages 6 to 12 months:	45 micrograms
Ages 1 to 3 years:	100 micrograms
Ages 4 to 6 years:	200 micrograms
Ages 7 to 10 years:	300 micrograms

Best dietary sources

Folic acid is available in green leafy vegetables such as broccoli, spinach, and romaine lettuce. It is important to note that cooking these vegetables reduces the amount of folic acid the body receives. Other natural sources of folic acid include: fruits—especially oranges and orange juice—calves' liver, brewer's yeast, wheat germ, rice, barley, beans, peas, split peas, chickpeas, lentils, soybeans, and sprouts.

One-half pound of fresh spinach contains 463 micrograms of folic acid; 1 tablespoon of brewer's yeast provides 308 micrograms. One-half cup of dry soybeans has 236 micrograms of folic acid; 1 cup of fresh orange juice provides 164 micrograms.

GAMMA-LINOLENIC ACID

What it is

Gamma-linolenic acid (GLA) is manufactured in the body from linolenic acid, one of the three essential fatty acids required in our diets. It is also found in oil expressed from the seeds of the evening primrose plant, and is available in a supplement called evening primrose oil.

What it does

Gamma-linolenic acid plays a role in the production of prostaglandins, hormone-like substances that, under some conditions, may help the body fight inflammation.

Why you need it

Some researchers believe that anti-inflammatory properties of certain prostaglandins that gamma-linolenic acid helps form may play a role in the body's ability to fight arthritis.

Can you take too much?
There is currently no evidence that gamma-linolenic acid is toxic.

Recommended daily allowances
No recommended allowance has been established for this substance.

Best dietary sources
Gamma-linolenic acid is found in fish.

GAMMA-TOCOPHEROL

See Vitamin E

GLA

See Gamma-Linolenic Acid

GLUTAMIC ACID

See Nonessential Amino Acids

GLUTAMINE

See Nonessential Amino Acids

GLYCINE

See Nonessential Amino Acids

HISTIDINE

See Nonessential Amino Acids

INOSITOL

What it is
Inositol is part of the vitamin B complex. The body manufactures its own supply of this substance, which it then uses to produce lecithin, a compound that aids in the body's utilization of fats. Inositol is found in many foods and is available both as a separate supplement and as a component of lecithin supplements.

What it does
As a component of lecithin, inositol is responsible for transferring needed fats from the liver to the body's cells.

Why you need it
By assisting in the proper utilization of fat and cholesterol, inositol lowers blood cholesterol levels, thus protecting the arteries and heart from excessive cholesterol build-up.

Can you take too much?
Inositol has not been found toxic at any dosage level.

Recommended daily allowances
The government has not yet established a recommended dietary allowance (RDA) for inositol, but doctors usually order no more than 500 to 1,000 milligrams daily when prescribing a supplement.

Best dietary sources
Inositol is found in dried beans, chickpeas, and lentils; cantaloupe and citrus fruit (other than lemons); calves' liver, pork, and veal; nuts; oats; rice; whole-grain products; lecithin granules, and wheat germ.

IODINE

What it is
Iodine, one of the minerals that we need in only trace amounts, appears in various fish and seafood products and is also available as a natural supplement. A physician's prescription is necessary for the larger dosage strengths.

What it does

Iodine is an important ingredient in the thyroid hormones that regulate many bodily functions.

Why you need it

Iodine is essential for proper functioning of the thyroid gland. Doctors use this mineral to shrink the thyroid prior to surgery and in tests to see how well the gland is working. Iodine is also useful in the treatment of goiter, an enlargement of the thyroid gland that appears as a swelling in the neck area. Iodine helps the cells function normally and keeps skin, hair, and nails healthy.

Can you take too much?

Warning signs that you may have too much iodine in your system include confusion, an irregular heartbeat, and stools that are either bloody or black and tarry. If you develop any of these symptoms of potential iodine toxicity, stop taking the supplement and call your doctor.

Recommended daily allowances

ADULTS

All adults:	150 micrograms

Women require an additional 25 micrograms of iodine each day during pregnancy. Women who are breastfeeding an infant need an extra 50 micrograms per day.

Although pregnant women need some additional iodine, too much can have serious consequences. Excessive amounts can give the baby an enlarged thyroid or an underactive thyroid. Cretinism, a form of dwarfism accompanied by mental deficiency, is another possible birth defect related to excessive iodine intake during pregnancy.

Breastfeeding mothers should avoid taking iodine supplements and megadoses while nursing an infant. The iodine that appears in breast milk may cause a skin rash, and can keep the baby's thyroid from functioning properly.

CHILDREN

Infants up to 6 months:	40 micrograms
Ages 6 to 12 months:	50 micrograms
Ages 1 to 3 years:	70 micrograms
Ages 4 to 6 years:	90 micrograms
Ages 7 to 10 years:	120 micrograms
Age 11 and older:	150 micrograms

Best dietary sources

Fish and seafood, including cod, haddock, herring, lobster, oysters, shrimp, and canned salmon are the primary sources of iodine. Other natural sources include cod-liver oil, sunflower seeds, iodized table salt, sea salt, and seaweed.

IRON

What it is

Although we've all heard that iron is essential for good blood, it is actually one of the minerals that we need in only trace amounts. Iron is supplied in a wide range of foods and in several different supplement formulations, including ferrous fumarate, ferrous gluconate, ferrous sulfate, and, for deep muscle injections, iron dextran.

What it does

Iron is an essential part of hemoglobin, the red part of red blood cells that carries oxygen throughout the body. Hemoglobin stores approximately 60 to 70 percent of the body's iron supply. Additional iron stored in the muscle tissue helps deliver the oxygen needed to make the muscles contract.

Why you need it

Iron deficiency leads to anemia—failure of the blood to supply sufficient oxygen to the body's cells. Signs of severe anemia include weakness, dizziness, headache, drowsiness, fatigue, and irritability.

Can you take too much?

Damage from a single dose of iron is unlikely. You would need to take more than 1,000 times the RDA for the dose to be fatal. However, iron can build up to toxic levels gradually within the body, especially in older men. Early signs that you may have too much iron in your system are abdominal pain, severe nausea, diarrhea, or vomiting with blood. As iron toxicity intensifies, you may begin to feel weak or even collapse. Your skin may look pale, while your lips, hands, and fingernails begin to take on a bluish tinge. Shallow breathing and a weak, rapid heartbeat are also among the later warning signs of iron overdose. Extreme toxicity can cause convulsions and coma.

When first taking an iron supplement, you may find your stools turning black or gray. This is not a problem. However, if you notice blood in the stool, seek treatment immediately.

Emergency treatment is also essential if you have chest pain, chills, hives, shortness of breath or a skin rash or if you lose consciousness. If you develop these symptoms, discontinue taking the supplement and call your doctor.

Recommended daily allowances

ADULTS

Males 11 to 18:	18 milligrams
Males 19 and older:	10 milligrams
Females 11 to 50:	18 milligrams
Females 51 and older:	10 milligrams

Women need an extra 30 to 60 milligrams of iron each day during pregnancy and while breastfeeding. However, pregnant women should not take an iron supplement during the first trimester unless prescribed by their physician. Nursing mothers who are healthy and eat a well-balanced diet may not need an iron supplement. In any event, do not take megadoses during pregnancy or while breastfeeding, and do not give your baby an iron supplement without first checking with the doctor.

CHILDREN

Infants up to 6 months:	10 milligrams
Ages 6 months to 3 years:	15 milligrams
Ages 4 to 10 years:	10 milligrams

Best dietary sources

Good sources of iron include enriched bread; prune juice; nuts, including cashews, pistachios, and walnuts; caviar; cheddar cheese, egg yolks; chickpeas; lentils; pumpkin seeds; black-strap molasses; mussels; wheat germ; whole-grain products; and seaweed.

One cup of prune juice contains 10.5 milligrams of iron, a cup of cooked chickpeas nearly 7 milligrams, and a cup of cooked spinach 4.2 milligrams. Cooking in iron pots and pans greatly increases the amount of iron in your food.

Humans have trouble absorbing iron, even from foods rich in the mineral. A person with normal iron levels will probably absorb only about 10 percent of the iron available in food. A person with an iron deficiency, however, will absorb from 20 to 30 percent of the available iron. Vitamin C increases the body's ability to absorb iron.

ISOLEUCINE

See Branched-Chain Amino Acids

L-CARNITINE

What it is

L-carnitine is a product of two of the essential amino acids that the body cannot produce on its own: lysine and methionine. It can be obtained from meat and dairy products and is also available as natural and synthetic supplements.

What it does

Lysine, methionine, and the other essential amino acids must all be on hand before the body can manufacture the proteins needed to repair and maintain its tissues.

Why you need it

Without the essential amino acids, including those in l-carnitine, normal growth and development is impossible. Unless you're a strict vegetarian, however, a deficiency is unlikely. Muscle weakness is the main sign that you may have a deficiency of l-carnitine in your system.

Can you take too much?

Like most amino acids, l-carnitine is rarely toxic, taken in large amounts.

Recommended daily allowances

No allowance has been established.

Best dietary sources

Natural sources of l-carnitine include dairy products, avocados, and lamb, beef, and other red meats. L-carnitine is also found in the soybean product called tempeh.

LECITHIN

What it is

Lecithin is a natural compound that includes choline, inositol, phosphorus, and various fatty acids. It is found throughout the body, and is available in a variety of foods, as well as natural and synthetic supplements.

What it does

The choline and inositol in lecithin both play important roles in the body's handling of fats. Choline is also an ingredient of acetylcholine, an essential chemical messenger in many parts of the nervous system.

Why you need it

By promoting the normal processing of fat and cholesterol, lecithin protects against hardening of the arteries and heart disease. It also helps maintain the health of the liver and kidneys.

If you are taking nicotinic acid (a form of niacin) to lower your cholesterol, you may be advised to take lecithin as a way of boosting your choline intake. High levels of niacin tend to deplete the choline in your system.

Can you take too much?

Excessive dose can cause dizziness, nausea, and vomiting. Follow manufacturers' recommendations, and, if you develop any of these symptoms, stop taking the supplement and call your physician.

Recommended daily allowances

There is no recommended dietary allowance (RDA) for lecithin. Two tablespoons daily is the usual dosage.

Best dietary sources

Good sources of lecithin include cabbage, cauliflower, chickpeas, green beans, lentils, soybeans, corn, split peas, calves' liver and eggs.

LEUCINE

See Branched-Chain Amino Acids

LYSINE

What it is
Lysine is one of the amino acids considered "essential" because they cannot be manufactured in the body and must be obtained through diet. Lysine is available in natural and synthetic supplement form.

What it does
Amino acids are the raw material used by the body to manufacture human proteins. These proteins are a vital component of all the body's cells.

Why you need it
Lysine plays an especially important role in the production of antibodies, hormones, and enzymes. It is also important for the repair of damaged tissue.

Can you take too much?
Amino acids are rarely toxic, even in large amounts.

Recommended daily allowances
There is no official recommended dietary allowance for lysine. The estimated adult daily requirement is approximately 5.5 milligrams per pound of body weight. Infants need 8 times that amount; children, 4 times that amount.

Women who are healthy and eat a well-balanced diet do not require lysine supplementation during pregnancy or while breastfeeding. If you do use a supplement, take it in moderation.

Best dietary sources
Good sources of lysine include red meat, milk, cheese, eggs, fish, lima beans, potatoes, soy products, and yeast.

MAGNESIUM

What it is
Magnesium is one of the minerals that we require in relatively large amounts. It is particularly abundant in green vegetables, and is also available in natural supplements—some of which require a physician's prescription.

What it does
Magnesium plays many roles in the body. It promotes absorption and use of other minerals such as calcium, helps move sodium and potassium across the cell membranes; is involved in the metabolism of proteins, and turns on essential enzymes.

Why you need it
Magnesium helps bones grow and teeth remain strong. It enables nerve impulses to travel through the body, keeps the body's metabolism in balance, and helps the muscles — including the heart — work properly. Small amounts of magnesium work as an antacid; large amounts of magnesium work as a laxative.

Can you take too much?
Although magnesium toxicity is rare, it can lead to serious problems, including severe nausea and vomiting, extreme muscle weakness, and difficulty breathing. The blood pressure can drop to an extremely low level, and the heartbeat may become irregular.

If your heartbeat seems irregular, seek emergency medical treatment immediately. Stop taking magnesium supplements and call your doctor if you notice any of the other signs of potential magnesium toxicity. You should also tell your physician if you lose your appetite, develop diarrhea, abdominal pain, mood changes, fatigue, or weakness; or if you experience discomfort when you urinate.

Recommended daily allowances

ADULTS

Males 11 to 14 years:	350 milligrams
Males 15 to 18 years:	400 milligrams
Males 18 and older:	350 milligrams
Females 11 and older:	300 milligrams

Women require an additional 150 milligrams of magnesium each day during pregnancy and while breastfeeding an infant. However, it is best to get the extra amount through your diet. Experts advise *against* taking magnesium supplements during pregnancy — the risk to the developing baby outweighs any benefits of supplementation.

You should also avoid taking large quantities of magnesium while you are breastfeeding. If magnesium supplements are necessary, your physician will recommend that you stop breastfeeding.

CHILDREN

Infants up to 6 months:	50 milligrams
Ages 6 to 12 months:	70 milligrams
Ages 1 to 3 years:	150 milligrams
Ages 4 to 6 years:	200 milligrams
Ages 7 to 10 years:	250 milligrams

Best dietary sources

Many foods are rich in magnesium. Good sources include fish and seafood, including bluefish, carp, cod, flounder, halibut, herring, mackerel, ocean perch, shrimp, and swordfish; fruits and fruit juice; leafy green vegetables; dairy products; nuts, including almonds; molasses; soybeans; sunflower seeds; wheat germ; and snails.

One-half cup of dry soybeans contains 278 milligrams of magnesium; 1/2 pound of spinach provides 200 milligrams. One-half of a medium avocado contains 51 milligrams; 1 cup of bottled grape juice has 30 milligrams, a cup of skim milk or buttermilk 34 milligrams, a cup of ice cream 19 milligrams.

MANGANESE

What it is

Manganese is one of the minerals needed by the body in relatively small (trace) amounts. Found in many beans, nuts, and grains, it is also available by prescription in natural and synthetic supplements.

What It Does

Manganese is concentrated in the pituitary gland, liver, pancreas, kidney, and bones. It is needed for proper utilization of several of the vitamins, including vitamin C; and it plays a role in the body's production of protein, sugar, fat, and cholesterol. It helps nourish the bones and nerves.

Why you need it

Without sufficient manganese, the body's system for processing blood sugar may falter, leading to diabetes. The nervous system may also be affected resulting in poor coordination and even seizures.

Can you take too much?

Signs of manganese toxicity include depression, trouble sleeping, and impotence. Some people may develop delusions or experience hallucinations following overdoses.

When taking manganese supplements, seek emergency treatment if you have trouble breathing or suffer leg cramps. Your doctor also needs to know if you lose your appetite, have headaches, or feel unusually tired.

Recommended daily allowances

The government has not yet established a recommended dietary allowance (RDA) for manganese. The estimated safe and adequate daily intake is as follows:

ADULTS

All adults:	2.5 to 5 milligrams

Women who are pregnant or breastfeeding should not take supplements that contain manganese unless prescribed by their physician and should never take megadoses of this mineral.

CHILDREN

Infants up to 6 months:	0.5 to 0.7 milligrams
Ages 6 to 12 months:	0.7 to 1 milligram
Ages 1 to 3 years:	1 to 1.5 milligrams
Ages 4 to 6 years:	1.5 to 2 milligrams
Ages 7 to 10 years:	2 to 3 milligrams
Age 11 and older:	2.5 to 5 milligrams

Best dietary sources
You can find manganese in vegetables, including dried beans, peas, and spinach; chestnuts, hazelnuts, peanuts, and pecans; buckwheat, bran, barley, and oatmeal; fruits, including avocados and blackberries; cloves and ginger; coffee; and seaweed.

MENADIOL

See Vitamin K

METHIONINE

What it is
Methionine is one of the amino acids considered "essential" because they cannot be manufactured in the body and must be obtained through diet. Worse yet for strict vegetarians, this particular amino acid is found only in meat and dairy products. However, natural and synthetic methionine supplements are available.

What it does
Amino acids are the raw material used by the body to manufacture human proteins. These proteins are a vital component of all the body's cells.

Why you need it
Methionine is thought to be necessary for effective use of two other amino acids, cystine and taurine.

Can you take too much?
Amino acids are rarely toxic, even in large amounts.

Recommended daily allowances
There is no official recommended dietary allowance for methionine. The estimated adult daily requirement for methionine and cystine combined is approximately 4.5 milligrams per pound of body weight. Infants need 5 times that amount; children require twice that amount.

Women who are healthy and eat a well-balanced diet do not require methionine supplementation during pregnancy or while breastfeeding. If you do use a supplement, take it in moderation.

Best dietary sources
Methionine is found only in meat, fish, eggs, and milk.

MOLYBDENUM

What it is
Molybdenum is one of the minerals that we need in only trace amounts. It is found in certain vegetables, organ meats, and cereal grains. A molybdenum supplement is available by prescription.

What it does
Molybdenum is part of the bones, teeth, kidney, and liver. It helps the body use its

iron reserves, and plays a role in the burning of fat.

Why you need it

Because it is an ingredient of tooth enamel, a shortage of molybdenum can contribute to tooth decay. A deficiency can also lead to anemia (oxygen starvation in the tissues), and even impotence.

Can you take too much?

Regular doses of 10 to 15 milligrams of molybdenum per day — 20 to 30 times the estimated safe amount—can cause the painfully swollen joints associated with gout. When people take even slightly more than the estimated safe intake of molybdenum, it can deplete the body of copper. Signs of moderate molybdenum toxicity include diarrhea and a depressed growth rate in children.

Recommended daily allowances

The government has not yet established a recommended dietary allowance (RDA) for molybdenum. The estimated safe and adequate daily intake is as follows:

ADULTS

All adults:	150 to 500 micrograms

CHILDREN

Infants up to 6 months:	30 to 60 micrograms
Ages 6 to 12 months:	40 to 80 micrograms
Ages 1 to 3 years:	50 to 100 micrograms
Ages 4 to 6 years:	60 to 150 micrograms
Ages 7 to 10 years:	100 to 300 micrograms
Age 11 and older:	150 to 500 micrograms

Best dietary sources

Molybdenum is found in dark green leafy vegetables; organ meats, including liver, kidney, and sweetbreads; beans, peas and other legumes; and cereal grains. The actual amount of molybdenum in grains and vegetables depends on the amount in the soil when the produce was growing.

MYO-INOSITOL

See Inositol

NIACIN

What it is

Niacin, also known as vitamin B₃, is one of the water-soluble vitamins that need constant replenishment.

Niacin supplements are available in two forms, nicotinic acid (the prescription drug Nicolar) and niacinamide, found in over-the-counter supplements. The nicotinic acid form of vitamin B₃ lowers the amount of cholesterol in the blood, thereby reducing the risk of heart disease. Niacinamide does not have this effect.

What it does

Niacin helps release the energy from food and aids the body in synthesizing DNA. It works with other compounds to help the body process fat and produce sugar while aiding the tissues to rid themselves of waste products. The nicotinic acid form of the vitamin lowers the amount of cholesterol and triglycerides in the blood.

Why you need it

Niacin helps the body's skin, nerves, and digestive system stay healthy. It is used to treat dizziness and ringing in the ears and to help prevent premenstrual headaches. Niacin supplements are also given to treat pellagra, a potentially fatal niacin deficiency disease characterized by diarrhea, mental disorders, depression, and skin problems. The nicotinic acid form of niacin is prescribed to reduce the amount of cholesterol and triglycerides in the blood.

Can you take too much?

Too much nicotinic acid—more than 2,000 milligrams a day—over a long period of time may damage the liver or cause a stomach ulcer to flare up. Nausea, vomiting, abdominal cramps or pain, faintness, and a yellowish color to the skin and eyes are warning signs of excessive dosage. The niacinamide form of the vitamin does not have these effects.

Recommended daily allowances

ADULTS

Males 11 to 18:	18 milligrams
Males 19 to 22:	19 milligrams
Males 23 to 50:	18 milligrams
Males 50 and older:	16 milligrams
Females 11 to 14:	15 milligrams
Females 15 to 22:	14 milligrams
Females 23 and older:	13 milligrams

Women need an additional 2 milligrams of niacin each day during pregnancy. Breastfeeding mothers need an extra 4 milligrams per day.

CHILDREN

Infants up to 6 months:	6 milligrams
Ages 6 to 12 months:	8 milligrams
Ages 1 to 3 years:	9 milligrams
Ages 4 to 6 years:	11 milligrams
Ages 7 to 10 years:	16 milligrams

Best dietary sources

Good sources are lean meats, fish, and poultry, including beef liver, pork, veal, turkey, chicken (white meat), salmon, swordfish, tuna, and halibut. Peanuts, brewer's yeast, and sunflower seeds also provide niacin.

A 4-ounce piece of tofu contains nearly 16 milligrams of niacin. One-half cup of dry soybeans provides 11.5 milligrams. One cup of cottage cheese contains 8 milligrams—about half of the adult RDA.

NIACINAMIDE

See Niacin

NICKEL

What it is

Nickel is one of the minerals that we require in only trace amounts. It is available in some types of food, and as a supplement.

What it does

Nickel appears to play only a minor role in human nutrition. It is thought to be involved in the body's use of fats and the blood sugar glucose.

Why you need it

Unlike deficiencies of most other vitamins and minerals, a lack of nickel causes few immediate symptoms. It may aggravate anemia, the condition that results when insufficient oxygen reaches the body's tissues.

Can you take too much?

Although it's difficult to develop a nickel deficiency, too much can definitely be a problem. Symptoms of toxic levels include headache, vertigo, nausea, vomiting, chest pain, and coughing.

Recommended daily allowances

No recommendation has been established. The amount found in a normal diet can range from a few micrograms to hundreds of milligrams, depending on the nickel content of the soil in which the food is grown.

Best dietary sources

Foods that may contain nickel include grains, beans, vegetables, and seafood.

NICOTINAMIDE

See Niacin

NICOTINIC ACID

See Niacin

NONESSENTIAL AMINO ACIDS

What they are
Amino acids are the raw materials used by the body to manufacture human protein—a vital component of all the body's cells. This group of amino acids is labeled "nonessential" because, when the acids are lacking in the diet, they can be manufactured in the body.

What they do
All the nonessential amino acids must be on hand before the body can synthesize protein; and several have additional, more specialized roles as well.

■**Arginine** turns on human growth hormone and is considered essential during childhood, when the body's production of this amino acid can't keep up with demand.

■**Cystine** is an ingredient of the body's major antioxidant, as substance called glutathione. It thereby plays an important role in neutralizing toxic pollutants and byproducts within the body.

■**Glutamic acid** is another component of glutathione. It is related to glutamate, one of the nervous system's chemical messengers. Glutamate appears in our diets as the flavor enhancer MSG.

■**Glutamine** is a derivative of glutamic acid.

■**Glycine** is yet another component of the antioxidant, glutathione.

■**Histidine** is needed for growth in children and is deemed essential during the childhood years, when demand outpaces the body's ability to produce this substance.

■**Taurine** helps regulate the nervous system and the muscles.

■**Tyrosine,** which is manufactured from the essential amino acid phenylalanine, plays a role in the production of three of the nervous system's messengers: dopamine, epinephrine, and norepinephrine.

Why you need them
Deficiencies of arginine and histidine can stunt growth in small children. Glutamine supplements are prescribed for certain digestive disorders and to treat alcoholism. Taurine is sometimes helpful in the treatment of epilepsy.

Can you take too much?
Large doses of arginine may cause nausea or diarrhea; and excessive amounts of tyrosine can lead to changes in blood pressure and migraine headaches. In general, however, even large amounts of these amino acids in your system are unlikely to cause any severe problems.

Recommended daily allowances
There are no official recommended daily allowances for these nutrients; and it is advisable to take supplements only under a doctor's supervision. Women taking supplements while pregnant or breastfeeding should be especially careful to avoid excessive doses.

Best dietary sources
A complete set of all the amino acids is available in most meat and dairy products. Arginine can also be found in cereals, whole-wheat products, brown rice, chocolate, popcorn, nuts, raisins, and pumpkin and sesame seeds. Other sources of

tyrosine include almonds, peanuts, bananas, avocados, lima beans, pickled herring, and pumpkin and sesame seeds.

OIL OF EVENING PRIMROSE

See Gamma-Linolenic Acid

OMEGA-3 FATTY ACIDS

What they are
This group of fatty acids, also known as fish oil, have gained popularity as a protective agent for the heart. Omega-3 supplements contain docosahexaenoic acid (DHA) and eicosapentaenoic acid (EPA).

What they do
The omega-3 fatty acids are believed to lower the levels of triglycerides (fats) and total cholesterol in the blood, while raising the amount of HDL (good) cholesterol. These acids also discourage unwanted clotting that can aggravate plaque build-up.

Why you need them
In people with a cholesterol problem, omega-3 fatty acids can help prevent the buildup of cholesterol-laden plaque that can clog the arteries and lead to heart attack and stroke.

Can you take too much?
Because omega-3 fatty acids discourage clotting, excessive levels can lead to bleeding problems in case of an accident or trauma. Women who menstruate are also in greater danger of developing anemia.

Recommended daily allowances
There is no recommended dietary allowance (RDA) for the omega-3 fatty acids.

To increase your intake of the omega-3 fatty acids, nutritionists generally recommend eating more fish (2 to 3 times a week), rather than taking large amounts of supplements. A 7-ounce serving of certain types of fish easily provides 2 to 4 grams of omega-3 fatty acids.

Best dietary sources
The omega-3 fatty acids are found in cold-water fish. Best sources include cod, tuna, salmon, halibut, shark, and mackerel. Herring, bluefish, shrimp, flounder, and swordfish also provide good amounts of these acids.

A 7-ounce portion of herring contains 3.2 grams of omega-3 acids. The same serving of salmon or bluefish provides 2.4 grams. Seven ounces of tuna has 1 gram.

PABA

What it is
Also known as para-aminobenzoic acid, this water-soluble member of the vitamin B complex is closely associated with folic acid. The body receives a constant supply of PABA from friendly bacteria residing in the intestines.

What it does
PABA plays a role in the breakdown and use of proteins, and in the formation of red blood cells. It also stimulates production of folic acid in the intestines, and helps maintain the health of the skin and hair.

Why you need it
Unless something—such as a sulfa drug—disrupts intestinal production, there appears to be no need for PABA in the diet. If a deficiency does develop, it is signaled by fatigue, depression, nervousness, headache, and digestive disorders. In ointment form, PABA provides burn relief. It is also used as a sunscreen.

Can you take too much?

Sustained megadosing can cause damage to the liver, heart, and kidneys. Symptoms of overdose include nausea and vomiting.

Recommended daily allowances

PABA is normally unneeded; and there is no recommended dietary allowance.

Best dietary sources

PABA can be obtained from liver, yeast, wheat germ, and molasses.

PANTETHINE

See Pantothenic Acid

PANTOTHENIC ACID

What it is

Pantothenic acid is a water-soluble vitamin also known as vitamin B_5 and pantethine. It is found in a variety of foods and is manufactured synthetically. Your physician can prescribe an injectable form.

What it does

Pantothenic acid helps the body release energy from carbohydrates, protein, and fat.

Why you need it

Pantothenic acid helps the body grow and develop normally. Some people believe that this vitamin also helps wounds heal more quickly by stimulating the cells to grow.

Can you take too much?

Even at doses hundreds of times the usual amount, pantothenic acid causes no problems. However, you may develop diarrhea or retain water if you ingest megadoses of 10 grams or more.

Recommended daily allowances

A recommended dietary allowance (RDA) has not yet been established for pantothenic acid.

ADULTS

The estimated adequate intake for males and females 10 years of age and older is 4 to 7 milligrams per day.

Women may need additional pantothenic acid during pregnancy or while breastfeeding.

CHILDREN

The estimated adequate daily intake for children is:

Infants up to 6 months:	2 milligrams
Ages 6 to 3 years:	3 milligrams
Ages 4 to 6 years:	3 to 4 milligrams
Ages 7 to 9 years:	4 to 5 milligrams

Best dietary sources

Pantothenic acid is found in all types of meats, including organ meats and especially liver. It is also available in eggs, lobster, whole-grain cereals, wheat germ, brewer's yeast, corn, peas, lentils, soybeans, peanuts, and sunflower seeds.

One-half cup of dry soybeans contains 1.8 milligrams of pantothenic acid; the same amount of lentils contains 1.3 milligrams. One tablespoon of brewer's yeast or 1 cup of fresh peas provides 1.2 milligrams.

PHENYLALANINE

What it is

Phenylalanine is one of the amino acids considered "essential" because they cannot be manufactured in the body and must be obtained through diet. Natural and synthetic phenylalanine supplements are also available.

What it does

Amino acids are the raw material used by the body to manufacture human proteins. These proteins are a vital component of all the body's cells.

Why you need it

Phenylalanine has a special role in the production of dopamine, epinephrine, and norepinephrine, three chemical messengers that aid in transmitting signals through the nervous system. However, extra phenylalanine can be both helpful and harmful. Do not take phenylalanine supplements without consulting your physician.

Can you take too much?

Potential side effects of excessive phenylalanine include high or low blood pressure and migraine headaches. If you think you may be having a reaction to phenylalanine, stop taking the supplement and call your doctor right away.

Children born without the ability to process phenylalanine can build up dangerous levels of this amino acid, resulting in mental retardation, seizures, extreme hyperactivity, and psychosis. Tests can uncover this condition, called phenylketonuria, in the newborn; and treatment is available.

Recommended daily allowances

There is no official recommended dietary allowance for phenylalanine. The estimated adult daily requirement for phenylalanine and the related amino acid tyrosine combined is approximately 7 milligrams per pound of body weight. Infants require almost 9 times that amount; children need 10 milligrams per pound.

Women who are healthy and eat a well-balanced diet do not require phenylalanine supplementation during pregnancy or while breastfeeding. If you do use a supplement take it in moderation.

Best dietary sources

Foods rich in phenylalanine include almonds and peanuts; bananas and avocados; cheese and cottage cheese; lima beans; non-fat dried milk; pumpkin and sesame seeds; and pickled herring.

PHOSPHORUS

What it is

Phosphorus is, after calcium, the body's second most plentiful mineral. It is a major component of the bones, and appears in every cell in the body. Supplements are available in the form of various phosphates.

What it does

Phosphorus participates in virtually all the chemical reactions in the body. It helps the body use many of the B vitamins, and plays an important role in the utilization of fats, proteins, and carbohydrates. It stimulates muscle contraction, supports cell division and growth, and participates in transmission of nerve impulses.

Why you need it

As one of the two major ingredients of bones and teeth, phosphorus is essential for normal growth, healing of fractures, and prevention of osteoporosis, the brittle bone disease. It helps the body produce energy and plays an important role in the growth, maintenance, and repair of all of the tissues. A deficiency can lead to ailments ranging from weight loss and fatigue to arthritis, gum disease, and tooth decay.

Can you take too much?

Phosphorus is not toxic. However potassium phosphate supplements often prescribed for kidney stones can cause side effects, including shortness of breath, an irregular heartbeat, or seizures.

When taking potassium phosphate, call your doctor immediately if you notice any of the following potential warning signs: headache; pain in the abdomen, bones or joints; confusion; diarrhea; muscle cramps; swelling in your feet or legs; numbness or tingling in your hands and feet; unusual fatigue or thirst; or a decline in urine output.

Recommended daily allowances

ADULTS

All adults:	800 milligrams

Women need an extra 400 milligrams of phosphorus each day during pregnancy and while breastfeeding an infant. See your doctor before taking a supplement. Do not take megadoses of this mineral.

CHILDREN

Infants up to 6 months:	240 milligrams
Ages 6 to 12 months:	360 milligrams
Ages 1 to 10 years:	800 milligrams
Ages 11 to 17 years:	1,200 milligrams

Best dietary sources
Potassium phosphate occurs naturally in meats, including red meat and calves liver; poultry; fish and seafood, including tuna, scallops, and canned sardines; milk and milk products; cheddar, pasteurized and processed cheese; eggs; almonds and peanuts; dried beans, peas, and soybeans; pumpkin and sunflower seeds; and whole-grain products.

POTASSIUM

What it is
Potassium is one of the key minerals required by the body to maintain its normal daily functions. Potassium supplements—often prescribed for people on blood

pressure medications—are available in a variety of forms including potassium acetate, potassium bicarbonate, potassium chloride, potassium citrate, and potassium gluconate.

What it does
Along with sodium, potassium regulates the water balance within the body and its cells. It also helps govern the body's acid balance and the electrical charge within the cells. It is essential to the healthy functioning of the brain, heart, muscles, and kidneys.

Why you need it
Potassium keeps the heart beating normally, helps the muscles contract, and feeds the cells by controlling the transfer of nutrients from surrounding fluids. It helps the kidneys remove waste products from the body, works with phosphorus to supply oxygen to the brain, and cooperates with calcium to regulate the nerves.

Can you take too much?
Too much potassium throws off the fluid and electrical balance in the cells and can lead to such serious problems as irregular or rapid heartbeat, a drop in blood pressure, and paralysis of the arms and legs. Convulsions, coma, and even cardiac arrest can follow a severe overdose. Never take more potassium than recommended or prescribed; and call your doctor if you become confused or extremely fatigued, develop nausea or diarrhea, or notice a heaviness in your legs or a numbness and tingling in your hands and feet. Seek emergency medical treatment if your stool is either bloody or black and tarry, if you are having trouble breathing, or if your heartbeat seems to be irregular.

Recommended daily allowances
The amount of salt you use affects your potassium requirements; and there is no standard recommended dietary allowance

(RDA) for this mineral. Nutritional experts currently advise cutting back on the amount of table salt you use and increasing the amount of potassium-rich foods you eat. Many experts peg the minimum daily requirement at roughly 2,000 to 2,500 milligrams. Since a normal diet supplies from 2,000 to 6,000 milligrams daily, supplements aren't necessary unless you are taking medications that deplete the body's potassium supply.

Best dietary sources
Potassium is found in fruits, including avocados, bananas, citrus fruits, raisins, and dried peaches; grapefruit, tomato, and orange juice; vegetables, including fresh spinach, parsnips, and potatoes; nuts, including almonds, Brazil nuts, cashews, peanuts, pecans, and walnuts; milk; molasses, dried lentils; canned sardines; and whole-grain cereals.

One cup of cooked spinach contains 1,160 milligrams of potassium. One-half cup of raisins or one-half of a medium avocado provides 650 milligrams. One cooked potato or 1 cup of orange juice contains 500 milligrams.

PYRIDOXAL PHOSPHATE

See Vitamin B₆

PYRIDOXINE

See Vitamin B₆

RETINOL

See Vitamin A

RIBOFLAVIN

What it is
Riboflavin, also called vitamin B₂, is a water-soluble vitamin commonly found in dairy products. It is also produced synthetically.

What it does
Riboflavin plays an important role in the body's production of energy. It helps tissues breathe and get rid of waste. It also helps activate vitamin B₆.

Why you need it
Riboflavin helps the body grow and develop. It keeps the mucous membranes healthy and protects the nervous system, skin, and eyes. Riboflavin is also useful in the treatment of various medical conditions, including infections, stomach and liver disorders, burns, and alcoholism. Researchers also believe that riboflavin helps the body absorb iron more efficiently. It is not uncommon for iron and riboflavin deficiencies to occur simultaneously.

Can you take too much?
Riboflavin appears to be harmless no matter how high the dose. However, too much riboflavin may darken the color of your urine.

Recommended daily allowances
ADULTS

Males 11 to 14 years:	1.6 milligrams
Males 15 to 22 years:	1.7 milligrams
Males 23 to 50 years:	1.6 milligrams
Males 51 and older:	1.4 milligrams
Females 11 to 22 years:	1.3 milligrams
Females 23 and older:	1.2 milligrams

Women require an additional 0.3 milligrams of riboflavin each day during pregnancy. Breastfeeding mothers need an extra 0.5 milligrams of riboflavin per day.

People who exercise a lot—especially women—probably need extra riboflavin as well.

CHILDREN

Infants up to 6 months:	0.4 milligrams
Ages 6 to 12 months:	0.6 milligrams
Ages 1 to 3 years:	0.8 milligrams
Ages 4 to 6 years:	1.0 milligrams
Ages 7 to 10 years:	1.4 milligrams

Best dietary sources
The body is not able to store riboflavin, so this vitamin must constantly be replenished to prevent a deficiency.

Milk is probably the single best source of riboflavin. One quart of milk contains 1.7 milligrams of riboflavin—enough riboflavin for almost any adult or child. Other good sources of riboflavin include cheese, yogurt, chicken, organ meats, leafy green vegetables, cereal, bread, wheat germ, brewer's yeast, and almonds.

SALT

See Sodium

SELENIUM

What it is
Selenium is one of the minerals required by the body in only trace amounts. It is a potent antioxidant. Supplements are available in several formulations.

What it does
Working with vitamin E, selenium helps fend off the damage that oxidation can cause to the cells.

Why you need it
Because selenium maintains tissue elasticity by preventing excessive cell damage, a deficiency can cause premature aging. A lack of selenium can also lead to male infertility.

Can you take too much?
Sustained dosages greater than 700 to 1,100 micrograms are not recommended. Toxic levels of selenium can lead to loss of hair, teeth, and nails, a decline in energy, and even paralysis.

Recommended daily allowances
The government has not yet established a recommended dietary allowance (RDA) for selenium. The estimated safe and adequate daily intake is as follows:

ADULTS

All adults:	50 to 200 micrograms

Women should not take megadoses of selenium during pregnancy or while breastfeeding.

CHILDREN

Infants up to 6 months:	10 to 40 micrograms
Ages 6 to 12 months:	20 to 60 micrograms
Ages 1 to 3 years:	20 to 80 micrograms
Ages 4 to 6 years:	30 to 120 micrograms
Ages 7 and older:	50 to 200 micrograms

Best dietary sources
The amount of selenium in the following foods varies according to the amount in the soil in which they grew. Selenium is found in: vegetables, including broccoli, cabbage, celery, cucumbers, garlic, mushrooms, and onions; kidney, liver, and chicken; whole-grain products, bran, and wheat germ; egg yolks; tuna and seafood; and milk.

SODIUM

What it is
Sodium pervades our food supply. As sodium chloride it is known as salt.

What it does
Sodium maintains the balance of water inside and outside of the body's cells. Together with potassium, it also regulates the body's acid balance and plays a role in governing the electrical charge in the nerves and muscles.

Why you need it
Sodium prevents dehydration and is essential for proper functioning of nerves and muscles. Deficiencies are almost unheard of, but could result in digestive problems, weight loss, and arthritis.

Can you take too much?
Excessive sodium levels can cause body tissue to retain water and swell. Extremely high levels of sodium can lead to dizziness, stupor, and even a coma.

For people with high blood pressure, the extra water retention caused by sodium can make the pressure worse. Blood pressure patients are therefore advised to keep their salt intake below average.

Recommended daily allowances
With other vitamins and minerals, the concern is a possible deficiency. With sodium, the problem is excess. The typical American diet contains as much as 12 grams of sodium per day, while we only need about 3. There is no official recommended dietary allowance (RDA) for sodium. Estimates of the minimum requirements are as follows:

ADULTS

All adults:	1.1 to 3.3 grams

According to current guidelines, healthy women need not restrict the amount of sodium in their diets during pregnancy or while breastfeeding.

CHILDREN

Infants up to 6 months:	0.11 to 0.35 gram
Ages 6 to 12 months:	0.25 to 0.75 gram
Ages 1 to 3 years:	0.32 to 1 gram
Ages 4 to 6 years:	0.45 to 1.35 grams
Ages 7 to 10 years:	0.6 to 1.8 grams
Ages 11 to 17 years:	0.9 to 2.3 grams

Best dietary sources
Table salt is the primary source. Other foods containing sodium include: bacon, dried and fresh beef, ham, and other meats; milk, butter, and margarine; clams and canned sardines; bread; green beans; and canned tomatoes.

Manufacturers typically add salt to improve the taste of canned vegetables and processed foods. Bouillon, soups, pickles, potato chips and many "snack" foods are especially high in salt.

One teaspoon of salt contains 2 grams of sodium. One cup of cottage cheese provides slightly more than 1/2 gram. One cup of canned corn, 1 cup of canned tomato juice, or 1 slice of pizza (1/6 of a 12-inch pie) each provide about 1/2 gram of sodium.

SODIUM FLUORIDE

See Fluoride

SULFUR

What it is
Sulfur is a component of several amino acids found naturally in protein. Our requirements are met fully through our normal diet. The

only people at risk of a deficiency are strict vegetarians.

What it does
Sulfur is one of the raw materials used by the liver to manufacture the bile required by the digestive system. It is also a component of the keratin in skin, nails, and hair.

Why you need it
Sulfur maintains a good complexion and glossy hair.

Can you take too much?
Sulfur is unlikely to cause any problems, even if your body has more than it needs.

Recommended daily allowances
There is no recommended dietary allowance (RDA) for sulfur and no reports of deficiency.

Best dietary sources
Eggs are the richest source of sulfur. It is also available in meat, fish, dried beans, cabbage, milk, and wheat germ.

TAURINE

See Nonessential Amino acids

TETRAHYDROFOLIC ACID

See Folic Acid

THIAMIN

What it is
Thiamin, one of the water-soluble vitamins, is also called vitamin B_1. Thiamin is widely available in foods and is also produced synthetically. An injectable form is available by prescription.

A well-balanced diet should generally provide enough thiamin for healthy people.

However, more adults are deficient in thiamin than in almost any other vitamin. One of the reasons this deficiency has become so common is the high rate of alcoholism. Alcohol impairs the absorption of many nutrients and is especially detrimental to the body's ability to process thiamin.

Very young children and elderly people who do not eat a well-balanced diet are also in danger of developing a serious thiamin deficiency. Although rare, an uncorrected thiamin deficiency can lead to symptoms of beriberi, a disorder that affects the nervous system and may involve the heart and circulatory systems.

What it does
Thiamin plays an important role in converting blood sugar (glucose) into the energy needed to fuel the body. It also helps release energy from fat, and together with adenosine triphosphate, it forms a compound needed to convert carbohydrates into energy.

Why you need it
Thiamin is important for normal growth and development. It keeps the mucous membranes healthy; and helps keep the nervous system, heart, and muscles working properly. Physicians prescribe thiamin supplements to treat beriberi. Thiamin supplements are also important for alcoholics. The mental confusion, vision disturbances, and staggering gait typically associated with alcoholism are also symptoms of beriberi.

Can you take too much?
Oral overdoses are extremely rare. People who take several hundred milligrams of thiamin daily—literally hundreds of times the recommended daily amount—may become drowsy. Large injections of thiamin

occasionally cause an allergic reaction similar to anaphylactic shock.

Recommended daily allowances

ADULTS

Males 11 to 18:	1.4 milligrams
Males 19 to 50:	1.5 milligrams
Males 51 and older:	1.2 milligrams

The RDA for females is:

Females 11 to 22:	1.1 milligrams
Females 23 and older:	1.0 milligrams

Women require an addition 0.4 milligrams of thiamin each day during pregnancy. Breastfeeding mothers need an extra 0.5 milligrams of thiamin per day.

CHILDREN

Infants up to 6 months:	0.3 milligrams
Ages 6 months to 12 months:	0.5 milligrams
Ages 1 to 3 years:	0.7 milligrams
Ages 4 to 6 years:	0.9 milligrams
Ages 7 to 10 years:	1.2 milligrams

Best dietary sources

The body is not able to store thiamin very well, so it is important to constantly replenish your thiamin supply. The best sources are whole grain cereals, rye and whole wheat flour, wheat germ, rice bran, dried sunflower seeds, soybeans, navy and kidney beans, meat, pork, and salmon steak.

A tablespoonful of brewer's yeast provides 1.2 milligrams of thiamin; one cup of cooked kidney beans contains 0.51 milligrams; two slices of whole wheat bread have 0.15 milligrams.

THREONINE

What it is

Threonine is one of the amino acids considered "essential" because they cannot be manufactured in the body and must be obtained through diet.

What it does

The body must have supplies of all the amino acids, including threonine, on hand in order to manufacture human proteins. These proteins are a vital component of all the body's cells and its many hormones and enzymes.

Why you need it

The body requires a continuing supply of fresh proteins to support normal functions and maintain the tissues in good repair. Without the amino acids, production of these proteins would slow to a halt.

Can you take too much?

Amino acids are rarely toxic, even in large amounts.

Recommended daily allowances

There is no official recommended allowance for threonine. The estimated adult daily requirement is approximately 3.5 milligrams per pound of body weight. Infants require 8 times that amount; children need about 3 times the adult requirement.

Best dietary sources

A complete set of all the amino acids is available in most meat and dairy products.

TRIBASIC CALCIUM PHOSPHATE

See Calcium

TRYPTOPHAN

What it is

Tryptophan is one of the amino acids considered "essential" because they cannot be manufactured in the body and must be obtained through diet. Natural and synthetic tryptophan supplements are also available, despite a recent incident in which contaminated supplements caused illness.

What it does
Tryptophan is the raw material for serotonin, one of the chemicals that regulate the transmission of nerve impulses in the brain.

Why you need it
The serotonin manufactured from tryptophan is one of the major chemicals governing mood and behavior. The well known antidepressant drug Prozac, for instance, works by boosting serotonin levels in the brain. Serotonin also has a calming affect; and a lack of serotonin may spark a headache.

Can you take too much?
When correctly manufactured, tryptophan supplements pose no danger.

Recommended daily allowances
There is no official recommended dietary allowance for tryptophan. The estimated adult daily requirement is less than 1.5 milligrams per pound of body weight. Infants require 7 times that amount; children need less than 2 milligrams per pound.

Best dietary sources
Tryptophan is particularly plentiful in bananas, dried dates, milk, cottage cheese, meat, fish, turkey, and peanuts.

TYROSINE

See Nonessential Amino Acids

VALINE

See Branched-Chain Amino Acids

VANADIUM

What it is
Vanadium, one of the minerals needed in only trace amounts, can be obtained from fish, meat, whole grain, oils, and vitamin supplements.

What it does
We do not yet know exactly how vanadium works in the body, but we do know that it's present in most body tissues.

Why you need it
Vanadium is needed for proper development of bones, cartilage, and teeth.

Can you take too much?
Megadoses can lead to anemia, eye irritation, and respiratory problems.

Recommended daily allowances
The government has not yet established a recommended dietary allowance (RDA) for vanadium. Adults probably need 100 to 300 micrograms of vanadium per day. Most people get more than 10 times that amount in their daily diet.

Best dietary sources
Vanadium is found in meat, seafood, grains, and vegetable oil.

VITAMIN A

What it is
Vitamin A, also known as retinol, is one of the fat-soluble vitamins that can be stored by the body. There are two ways of getting this vitamin from your diet: either as vitamin A itself (especially plentiful in liver) or as beta-carotene, a plant-based substance that the body can convert into vitamin A. Megadoses of vitamin A itself can be toxic. Megadoses of beta-carotene are not, since

the body converts only as much as needed into Vitamin A.

What it does

Vitamin A helps regulate cell development, promotes bone growth and tooth development, and boosts the body's immune system and resistance to respiratory infections. By helping to form rhodopsin, a substance the eyes need to function in partial darkness, vitamin A enables us to see at night.

Why you need it

Vitamin A is essential for good vision, especially night vision. It helps keep the skin, hair, and mucous membranes healthy. It also promotes reproduction by helping testicles and ovaries to function properly and aiding in the development of the embryo.

Can you take too much?

A large overdose of vitamin A—500,000 IU or more—can cause headache, vomiting, bone pain, weakness, blurred vision, irritability, and flaking of the skin. Long-term intake of 100,000 IU or more per day can also lead to toxicity. Symptoms include hair loss, headache, bone thickening, an enlarged liver and spleen, anemia, menstrual problems, stiffness, joint pain, weakness, and dry skin. High doses of beta-carotene, on the other hand, have no toxic effects.

Authorities recommend that pregnant women take no more than 5,000 IU of vitamin A per day. The same is true for women taking birth control pills, which tend to increase the amount of retinol in the blood. Regular doses of 25,000 to 50,000 IU or more per day may cause birth defects.

Recommended daily allowances

The recommended dietary allowance (RDA) for vitamin A is expressed in International

Units (IU). One IU contains approximately 5 micrograms of retinol or 30 micrograms of beta-carotene.

ADULTS

Males 11 years and older:	5,000 IU.
Females 11 years and older:	4,000 IU.

Women need an additional 1,000 IU each day during pregnancy. Breastfeeding mothers need an extra 2,000 IU per day.

It is important to note that a daily intake of 5,000 IU may not be enough for many people. For example, people who smoke, eat a lot of junk food, or have diabetes or an infection may need more.

CHILDREN

Infants up to 12 months:	1,875 IU
Ages 1 to 3 years:	2,000 IU
Ages 4 to 6 years:	2,500 IU
Ages 7 to 10 years:	3,300 IU

Best dietary sources

The average person has up to a two-year supply of vitamin A stored in the liver. However, you need to constantly replenish this supply to prevent a deficiency—and thus night blindness—from developing.

Beta-carotene, the vitamin A precursor, is available in many fruits and vegetables. Good sources include carrots, sweet potatoes, broccoli, spinach, tomatoes, lettuce, winter squash, apricots, cantaloupe, and watermelon.

One sweet potato provides almost 10,000 IU. A single carrot contains almost 5,000 IU, a cup of cooked carrots provides 15,000 IU. Liver is an excellent source of vitamin A itself. One-half pound of calves' liver provides almost 75,000 IU.

VITAMIN B$_1$

See Thiamin

VITAMIN B$_2$

See Riboflavin

VITAMIN B$_3$

See Niacin

VITAMIN B$_5$

See Pantothenic Acid

VITAMIN B$_6$

What it is

Vitamin B$_6$, also known as pyridoxine and pyridoxal phosphate is one of the water-soluble vitamins that the body can't store. You need a continued daily supply from food or supplements. A synthetic form is available.

What it does

Vitamin B$_6$ helps the body process the protein, fat, and carbohydrates in our diet. It works with other vitamins and minerals to supply the energy used in our muscles, and plays a role in cell growth, including the body's production of red blood cells and cells of the immune system.

Why you need it

Vitamin B$_6$ plays a crucial role in maintaining the body's immune system. It helps the brain work properly and assists in maintaining the proper chemical balance in the body's fluids. It also helps the body resist stress. Physicians prescribe this vitamin to treat certain types of anemia and to counteract poisoning from the prescription drugs cycloserine and isoniazid.

Can you take too much?

There is currently little evidence that more than 50 milligrams of vitamin B$_6$ per day will do the body any extra good. However, a total daily intake of more than 500 milligrams can lead to serious nerve damage. Clumsiness and numbness in the hands and feet are signs that you may be getting too much vitamin B$_6$. To be on the safe side, experts recommend that you avoid taking supplements of more than 200 milligrams per day.

Recommended daily allowances

ADULTS

Males 11 years and older:	2.2 milligrams
Females 11 years and older:	2.0 milligrams

Women need an additional 0.6 milligrams of vitamin B$_6$ each day during pregnancy. Breastfeeding mothers need an extra 0.5 milligrams per day.

CHILDREN

Infants up to 6 months:	0.3 milligrams
Ages 6 months to 12 months:	0.6 milligrams
Ages 1 to 3 years:	0.9 milligrams
Ages 4 to 6 years:	1.3 milligrams
Ages 7 to 10 years:	1.8 milligrams

Best dietary sources

Vitamin B$_6$ is available in meats; fish, including salmon, shrimp, and tuna; whole grains, including bran, whole wheat flour, wheat germ, and rice; bananas; vegetables, including avocados and carrots; and brewer's yeast, hazelnuts, lentils, soybeans, and sunflower seeds.

One-half cup of soybeans provides 0.85 milligrams of vitamin B$_6$; a medium banana has 0.61 milligrams; one-half of a medium avocado has 0.46 milligrams; and one-quarter cup of wheat germ provides 0.3 milligrams.

VITAMIN B₉

See Folic Acid

VITAMIN B₁₂

What it is

Vitamin B₁₂, a water-soluble vitamin, is also called cobalamin and cyanocobalamin. It is found in meat, fish, dairy products, and eggs—but cannot be obtained from plant-based foods. People who follow a strict vegetarian or macrobiotic diet are at serious risk of developing a vitamin B₁₂ deficiency. This is of particular concern for children. A synthetic form of vitamin B₁₂ is available, but a prescription is necessary if your physician decides you need high doses or must take it by injection.

What it does

Vitamin B₁₂ helps the body process and burn fats and carbohydrates. It also helps the nervous system work properly and aids in growth and cell development—especially bloodcells. It is also necessary for production of the protective sheath that covers nerve cells, and helps the body process DNA.

Why you need it

Vitamin B₁₂ is essential to the body's growth and development. This vitamin is also useful in the treatment of some types of nerve damage and pernicious anemia. Supplements can help prevent a deficiency in strict vegetarians. Vitamin B₁₂ supplementation is particularly important to assure normal growth and development in children who follow a vegetarian diet.

Can you take too much?

Very few problems have been reported with vitamin B₁₂—even when people take as much as 1,000 milligrams per day. However, if you take vitamin B₁₂ along with large amounts of vitamin C, you may develop a nosebleed, bleeding from the ears, or a dry mouth.

Recommended daily allowances

ADULTS

The RDA for everyone 11 years and older is 3 micrograms. Women need an extra 1 microgram of vitamin B₁₂ each day during pregnancy and while they are breastfeeding an infant.

CHILDREN

Infants up to 6 months:	0.5 micrograms
Ages 6 to 12 months:	1.5 micrograms
Ages 1 to 3 years:	2 micrograms
Ages 4 to 6 years:	2.5 micrograms
Ages 7 to 10 years:	3 micrograms

Best dietary sources

The best sources of vitamin B₁₂ are fish, including clams, flounder, herring, mackerel, sardines, and snapper; dairy foods, including milk and milk products, blue cheese, and swiss cheese; organ meats, especially kidney and liver; other meats, such as beef, pork, and liverwurst; and eggs.

One-half cup of cottage cheese, packed, provides 1 microgram of vitamin B₁₂ . One cup of whole or skim milk or one large egg contains 1 microgram. One ounce of cheddar, brick, or mozzarella cheese has 0.28 microgram.

VITAMIN C

What it is

Vitamin C, one of the water-soluble vitamins, is also called ascorbic acid.

Some nutritionists have extolled vitamin C as a "cure" for the common cold. While there is no proof for this claim, some studies have indicated that vitamin C can help prevent colds from developing and also ease the symptoms if you do get one.

Researchers may not be convinced, but a great many people believe in vitamin C—it is estimated that more than half of all adults take vitamin C supplements. Taking large doses once a day could, however, be a waste of money, since the body tends to get rid of supplemental vitamin C very quickly. Taking smaller doses several times a day could prove to be more effective.

What it does
Vitamin C plays an essential role in the manufacture of collagen, a substance in connective tissue that essentially holds the bones together. Vitamin C also helps repair damaged tissue and has antioxidant properties.

Why you need it
Vitamin C may or may not cure the common cold, but it is definitely valuable in many other ways. This vitamin helps the body absorb more iron and is, therefore, useful in the treatment of iron-deficiency and other types of anemia. Vitamin C plays a role in the production of hemoglobin and red blood cells, works to keep the gums and teeth healthy, helps heal broken bones and wounds, and is one of the substances physicians choose to treat urinary tract infections.

Vitamin C continues to be used to treat the deficiency disease scurvy. Although scurvy was much more common in the nineteenth century, it has not disappeared. Symptoms include muscle weakness or wasting, bleeding or swollen gums, loss of teeth, rough skin, delayed wound healing, fatigue, and depression.

Can you take too much?
The body rids itself of extra vitamin C very quickly. Daily doses of as much as 5,000 to 10,000 milligrams taken for several years have failed to produce any serious side effects. However, if too much vitamin C accumulates in the body, facial flushing, headaches, stomach cramps, nausea, or vomiting are possibilities. At a dose of more than 1,000 milligrams per day, you may also notice that you have to urinate more frequently or start having mild diarrhea. Dizziness and faintness may occur following a vitamin C injection.

Recommended daily allowances
ADULTS

The RDA for everyone 15 years of age and older is 60 milligrams.

Women need an additional 20 milligrams of vitamin C each day during pregnancy—a developing baby needs the vitamin to support the growth and formation of its bones, teeth and connective tissue. Breastfeeding mothers need an extra 40 milligrams of vitamin C per day to pass on to their rapidly growing babies. If you are pregnant or breastfeeding, your physician will determine the exact amount of vitamin C that you need to take.

People over the age of 55 and smokers may also need a vitamin C supplement.

CHILDREN

Infants up to 12 months:	35 milligrams
Ages 1 to 10 years:	45 milligrams
Ages 11 to 14 years:	50 milligrams

Best dietary sources
Most people know that oranges and orange juice contain vitamin C, but the vitamin is also available in many other fruits, and even in vegetables. Sources of vitamin C include

broccoli, brussels sprouts, cabbage, grapefruit, green peppers, lemons, potatoes, spinach, strawberries, sweet and hot peppers, tangerines, and tomatoes.

One cup of orange juice provides 120 milligrams of vitamin C; a medium orange contains 66 milligrams. One stalk of raw broccoli has 160 milligrams of vitamin C; a medium green pepper, raw, provides 70 milligrams.

VITAMIN D

What it is

There are two forms of vitamin D: ergocalciferol, which is found in a relatively small selection of foods; and cholecalciferol, which the body manufactures when exposed to the sun. Vitamin D is fat-soluble, can build up inside the body, and therefore is highly toxic when taken in large doses for a long time. Milk fortified with vitamin D is our major dietary source.

What it does

Vitamin D helps to control the formation of bone tissue. It increases the amount of calcium and phosphorus the body absorbs from the small intestine and thus helps regulate the growth, hardening, and repair of the bones.

Why you need it

Vitamin D is essential for the normal growth and development of the teeth, bones, and cartilage in children. It's also needed to keep adult teeth and bones in good repair. Vitamin D prevents rickets, a deficiency disease characterized by malformations of bones and teeth in children and by brittle, easily broken bones in adults.

Can you take too much?

For adults, doses of 50,000 IU per day can prove toxic; and doses of 25,000 IU daily are risky. For a small child, as little as 1,800 IU per day can cause harm. Long-term overdose of vitamin D can cause *irreversible* damage to the kidneys and cardiovascular system, and can retard growth in children. Excessive amounts of the vitamin may lead to high blood pressure and premature hardening of the arteries. Nausea, abdominal pain, loss of appetite, weight loss, seizures, and an irregular heartbeat may be signs that you are taking too much. If you have any concerns, stop taking the vitamin right away and consult your physician.

Vitamin D produced by sunlight is not a concern. Overexposure to the sun does not cause vitamin D toxicity among healthy people.

Recommended daily allowances

ADULTS

Ages 19 to 22 years:	600 IU
Ages 23 years and older:	400 IU

Women need an extra 400 IU each day during pregnancy and while they are breastfeeding an infant. The additional vitamin D is important for the baby's normal growth. Do not increase dosage beyond this point, however. Too much vitamin D during pregnancy may cause abnormalities.

People over the age of 55 may also need to take a vitamin D supplement—especially women who have completed menopause.

The increasing use of sunscreens protects against the harmful ultraviolet rays that cause skin cancer; unfortunately, this sensible practice also limits the body's production of vitamin D. If you live in an area that does not typically have a lot of sunshine, you may want to check with your doctor about the possible need for extra vitamin D. This is especially important for children, whose bones and teeth need vitamin D to grow properly.

CHILDREN

Through age 18:	800 IU

Best dietary sources
Sunlight is the best source of vitamin D, but you can also boost your body's supply by drinking fortified milk. Other sources include herring, mackerel, salmon, sardines and cod- and halibut-liver oils.

VITAMIN E

What it is
Vitamin E, also known as alpha-tocopherol, is a leading antioxidant. Although it is one of the fat soluble vitamins that can build up in the body, it has proven safe in much larger than standard doses. A synthetic form of vitamin E is available, and your doctor can also prescribe vitamin E injections.

What it does
Vitamin E protects the fats found in cell membranes throughout the body from oxidation, or spoilage. Because of this ability to inhibit the natural cell destruction that occurs with age, vitamin E is being tested as a treatment for many of the chronic diseases of the elderly.

Why you need it
In addition to preventing the oxidation of cells and tissue, vitamin E helps to prevent blood clots, thereby reducing the risk of heart disease. It may also discourage development of some types of cancer; and it is needed for production of normal red blood cells. It helps children grow and develop normally and is used to treat

vitamin E deficiency in premature or low-birthweight babies.

Can you take too much?
Even at doses of 1,500 IU per day (50 times the RDA), vitamin E has no harmful effects. However, at doses of 2,400 IU per day, it may cause bleeding problems due to its clot-preventing ability. Too much vitamin E may also reduce your body's supply of vitamin A, alter the immune system, and impair sexual function.

Because they can impede formation of blood clots, vitamin E supplements should be avoided for 2 weeks before and after surgery. You should also forego large doses when taking anticoagulant medications.

Recommended daily allowances
ADULTS

Males 18 or older:	30 IU
Females 18 or older:	24 IU

Women need an additional 6 IU each day during pregnancy. Breastfeeding mothers need an extra 9 IU per day.

People over the age of 55, smokers, and people who abuse alcohol may need to take vitamin E supplements.

CHILDREN

Infants up to 12 months:	9 to 12 IU
Ages 1 to 7 years:	15 to 21 IU
Ages 11 to 18 years:	24 IU

Best dietary sources
Vegetable oils, including corn, cottonseed, and peanut oils, are the best source of vitamin E. Almonds, hazelnuts, safflower nuts, sunflower seeds, walnuts, wheat germ, whole-wheat flour, and margarine are also rich in vitamin E. Various fruits and vegetables—spinach, lettuce, onions,

blackberries, apples, and pears—also contain this vitamin.

VITAMIN H

See Biotin

VITAMIN K

What it is
There are two forms of vitamin K: phylloquinone, which is found in green leafy vegetables; and menaquinone, which is produced within the body by "friendly" bacteria that reside in the intestinal tract. A deficiency may result if antibiotics or an intestinal disease destroy these bacteria.

What it does
Vitamin K is an essential element in the blood's normal clotting process. It promotes production of the clotting factors, such as prothrombin, that stop us from bleeding.

Why you need it
Vitamin K helps prevent abnormal bleeding, and is given to newborns as a precaution against hemorrhagic (bleeding) disease. It is also prescribed to correct deficiencies that result in bleeding disorders.

Can you take too much?
Doses as high as 500 times the usual recommendation have failed to cause any ill effect. However, allergic-type reactions have been reported; and the vitamin could interfere with the liver's ability to function, although liver problems are not very common. Infants who receive an excessive amount may suffer brain damage.

Recommended daily allowances
The government has not yet established the recommended dietary allowance (RDA) for vitamin K.

ADULTS
The estimated adequate daily intake for everyone 18 years of age and older is 70 to 140 micrograms.

There is currently no information on the safety and effectiveness of vitamin K supplements during pregnancy. If you are pregnant or are breastfeeding, do not take vitamin K without consulting your physician.

CHILDREN
The estimated adequate daily intake of vitamin K for children is as follows:

Infants up to 6 months:	12 micrograms
Ages 6 to 12 months:	10 to 20 micrograms
Ages 1 to 3 years:	15 to 30 micrograms
Ages 4 to 6 years:	20 to 40 micrograms
Ages 7 to 10 years:	30 to 60 micrograms
Ages 11 to 17 years:	50 to 100 micrograms

Best dietary sources
Vitamin K is found in brussels sprouts, cabbage, cauliflower, oats, soybeans, spinach, cheddar cheese, egg yolks, and green tea.

ZINC

What It Is
Zinc is one of the minerals that we require in just trace amounts. It is found in a variety of meat and grain products. Supplements are available as well.

What It Does
Zinc is part of the molecular structure of more than 80 enzymes, and works with the red blood cells to transport waste carbon dioxide from body tissue to the lungs for exhalation. It is essential for the production of the RNA and DNA that governs the division, growth, and repair of the body's cells.

Why you need it

Zinc is an extremely important mineral: It helps the body grow and develop, and also promotes normal fetal growth. It preserves our sense of taste and smell, helps wounds heal, and keeps the right amount of vitamin A in our blood. It is also a component of the insulin that regulates our energy supply.

Can you take too much?

Doses of more than 40 times the RDA cause few, if any, problems. Nausea, vomiting, and diarrhea may follow sustained overdosage. Other consequences include drowsiness, sluggishness, light-headedness, and restlessness. Difficulty writing or walking can also be warning signs of zinc toxicity.

Recommended daily allowances

ADULTS

All adults:	15 milligrams

Women need an additional 5 milligrams of zinc each day during pregnancy. Women who are breastfeeding an infant should take an extra 10 milligrams per day. Since women may not get all the zinc they need from their diet, it is important that they discuss the possibility of supplementation with a physician.

CHILDREN

Infants up to 6 months:	3 milligrams
Ages 6 to 12 months:	5 milligrams
Ages 1 to 10 years:	10 milligrams
Age 11 and older:	15 milligrams

Best dietary sources

Zinc can be obtained from meat, including beef, lamb, and pork; poultry; seafood, including herring and oysters; egg yolk; milk; maple syrup and black-strap molasses; sesame and sunflower seeds; soybeans; whole-grain products; wheat bran; wheat germ; and yeast.

PART FOUR

Medications in Nutrition

Brand name:

ACUTRIM

Pronounced: AK-you-trim
Generic name: Phenylpropanolamine

Why is this drug prescribed?

Acutrim is a nonprescription appetite suppressant medication to be used with a weight loss and exercise program.

Most important fact about this drug

Do not take more than 1 tablet each 24 hours. Taking more than the recommended dose will not speed weight loss and could cause serious health problems.

How should you take this medication?

Take this medication exactly as recommended on the package labeling: 1 tablet at mid-morning with a full glass of water. Swallow the tablet whole; do not crush, divide, chew, or dissolve. Do not take Acutrim for longer than 3 months; this should be enough time to establish the new eating habits necessary to maintain weight loss.

Read the diet plan enclosed in the package.

■ *If you miss a dose...*
  If you miss a dose and remember it late in the day, skip the dose and go back to your regular schedule the next day. Do not take double doses.

■ *Storage instructions...*
  Protect from extreme heat and moisture.

What side effects may occur?

If you experience nervousness, dizziness, sleeplessness, throbbing heartbeat, or headaches, stop using Acutrim and contact your doctor.

Why should this drug not be prescribed?

If you are being treated for high blood pressure, depression, or an eating disorder, or if you have heart disease, diabetes, or a thyroid disorder, do not take Acutrim unless you will be monitored by your doctor.

Special warnings about this medication

Acutrim is for adult use only. Do not give Acutrim to children under 12 years of age. Consult your doctor before taking Acutrim if you are under 18.

Possible food and drug interactions when taking this medication

If Acutrim is taken with certain other drugs, the effects of either could be increased, decreased, or altered. It is especially important to check with your doctor or pharmacist before combining Acutrim with the following:

Any cough/cold or allergy preparation containing phenylpropanolamine or any type of nasal decongestant.
Antidepressants classified as monoamine oxidase inhibitors, such as Nardil, Marplan, and Parnate.

Special information if you are pregnant or breastfeeding

As with any medication, if you are pregnant or nursing a baby, seek the advice of a health care professional before using Acutrim.

Recommended dosage

ADULTS

1 tablet at mid-morning with a full glass of water.

Overdosage

Any medication taken in excess can have serious consequences. If you suspect an overdose, seek medical attention immediately.

Generic name:

ALLOPURINOL

See Zyloprim, page 697.

Brand name:

ANASPAZ

See Levsin, page 636.

Category:

ANTACIDS

Brand names: Gaviscon, Gelusil, Maalox, Mylanta, Rolaids, Tums

Why is this drug prescribed?

Available under a number of brand names, antacids are used to relieve the uncomfortable symptoms of acid indigestion, heartburn, gas, and sour stomach.

Most important fact about this drug

Do not take antacids for longer than 2 weeks or in larger than recommended doses unless directed by your doctor. If your symptoms persist, contact your doctor. Antacids should be used only for occasional relief of stomach upset.

How should you take this medication?

If you take a chewable antacid tablet, chew thoroughly before swallowing so that the medicine can work faster and be more effective. Allow Mylanta Soothing Lozenges to completely dissolve in your mouth. Shake liquids well before using.

■ If you miss a dose...
Take this medication only as needed or as instructed by your doctor.

■ Storage instructions...
Store at room temperature. Keep liquids tightly closed and protect from freezing.

What side effects may occur?

When taken as recommended, antacids are relatively free of side effects. Occasionally, one of the following symptoms may develop.

■ Side effects may include:
Chalky taste
Constipation
Diarrhea
Increased thirst
Stomach cramps

Why should this drug not be prescribed?

Do not take antacids if you have signs of appendicitis or an inflamed bowel; symptoms include stomach or lower abdominal pain, cramping, bloating, soreness, nausea, or vomiting.

If you are sensitive to or have ever had an allergic reaction to aluminum, calcium, magnesium, or simethicone, do not take an antacid containing these ingredients. If you are elderly and have bone problems or if you are taking care of an elderly person with Alzheimer's disease, do not use an antacid containing aluminum.

Special warnings about this medication

If you are taking any prescription drug, check with your doctor before you take an antacid. Also, tell your doctor or pharmacist about any drug allergies or medical conditions you have.

If you have kidney disease, do not take an antacid containing aluminum or magnesium. If you are on a sodium-restricted diet, do not take Gaviscon without checking first with your doctor or pharmacist.

Possible food and drug interactions when taking this medication

If antacids are taken with certain other medications, the effects of either could be increased, decreased, or altered. It is especially important to check with your doctor before combining antacids with the following:

Cellulose sodium phosphate (Calcibind)
Isoniazid (Rifamate)
Ketoconazole (Nizoral)
Mecamylamine (Inversine)
Methenamine (Mandelamine)
Sodium polystyrene sulfonate resin
  (Kayexalate)
Tetracycline antibiotics (Achromycin,
  Minocin)

Special information if you are pregnant or breastfeeding

As with all medications, ask your doctor or health care professional whether it is safe for you to use antacids while you are pregnant or breastfeeding.

Recommended dosage

ADULTS

Take antacids according to the following schedules, or as directed by your doctor.

Gaviscon and Gaviscon Extra Strength Relief Formula Chewable Tablets
Chew 2 to 4 tablets 4 times a day after meals and at bedtime or as needed. Follow with half a glass of water or other liquid. Do not swallow the tablets whole.

Gaviscon Extra Strength Relief Formula Liquid
Take 2 to 4 teaspoonfuls 4 times a day after meals and at bedtime. Follow with half a glass of water or other liquid.

Gaviscon Liquid
Take 1 or 2 tablespoonfuls 4 times a day after meals and at bedtime. Follow with half a glass of water.

Gelusil Liquid and Chewable Tablets
Take 2 or more teaspoonfuls or tablets 1 hour after meals and at bedtime. The tablets should be chewed.

Maalox Antacid Caplets
Take 1 caplet as needed. Swallow the tablets whole; do not chew them.

Maalox Heartburn Relief Chewable Tablets
Chew 2 to 4 tablets after meals and at bedtime. Follow with half a glass of water or other liquid.

Maalox Heartburn Relief Suspension, Maalox Magnesia and Alumina Oral Suspension, and Extra Strength Maalox Antacid Plus Anti-Gas Suspension
Take 2 to 4 teaspoonfuls 4 times a day, 20 minutes to 1 hour after meals and at bedtime.

Maalox Plus Chewable Tablets
Chew 1 to 4 tablets 4 times a day, 20 minutes to 1 hour after meals and at bedtime.

Extra Strength Maalox Antacid Plus Anti-Gas Chewable Tablets
Chew 1 to 3 tablets 20 minutes to 1 hour after meals and at bedtime.

Mylanta and Mylanta Double Strength Liquid and Chewable Tablets Antacid/Anti-Gas
Take 2 to 4 teaspoonfuls of liquid or chew 2 to 4 tablets between meals and at bedtime.

Mylanta Gelcaps
Take 2 to 4 gelcaps as needed.

Mylanta Soothing Lozenges
Dissolve 1 lozenge in your mouth. If
needed, follow with a second. Repeat as
needed.

*Rolaids, Calcium-Rich/Sodium Free Rolaids,
and Extra Strength Rolaids*
Chew 1 or 2 tablets as symptoms occur.
Repeat hourly if symptoms return.

*Tums, Tums E-X, and Tums Anti-Gas
Formula*
Chew 1 or 2 tablets as symptoms occur.
Repeat hourly if symptoms return. You may
also hold the tablet between your gum and
cheek and let it dissolve gradually.

CHILDREN

Do not give to children under 6 years of
age, unless directed by your doctor.

Overdosage
Any medication taken in excess can have
serious consequences. If you suspect an
overdose, seek medical attention
immediately.

■ *Symptoms of antacid overdose may
include:*

For *aluminum-containing antacids (Gaviscon,
Gelusil, Maalox, Mylanta)*
Bone pain, constipation (severe and
continuing), feeling of discomfort
(continuing), loss of appetite (continuing),
mood or mental changes, muscle
weakness, swelling of wrists or ankles,
weight loss (unusual)

For *calcium-containing antacids (Mylanta,
Rolaids, Tums)*
Constipation (severe and continuing),
difficult or painful urination, frequent urge
to urinate, headache (continuing), loss of
appetite (continuing), mood or mental
changes, muscle pain or twitching, nausea
or vomiting, nervousness or restlessness,

slow breathing, unpleasant taste, unusual
tiredness or weakness

For *magnesium-containing antacids
(Gaviscon, Gelusil, Maalox, Mylanta)*
Difficult or painful urination, dizziness or
light-headedness, irregular heartbeat, mood
or mental changes, unusual tiredness or
weakness

Brand name:

ASACOL

See Rowasa, page 681.

Brand name:

AXID

Pronounced: AK-sid
Generic name: Nizatidine

Why is this drug prescribed?
Axid is prescribed for the treatment of
duodenal ulcers and noncancerous stomach
ulcers. Full-dose therapy for these problems
lasts no longer than 8 weeks. However, your
doctor may prescribe Axid at a reduced
dosage after a duodenal ulcer has healed.
The drug is also prescribed for the
heartburn and the inflammation that result
when acid stomach contents flow backward
into the esophagus. Axid belongs to a class
of drugs known as histamine H_2 blockers.

Most important fact about this drug
Although Axid can be used for up to 8-12
weeks, most ulcers are healed within 4
weeks of therapy.

How should you take this medication?
Take this medication exactly as prescribed
by your doctor.

■ *If you miss a dose...*
Take it as soon as you remember. If it is almost time for your next dose, skip the one you missed and go back to your regular schedule. Do not take 2 doses at once.

■ *Storage instructions...*
Store at room temperature.

What side effects may occur?

Side effects cannot be anticipated. If any develop or change in intensity, inform your doctor as soon as possible. Only your doctor can determine if it is safe for you to continue taking Axid.

■ *More common side effects may include:*
Abdominal pain
Diarrhea
Dizziness
Gas
Headache
Indigestion
Inflammation of the nose
Nausea
Pain
Sore throat
Vomiting
Weakness

■ *Less common or rare side effects may include:*
Abnormal dreams, anxiety, back pain, chest pain, constipation, dimmed vision, dry mouth, fever, inability to sleep, increased cough, infection, itching, loss of appetite, muscle pain, nervousness, rash, sleepiness, stomach/intestinal problems, tooth problems

Why should this drug not be prescribed?

If you are sensitive to or have ever had an allergic reaction to Axid or similar drugs such as Zantac, you should not take this medication. Make sure your doctor is aware of any drug reactions you have experienced.

Special warnings about this medication

Axid could mask a stomach malignancy. If you continue to have any problems, notify your doctor.

If you have moderate to severe kidney disease, your doctor will reduce your dosage.

Possible food and drug interactions when taking this medication

If Axid is taken with certain other drugs, the effects of either could be increased, decreased, or altered. It is especially important to check with your doctor before combining Axid with aspirin, especially in high doses.

Special information if you are pregnant or breastfeeding

The effects of Axid during pregnancy have not been adequately studied. If you are pregnant or plan to become pregnant, inform your doctor immediately. Axid appears in breast milk and could affect a nursing infant. If this medication is essential to your health, your doctor may advise you to discontinue breastfeeding until your treatment with this medication is finished.

Recommended dosage

ADULTS

Active Duodenal Ulcer:
The usual dose is 300 milligrams once a day at bedtime, but your doctor may have you take 150 milligrams twice a day.

Active Noncancerous Stomach Ulcer:
The usual dose is 150 milligrams twice a day or 300 milligrams once a day at bedtime.

Maintenance of a Healed Duodenal Ulcer:
The usual dose is 150 milligrams once a day at bedtime.

If you have moderate to severe kidney disease, your doctor will prescribe a lower dose.

CHILDREN

The safety and effectiveness of Axid have not been established in children.

ELDERLY

Your doctor will determine the dosage based on your needs.

Overdosage

No specific information on Axid overdose is available. However, any medication taken in excess can have serious consequences. If you suspect an overdose of Axid, seek medical attention immediately.

Brand name:

AZULFIDINE

Pronounced: A-ZUL-fi-deen
Generic name: Sulfasalazine

Why is this drug prescribed?

Azulfidine, an anti-inflammatory medicine, is prescribed for the treatment of mild to moderate ulcerative colitis (a long-term, progressive bowel disease) and as an added treatment in severe ulcerative colitis (chronic inflammation and ulceration of the lining of large bowel and rectum, the main symptom of which is bloody diarrhea). This medication is also prescribed to decrease severe attacks of ulcerative colitis.

Azulfidine EN-tabs are prescribed for people who cannot take the regular Azulfidine tablet because of symptoms of stomach and intestinal irritation such as nausea and vomiting when taking the first few doses of the drug, or for those in whom a reduction in dosage does not lessen the stomach or intestinal side effects.

Most important fact about this drug

Although ulcerative colitis rarely disappears completely, the risk of recurrence can be substantially reduced by the continued use of this drug.

How should you take this medication?

Take this medication in evenly spaced, equal doses, as determined by your doctor, preferably after meals or with food to avoid stomach upset.

It is important that you drink plenty of fluids while taking this medication to avoid kidney stones.

■ *If you miss a dose...*
Take it as soon as you remember. If it is almost time for your next dose, skip the one you missed and go back to your regular schedule. Do not take 2 doses at once.

■ *Storage instructions...*
Store at room temperature.

What side effects may occur?

Side effects cannot be anticipated. If any develop or change in intensity, inform your doctor as soon as possible. Only your doctor can determine if it is safe for you to continue taking Azulfidine.

■ *More common side effects may include:*
Headache
Lack or loss of appetite
Nausea
Stomach distress
Vomiting

■ *Less common side effects may include:*
Anemia, bluish discoloration of the skin, fever, hives, itching, skin rash

■ *Rare side effects may include:*
Abdominal pain, blood disorders, blood in
the urine, bloody diarrhea, convulsions,
diarrhea, drowsiness, hallucinations,
hearing loss, hepatitis, inability to fall or
stay asleep, inflammation of the mouth,
intestinal inflammation, itchy skin
eruptions, joint pain, kidney disorders,
lack of muscle coordination, loss of hair,
mental depression, red, raised rash, ringing
in the ears, sensitivity to light, severe
allergic reaction, skin discoloration, skin
disorders, spinal cord defects, swelling
around the eye, urine discoloration,
vertigo

Why should this drug not be prescribed?

If you are sensitive to or have ever had an
allergic reaction to Azulfidine, salicylates
(aspirin), or other sulfa drugs, you should
not take this medication. Make sure your
doctor is aware of any drug reactions you
have experienced.

Unless you are directed to do so by your
doctor, do not take Azulfidine if you have
an intestinal or urinary obstruction or if you
have porphyria (an inherited disorder
involving the substance that gives color to
the skin and iris of the eyes).

Special warnings about this medication

If you have kidney or liver damage or any
blood disease, your doctor will check you
very carefully before prescribing Azulfidine.
Deaths have been reported from allergic
reactions, blood diseases, kidney or liver
damage, changes in nerve and muscle
impulses, and fibrosing alveolitis
(inflammation of the lungs due to a
thickening or scarring of tissue). Signs such
as sore throat, fever, abnormal paleness of
the skin, purple or red spots on the skin, or
jaundice (yellowing of the skin) may be an
indication of a serious blood disorder. Your
doctor will do frequent blood counts and

urine tests. Use caution taking Azulfidine if
you have a severe allergy or bronchial
asthma.

If Azulfidine EN-tabs are eliminated
undisintegrated, stop taking the drug and
notify your doctor immediately. (You may
lack the intestinal enzymes necessary to
dissolve this medication.)

Men taking Azulfidine may experience
temporary infertility and a low sperm count.

Skin and urine may become yellow-orange in
color while taking Azulfidine.

In addition, prolonged exposure to the sun
should be avoided.

Possible food and drug interactions when taking this medication

If Azulfidine is taken with certain other
drugs, the effects of either could be
increased, decreased, or altered. It is
especially important to check with your
doctor before combining Azulfidine with the
following:

Digoxin (Lanoxin)
Folic acid (a B-complex vitamin)

Special information if you are pregnant or breastfeeding

The effects of Azulfidine during pregnancy
have not been adequately studied. If you are
pregnant or plan to become pregnant,
inform your doctor immediately. Azulfidine
is secreted in breast milk and could affect a
nursing infant. If this medication is essential
to your health, your doctor may advise you
to discontinue breastfeeding until your
treatment is finished.

Recommended dosage

Your doctor will carefully individualize your
dosage and monitor your response
periodically.

ADULTS

The usual recommended initial dose is 3 to 4 grams daily divided into smaller doses (intervals between nighttime doses should not exceed 8 hours). In some cases the initial dosage is 1 to 2 grams daily to lessen side effects.

Maintenance Therapy
The usual maintenance dose is 2 grams daily.

CHILDREN AGED 2 AND OLDER

The usual recommended initial dose is 40 to 60 milligrams per 2.2 pounds of body weight in each 24-hour period, divided into 3 to 6 doses.

Maintenance Therapy
The usual maintenance dose is 30 milligrams per 2.2 pounds of body weight in each 24-hour period, divided into 4 doses.

Overdosage

Any medication taken in excess can have serious consequences. If you suspect an Azulfidine overdose, seek emergency medical attention immediately.

■ *Symptoms of Azulfidine overdose may include:*
Abdominal pain
Convulsions
Drowsiness
Nausea
Stomach upset
Vomiting

Generic name:

BELLATAL

See Donnatal, page 621.

Brand name:

BENTYL

Pronounced: BEN-til
Generic name: Dicyclomine hydrochloride

Why is this drug prescribed?
Bentyl is prescribed for the treatment of functional bowel/irritable bowel syndrome (abdominal pain, accompanied by diarrhea and constipation associated with stress).

Most important fact about this drug
Heat prostration (fever and heat stroke due to decreased sweating) can occur with use of this drug in hot weather. If symptoms occur, stop taking the drug and notify your doctor immediately.

How should you take this medication?
Take this medication exactly as prescribed.

■ *If you miss a dose...*
Take it as soon as you remember. If it is almost time for your next dose, skip the one you missed and go back to your regular schedule. Do not take 2 doses at once.

■ *Storage instructions...*
Store at room temperature. Keep tablets out of direct sunlight. Keep syrup away from excessive heat.

What side effects may occur?
Side effects cannot be anticipated. If any develop or change in intensity, inform your doctor as soon as possible. Only your doctor can determine if it is safe for you to continue taking Bentyl.

■ *Side effects may include:*
Blurred vision
Dizziness
Drowsiness
Dry mouth
Light-headedness

Nausea
Nervousness
Weakness

Not all of the following side effects have been reported with dicyclomine hydrochloride, but they have been reported for similar drugs with antispasmodic action; contact your doctor if they occur.

Abdominal pain, bloated feeling, constipation, decreased sweating, difficulty in urinating, double vision, enlargement of the pupil of the eye, eye paralysis, fainting, headache, hives, impotence, inability to urinate, increased pressure in the eyes, itching, labored, difficult breathing, lack of coordination, lack or loss of appetite, nasal stuffiness or congestion, numbness, rapid heartbeat, rash, severe allergic reaction, sluggishness, sneezing, suffocation, suppression of breast milk, taste loss, temporary cessation of breathing, throat congestion, tingling, vomiting

Why should this drug not be prescribed?

If you are sensitive to or have ever had an allergic reaction to Bentyl, you should not take this medication. Make sure your doctor is aware of any drug reactions you have experienced.

Unless you are directed to do so by your doctor, do not take this drug if you have a blockage of the urinary tract, stomach, or intestines; severe ulcerative colitis (inflammatory disease of the large intestine); reflux esophagitis (inflammation of the esophagus usually caused by the backflow of acid stomach contents); glaucoma; or myasthenia gravis (a disease characterized by long-lasting fatigue and muscle weakness).

This drug should not be given to infants less than 6 months of age or used by women who are nursing an infant.

Special warnings about this medication

Bentyl may produce drowsiness or blurred vision. Therefore, driving a car, operating machinery, or participating in any activity that requires full mental alertness is not recommended.

Diarrhea may be an early symptom of a partial intestinal blockage, especially in people who have had bowel removals and an ileostomy or colostomy. If this occurs, notify your doctor immediately.

You should use this medication with caution if you have autonomic neuropathy (a nerve disorder); liver or kidney disease; hyperthyroidism; high blood pressure; coronary heart disease; congestive heart failure; rapid, irregular heartbeat; hiatal hernia (protrusion of part of the stomach through the diaphragm); or enlargement of the prostate gland.

Possible food and drug interactions when taking this medication

If Bentyl is taken with certain other drugs, the effects of either could be increased, decreased, or altered. It is especially important to check with your doctor before combining Bentyl with the following:

Airway-opening drugs such as Proventil and
    Ventolin
Amantadine (Symmetrel)
Antacids such as Maalox
Antiarrhythmics such as quinidine (Quinidex)
Antiglaucoma drugs such as Pilopine
Antihistamines such as Tavist
Benzodiazepines (tranquilizers) such as
    Valium and Xanax
Corticosteroids such as prednisone
    (Deltasone)
Digoxin (the heart failure medication
    Lanoxin)
Major tranquilizers such as Mellaril and
    Thorazine

MAO inhibitors (antidepressants such as Nardil and Parnate)

Metoclopramide (the gastrointestinal stimulant Reglan)

Narcotic analgesics (pain relievers such as Demerol)

Nitrates and nitrites (heart medications such as nitroglycerin)

Tricyclic antidepressant drugs such as Elavil and Tofranil

Special information if you are pregnant or breastfeeding

The effects of Bentyl during pregnancy have not been adequately studied. If you are pregnant or plan to become pregnant, notify your doctor. Bentyl does appear in breast milk and could affect a nursing infant. Do not use it when breastfeeding.

Recommended dosage

ADULTS

The usual dosage is 160 milligrams per day divided into 4 equal doses. Since this dose is associated with a significant incidence of side effects, your doctor may recommend a starting dose of 80 milligrams per day divided into 4 equal doses. If no side effects appear, the doctor will then increase the dose.

If this drug is not effective within 2 weeks or side effects require doses below 80 milligrams per day, your doctor may discontinue it.

Overdosage

Any medication taken in excess can have serious consequences. If you suspect an overdose, seek medical attention immediately.

■ *Symptoms of a Bentyl overdose include:* Blurred vision, difficulty in swallowing, dilated pupils, dizziness, dryness of the mouth, headache, hot, dry skin, nausea,

nerve blockage causing weakness and possible paralysis, vomiting

Generic name:

CALCIUM CARBONATE

See Caltrate 600, page 608.

Brand name:

CALTRATE 600

Pronounced: CAL-trait
Generic name: Calcium carbonate
Other brand names: Os-Cal 500, Oystercal 500

Why is this supplement prescribed?

Caltrate is a supplement for women who do not get enough calcium in their diets or have a need for more calcium. Calcium supplements may reduce the rate of bone loss and help prevent osteoporosis (brittle bones). Calcium is also needed for the heart, muscles, and nervous system to work properly. The vitamin D in Caltrate + Vitamin D helps the body absorb calcium, while the extra iron in Caltrate + Iron & Vitamin D supplements diets deficient in iron.

Most important fact about this supplement

If you do not get enough calcium in your diet, a calcium supplement may help prevent serious bone disease, especially later in life.

How should you take this supplement?

Follow the dosing instructions on the bottle. Do not take more than the recommended dose. Take calcium with meals, even if only a light snack. Drink a full glass of water or juice when taking a calcium supplement.

Certain foods, such as spinach, rhubarb, bran, whole cereals, and dairy products reduce absorption of calcium supplements. Allow 2 to 3 hours between taking calcium and eating any of these foods.

■ *If you miss a dose...*
 If you are taking the calcium supplement on a regular schedule, take the dose you missed as soon as possible and then go back to your regular dosing schedule.

■ *Storage instructions...*
 Store at room temperature.

What side effects may occur?
No side effects have been reported.

Why should this supplement not be used?
If you have any medical problems, check with your doctor before starting on a calcium supplement.

Special warnings about this supplement
Do not take more calcium than suggested on the packaging, as too much may cause excessive levels of calcium in the blood or increase the chance of kidney stones.

Possible food and drug interactions when taking this supplement
Be sure to tell your doctor if you are taking any medications, because dietary supplements and certain medications should not be used together. For example, if you are taking a tetracycline antibiotic, take your calcium supplement at least 1 hour before or 3 hours after you take the antibiotic.

Certain other drugs also may interact with calcium. Check with your doctor before combining calcium with the following:

Atenolol (Tenormin)
Iron preparations such as Feosol
Quinolone antibiotics such as Cipro and
 Floxin

Special information if you are pregnant or breastfeeding
Ask your doctor whether you should take a calcium supplement while you are pregnant or breastfeeding. Taking too much of any supplement may be harmful to you or your unborn child.

Recommended dosage
For Caltrate 600, Caltrate 600 + Iron & Vitamin D, and Caltrate 600 + Vitamin D tablets, use the following dosage recommendations:

ADULTS

The usual dose is 1 or 2 tablets daily or as directed by your doctor.

Overdosage
Mega doses of any dietary supplement can be harmful. If you have unexplained symptoms and suspect an overdose, check with your doctor.

Brand name:

CARAFATE

Pronounced: CARE-uh-fate
Generic name: Sucralfate

Why is this drug prescribed?
Carafate Tablets and Suspension are used for the short-term treatment (up to 8 weeks) of an active duodenal ulcer; Carafate Tablets are also used for longer-term therapy at a reduced dosage after a duodenal ulcer has healed.

Carafate helps ulcers heal by forming a protective coating over them.

Some doctors also prescribe Carafate for ulcers in the mouth and esophagus that develop during cancer therapy, for digestive tract irritation caused by drugs, for long-term treatment of stomach ulcers, and to relieve pain following tonsil removal.

Most important fact about this drug

A duodenal ulcer is a recurring illness. While Carafate can cure an acute ulcer, it cannot prevent other ulcers from developing or lessen their severity.

How should you take this medication?

Carafate works best when taken on an empty stomach. If you take an antacid to relieve pain, avoid doing it within one-half hour before or after you take Carafate. Always take Carafate exactly as prescribed.

■ *If you miss a dose...*
Take it as soon as you remember. If it is almost time for your next dose, skip the one you missed and go back to your regular schedule. Never take 2 doses at the same time.

■ *Storage instructions...*
Store at room temperature. Protect the suspension from freezing.

What side effects may occur?

Side effects cannot be anticipated. If any develop or change in intensity, inform your doctor as soon as possible. Only your doctor can determine if it is safe for you to continue taking Carafate.

■ *More common side effects may include:*
Constipation

■ *Less common or rare side effects may include:*
Back pain, diarrhea, dizziness, dry mouth, gas, headache, indigestion, insomnia, itching, nausea, possible allergic reactions, including hives and breathing difficulty, rash, sleepiness, stomach upset, vertigo, vomiting

Why should this drug not be prescribed?

There are no restrictions on the use of this drug.

Special warnings about this medication

If you have kidney failure or are on dialysis, the doctor will be cautious about prescribing this drug. Use of Carafate while taking aluminum-containing antacids may increase the possibility of aluminum poisoning in those with kidney failure.

Possible food and drug interactions when taking this medication

If Carafate is taken with certain other drugs, the effects of either could be increased, decreased, or altered. It is especially important to check with your doctor before combining Carafate with the following:

Antacids such as Mylanta and Maalox
Blood-thinning drugs such as Coumadin
Cimetidine (Tagamet)
Digoxin (Lanoxin)
Drugs for controlling spasms, such as Bentyl
Ketoconazole (Nizoral)
Phenytoin (Dilantin)
Quinidine (Quinidex)
Quinilone antibiotics such as Cipro and Floxin
Ranitidine (Zantac)
Tetracycline (Achromycin V)
Theophylline (Theo-Dur)

Special information if you are pregnant or breastfeeding

The effects of Carafate during pregnancy have not been adequately studied. If you are pregnant or plan to become pregnant, inform your doctor immediately. Carafate may appear in breast milk and could affect a nursing infant. If this medication is essential to your health, your doctor may advise you to discontinue breastfeeding until your treatment with this medication is finished.

Recommended dosage

ADULTS

Active Duodenal Ulcer:
The usual dose is 1 gram (1 tablet or 2 teaspoonfuls of suspension) 4 times a day on an empty stomach. Although your ulcer may heal during the first 2 weeks of therapy, Carafate should be continued for 4 to 8 weeks.

Maintenance Therapy:
The usual dose is 1 gram (1 tablet) 2 times a day.

CHILDREN

The safety and effectiveness of Carafate in children have not been established.

Overdosage

Although the risk of overdose with Carafate is low and no specific symptoms of overdose have been reported, any medication taken in excess can have serious consequences. If you suspect an overdose, seek medical attention immediately.

Generic name:

CENTRUM

See *Multivitamins, page 655.*

Generic name:

CHLORDIAZEPOXIDE WITH CLIDINIUM

See *Librax, page 639.*

Generic name:

CHLORPROPAMIDE

See *Diabinese, page 618.*

Generic name:

CHOLESTYRAMINE

See *Questran, page 678.*

Brand name:

CHRONULAC SYRUP

Pronounced: KRON-yoo-lak
Generic name: Lactulose
Other brand name: Duphalac

Why is this drug prescribed?

Chronulac treats constipation. In people who are chronically constipated, Chronulac increases the number and frequency of bowel movements.

Most important fact about this drug

It may take 24 to 48 hours to produce a normal bowel movement.

How should you take this medication?

Take this medication exactly as prescribed. If you find the taste of Chronulac unpleasant, it can be taken with water, fruit juice, or milk.

■ *If you miss a dose...*
Take the forgotten dose as soon as you remember; but do not try to "catch up" by taking a double dose.

■ *Storage instructions...*
Store at room temperature. Avoid excessive heat or direct light. The liquid may darken in color, which is normal.

What side effects may occur?

Side effects cannot be anticipated. If any develop or change in intensity, inform your doctor as soon as possible. Only your doctor can determine if it is safe for you to continue taking Chronulac.

■ *Side effects may include:*
Diarrhea
Gas (temporary, at the beginning of use)
Intestinal cramps (temporary, at the
   beginning of use)
Nausea
Potassium and fluid loss
Vomiting

Why should this drug not be prescribed?

Chronulac contains galactose, a simple sugar.
If you are on a low-galactose diet, do not
take this medication.

Special warnings about this medication

Because of its sugar content, this medication
should be used with caution if you have
diabetes.

If unusual diarrhea occurs, contact your
doctor.

Possible food and drug interactions when taking this medication

If Chronulac is taken with certain other
drugs, the effects of either could be
increased, decreased, or altered. It is
especially important to check with your
doctor before combining Chronulac with
non-absorbable antacids such as Maalox and
Mylanta.

Special information if you are pregnant or breastfeeding

The effects of Chronulac during pregnancy
have not been adequately studied. If you are
pregnant or plan to become pregnant,
inform your doctor immediately. Chronulac
may appear in breast milk and could affect
a nursing infant. If this medication is
essential to your health, your doctor may
advise you to stop breastfeeding until your
treatment is finished.

Recommended dosage

The usual dose is 1 to 2 tablespoonfuls (15
to 30 milliliters) daily. Your doctor may
increase the dose to 60 milliliters a day, if
necessary.

Overdosage

Any medication taken in excess can have
serious consequences. If you suspect an
overdose, seek medical treatment
immediately.

■ *Symptoms of Chronulac overdose may
   include:*
Abdominal cramps
Diarrhea

Generic name:

CIMETIDINE

See Tagamet, page 685.

Generic name:

CISAPRIDE

See Propulsid, page 673.

Brand name:

CLINDEX

See Librax, page 639.

Brand name:

COLACE

Pronounced: KOH-lace
Generic name: Docusate sodium

Why is this drug prescribed?

Colace, a stool softener, promotes easy
bowel movements without straining. It
softens the stool by mixing in fat and water.
Colace is helpful for people who have had
recent rectal surgery, people with heart

problems or high blood pressure, patients with hernias, and women who have just had babies.

Most important fact about this drug
Colace is for short-term relief only, unless your doctor directs otherwise. It usually takes a day or two for the drug to achieve its laxative effect; some people may need to wait 4 or 5 days.

How should you take this medication?
To conceal the drug's bitter taste, take Colace liquid in half a glass of milk or fruit juice; it can be given in infant formula. The proper dosage of this medication may also be added to a retention or flushing enema.

■ *If you miss a dose...*
Take this medication only as needed.

■ *Storage instructions...*
Store at room temperature. Keep from freezing.

What side effects may occur?
Side effects are unlikely. The main ones reported are bitter taste, throat irritation, and nausea (mainly associated with use of the syrup and liquid). Rash has occurred.

Why should this drug not be prescribed?
There are no known reasons this drug should not be prescribed.

Possible food and drug interactions when taking this medication
No interactions have been reported with Colace.

Special information
if you are pregnant or breastfeeding
If you are pregnant, plan to become pregnant, or are breastfeeding your baby, notify your doctor before using this medication.

Recommended dosage
Your doctor will adjust the dosage according to your needs.

You will be using higher doses at the start of treatment with Colace. You should see an effect on stools 1 to 3 days after the first dose.

ADULTS AND CHILDREN 12 AND OLDER

The suggested daily dosage is 50 to 200 milligrams.

In enemas, add 50 to 100 milligrams of Colace or 5 to 10 milliliters of Colace liquid to a retention or flushing enema, as prescribed by your doctor.

CHILDREN UNDER 12

The suggested daily dosage for children 6 to 12 years of age is 40 to 120 milligrams; for children 3 to 6 years of age, it is 20 to 60 milligrams; for children under 3 years of age, it is 10 to 40 milligrams.

Overdosage
Overdose is unlikely with the normal use of Colace.

Brand name:

COLBENEMID

Pronounced: Kol-BEN-e-mid
Generic ingredients: Probenecid, Colchicine
Other brand name: Col-Probenecid

Why is this drug prescribed?
ColBENEMID is prescribed for the treatment of long-term gouty arthritis (a disease that produces pain and swelling of the joints accompanied by fever and chills) when complicated by frequent, recurrent severe attacks of gout.

Most important fact about this drug

Therapy with ColBENEMID should not be started until an acute gout attack (symptoms that come on suddenly) has subsided. However, if an acute attack occurs during therapy, your doctor may ask you to use additional colchicine or take other appropriate measures to control the attack. You should not alter the dose of ColBENEMID.

How should you take this medication?

Take this medication exactly as prescribed.

Drink plenty of fluids to prevent blood in the urine, renal colic (sharp lower back pain produced by the passage of kidney stones), rib or backbone pain, and uric acid stones (crystallized urinary byproducts), which are sometimes caused by ColBENEMID. Sufficient sodium bicarbonate (antacid) or potassium citrate (a supplement) should also be taken to make the urine less acid.

- *If you miss a dose...*
  Take it as soon as you remember. If it is almost time for your next dose, skip the one you missed and go back to your regular schedule. Do not take 2 doses at once.

- *Storage instructions...*
  Store away from light.

What side effects may occur?

Side effects cannot be anticipated. If any develop or change in intensity, inform your doctor as soon as possible. Only your doctor can determine if it is safe for you to continue taking ColBENEMID.

- *Side effects may include:*
  Abdominal pain, anaphylactic shock (an allergic reaction including shortness of breath, increased heart rate, tingling in throat, and collapse), anemia, attack of sharp gouty arthritis, backbone or rib

pain, blood in the urine, diarrhea, dizziness, fever, flushing, frequent urination, hair loss, headache, hives, itching, lack or loss of appetite, liver damage, muscular weakness, nausea, nerve inflammation, reddish or purplish spots, scant urine, sharp back pain traveling to groin, skin inflammation, sore gums, uric acid kidney stones, vomiting

Why should this drug not be prescribed?

If you are sensitive to or have ever had an allergic reaction to probenecid (antigout medication), colchicine (gout pain reliever), or similar drugs, you should not take this medication. Be sure your doctor is aware of any drug reactions you have experienced.

Unless you are directed to do so by your doctor, do not take this medication if you have any abnormal condition of the blood or uric acid kidney stones.

Special warnings about this medication

Treatment with ColBENEMID may aggravate gout. If this occurs, your doctor may increase your dosage of colchicine or prescribe another treatment.

Do not use salicylates (aspirin) while taking ColBENEMID for pain relief; use acetaminophen (Tylenol, Anacin-3, for example).

Severe allergic reactions have occurred, rarely, with the use of this medication. Most of these reactions have been seen within several hours after restarting treatment following previous use of the drug. Notify your doctor if you experience an allergic reaction.

If you have ever had a peptic (stomach) ulcer, you should use this medication cautiously.

If your kidney has lost some of its function, your doctor may prescribe an increased dosage of this medication.

Possible food and drug interactions when taking this medication

If ColBENEMID is taken with certain other drugs, the effects of either could be increased, decreased, or altered. It is especially important to check with your doctor before combining ColBENEMID with the following:

Acetaminophen (Tylenol, others)
Indomethacin (Indocin), an anti-inflammatory drug
Ketamine, a non-barbiturate general anesthetic
Ketoprofen (Orudis), an anti-inflammatory drug
Lorazepam (Ativan), a tranquilizer
Meclofenamate (Meclomen), an anti-inflammatory drug
Methotrexate, a cancer drug
Naproxen (Naprosyn), an anti-inflammatory drug
Penicillin (Pen Veck), an antibiotic
Pyrazinamide
Rifampin (Rifadin), an antibacterial drug
Salicylates (aspirin)
Sulfonamides (antibacterial drugs such as Bactrim and Septra)
Sulfonylureas such as Micronase, an oral diabetes medication
Sulindac (Clinoril), an anti-inflammatory drug
Theophylline (in airway-opening drugs such as Theo-Dur)
Thiopental, a general anesthetic

Special information if you are pregnant or breastfeeding

ColBENEMID may cause birth defects. If you are pregnant, plan to become pregnant, or are breastfeeding your baby, inform your doctor immediately.

Recommended dosage

ADULTS

The recommended dosage is 1 tablet daily for 1 week, followed by 1 tablet twice a day thereafter.

If you have decreased kidney function, a daily dosage of 2 tablets may be adequate. However, if necessary, your doctor may increase your daily dosage by 1 tablet every 4 weeks if symptoms of gouty arthritis are not controlled. Usually, you should take no more than 4 tablets per day. When you have had no severe attacks for 6 months or more, your doctor may decrease the daily dosage by 1 tablet every 6 months. Laboratory blood tests may be required to determine uric acid levels in the urine before your doctor lowers the dosage.

ColBENEMID should not be given to children under 2 years of age.

Overdosage

Any medication taken in excess can have serious consequences. Overdosage with colchicine may result in severe, even fatal, reactions.

If you suspect a ColBENEMID overdose, seek emergency medical treatment immediately.

■ *Symptoms of a ColBENEMID overdose may include:*
Bacterial infection, blood in stools, blood in urine, bone marrow failure (decreased formation of red and white blood cells), coma, difficulty breathing, epilepsy, fluid in the lungs, heart damage, kidney damage, low blood pressure, muscle weakness, severe diarrhea, stomach pain

Brand name:

COLESTID

Pronounced: Koh-LESS-tid
Generic name: Colestipol hydrochloride

Why is this drug prescribed?

Colestid, in conjunction with diet, is used to help lower high levels of cholesterol in the blood. It is available in plain and orange-flavored varieties.

Most important fact about this drug

Accidentally inhaling Colestid may cause serious effects. To avoid this, NEVER take it in its dry form. Colestid should always be mixed with water or other liquids BEFORE you take it.

How should you take this medication?

Colestid should be mixed with liquids such as:

Carbonated beverages (may cause stomach or intestinal discomfort)
Flavored drinks
Milk
Orange juice
Pineapple juice
Tomato juice
Water

Colestid may also be mixed with:

Milk used on breakfast cereals
Pulpy fruit (such as crushed peaches, pears, or pineapple) or fruit cocktail
Soups with a high liquid content (such as chicken noodle or tomato)

To take Colestid with beverages:

1. Measure at least 3 ounces of liquid into a glass.
2. Add the prescribed dose of Colestid to the liquid.

3. Stir until Colestid is completely mixed (it will not dissolve) and then drink the mixture.
4. Pour a small amount of the beverage into the glass, swish it around, and drink it. This will help make sure you have taken all the medication.

■ *If you miss a dose...*
Take the forgotten dose as soon as you remember. If it is almost time for the next dose, skip the one you missed and go back to your regular schedule. Never try to "catch up" by doubling the dose.

■ *Storage instructions...*
Store Colestid at room temperature.

What side effects may occur?

Side effects cannot be anticipated. If any develop or change in intensity, inform your doctor as soon as possible. Only your doctor can determine if it is safe for you to continue taking Colestid.

■ *Most common side effects:*
Constipation
Worsening of hemorrhoids

■ *Less common or rare side effects may include:*
Abdominal bloating or distention/cramping/pain, arthritis, diarrhea, dizziness, fatigue, gas, headache, hives, joint pain, loss of appetite, muscle pain, nausea, shortness of breath, skin inflammation, vomiting, weakness

■ *Additional side effects from regular Colestid may include:*
Anxiety, belching, drowsiness, vertigo

■ *Additional side effects from Flavored Colestid may include:*
Aches and pains in arms and legs, angina (crushing chest pain), backache, bleeding hemorrhoids, blood in the stool, bone

pain, chest pain, indigestion, insomnia, light-headedness, loose stools, migraine, rapid heartbeat, rash, sinus headache, swelling of hands or feet

Why should this drug not be prescribed?
You should not be using Colestid if you are allergic to it or any of its components.

Special warnings about this medication
Before starting treatment with Colestid, you should:

■ Be tested (and treated) for diseases that may contribute to increased blood cholesterol, such as an underactive thyroid gland, diabetes, nephrotic syndrome (a kidney disease), dysproteinemia (a blood disease), obstructive liver disease, and alcoholism.
■ Be on a diet plan (approved by your doctor) that stresses low-cholesterol foods and weight loss (if necessary).

Because certain medications may increase cholesterol, you should tell your doctor all of the medications you use.

Colestid may prevent the absorption of vitamins such as A, D, K, and folic acid. Long-term use of Colestid may be connected to increased bleeding from a lack of vitamin K. Taking vitamin K_1 will help relieve this condition and prevent it in the future.

Your cholesterol and triglyceride levels should be checked regularly while you are taking Colestid.

Colestid may cause or worsen constipation. Dosages should be adjusted by your doctor. You may need to increase your intake of fiber and fluid. A stool softener also may be needed occasionally. People with coronary artery disease should be especially careful to avoid constipation. Hemorrhoids may be worsened by constipation related to Colestid.

If you have phenylketonuria (a hereditary disease caused by your body's inability to handle the amino acid phenylalanine), be aware that Flavored Colestid contains phenylalanine.

Possible food and drug interactions when taking this medication
Colestid may delay or reduce the absorption of other drugs. The time period between taking Colestid and taking other medications should be as long as possible. Other drugs should be taken at least 1 hour before or 4 hours after taking Colestid.

If Colestid is taken with certain other drugs, the effects of either could be increased, decreased, or altered. It is especially important to check with your doctor before combining Colestid with the following:

Chlorothiazide (Diuril)
Digitalis (Lanoxin)
Furosemide (Lasix)
Gemfibrozil (Lopid)
Hydrochlorothiazide (HydroDIURIL)
Penicillin G, including brands such as Pentids
Phosphate supplements
Propranolol (Inderal)
Tetracycline drugs such as Sumycin
Vitamins such as A, D, and K

Special information if you are pregnant or breastfeeding
The effects of Colestid during pregnancy have not been adequately studied. If you are pregnant or planning to become pregnant, or plan to breastfeed, check with your doctor.

Recommended dosage

ADULTS

One packet or 1 level scoopful of Flavored Colestid contains 5 grams of Colestipol.

The usual starting dose is 1 packet or 1 level scoopful once or twice a day. Your doctor may increase this by 1 dose a day every month or every other month, up to 6 packets or 6 level scoopfuls taken once a day or divided into smaller doses.

CHILDREN

The safety and effectiveness of Colestid have not been established for children.

Overdosage

Overdoses of Colestid have not been reported. If an overdose occurred, the most likely harmful effect would be obstruction of the stomach and/or intestines. If you suspect an overdose, seek medical help immediately.

Generic name:

COLESTIPOL

See Colestid, page 616.

Brand name:

COL-PROBENECID

See ColBENEMID, page 613.

Brand name:

DIABETA

See Micronase, page 652.

Brand name:

DIABINESE

Pronounced: dye-AB-in-eez
Generic name: Chlorpropamide

Why is this drug prescribed?

Diabinese is an oral antidiabetic medication used to treat Type II (non-insulin-dependent) diabetes. Diabetes occurs when the body fails to produce enough insulin or is unable to use it properly. Insulin is believed to work by helping sugar penetrate the cell wall so it can be used by the cell.

There are two forms of diabetes: Type I insulin-dependent and Type II non-insulin-dependent. Type I usually requires insulin injection for life, while Type II diabetes can usually be treated by dietary changes and oral antidiabetic medications such as Diabinese. Apparently, Diabinese controls diabetes by stimulating the pancreas to secrete more insulin. Occasionally, Type II diabetics must take insulin injections on a temporary basis, especially during stressful periods or times of illness.

Most important fact about this drug

Always remember that Diabinese is an aid to, not a substitute for, good diet and exercise. Failure to follow a sound diet and exercise plan can lead to serious complications, such as dangerously high or low blood sugar levels. Remember, too, that Diabinese is *not* an oral form of insulin, and cannot be used in place of insulin.

How should you take this medication?

Ordinarily, your doctor will ask you to take a single daily dose of Diabinese each morning with breakfast. However, if this upsets your stomach, he or she may ask you to take Diabinese in smaller doses throughout the day.

To prevent low blood sugar levels (hypoglycemia):

■ You should understand the symptoms of hypoglycemia
■ Know how exercise affects your blood sugar levels
■ Maintain an adequate diet
■ Keep a source of quick-acting sugar with you all the time

■ *If you miss a dose...*
Take it as soon as you remember. If it is almost time for the next dose, skip the one you missed and go back to your regular schedule. Do not take 2 doses at the same time.

■ *Storage instructions...*
Store at room temperature.

What side effects may occur?

Side effects cannot be anticipated. If any develop or change in intensity, inform your doctor as soon as possible. Only your doctor can determine if it is safe for you to continue taking Diabinese.

Side effects from Diabinese are rare and seldom require discontinuation of the medication.

■ *More common side effects include:*
Diarrhea
Hunger
Itching
Loss of appetite
Nausea
Stomach upset
Vomiting

■ *Less common or rare side effects may include:*
Anemia and other blood disorders, hives, inflammation of the rectum and colon, sensitivity to light, yellowing of the skin and eyes

Diabinese, like all oral antidiabetics, can cause hypoglycemia (low blood sugar). The risk of hypoglycemia is increased by missed meals, alcohol, other medications, and excessive exercise. To avoid hypoglycemia, closely follow the dietary and exercise regimen suggested by your physician.

■ *Symptoms of mild hypoglycemia may include:*
Cold sweat
Drowsiness
Fast heartbeat
Headache
Nausea
Nervousness

■ *Symptoms of more severe hypoglycemia may include:*
Coma
Pale skin
Seizures
Shallow breathing

Contact your doctor immediately if these symptoms of severe low blood sugar occur.

Why should this drug not be prescribed?

You should not take Diabinese if you have ever had an allergic reaction to it.

Do not take Diabinese if you are suffering from diabetic ketoacidosis (a life-threatening medical emergency caused by insufficient insulin and marked by excessive thirst, nausea, fatigue, pain below the breastbone, and a fruity breath).

Special warnings about this medication

It's possible that drugs such as Diabinese may lead to more heart problems than diet treatment alone, or diet plus insulin. If you have a heart condition, you may want to discuss this with your doctor.

If you are taking Diabinese, you should check your blood and urine periodically for the presence of abnormal sugar levels.

Remember that it is important that you closely follow the diet and exercise regimen established by your doctor.

Even people with well-controlled diabetes may find that stress, illness, surgery, or fever results in a loss of control. If this happens, your doctor may recommend that Diabinese be discontinued temporarily and insulin used instead.

In addition, the effectiveness of any oral antidiabetic, including Diabinese, may decrease with time. This may occur because of either a diminished responsiveness to the medication or a worsening of the diabetes.

Possible food and drug interactions when taking this medication

When you take Diabinese with certain other drugs, the effects of either could be increased, decreased, or altered. It is important that you consult with your doctor before taking Diabinese with the following:

Anabolic steroids
Aspirin in large doses
Barbiturates such as Seconal
Beta-blocking blood pressure medications such as Inderal and Tenormin
Calcium-blocking blood pressure medications such as Cardizem and Procardia
Chloramphenicol (Chloromycetin)
Coumarin (Coumadin)
Diuretics such as Diuril and HydroDIURIL
Epinephrine (Epipen)
Estrogen medications such as Premarin
Isoniazid (Nydiazid)
Major tranquilizers such as Mellaril and Thorazine
MAO inhibitor-type antidepressants such as Nardil and Parnate

Nicotinic acid (Nicobid, Nicolar)
Nonsteroidal anti-inflammatory agents such as Advil, Motrin, Naprosyn, and Nuprin
Oral contraceptives
Phenothiazines
Phenylbutazone (Butazolidin)
Phenytoin (Dilantin)
Probenecid (Benemid, ColBENEMID)
Steroids such as prednisone
Sulfa drugs such as Bactrim and Septra
Thyroid medications such as Synthroid

Avoid alcohol since excessive alcohol consumption can cause low blood sugar, breathlessness, and facial flushing.

Special information if you are pregnant or breastfeeding

The effects of Diabinese during pregnancy have not been adequately established. If you are pregnant or plan to become pregnant you should inform your doctor immediately. Since studies suggest the importance of maintaining normal blood sugar (glucose) levels during pregnancy, your physician may prescribe injected insulin.

To minimize the risk of low blood sugar (hypoglycemia) in newborn babies, Diabinese, if prescribed during pregnancy, should be discontinued at least 1 month before the expected delivery date.

Since Diabinese appears in breast milk, it is not recommended for nursing mothers. If diet alone does not control glucose levels, then insulin should be considered.

Recommended dosage

Dosage levels are determined by each individual's needs.

ADULTS

Usually, an initial daily dose of 250 milligrams is recommended for stable, middle-aged, non-insulin-dependent diabetics.

After 5 to 7 days, your doctor may adjust this dosage in increments of 50 to 125 milligrams every 3 to 5 days to achieve the best benefit. People with mild diabetes may respond well to daily doses of 100 milligrams or less of Diabinese, while those with severe diabetes may require 500 milligrams daily. Maintenance doses above 750 milligrams are not recommended.

ELDERLY

People who are elderly, malnourished, or debilitated and those with impaired kidney and liver function usually take an initial dose of 100 to 125 milligrams.

CHILDREN

Safety and effectiveness have not been established.

Overdosage

An overdose of Diabinese can cause low blood sugar (see "What side effects may occur?" for symptoms).

Eating sugar or a sugar-based product will often correct the condition. If you suspect an overdose, seek medical attention immediately.

Generic name:

DICYCLOMINE

See Bentyl, page 606.

Generic name:

DIETHYLPROPION

See Tenuate, page 688.

Generic name:

DOCUSATE

See Colace, page 612.

Brand name:

DONNATAL

Pronounced: DON-nuh-tal
Generic ingredients: Phenobarbital,
    Hyoscyamine sulfate, Atropine sulfate,
    Scopolamine hydrobromide
Other brand name: Bellatal

Why is this drug prescribed?

Donnatal is a mild antispasmodic medication; it has been used with other drugs for relief of cramps and pain associated with various stomach, intestinal, and bowel disorders, including irritable bowel syndrome, acute colitis, and duodenal ulcer.

One of its ingredients, phenobarbital, is a mild sedative.

Most important fact about this drug

Phenobarbital, one of the ingredients of Donnatal, can be habit-forming. If you have ever been dependent on drugs, do not take Donnatal.

How should you take this medication?

Take Donnatal one-half hour to 1 hour before meals. Use it exactly as prescribed.

■ *If you miss a dose...*
    Take it as soon as you remember. If it is almost time for your next dose, skip the one you missed and go back to your regular schedule. Never take 2 doses at the same time.

■ *Storage instructions...*
Store at room temperature in a tightly closed container. Protect from light.

What side effects may occur?

Side effects cannot be anticipated. If any develop or change in intensity, inform your doctor as soon as possible. Only your doctor can determine if it is safe for you to continue taking Donnatal.

■ *Side effects may include:*
Agitation, allergic reaction, bloated feeling, blurred vision, constipation, decreased sweating, difficulty sleeping, difficulty urinating, dilation of the pupil of the eye, dizziness, drowsiness, dry mouth, excitement, fast or fluttery heartbeat, headache, hives, impotence, muscular and bone pain, nausea, nervousness, rash, reduced sense of taste, suppression of lactation, vomiting, weakness

Why should this drug not be prescribed?

Do not take Donnatal if you suffer from the eye condition called glaucoma, diseases that block the urinary or gastrointestinal tracts, or myasthenia gravis, a condition in which the muscles become progressively paralyzed. Also, you should not use Donnatal if you have intestinal atony (loss of strength in the intestinal muscles), unstable cardiovascular status, severe ulcerative colitis (chronic inflammation and ulceration of the bowel), or hiatal hernia (a rupture in the diaphragm above the stomach). You should also avoid Donnatal if you have acute intermittent porphyria—a disorder of the metabolism in which there is severe abdominal pain and sensitivity to light.

If you are sensitive to or have ever had an allergic reaction to Donnatal, its ingredients, or similar drugs, you should not take this medication. Also avoid Donnatal if

phenobarbital makes you excited or restless, instead of calming you down. Make sure your doctor is aware of any drug reactions you have experienced.

Special warnings about this medication

Be cautious in using Donnatal if you suffer from high blood pressure, overactive thyroid (hyperthyroidism), irregular or rapid heartbeat, or heart, kidney, or liver disease.

Donnatal can decrease sweating. If you are exercising or are subjected to high temperatures, be alert for heat prostration.

If you develop diarrhea, especially if you have an ileostomy or colostomy (artificial openings to the bowel), check with your doctor.

If you have a gastric ulcer, use this medication with caution.

Donnatal may cause you to become drowsy or less alert. You should not drive or operate dangerous machinery or participate in any hazardous activity that requires full mental alertness until you know how this drug affects you.

Possible food and drug interactions when taking this medication

Donnatal may intensify the effects of alcohol. Check with your doctor before using alcohol with this medication.

Avoid taking antacids within 1 hour of a dose of Donnatal; they may reduce its effectiveness.

If Donnatal is taken with certain other drugs, the effects of either could be increased, decreased, or altered. It is especially important to check with your doctor before combining Donnatal with the following:

Antidepressants such as Elavil and Tofranil
Antidepressants known as MAO inhibitors,
  including Nardil and Parnate
Antihistamines such as Benadryl
Antispasmodic drugs such as Bentyl and
  Cogentin
Barbiturates such as Seconal
Blood-thinning drugs such as Coumadin
Diarrhea medications containing Kaolin or
  attapulgite
Digitalis (Lanoxin)
Narcotics such as Percocet
Potassium (Slow-K, K-Dur, others)
Steroids such as Medrol and Deltasone
Tranquilizers such as Valium

Special information
if you are pregnant or breastfeeding

The effects of Donnatal during pregnancy
have not been adequately studied. If you are
pregnant or plan to become pregnant, this
drug should be used only when prescribed
by your doctor. It is not known whether
Donnatal appears in breast milk. If this
medication is essential to your health, your
doctor may advise you to discontinue
breastfeeding until your treatment is
finished.

Recommended dosage

ADULTS

Your doctor will adjust the dosage to your
needs.

Tablets or Capsules
The usual dosage is 1 or 2 tablets or
capsules, 3 or 4 times a day.

Liquid
The usual dosage is 1 or 2 teaspoonfuls, 3
or 4 times a day.

Donnatal Extentabs
The usual dosage is 1 tablet every 12 hours.
Your doctor may tell you to take 1 tablet
every 8 hours, if necessary.

CHILDREN

Dosage of the elixir is determined by body
weight; it can be given every 4 to 6 hours.
Follow your doctor's instructions carefully
when giving this medication to a child.

Overdosage

Any medication taken in excess can cause
symptoms of overdose. If you suspect an
overdose, seek medical attention
immediately.

■ *The symptoms of Donnatal overdose may
include:*
Blurred vision
Central nervous system stimulation
Difficulty swallowing
Dilated pupils
Dizziness
Dry mouth
Headache
Hot and dry skin
Nausea
Vomiting

Brand name:

DUPHALAC

See Chronulac Syrup, page 611.

Brand name:

EFFER-SYLLIUM

See Metamucil, page 646.

Generic name:

FAMOTIDINE

See Pepcid, page 664.

Brand name:

FASTIN

Pronounced: FAS-tin
Generic name: Phentermine hydrochloride
Other brand names: Ionamin, Oby-Cap

Why is this drug prescribed?

Fastin, an appetite suppressant, is prescribed for short-term use (a few weeks) as part of an overall diet plan for weight reduction. Fastin should be used along with a behavior modification program.

Most important fact about this drug

Always remember that Fastin is an aid to, not a substitute for, good diet and exercise. Take Fastin only as directed by your doctor. Do not take it more often or for a longer time than your doctor has ordered. Fastin can lose its effectiveness after a few weeks.

How should you take this medication?

Take Fastin about 2 hours after breakfast. Do not take it late in the evening because it may keep you from sleeping.

Take Ionamin before breakfast or 10 to 14 hours before you go to bed. Ionamin capsules should be swallowed whole.

■ *If you miss a dose...*
Skip the missed dose completely; then take the next dose at the regularly scheduled time.

■ *Storage instructions...*
Store away from heat, light, and moisture.

What side effects may occur?

Side effects cannot be anticipated. If any develop or change in intensity, inform your doctor as soon as possible. Only your doctor can determine if it is safe for you to continue taking this medication.

■ *Side effects may include:*
Changes in sex drive, constipation, diarrhea, dizziness, dry mouth, exaggerated feelings of depression or elation, headache, high blood pressure, hives, impotence, inability to fall or stay asleep, increased heart rate, overstimulation, restlessness, stomach or intestinal problems, throbbing heartbeat, tremors, unpleasant taste

Why should this drug not be prescribed?

If you are sensitive to or have ever had an allergic reaction to phentermine hydrochloride or other drugs that stimulate the nervous system, you should not take this medication. Make sure your doctor is aware of any drug reactions you have experienced.

Do not take this drug if you have hardening of the arteries, symptoms of heart or blood vessel disease, an overactive thyroid gland, the eye condition known as glaucoma, or moderate to severe high blood pressure. Also avoid this drug if you are agitated, have ever abused drugs, or have taken an MAO inhibitor, including antidepressant drugs such as Nardil and Parnate, within the last 14 days.

Special warnings about this medication

Fastin may affect your ability to perform potentially hazardous activities. Therefore, you should be extremely careful if you have to drive a car or operate machinery.

You can become psychologically dependent on this drug. Consult your doctor if you rely on this drug to maintain a state of well-being.

If you stop taking Fastin suddenly after you have taken high doses for a long time, you may find you are extremely fatigued or depressed, or that you have trouble sleeping.

If you continually take too much of any appetite suppressant it can cause severe skin disorders, a pronounced inability to fall or stay asleep, irritability, hyperactivity, and personality changes.

Even if your blood pressure is only mildly high, be careful taking this drug.

Possible food and drug interactions when taking this medication

This drug may intensify the effects of alcohol. Avoid alcoholic beverages while you are taking it.

If Fastin is taken with certain other drugs, the effects of either can be increased, decreased, or altered. It is especially important that you check with your doctor before combining Fastin with the following:

Antidepressants classified as MAO inhibitors, including Nardil and Parnate
Diabetes medications such as insulin and Micronase
High blood pressure medications such as guanethidine (Ismelin)

Special information if you are pregnant or breastfeeding

The effects of Fastin during pregnancy have not been adequately studied. If you are pregnant, plan to become pregnant, or are breastfeeding, notify your doctor immediately.

Recommended dosage

ADULTS

Fastin or Oby-Cap
The usual dosage is 1 capsule approximately 2 hours after breakfast. One capsule should suppress your appetite for 12 to 14 hours.

Ionamin
The usual dose is 1 capsule a day, taken before breakfast or 10 to 14 hours before bedtime.

CHILDREN

This drug is not recommended for use in children under 12 years of age.

Overdosage

Any medication taken in excess can have serious consequences. An overdose of Fastin can be fatal. If you suspect an overdose, seek emergency medical treatment immediately.

■ *Symptoms of Fastin overdose may include:* Abdominal cramps, aggressiveness, confusion, diarrhea, exaggerated reflexes, hallucinations, high or low blood pressure, irregular heartbeat, nausea, panic states, rapid breathing, restlessness, tremors, vomiting

Fatigue and depression may follow the stimulant effects of Fastin.

In cases of fatal poisoning, convulsions and coma usually precede death.

Generic name:

FENFLURAMINE

See Pondimin, page 667.

Brand name:

FIBERALL NATURAL

See Metamucil, page 646.

Generic name:

FLUOXETINE

See Prozac, page 675.

Generic name:

FLUVASTATIN

See Lescol, page 634.

Generic name:

GAVISCON

See Antacids, page 600.

Generic name:

GELUSIL

See Antacids, page 600.

Generic name:

GEMCOR

See Lopid, page 640.

Generic name:

GEMFIBROZIL

See Lopid, page 640.

Generic name:

GLIPIZIDE

See Glucotrol, page 626.

Brand name:

GLUCOTROL

Pronounced: GLUE-kuh-troll
Generic name: Glipizide

Why is this drug prescribed?

Glucotrol is an oral antidiabetic medication used to treat Type II (non-insulin-dependent) diabetes. In diabetics the body either does not make enough insulin or the insulin that is produced no longer works properly.

There are actually two forms of diabetes: Type I insulin-dependent and Type II non-insulin-dependent. Type I usually requires insulin injections for life, while Type II diabetes can usually be treated by dietary changes and/or oral antidiabetic medications such as Glucotrol. Apparently, Glucotrol controls diabetes by stimulating the pancreas to secrete more insulin. Occasionally, Type II diabetics must take insulin injections on a temporary basis, especially during stressful periods or times of illness.

Most important fact about this drug

Always remember that Glucotrol is an aid to, not a substitute for, good diet and exercise. Failure to follow a sound diet and exercise plan can lead to serious complications, such as dangerously high or low blood sugar levels. Remember, too, that Glucotrol is *not* an oral form of insulin, and cannot be used in place of insulin.

How should you take this medication?

In general, to achieve the best control over blood sugar levels, Glucotrol should be taken 30 minutes before a meal. However, the exact dosing schedule as well as the dosage amount must be determined by your physician.

■ *If you miss a dose...*
Take it as soon as you remember. If it is
almost time for your next dose, skip the
one you missed and go back to your
regular schedule. Never take 2 doses at
the same time.

■ *Storage instructions...*
Glucotrol should be stored at room
temperature.

What side effects may occur?
Side effects from Glucotrol are rare and
seldom require discontinuation of the
medication.

■ *More common side effects may include:*
Constipation, diarrhea, dizziness,
drowsiness, headache, hives, itching, low
blood sugar, nausea, sensitivity to light,
skin rash and eruptions, stomach pain

■ *Less common or rare side effects may
include:*
Anemia and other blood disorders, yellow
eyes and skin

Glucotrol, like all oral antidiabetic drugs,
can cause low blood sugar. This risk is
increased by missed meals, alcohol, other
medications, and/or excessive exercise. To
avoid low blood sugar, you should closely
follow the dietary and exercise regimen
suggested by your physician.

■ *Symptoms of mild low blood sugar may
include:*
Blurred vision
Cold sweats
Dizziness
Fast heartbeat
Fatigue
Headache
Hunger
Light-headedness
Nausea
Nervousness

■ *Symptoms of more severe low blood sugar
may include:*
Coma
Disorientation
Pale skin
Seizures
Shallow breathing

Ask your doctor what steps you should take
if you experience mild hypoglycemia. If
symptoms of severe low blood sugar occur,
contact your doctor immediately. Severe
hypoglycemia should be considered a
medical emergency, and prompt medical
attention is essential.

Why should this drug not be prescribed?
You should not take Glucotrol if you have
had an allergic reaction to it previously.

Glucotrol will be stopped if you are
suffering from diabetic ketoacidosis (a life-
threatening medical emergency caused by
insufficient insulin and marked by excessive
thirst, nausea, fatigue, pain below the
breastbone, and a fruity breath).

Special warnings about this medication
It's possible that drugs such as Glucotrol
may lead to more heart problems than diet
treatment alone, or diet plus insulin. If you
have a heart condition, you may want to
discuss this with you doctor.

If you are taking Glucotrol, you should
check your blood and urine periodically for
the presence of abnormal sugar (glucose)
levels.

Even people with well-controlled diabetes
may find that injury, infection, surgery, or
fever results in a lack of control over their
diabetes. In these cases, the physician may
recommend that you stop taking Glucotrol
temporarily and use insulin instead.

In addition, the effectiveness of any oral antidiabetic, including Glucotrol, may decrease with time. This may occur because of either a diminished responsiveness to the medication or a worsening of the diabetes.

Possible food and drug interactions when taking this medication

It is essential that you closely follow your physician's dietary guidelines and that you inform your physician of any medication, either prescription or nonprescription, that you are taking. Specific medications that affect Glucotrol include:

Airway-opening drugs such as Sudafed
Antacids such as Mylanta
Aspirin
Chloramphenicol (Chloromycetin)
Cimetidine (Tagamet)
Clofibrute (Atromid-S)
Corticosteroids such as prednisone
    (Deltasone)
Coumarin (Coumadin)
Diuretics such as HydroDIURIL
Estrogens such as Premarin
Fluconazole (Diflucan)
Gemfibrozil (Lupid)
Heart and blood pressure medications called
    beta blockers such as Tenormin and
    Lopressor
Heart medications called calcium channel
    blockers such as Cardizem and Procardia
    XL
Isoniazid (Nydrazid)
Itraconazole (Sponanox)
MAO inhibitors (antidepressant drugs such as
    Nardil)
Major tranquilizers such as Thorazine and
    Mellavil
Miconazole (Monistat)
Nicotinic acid (Nicobid)
Nonsteroidal anti-inflammatory drugs such
    as Motrin
Oral contraceptives
Phenytoin (Dilantin)

Probenecid (Benemid)
Rifampin (Rifadin)
Sulfa drugs such as Bactrim
Thyroid medications such as Synthroid

Alcohol must be used carefully, since excessive alcohol consumption can cause low blood sugar.

Special information if you are pregnant or breastfeeding

The effects of Glucotrol during pregnancy have not been adequately studied. Therefore, if you are pregnant, or planning to become pregnant, you should take Glucotrol only on the advice of your physician. Since studies suggest the importance of maintaining normal blood sugar (glucose) levels during pregnancy, your physician may prescribe insulin during pregnancy. To minimize the risk of low blood sugar in newborn babies, Glucotrol, if taken during pregnancy, should be discontinued at least one month before the expected delivery date. Although it is not known if Glucotrol appears in breast milk, other oral antidiabetics do. Because of the potential for hypoglycemia in nursing infants, your doctor may advise you either to discontinue Glucotrol or to stop nursing. If Glucotrol is discontinued and if diet alone does not control glucose levels, your doctor may prescribe insulin.

Recommended dosage

Dosage levels must be determined by each patient's needs.

ADULTS

The usual recommended starting dose is 5 milligrams taken before breakfast. Depending upon blood glucose response, this initial dose may be increased in increments of 2.5 to 5 milligrams. The maximum recommended daily dose is 40 milligrams; total daily dosages above 15 milligrams are usually divided into 2 equal doses that are taken before meals.

CHILDREN

The safety and effectiveness of this drug in children have not been established.

ELDERLY

The elderly or those with liver disease usually start with 2.5 milligrams.

Overdosage

An overdose of Glucotrol can cause low blood sugar.

- *Symptoms of mild low blood sugar include:*
  Blurred vision
  Cold sweats
  Dizziness
  Fatigue
  Headache
  Hunger
  Light-headedness
  Nausea
  Nervousness
  Rapid heartbeat

Eating sugar or a sugar-based product will often correct the condition. Otherwise, seek medical attention immediately.

- *Symptoms of more severe low blood sugar include:*
  Coma
  Disorientation
  Pale skin
  Seizures
  Shallow breathing

Contact your doctor immediately if these symptoms occur.

Generic name:

GLYBURIDE

See Micronase, page 652.

Brand name:

GLYNASE

See Micronase, page 652.

Brand name:

HUMULIN

See Insulin, page 629.

Brand name:

HYDROCIL INSTANT

See Metamucil, page 646.

Generic name:

HYOSCYAMINE

See Levsin, page 636.

Brand name:

ILETIN

See Insulin, page 629.

Generic name:

INSULIN

Pronounced: IN-suh-lin
Available formulations:
Insulin, Human:
  Humulin

Insulin, Human Isophane Suspension:
  Humulin N
Insulin, Human NPH:
  Insulatard NPH Human
  Novolin N
Insulin, Human Regular:
  Novolin R
  Humulin BR & R
  Velosulin Human
Insulin, Human Regular and Human NPH mixture:
  Humulin 70/30
  Mixtard Human 70/30
  Novolin 70/30
Insulin, Human, Zinc Suspension:
  Humulin L & U
  Novolin L
Insulin, NPH:
  NPH Iletin I (also II, Beef; II, Pork)
  Insulatard NPH
  NPH Insulin
Insulin Regular and NPH mixture:
  Mixtard 70/30
Insulin, Zinc Crystals:
  NPH Iletin I
Insulin, Regular:
  Iletin I Regular (also II, Beef; II, Pork)
  Regular Insulin
  Velosulin
Insulin, Zinc Suspension:
  Iletin I, Lente
  Protamine, Zinc and Iletin
  Iletin I, Semilente
  Iletin I
  Lente Insulin
  Ultralente Insulin

Why is this drug prescribed?

Insulin is prescribed for diabetes mellitus when this condition does not improve with oral medications or by modifying your diet. Insulin is a hormone produced by the pancreas, a large gland that lies near the stomach. This hormone is necessary for the body's correct use of food, especially sugar.

Insulin apparently works by helping sugar penetrate the cell wall, where it is then utilized by the cell. In people with diabetes, the body either does not make enough insulin, or the insulin that is produced cannot be used properly.

There are actually two forms of diabetes: Type I insulin-dependent and Type II non-insulin-dependent. Type I usually requires insulin injection for life, while Type II diabetes can usually be treated by dietary changes and/or oral antidiabetic medications such as Diabinese and Glucotrol. Occasionally, Type II diabetics must take insulin injections on a temporary basis, especially during stressful periods or times of illness.

The various insulin brands above differ in several ways: in the source (animal, human, or genetically engineered), in the time requirements for the insulin to take effect, and in the length of time the insulin remains working.

Regular insulin is manufactured from beef and pork pancreas, begins working within 30 to 60 minutes, and lasts for 6 to 8 hours. Variations of insulin have been developed to satisfy the needs of individual patients. For example, zinc suspension insulin is an intermediate-acting insulin that starts working within 1 to 1½ hours and lasts approximately 24 hours. Insulin combined with zinc and protamine is a longer-acting insulin that takes effect within 4 to 6 hours and lasts up to 36 hours. The time and course of action may vary considerably in different individuals or at different times in the same individual.

Animal-based insulin is a very safe product. However, some components may cause an allergic reaction (see "What side effects may occur?"). Therefore, genetically engineered human insulin has been developed to lessen the chance of an allergic reaction. It is structurally identical to the insulin produced by your body's pancreas. However, some human insulin may be produced in a semi-synthetic process that begins with animal-based ingredients, which may cause an allergic reaction.

Most important fact about this drug

Regardless of the type of insulin your doctor has prescribed, you should follow carefully the dietary and exercise guidelines he or she has recommended. Failure to follow these guidelines or to take your insulin as prescribed may result in serious and potentially life-threatening complications such as hypoglycemia (lowered blood sugar levels).

How should you take this medication?

Take your insulin exactly as prescribed, being careful to follow your doctor's dietary and exercise recommendations.

■ *If you miss a dose...*
Your doctor should tell you what to do if you miss an insulin injection or meal.

■ *Storage instructions...*
Store insulin in a refrigerator (but not in the freezer) or in another cool, dark place. Do not expose insulin to heat or direct sunlight.

Some brands of prefilled syringes can be kept at room temperature for a week or a month. Check your product's label. Never use insulin after the expiration date which is printed on the label and carton.

What side effects may occur?

While side effects from insulin use are rare, allergic reactions or low blood sugar (sometimes called "an insulin reaction") may pose significant health risks. Your doctor should be notified if any of the following occur:

■ *Mild allergic reactions:*
Swelling, itching or redness at the injection site (usually disappears within a few days or weeks)

■ *More serious allergic reactions:*
Fast pulse
Low blood pressure
Perspiration
Rash over the entire body
Shortness of breath, shallow breathing, or wheezing

Other side effects are virtually eliminated when the correct dose of insulin is matched with the proper diet and level of physical activity. Low blood sugar may develop in poorly controlled or unstable diabetes. Consuming sugar or a sugar-containing product will usually correct the condition, which can be brought about by taking too much insulin, missing or delaying meals, exercising or working more than usual, an infection or illness, a change in the body's need for insulin, drug interactions, or consuming alcohol.

■ *Symptoms of low blood sugar include:*
Abnormal behavior, anxiety, blurred vision, cold sweat, confusion, depressed mood, dizziness, drowsiness, fatigue, headache, hunger, inability to concentrate, light-headedness, nausea, nervousness, personality changes, rapid heartbeat, restlessness, sleep disturbances, slurred speech, sweating, tingling in the hands, feet, lips, or tongue, tremor, unsteady movement

Contact your physician if these symptoms persist.

■ *Symptoms of more severe low blood sugar include:*
Coma
Disorientation

Remember, too, the symptoms associated with an under-supply of insulin, which can be brought on by taking too little of it, overeating, or fever and infection.

■ *Symptoms of insufficient insulin include:*
Drowsiness
Flushing
Fruity breath
Heavy breathing
Loss of appetite
Rapid pulse
Thirst

If you are ill, you should check your urine for ketones (acetone), and notify your doctor if the test is positive. This condition can be life-threatening.

Why should this drug not be prescribed?
Insulin should be used only to correct diabetic conditions.

Special warnings about this medication
Wear personal identification that states clearly that you are diabetic. Carry a sugar-containing product such as hard candy to offset any symptoms of low blood sugar.

Do not change the type of insulin or even the model and brand of syringe or needle you use without your physician's instruction. Failure to use the proper syringe may lead to improper dosage levels of insulin.

If you become ill from any cause, especially with nausea and vomiting or fever, your insulin requirements may change. It is important to eat as normally as possible. If you have trouble eating, drink fruit juices, soda, or clear soups, or eat small amounts of bland foods. Test your urine and/or

blood sugar and tell your doctor at once. If you have severe and prolonged vomiting, seek emergency medical care.

If you are taking insulin, you should check your glucose levels with home blood and urine testing devices. If your blood tests consistently show above-normal sugar levels or your urine tests consistently show the presence of sugar, your diabetes is not properly controlled, and you should tell your doctor.

To avoid infection or contamination, use disposable needles and syringes or sterilize your reusable syringe and needle carefully.

Always keep handy an extra supply of insulin as well as a spare syringe and needle.

Possible food and drug interactions when taking this medication
Follow your physician's dietary guidelines as closely as you can and inform your physician of any medication, either prescription or non-prescription, that you are taking. Specific medications, depending on the amount present, that affect insulin levels or its effectiveness include:

Anabolic steroids such as Androl-50
Appetite suppressants such as Tenuate
Aspirin
Beta-blocking blood pressure medicines such as Tenormin and Lopressor
Diuretics such as Lasix and Dyazide
Epinephrine (EpiPen)
Estrogens such as Premarin
MAO inhibitors (antidepressant drugs such as Nardil and Parnate)
Phenytoin (Dilantin)
Steroid medications such as prednisone
Thyroid medications such as Synthroid and Proloid

Use alcohol carefully, since excessive alcohol consumption can cause low blood sugar.

Don't drink unless your doctor has approved it.

Special information if you are pregnant or breastfeeding

Insulin is considered safe for pregnant women, but pregnancy may make managing your diabetes more difficult.

Properly controlled diabetes is essential for the health of the mother and the developing baby; therefore, it is extremely important that pregnant women follow closely their physician's dietary and exercise guidelines and prescribing instructions.

Since insulin does not pass into breast milk, it is safe for nursing mothers.

Recommended dosage

Your doctor will specify which insulin to use, how much, when, and how often to inject it. Your dosage may be affected by changes in food, activity, illness, medication, pregnancy, exercise, travel, or your work schedule. Proper control of your diabetes requires close and constant cooperation with your doctor. Failure to use your insulin as prescribed may result in serious and potentially fatal complications.

Some insulins should be clear, and some have a cloudy precipitate. Find out what your insulin should look like and check it carefully before using.

Overdosage

An overdose of insulin can cause low blood sugar (hypoglycemia). Symptoms include:

Depressed mood, dizziness, drowsiness, fatigue, headache, hunger, inability to concentrate, irritability, nausea, nervousness, personality changes, rapid heartbeat, restlessness, sleep disturbances, slurred speech, sweating, tingling, tremor, unsteady movements

■ *Symptoms of more severe low blood sugar include:*
Coma
Disorientation
Pale skin
Seizures

Your doctor should be contacted immediately if these symptoms of severe low blood sugar occur.

Eating sugar or a sugar-based product will often correct the condition. If you suspect an overdose, seek medical attention immediately.

Brand name:

IONAMIN

See Fastin, page 624.

Brand name:

KAON-CL

See Micro-K, page 650.

Brand name:

K-DUR

See Micro-K, page 650.

Brand name:

KLOR-CON

See Micro-K, page 650.

Brand name:

KONSYL

See Metamucil, page 646.

Generic name:

LACTULOSE

See Chronulac Syrup, page 611.

Brand name:

LESCOL

Pronounced: LESS-cahl
Generic name: Fluvastatin sodium

Why is this drug prescribed?

Lescol is a cholesterol-lowering drug. Your doctor may prescribe Lescol if you have been unable to reduce your blood cholesterol level sufficiently with a low-fat, low-cholesterol diet alone.

Most important fact about this drug

Lescol is usually prescribed only if diet, exercise, and weight-loss fail to bring your cholesterol levels under control. It's important to remember that Lescol is a supplement—not a substitute—for those other measures. To get the full benefit of the medication, you need to stick to the diet and exercise program prescribed by your doctor. All these efforts to keep your cholesterol levels normal are important because together they may lower your risk of heart disease.

How should you take this medication?

Take Lescol at bedtime; you may take it with or without food.

■ If you miss a dose...
If you miss a dose of this medication, take it as soon as you remember. However, if it is almost time for your next dose, skip the one you missed and go back to your regular schedule. Do not take 2 doses at the same time.

■ Storage instructions...
Store at room temperature. Protect from direct light and excessive heat. Keep out of reach of children.

What side effects may occur?

Side effects cannot be anticipated. If any develop or change in intensity, tell your doctor as soon as possible. Only your doctor can determine if it is safe for you to continue taking Lescol.

■ More common side effects may include:
Abdominal pain, accidental injury, back pain, diarrhea, fatigue, flu-like symptoms, headache, indigestion, joint disease, muscle pain, nasal inflammation, nausea, sour throat, upper respiratory infection

■ Less common side effects may include:
Allergy, bronchitis, constipation, coughing, dizziness, dental problems, gas, inflamed sinuses, insomnia, rash

Why should this drug not be prescribed?

Do not take Lescol while pregnant or nursing. Also avoid Lescol if you are experiencing liver problems, or if you have ever been found to be sensitive to it.

Special warnings about this medication

Because Lescol may damage the liver, your doctor may order a blood test to check your liver enzyme levels before you start taking this medication. Blood tests will probably be done at 6 and 12 weeks after you start Lescol therapy and periodically after that. If your liver enzymes rise too high, your doctor may tell you to stop taking Lescol. Your doctor will monitor you especially closely if you have ever had liver disease or if you are, or have ever been, a heavy drinker.

Since Lescol may cause damage to muscle tissue, be sure to tell your doctor of any unexplained muscle pain, tenderness, or weakness right away, especially if you also have a fever or feel sick. Your doctor may want to do a blood test to check for signs of muscle damage. If your blood test shows signs of muscle damage, your doctor may suggest discontinuing this medication.

If your risk of muscle and/or kidney damage suddenly increases because of major surgery or injury, or conditions such as low blood pressure, severe infection, or seizures, your doctor may tell you to stop taking Lescol for a while.

Be sure to tell your doctor about any medical conditions you may have before starting therapy with Lescol.

Possible food and drug interactions when taking this medication

If you take Lescol with certain drugs, the effects of either could be increased, decreased, or altered. It is especially important to check with your doctor before combining Lescol with the following:

Cholestyramine (Questran)
Cimetidine (Tagamet)
Clofibrate (Atromid-S)
Cyclosporine (Sandimmune)
Digoxin (Lanoxin, Lanoxicaps)
Erythromycin (E-Mycin, E.E.S.)
Gemfibrozil (Lopid)
Ketoconazole (Nizoral)
Omeprazole (Prilosec)
Ranitidine (Zantac)
Rifampin (Rifadin)
Spironolactone (Aldactone, Aldactazide)

Special information if you are pregnant or breastfeeding

You must not become pregnant while taking Lescol. This medication lowers cholesterol, and cholesterol is needed for a baby to develop properly. Because of the possible risk of birth defects, your doctor will prescribe Lescol only if you are highly unlikely to get pregnant while taking this medication. If you do become pregnant while taking Lescol, stop taking the drug and notify your doctor right away.

Lescol does appear in breast milk. Therefore, Lescol could cause severe side effects in a nursing baby. Do not take Lescol while breastfeeding your baby.

Recommended dosage

Your doctor will put you on a cholesterol-lowering diet before starting treatment with Lescol. You should continue on this diet while you are taking Lescol.

ADULTS

The usual starting dose is 20 milligrams per day, taken as a single dose at bedtime. The usual range after that is 20 to 40 milligrams per day as a single dose at bedtime. After 4 weeks of therapy with Lescol, your doctor will check your cholesterol level and adjust your dosage if necessary.

Combined Drug Therapy
If you are taking Lescol with another cholesterol medication such as Questran, make sure you take the other drug at least 2 hours before your dose of Lescol.

CHILDREN

The safety and effectiveness of Lescol in children under 18 years old have not been established. Do not give Lescol to children under 18 years of age.

Overdosage

Although no specific information about Lescol overdose is available, any medication taken in excess can have serious consequences. If you suspect an overdose of Lescol, seek medical attention immediately.

Brand name:

LEVSIN

Pronounced: LEV-sin
Generic name: Hyoscyamine sulfate
Other brand name: Anaspaz

Why is this drug prescribed?

Levsin is an antispasmodic medication given to help treat various stomach, intestinal, and urinary tract disorders that involve cramps, colic, or other painful muscle contractions. Because Levsin has a drying effect, it may also be used to dry a runny nose or to dry excess secretions before anesthesia is administered.

For inflammation of the pancreas, Levsin may be used to help control excess secretions and reduce pain. Levsin may also be taken in Parkinson's disease to help reduce muscle rigidity and tremors and to help control drooling and excess sweating.

Doctors also give Levsin as part of the preparation for certain diagnostic x-rays (for example, of the stomach, intestines, or kidneys).

Levsin comes in several forms, including regular tablets, tablets to be dissolved under the tongue, sustained-release capsules, liquid, drops, and an injectable solution.

Most important fact about this drug

Levsin may make you sweat less, causing your body temperature to increase and putting you at the risk of heatstroke. Try to stay inside as much as possible on hot days, and avoid warm places such as very hot baths and saunas.

How should you take this medication?

If you take Levsin for a stomach disorder, you may also need to take antacid medication. However, antacids make Levsin more difficult for the body to absorb. To minimize this problem, take Levsin before meals and the antacids after meals.

Take Levsin exactly as prescribed. Although the sublingual tablets (Levsin/SL) are designed to be dissolved under the tongue, they may also be chewed or swallowed. The regular tablets may also be dissolved under the tongue or swallowed.

Levsin can cause dry mouth. For temporary relief, suck on a hard candy or chew gum.

■ *If you miss a dose...*
Take it as soon as you remember. If it is almost time for your next dose, skip the one you missed and go back to your regular schedule. Do not take 2 doses at once.

■ *Storage instructions...*
Store at room temperature.

What side effects may occur?

Side effects cannot be anticipated. If any side effects develop or change in intensity, tell your doctor immediately. Only your doctor can determine whether it is safe for you to continue taking Levsin.

■ *Side effects may include:*
Allergic reactions, bloating, blurred vision, confusion, constipation, decreased sweating, dilated pupils, dizziness, drowsiness, dry mouth, excitement, headache, hives, impotence, inability to urinate, insomnia, itching, heart palpitations, lack of coordination, loss of

sense of taste, nausea, nervousness, rapid heartbeat, skin reactions, speech problems, vomiting, weakness

Why should this drug not be prescribed?
Do not take Levsin if you have ever had an allergic reaction to it or similar drugs such as scopolamine. Also, you should not be given Levsin if you have any of the following:

Bowel or digestive tract obstruction or paralysis
Glaucoma (excessive pressure in the eyes)
Myasthenia gravis (a disorder in which muscles become weak and tire easily)
Ulcerative colitis (severe bowel inflammation)
Urinary obstruction

Levsin is not appropriate if you have diarrhea, especially if you have a surgical opening to the bowels (an ileostomy or colostomy).

Special warnings about this medication
Be careful using Levsin if you have an overactive thyroid gland, heart disease, congestive heart failure, irregular heartbeats, high blood pressure, or kidney disease.

Because Levsin may make you dizzy or drowsy, or blur your vision, do not drive, operate other machinery, or do any other hazardous work while taking this medication.

While you are taking Levsin, you may experience confusion, disorientation, short-term memory loss, hallucinations, difficulty speaking, lack of coordination, coma, an exaggerated sense of well-being, decreased anxiety, fatigue, sleeplessness and agitation. These symptoms should disappear 12 to 48 hours after you stop taking the drug.

Possible food and drug interactions when taking this medication
If Levsin is taken with certain other drugs, the effects of either drug could be increased, decreased, or altered. It is especially important to check with your doctor before combining Levsin with the following:

Amantadine (Symmetrel)
Antacids
Antidepressant drugs such as Elavil, Nardil, Parnate, and Tofranil
Antihistamines such as Benadryl
Major tranquilizers such as Thorazine and Haldol
Other antispasmodic drugs such as Bentyl
Potassium supplements such as Slow-K

Special information if you are pregnant or breastfeeding
If you are pregnant or plan to become pregnant, inform your doctor immediately. Although it is not known whether Levsin can cause birth defects, pregnant women should avoid all drugs except those necessary to health.

Levsin appears in breast milk. Your doctor may ask you to forego breastfeeding when taking this drug.

Recommended dosage
LEVSIN/SL AND LEVSIN TABLETS

The tablets may be swallowed or placed under the tongue. Levsin/SL tablets may also be chewed.

Adults and Children 12 Years of Age and Older
The usual dose is 1 to 2 tablets every four hours or as needed. Do not take more than 12 tablets in 24 hours.

Children 2 to Under 12 Years of Age
The usual dose is one-half to 1 tablet every four hours or as needed. Do not give a child more than 6 tablets in 24 hours.

LEVSIN ELIXIR

Adults and Children 12 Years of Age and Older
The recommended dosage is 1 to 2 teaspoonfuls every four hours or as needed, but no more than 12 teaspoonfuls in 24 hours.

Children 2 to 12 Years of Age
The usual dosage is one-quarter to 1 teaspoonful every 4 hours or as needed. Do not give a child more than 6 teaspoonfuls in 24 hours.

LEVSIN DROPS

Adults and Children 12 Years of Age and Older
The recommended dosage is 1 to 2 milliliters every 4 hours or as needed, but no more than 12 milliliters in 24 hours.

Children 2 to 12 Years of Age
The usual dosage is one-quarter to 1 milliliter every 4 hours or as needed. Do not give a child more than 6 milliliters in 24 hours.

Children under 2 Years of Age
Your doctor will determine the dosage based on body weight. The doses may be repeated every 4 hours or as needed.

WEIGHT	USUAL DOSE	DO NOT EXCEED IN 24 HOURS
2.3 kilograms (5 lbs)	3 drops	18 drops
3.4 kilograms (7.5 lbs)	4 drops	24 drops
5 kilograms (11 lbs)	5 drops	30 drops
7 kilograms (15 lbs)	6 drops	36 drops
10 kilograms (22 lbs)	8 drops	48 drops
15 kilograms (33 lbs)	11 drops	66 drops

LEVSINEX TIMECAPS

Adults and Children 12 Years of Age and Older
The recommended dosage is 1 to 2 Timecaps every 12 hours. Your doctor may adjust the dosage to 1 Timecap every 8 hours if needed. Do not take more than 4 Timecaps in 24 hours.

Children 2 to 12 Years of Age
The usual dosage is 1 Timecap every 12 hours. Do not give a child more than 2 Timecaps in 24 hours.

Overdosage
Any medication taken in excess can have serious consequences. If you suspect an overdose, seek medical attention immediately.

■ *Symptoms of Levsin overdose may include:*
Blurred vision
Dilated pupils
Dizziness
Dry mouth
Excitement
Headache
Hot, dry skin
Nausea
Swallowing difficulty
Vomiting

Brand name:

LIBRAX

Pronounced: LIB-racks
Generic ingredients: Chlordiazepoxide
  hydrochloride, Clidinium bromide
Other brand name: Clindex

Why is this drug prescribed?

Librax is used, in combination with other
therapy, for the treatment of peptic ulcer,
irritable bowel syndrome (spastic colon), and
acute enterocolitis (inflammation of the
colon and small intestine). Librax is a
combination of a benzodiazepine
(chlordiazepoxide) and an antispasmodic
medication (clidinium).

Most important fact about this drug

Because of its sedative effects, you should
not operate heavy machinery, drive, or
engage in other hazardous tasks that require
you to be mentally alert while you are
taking Librax.

How should you take this medication?

Take Librax as directed by your doctor.
Other therapy may be prescribed to be used
at the same time.

Librax can make your mouth dry. For
temporary relief, suck a hard candy or chew
gum.

Take Librax before meals and at bedtime.

- *If you miss a dose...*
  Take it as soon as you remember. If it is
  almost time for your next dose, skip the
  one you missed and go back to your
  regular schedule. Do not take 2 doses at
  once.

- *Storage instructions...*
  Store away from heat, light, and moisture.

What side effects may occur?

Side effects cannot be anticipated. If any
develop or change in intensity, inform your
doctor as soon as possible. Only your
doctor can determine if it is safe for you to
continue taking Librax.

- *Side effects may include:*
  Blurred vision, changes in sex drive,
  confusion, constipation, drowsiness, dry
  mouth, fainting, lack of coordination, liver
  problems, minor menstrual irregularities,
  nausea, skin eruptions, swelling due to
  fluid retention, urinary difficulties,
  yellowing of skin and eyes

Why should this drug not be prescribed?

You should not take this drug if you have
glaucoma (elevated pressure in the eye),
prostatic hypertrophy (enlarged prostate), or
a bladder obstruction. If you are sensitive to
or have ever had an allergic reaction to
Librax or any of its ingredients, you should
not take this medication. Make sure your
doctor is aware of any drug reactions you
have experienced.

Special warnings about this medication

Librax can be habit-forming and has been
associated with drug dependence and
addiction. Be very careful taking this
medication if you have ever had problems
with alcohol or drug abuse. Never take
more than the prescribed amount.

In addition, you should not stop taking
Librax suddenly, because of the risk of
withdrawal symptoms (convulsions, cramps,
tremors, vomiting, sweating, feeling
depressed, and insomnia). If you have been
taking Librax over a long period of time,
your doctor will have you taper off
gradually.

The elderly are more likely to develop side
effects such as confusion, excessive

drowsiness, and uncoordinated movements when taking Librax. The doctor will probably prescribe a low dose.

Long-term treatment with Librax may call for periodic blood and liver function tests.

Possible food and drug interactions when taking this medication

If Librax is taken with certain other drugs, the effects of either can be increased, decreased, or altered. It is especially important to check with your doctor before combining Librax with the following:

Antidepressant drugs known as MAO
   inhibitors, such as Nardil and Parnate
Blood-thinning drugs such as Coumadin
Certain diarrhea medications such as
   Donnagel and Kaopectate
Ketoconazole (Nizoral)
Major tranquilizers such as Stelazine and
   Thorazine
Potassium supplements such as Micro-K

In addition, you may experience excessive drowsiness and other potentially dangerous side effects if you combine Librax with alcohol or other drugs, such as Benadryl and Valium, that make you drowsy.

Special information
if you are pregnant or breastfeeding

Several studies have found an increased risk of birth defects if Librax is taken during the first 3 months of pregnancy. Therefore, Librax is rarely recommended for use by pregnant women. If you are pregnant, plan to become pregnant, or are breastfeeding, inform your doctor immediately.

Recommended dosage

ADULTS

The usual dose is 1 or 2 capsules, 3 or 4 times a day before meals and at bedtime.

ELDERLY

Your doctor will have you take the lowest dose that is effective.

Overdosage

Any medication taken in excess can have serious consequences. A severe overdose of Librax can be fatal. If you suspect an overdose, seek medical help immediately.

■ *Symptoms of Librax overdose may include:*
  Blurred vision
  Coma
  Confusion
  Constipation
  Excessive sleepiness
  Excessively dry mouth
  Slow reflexes
  Urinary difficulties

Brand name:

LOPID

Pronounced: LOH-pid
Generic name: Gemfibrozil
Other brand name: Gemcor

Why is this drug prescribed?

Lopid is prescribed, along with a special diet, for treatment of people with very high levels of serum triglycerides (a fatty substance in the blood) who are at risk of developing pancreatitis (inflammation of the pancreas) and who do not respond adequately to a strict diet.

This drug can also be used to reduce the risk of coronary heart disease in people who have failed to respond to weight loss, diet, exercise, and other triglyceride- or cholesterol-lowering drugs.

Most important fact about this drug

Lopid is usually prescribed only if diet, exercise, and weight-loss fail to bring your cholesterol levels under control. It's important to remember that Lopid is a supplement—not a substitute—for these other measures. To get the full benefit of the medication, you need to stick to the diet and exercise program prescribed by your doctor. All these efforts to keep your cholesterol levels normal are important because together they may lower your risk of heart disease.

How should you take this medication?

Take this medication 30 minutes before the morning and evening meal, exactly as prescribed.

■ *If you miss a dose...*
Take it as soon as you remember. If it is almost time for the next dose, skip the one you missed and go back to your regular schedule. Do not take 2 doses at the same time.

■ *Storage instructions...*
Store at room temperature.

What side effects may occur?

Side effects cannot be anticipated. If any develop or change in intensity, inform your doctor as soon as possible. Only your doctor can determine if it is safe for you to continue taking Lopid.

■ *More common side effects may include:*
Abdominal pain, acute appendicitis, constipation, diarrhea, eczema, fatigue, headache, indigestion, nausea/vomiting, rash, vertigo

■ *Less common or rare side effects may include:*
Anemia, blood disorders, blurred vision, confusion, convulsions, decreased male fertility, decreased sex drive, depression, dizziness, fainting, hives, impotence, inflammation of the colon, irregular heartbeat, itching, joint pain, laryngeal swelling, muscle disease, muscle pain, muscle weakness, painful extremities, sleepiness, tingling sensation, weight loss, yellow eyes and skin

Why should this drug not be prescribed?

There is a slight possibility that Lopid may cause malignancy, gallbladder disease, abdominal pain leading to appendectomy, or other serious, possibly fatal, abdominal disorders. This drug should not be used by those who have only mildly elevated cholesterol levels, since the benefits do not outweigh the risk of these severe side effects.

If you are sensitive to or have ever had an allergic reaction to Lopid or similar drugs such as Atromid-S, you should not take this medication. Make sure your doctor is aware of any drug reactions you have experienced.

Unless you are directed to do so by your doctor, do not take this medication if you are being treated for severe kidney or liver disorders or gallbladder disease.

Special warnings about this medication

Excess body weight and excess alcohol intake may be important risk factors leading to unusually high levels of fats in the body. Your doctor will probably want you to lose weight and stop drinking before he or she tries to treat you with Lopid.

Your doctor will probably do periodic blood level tests during the first 12 months of therapy with Lopid because of blood diseases associated with the use of this medication.

Liver disorders have occurred with the use of this drug. Therefore, your doctor will probably test your liver function periodically.

If you are being treated for any disease that contributes to increased blood cholesterol, such as an overactive thyroid, diabetes, nephrotic syndrome (kidney and blood vessel disorder), dysproteinemia (excess of protein in the blood), or obstructive liver disease, consult with your doctor before taking Lopid.

Lopid should begin to reduce cholesterol levels during the first 3 months of therapy. If your cholesterol is not lowered sufficiently, this medication should be discontinued. Therefore, it is important that your doctor check your progress regularly.

The use of this medication may cause gallstones leading to possible gallbladder surgery. If you develop gallstones, your doctor will have you stop taking the drug.

The use of this drug may be associated with myositis, a muscle disease. If you have muscle pain, tenderness, or weakness, consult with your doctor. If myositis is suspected, your doctor will stop treating you with this drug.

Possible food and drug interactions when taking this medication

If Lopid is taken with certain other drugs, the effects of either could be increased, decreased, or altered. It is especially important to check with your doctor before combining Lopid with the following:

Blood-thinning drugs such as Coumadin
Fluvastatin (Lescol)
Lovastatin (Mevacor)
Pravastatin (Pravachol)
Simvastatin (Zocor)

Special information if you are pregnant or breastfeeding

The effects of Lopid during pregnancy have not been adequately studied. If you are pregnant or plan to become pregnant,

inform your doctor immediately. Because this medication causes tumors in animals, it may have an effect on nursing infants. If Lopid is essential to your health, your doctor may advise you to discontinue breastfeeding until your treatment with Lopid is finished.

Recommended dosage

ADULTS

The recommended dose is 1,200 milligrams divided into 2 doses, given 30 minutes before the morning and evening meals.

CHILDREN

Safety and effectiveness of Lopid have not been established for use in children.

ELDERLY

This drug should be used with caution by the elderly.

Overdosage

There have been no reported cases of overdose with Lopid. However, should you suspect a Lopid overdose, seek medical attention immediately.

Brand name:

LOPURIN

See Zyloprim, page 697.

Brand name:

LORELCO

Pronounced: Lore-ELL-Koh
Generic name: Probucol

Why is this drug prescribed?

Lorelco is used, along with diet, to lower cholesterol levels in the blood of people with primary hypercholesterolemia (a genetic defect that causes a lack of low-density lipoprotein [LDL] receptors, which remove cholesterol from the bloodstream). Lorelco lowers *total serum cholesterol*, which means that it not only reduces LDL, or "bad," cholesterol but may reduce HDL (high-density lipoprotein), or "good," cholesterol. The risk of lowering HDL cholesterol while lowering LDL cholesterol is unknown.

Most important fact about this drug

Lorelco is usually prescribed only if diet, exercise, and weight-loss fail to bring your cholesterol levels under control. It's important to remember that Lorelco is a supplement—not a substitute—for these other measures. To get the full benefit of the medication, you need to stick to the diet and exercise program prescribed by your doctor. All these efforts to keep your cholesterol levels normal are important because together they may lower your risk of heart disease.

How should you take this medication?

Take Lorelco with meals, exactly as prescribed.

■ *If you miss a dose...*
Take it as soon as you remember. If it is almost time for the next dose, skip the one you missed and go back to your regular schedule. Do not take 2 doses at the same time.

■ *Storage instructions...*
Store in a tightly closed container away from excessive heat and moisture.

What side effects may occur?

Side effects cannot be anticipated. If any develop or change in intensity, inform your doctor as soon as possible. Only your doctor can determine if it is safe for you to continue taking Lorelco.

■ *Side effects when treatment with Lorelco begins may include:*
Brief loss of consciousness or fainting
Chest pain
Dizziness
Nausea
Rapid, strong heartbeat
Vomiting

■ *Side effects during treatment may include:*
Abdominal pain, blurred vision, bruising, diarrhea, diminished sense of taste and smell, dizziness, excessive nighttime urination, excessive perspiration, fainting, gas, headache, impotence, inability to fall or stay asleep, indigestion, inflammation of the eyelid, irregular heartbeat, itching, loss of appetite, nausea, rash, ringing in the ears, stomach or intestinal bleeding, swelling due to fluid retention, tearing, tingling sensation, vomiting

Why should this drug not be prescribed?

If you are sensitive to or have ever had an allergic reaction to Lorelco or similar drugs, you should not use this medication. Make sure that your doctor is aware of any drug reactions you have experienced.

Unless you are directed to do so by your doctor, do not take this medication if you have had recent heart damage, have progressive heart disease, have serious abnormal heart rhythm, or experience unexplained fainting spells or other conditions that your doctor considers dangerous.

Special warnings about this medication

If you are being treated for any disease that contributes to increased blood cholesterol, such as hyperthyroidism, diabetes, nephrotic syndrome (kidney and blood vessel disorder), or obstructive liver disease, consult with your doctor before taking this medication.

Lorelco should begin to reduce cholesterol levels during the first 3 to 4 months of therapy. If your cholesterol is not lowered sufficiently, your doctor will have you stop taking this medication. Therefore, it is important that your doctor check your progress regularly.

Possible food and drug interactions when taking this medication

If Lorelco is taken with certain other drugs, the effects of either could be increased, decreased, or altered. It is especially important to check with your doctor before combining Lorelco with the following:

Certain antidepressants such as Elavil and Norpramin
Clofibrate (Atromid-S)
Drugs for irregular heartbeat such as Norpace and Quinidex
Major tranquilizers such as Mellaril and Thorazine

Special information if you are pregnant or breastfeeding

The effects of Lorelco during pregnancy have not been adequately studied. If you are pregnant or plan to become pregnant, inform your doctor immediately. It is recommended that women who plan to become pregnant stop taking this drug and delay the pregnancy with some form of birth control for at least six months. Lorelco may appear in breast milk and could affect a nursing infant. If this medication is essential to your health, your doctor may advise you to discontinue breastfeeding until your treatment is finished.

Recommended dosage

ADULTS

The recommended and maximum dose is 1,000 milligrams per day, divided into 2 doses of 500 milligrams each (two 250-

milligram tablets or one 500-milligram tablet), taken with the morning and evening meals.

CHILDREN

The safety and effectiveness of this drug have not been established in children.

ELDERLY

This drug should be used with caution by the elderly.

Overdosage

Any medication taken in excess can cause symptoms of overdose. If you suspect a Lorelco overdose, seek medical attention immediately.

Brand name:

LOVASTATIN

See Mevacor, page 648.

Brand name:

LURIDE

Pronounced: LUHR-ide
Generic name: Sodium fluoride

Why is this drug prescribed?

Luride is prescribed to strengthen children's teeth against decay during the period when the teeth are still developing.

Studies have shown that children who live where the drinking water contains a certain level of fluoride have fewer cavities than others. Fluoride helps prevent cavities in three ways: by increasing the teeth's resistance to dissolving on contact with acid, by strengthening teeth, and by slowing down the growth of mouth bacteria.

Luride may be given to children who live where the water fluoride level is 0.6 parts per million or less.

Most important fact about this drug

Before Luride is prescribed, it is important for the doctor to know the fluoride content of the water your child drinks every day. Your water company, or a private laboratory, can tell you the level of fluoride in your water.

How should you take this medication?

Give your child Luride exactly as prescribed by your doctor. It is preferable to give the tablet at bedtime after the child's teeth have been brushed. The youngster may chew and swallow the tablet or simply suck on it until it dissolves. The liquid form of this medicine is to be taken by mouth. It may be dropped directly into the mouth or mixed with water or fruit juice. Always store Luride drops in the original plastic dropper bottle.

■ *If you miss a dose...*
Take it as soon as you remember. If it is almost time for your next dose, skip the one you missed and go back to your regular schedule. Do not take 2 doses at once.

■ *Storage instructions...*
Store away from heat, light, and moisture. Keep the liquid from freezing.

What side effects may occur?

Side effects cannot be anticipated. If any develop, tell your doctor immediately. Only your doctor can determine whether it is safe for your child to continue taking Luride.

In rare cases, Luride may cause an allergic rash or some other unexpected effect.

Why should this drug not be prescribed?

Your child should not take Luride if he or she is sensitive to it or has had an allergic reaction to it in the past.

Your child should not take the 1-milligram strength of Luride if the drinking water in your area contains 0.3 parts per million of fluoride or more. He or she should not take the other forms of Luride if the water contains 0.6 parts per million of fluoride or more.

Special warnings about this medication

Do not give full-strength tablets (1 milligram) to children under the age of 6.

Possible food and drug interactions when taking this medication

Avoid giving your child Luride with dairy products. The calcium in dairy products may interact with the fluoride to create calcium fluoride, which the body cannot absorb well.

Recommended dosage

Since this drug is used to supplement water with low fluoride content, consult your physician to determine the proper amount based on the local water content. Also check with your doctor if you move to a new area, change to bottled water, or begin using a water-filtering device. Dosages are determined by both age and the fluoride content of the water.

INFANTS AND CHILDREN

The following daily dosages are recommended for areas where the drinking water contains fluoride at less than 0.3 parts per million:

Children 6 Months to 3 Years of Age
1 quarter-strength (0.25 milligram) tablet or ½ dropperful of liquid

3 to 6 Years of Age
1 half-strength (0.5 milligram) tablet or 1 dropperful of liquid

6 to 16 Years of Age
1 full-strength (1 milligram) tablet or 2 droppersful of liquid

For areas where the fluoride content of drinking water is between 0.3 and 0.6 parts per million, the recommended daily dosage of the tablets is one-half the above dosages. Dosage of the liquid should be reduced to ½ dropperful for children ages 3 to 6 and 1 dropperful for children over 6.

Overdosage

Any medication taken in excess can have serious consequences. Taking too much fluoride for a long period of time may cause discoloration of the teeth. Notify your doctor or dentist if you notice white, brown, or black spots on the teeth.

Generic name:

MAALOX

See Antacids, page 600.

Brand name:

MAALOX DAILY FIBER THERAPY

See Metamucil, page 646.

Brand name:

MATERNA

See Stuartnatal Plus, page 684.

Generic name:

MESALAMINE

See Rowasa, page 681.

Brand name:

METAMUCIL

Pronounced: MET-uh-MEW-sil
Generic name: Psyllium
Other brand names: Effer-Syllium, Fiberall Natural, Hydrocil Instant, Konsyl, Maalox Daily Fiber Therapy, Perdiem Fiber, Reguloid, Serutan, Syllact

Why is this drug prescribed?

Metamucil is used to treat constipation and irritable bowel syndrome (pain in the lower abdomen accompanied by diarrhea, usually stress-related). Metamucil is also prescribed to help treat the constipation of diverticular disease (development of pouches in the wall of the lower bowel). It is also used to clean the bowel in people with hemorrhoids and to treat the constipation that can accompany convalescence, old age, and pregnancy.

Some doctors also prescribe Metamucil to aid in reducing high cholesterol levels.

Most important fact about this drug

Contact your doctor before using Metamucil if you have any of the following conditions:

Abdominal pain
Difficulty in swallowing
Nausea
Sudden change in bowel habits that has lasted at least 2 weeks
Rectal bleeding
Vomiting

How should you take this medication?

If you are just starting on Metamucil, take 1 dose per day, gradually increasing to 3 times a day if needed or recommended by your doctor. If you experience any gas or bloating, slightly reduce the amount of Metamucil until your system adjusts to the additional fiber in your diet. Never attempt to swallow dry powder or wafers; mix Metamucil with an 8-ounce glass of water, fruit juice, or milk. Drink an additional glass of liquid if you can, and try to drink at least 6 to 8 full glasses of liquid daily to aid in stool softening. You may have to take Metamucil for 2 to 3 days to get the most benefit from it.

To avoid creating too much dust from the dry psyllium, which can cause an allergic reaction if you are sensitive to it, be careful when spooning powder into a glass.

■ *If you miss a dose...*
Resume your regular schedule with the next dose.

■ *Storage instructions...*
Store at room temperature. Protect from heat, light, and moisture.

What side effects may occur?
Side effects are unlikely.

Why should this drug not be prescribed?
If you are sensitive to or have ever had an allergic reaction to psyllium, you should not take this medication. Also avoid Metamucil if you have either of the following conditions:

Intestinal obstruction
Fecal impaction (an accumulation of hardened stool in the rectum or colon that cannot be passed)

Special warnings about this medication
If your constipation lasts longer than 1 week, call your doctor. This could be a sign of a more serious condition.

Metamucil swallowed dry or without enough liquid may swell and block your throat or esophagus, causing you to choke. Be sure to take this product with at least 8 ounces of liquid.

If you experience chest pain, vomiting, or difficulty in swallowing or breathing after taking Metamucil, seek medical attention immediately.

If you suffer from phenylketonuria (an enzyme-deficit disorder preventing the body's use of phenylalanine and resulting in harmful levels of this amino acid), avoid taking Sugar-Free Metamucil which contains phenylalanine.

Metamucil wafers contain gluten; do not take the wafers if you are allergic to this substance.

Possible food and drug interactions when taking this medication
None have been reported.

Special information if you are pregnant or breastfeeding
If you are pregnant or plan to become pregnant, or if you are breastfeeding, consult your doctor before starting on Metamucil.

Recommended dosage

ADULTS

Metamucil is generally taken 1 to 3 times daily, mixed with an 8-ounce glass of liquid. The amount per dose depends on the flavor type, and form of Metamucil you are using. Follow the package directions.

CHILDREN

For children 6 to 12 years old, use one-half the adult dose with 8 ounces of liquid, 1 to 3 times daily.

For children under age 6, consult your doctor.

Overdosage

An overdose of Metamucil is unlikely. However, any medication taken in excess can have serious consequences. If you suspect an overdose, seek medical attention immediately.

Brand name:

MEVACOR

Pronounced: MEV-uh-core
Generic name: Lovastatin

Why is this drug prescribed?

Mevacor is used, along with diet, to lower cholesterol levels in the blood of patients with primary hypercholesterolemia (too much cholesterol), a condition caused by a lack of the low-density lipoprotein (LDL) receptors that remove cholesterol from the bloodstream. However, Mevacor is usually prescribed only when a low-fat, low-cholesterol diet does not lower cholesterol levels enough.

Most important fact about this drug

Mevacor is usually prescribed only if diet, exercise, and weight-loss fail to bring your cholesterol levels under control. It's important to remember that Mevacor is a supplement—not a substitute—for these other measures. To get the full benefit of the medication, you need to stick to the diet and exercise program prescribed by your doctor. All these efforts to keep your cholesterol levels normal are important because together they may lower your risk of heart disease.

How should you take this medication?

Take Mevacor exactly as prescribed by your doctor.

Mevacor should be taken with meals.

■ *If you miss a dose...*
Take it as soon as you remember. If it is almost time for your next dose, skip the one you missed and go back to your regular schedule. Never take 2 doses at the same time.

■ *Storage instructions...*
Protect Mevacor from light. Store at room temperature. Keep container tightly closed.

What side effects may occur?

Mevacor is generally well tolerated. Any side effects that have occurred have usually been mild and short-lived. If any side effects develop or change in intensity, inform your doctor as soon as possible. Only your doctor can determine if it is safe for you to continue taking Mevacor.

■ *Side effects may include:*
Abdominal pain/cramps, altered sense of taste, blurred vision, constipation, diarrhea, dizziness, gas, headache, heartburn, indigestion, itching, muscle cramps, muscle pain, nausea, rash, weakness

Why should this drug not be prescribed?

If you are sensitive to or have ever had an allergic reaction to Mevacor or similar anticholesterol drugs, you should not take this medication. Make sure that your doctor is aware of any drug reactions that you have experienced.

Unless you are directed to do so by your doctor, do not take this medication if you are being treated for liver disease.

Do not take this drug if you are pregnant or nursing.

Special warnings about this medication

If you are being treated for any disease that contributes to increased blood cholesterol, such as hypothyroidism, diabetes, nephrotic syndrome (kidney and blood vessel disorder), dysproteinemia (an excess of protein in the blood), or liver disease, your doctor will closely monitor your reaction to Mevacor.

It is recommended that liver function tests be performed by your doctor before treatment with Mevacor begins, every 6 weeks during the first 3 months of therapy, every 8 weeks during the rest of the first year, and periodically (about 6-month intervals) thereafter.

This drug should be used with caution if you consume substantial quantities of alcohol or have a past history of liver disease.

Possible food and drug interactions when taking this medication

If Mevacor is taken with certain other drugs, the effects of either could be increased, decreased, or altered. It is especially important to check with your doctor before combining Mevacor with the following:

Blood-thinning drugs such as Coumadin
Cyclosporine (Sandimmune) and other immunosuppressive drugs (medication that lowers the body's defense reaction to a foreign or invading substance)
Erythromycin (E.E.S., PCE, others)
Gemfibrozil (Lopid)
Itraconazole (Sporanox)
Nicotinic acid or niacin (Nicobid)

If you are taking Mevacor in combination with nicotinic acid, Lopid, or immunosuppressive drugs such as cyclosporine, alert your doctor immediately if you experience muscle pain, tenderness, or weakness, especially with fever or general bodily discomfort. This could be the first sign of impending kidney damage.

If you are taking cyclosporine and need to take Sporanox as well, the doctor will temporarily take you off Mevacor.

Special information if you are pregnant or breastfeeding

You should take Mevacor only if pregnancy is highly unlikely. If you become pregnant while taking this drug, discontinue using it and notify your physician immediately. There may be a potential hazard to the developing baby. This medication may appear in breast milk and may have an effect on nursing infants. If this medication is essential to your health, you should discontinue breastfeeding until your treatment with this medication is finished.

Recommended dosage

ADULTS

The recommended starting dose is 20 milligrams once a day, taken with the evening meal. The maximum recommended dose is 80 milligrams per day, taken as a single dose or divided into smaller doses, as determined by your doctor. Adjustments to any dose, as determined by your doctor, should be made at intervals of 4 weeks or more.

If you are taking immunosuppressive drugs in combination with Mevacor, your dose of Mevacor should begin with 10 milligrams and should not exceed 20 milligrams per day.

Cholesterol levels should be monitored periodically by your doctor, who may decide to reduce the dose if your cholesterol level falls below the targeted range.

If you have reduced kidney function, your doctor will be cautious about increasing your dosage.

CHILDREN

The safety and effectiveness of this drug have not been established in children.

Overdosage

There have been no reported cases of overdose with Mevacor. However, if you suspect an overdose, seek medical attention immediately.

Brand name:

MICRO-K

Pronounced: MY-kroe kay
Generic name: Potassium chloride
Other brand names: Klor-Con, K-DUR,
  KAON-CL, Slow-K, Ten-K

Why is this drug prescribed?

Micro-K is used to treat or prevent low potassium levels in people who may face potassium loss caused by digitalis (Lanoxin) and non-potassium-sparing diuretics (such as Diuril and Dyazide) and certain diseases.

Potassium plays an essential role in the proper functioning of a wide range of systems in the body, including the kidneys, muscles, and nerves. As a result, a potassium deficiency may have a wide range of effects, including dry mouth, thirst, reduced urination, weakness, fatigue, drowsiness, low blood pressure, restlessness, muscle cramps, abnormal heart rate, nausea, and vomiting.

Micro-K, Klor-Con, K-DUR, KAON-CL, Slow-K and Ten-K are slow-release potassium formulations.

Most important fact about this drug

There have been reports of intestinal and gastric ulcers and bleeding associated with use of slow-release potassium chloride medications. Micro-K should be used only

by people who cannot take potassium chloride in liquid or effervescent forms.

Do not change from one brand of potassium chloride to another without consulting your doctor or pharmacist.

How should you take this medication?

Take Micro-K with meals and with water or some other liquid.

Tell your doctor if you have difficulty swallowing Micro-K. You may sprinkle the contents of the capsule onto a spoonful of soft food. Capsules should not be crushed, chewed, or sucked.

■ *If you miss a dose...*
 If it is within 2 hours of the scheduled time, take it as soon as you remember. If you do not remember until later, skip the dose you missed and go back to your regular schedule. Do not take 2 doses at once.

■ *Storage instructions...*
 Store at room temperature in a tightly closed container.

What side effects may occur?

Side effects cannot be anticipated. If any develop or change in intensity, inform your doctor as soon as possible. Only your doctor can determine if it is safe for you to continue taking Micro-K.

■ *Side effects may include:*
 Abdominal pain or discomfort
 Diarrhea
 Nausea
 Stomach and intestinal ulcers and bleeding,
  blockage, or perforation
 Vomiting

Why should this drug not be prescribed?

You should not be using Micro-K in a solid form if you are taking any drug or have any condition that could stop or slow Micro-K as it goes through the gastrointestinal tract.

If you have high potassium levels, you should not use Micro-K.

Special warnings about this medication

Before taking Micro-K, tell your doctor if you have ever had acute dehydration, heat cramps, adrenal insufficiency, diabetes, heart disease, kidney disease, liver disease, ulcers, or severe burns.

Tell your doctor immediately if you notice that your stools are black or tarry.

Possible food and drug interactions when taking this medication

If Micro-K is taken with certain other drugs, the effects of either could be increased, decreased, or altered. It is important to check with your doctor before combining Micro-K with the following:

Antispasmodic drugs such as Bentyl
Blood pressure medications classified as ACE
    inhibitors, such as Vasotec and Capoten
Digitalis (Lanoxin)
Potassium-sparing diuretics such as Midamor
    and Aldactone

Also tell your doctor if you use salt substitutes.

Special information
if you are pregnant or breastfeeding

Micro-K is generally considered safe for pregnant women or women who breastfeed their babies.

Recommended dosage

Dosages must be adjusted for each individual. Safety and effectiveness in children have not been established. The following are typical dosages for Micro-K and other leading slow-release potassium supplements.

TO TREAT LOW POTASSIUM LEVELS

Micro-K, Klor-Con 8, Slow-K
The usual dosage is 5 to 12 tablets or capsules per day.

Micro-K 10, Klor-Con 10, K-DUR 10, KAON-CL 10, Ten-K
The usual dose is 4 to 10 tablets or capsules per day.

K-DUR 20
The usual dose is 2 to 5 tablets per day.

TO PREVENT LOW POTASSIUM LEVELS

Micro-K, Klor-Con 8, Slow-K, K-DUR 10, KAON-CL 10, Ten-K
The usual dosage is 2 or 3 tablets or capsules per day.

Micro-K 10, Klor-Con 10
The usual dose is 2 tablets or capsules per day.

If you are taking more than 2 tablets or capsules per day, your total daily dose will be divided into smaller doses.

Overdosage

Any medication taken in excess can have serious consequences. Overdoses of these supplements can result in potentially fatal levels of potassium. Overdose symptoms may not be noticeable in their early stages. Therefore, if you have any reason to suspect an overdose, seek medical help immediately.

■ *Symptoms of potassium overdose may include:*
Blood in stools
Cardiac arrest
Irregular heartbeat
Muscle paralysis
Muscle weakness

Brand name:

MICRONASE

Pronounced: MIKE-roh-naze
Generic name: Glyburide
Other brand names: DiaBeta, Glynase

Why is this drug prescribed?

Micronase is an oral antidiabetic medication used to treat Type II (non-insulin-dependent) diabetes. Diabetes occurs either when the body does not make enough insulin or when the insulin that is produced no longer works properly. Insulin works by helping sugar get inside the cell, where it is then used for energy.

There are two forms of diabetes: Type I (insulin-dependent) and Type II (non-insulin-dependent). Type I diabetes usually requires insulin injections for life, while Type II diabetes can usually be treated by dietary changes, exercise, and/or oral antidiabetic medications such as Micronase. This medication controls diabetes by stimulating the pancreas to secrete more insulin and by helping insulin to work better. Type II diabetics may need insulin injections, sometimes only temporarily during stressful periods such as illness, or if an oral antidiabetic medication fails to control blood sugars, on a long-term basis.

Most important fact about this drug

Always remember that Micronase is an aid to, not a substitute for, good diet and exercise. Failure to follow a sound diet and exercise plan can lead to serious complications, such as dangerously high or low blood sugar levels. Remember, too, that Micronase is *not* an oral form of insulin, and cannot be used in place of insulin.

How should you take this medication?

In general, Micronase should be taken with breakfast or the first main meal of the day.

■ *If you miss a dose...*
Take it as soon as you remember. If it is almost time for your next dose, skip the one you missed and go back to your regular schedule. Never take 2 doses at the same time.

■ *Storage instructions...*
Keep this medication in the container it came in, tightly closed. Store it at room temperature.

What side effects may occur?

Side effects cannot be anticipated. If any develop or change in intensity, inform your doctor as soon as possible. Only your doctor can determine if it is safe for you to continue taking Micronase.

Many side effects from Micronase are rare and seldom require discontinuation of the medication.

■ *More common side effects may include:*
Bloating
Heartburn
Nausea

■ *Less common or rare side effects may include:*
Anemia and other blood disorders, blurred vision, changes in taste, headache, hives, itching, joint pain, liver problems, muscle pain, reddening of the skin, skin eruptions, skin rash, yellowing of the skin

Micronase, like all oral antidiabetics, may cause hypoglycemia (low blood sugar) especially in elderly, weak, and undernourished people, and those with kidney, liver, adrenal, or pituitary gland problems. The risk of hypoglycemia can be increased by missed meals, alcohol, other medications, fever, trauma, infection, surgery, or excessive exercise. To avoid hypoglycemia, you should closely follow the dietary and exercise plan suggested by your physician.

- *Symptoms of mild hypoglycemia may include:*
  Cold sweat
  Drowsiness
  Fast heartbeat
  Headache
  Nausea
  Nervousness

- *Symptoms of more severe hypoglycemia may include:*
  Coma
  Pale skin
  Seizures
  Shallow breathing

Eating sugar or a sugar-based product will often correct mild hypoglycemia.

Severe hypoglycemia should be considered a medical emergency, and prompt medical attention is essential.

Why should this drug not be prescribed?
You should not take Micronase if you have had an allergic reaction to it or to similar drugs such as Glucotrol or Diabinese.

Micronase should not be taken if you are suffering from diabetic ketoacidosis (a life-threatening medical emergency caused by insufficient insulin and marked by excessive thirst, nausea, fatigue, pain below the breastbone, and fruity breath).

Special warnings about this medication
It's possible that drugs such as Micronase may lead to more heart problems than diet treatment alone, or diet plus insulin. If you have a heart condition, you may want to discuss this with your doctor.

If you are taking Micronase, you should check your blood or urine periodically for abnormal sugar (glucose) levels.

It is important that you closely follow the diet and exercise plan recommended by your doctor.

The effectiveness of any oral antidiabetic, including Micronase, may decrease with time. This may occur either because of a diminished responsiveness to the medication or a worsening of the diabetes.

Possible food and drug interactions when taking this medication
If Micronase is taken with certain other drugs, the effects of either could be increased, decreased, or altered. It is especially important to check with your doctor before combining Micronase with the following:

Airway-opening drugs such as Proventil and Ventolin
Anabolic steroids such as testosterone and Danazol
Antacids such as Mylanta
Aspirin
Beta blockers such as Inderal and Tenormin
Blood thinners such as Coumadin
Calcium channel blockers such as Cardizem and Procardia
Certain antibiotics such as Cipro
Chloramphenicol (Chloromycetin)
Cimetidine (Tagamet)
Clofibrate (Atromid-S)
Estrogens such as Premarin
Fluconazole (Diflucan)
Furosemide (Lasix)
Gemfibrozil (Lopid)
Isoniazid (a drug used for tuberculosis)
Itraconazole (Sporanox)
Major tranquilizers such as Stelazine and Mellaril
MAO inhibitors (antidepressants such as

Nardil and Parnate)
Niacin (Nicolar, Nicobid)
Nonsteroidal anti-inflammatory drugs such
   as Advil, Motrin, Naprosyn, and Voltaren
Oral contraceptives
Phenytoin (Dilantin)
Probenecid (Benemid, ColBENEMID)
Steroids such as prednisone
Sulfa drugs such as Gantrisin
Thiazide diuretics such as Diuril and
   HydroDIURIL
Thyroid medications such as Synthroid

Be careful about drinking alcohol, since
excessive alcohol consumption can cause
low blood sugar.

Special information
if you are pregnant or breastfeeding

The effects of Micronase during pregnancy
have not been adequately studied in humans.
This drug should be used during pregnancy
only if the benefit outweighs the potential
risk to the unborn baby. Since studies
suggest the importance of maintaining
normal blood sugar (glucose) levels during
pregnancy, your physician may prescribe
insulin injections during pregnancy.

While it is not known if Micronase appears
in breast milk, other oral diabetes
medications do. Therefore, women should
discuss with their doctors whether to
discontinue the medication or to stop
breastfeeding. If the medication is
discontinued, and if diet alone does not
control glucose levels, then your doctor may
consider insulin injections.

Recommended dosage

Your doctor will tailor your dosage to your
individual needs.

ADULTS

Usually the doctor will prescribe an initial
daily dose of 2.5 to 5 milligrams.

Maintenance therapy usually ranges from
1.25 to 20 milligrams daily. Daily doses
greater than 20 milligrams are not
recommended. In most cases, Micronase is
taken once a day; however, people taking
more than 10 milligrams a day may respond
better to twice-a-day dosing.

CHILDREN

The safety and effectiveness of Micronase
have not been established in children.

ELDERLY

Elderly, malnourished or debilitated
individuals, or those with impaired kidney
and liver function, usually receive lower
initial and maintenance doses to minimize
the risk of low blood sugar (hypoglycemia).

Overdosage

An overdose of Micronase can cause low
blood sugar (hypoglycemia).

■ *Symptoms of severe hypoglycemia include:*
Coma
Pale skin
Seizure
Shallow breathing

If you suspect a Micronase overdose, seek
medical attention immediately.

Brand name:

MIXTARD

See Insulin, page 629.

Category:

MULTIVITAMINS

Brand names: Centrum, Theragran, Vi-Daylin

Why is this supplement prescribed?
Multivitamins are nutritional supplements for people whose diet may be deficient in certain vitamins and minerals. You may need a supplement if you are on a special diet, or don't eat the right foods. A supplement may also be necessary if you are a strict vegetarian, take medications that prevent the body from using certain nutrients, or have an illness that affects your appetite. In addition, special formulas are available for use during pregnancy.

Vitamin/mineral supplements come in a wide range of formulations. Three of the most widely used are Centrum, Theragran, and Vi-Daylin. Each of these brands offers a variety of formulas tailored to the needs of different groups.

Centrum is a multivitamin/multimineral supplement that includes all antioxidants, the vitamins that strengthen the body's natural defenses against cell damage. *Centrum Silver* contains higher strengths of the vitamins that people 50 years of age or older need the most. *Centrum, Jr.,* formulations are geared to children's needs.

Theragran is a multivitamin supplement. *Theragran-M* adds minerals to the formulation. *Theragran Stress Formula* contains higher strengths of the B vitamins that may be needed for people under stress, plus extra vitamin C.

Vi-Daylin is a multivitamin supplement; *Vi-Daylin + Iron* is a multivitamin plus iron, which may be needed by women who have heavy menstrual periods. Some Vi-Daylin formulations also contain fluoride. *Vi-Daylin*

drops are be given to infants and young children.

Most important fact about this supplement
Do not use supplements as a replacement for a diet rich in essential vitamins and minerals. Food contains many important ingredients not available in supplements.

How should you take this supplement?
Follow the dosing instructions on the bottle, or use as directed by your doctor.

Do not take more than suggested.

■ *If you miss a dose...*
If you forget to take your multivitamin for a day, don't be concerned. Resume your regular schedule the following day.

■ *Storage instructions...*
Keep out of the reach of children. Store at room temperature, and keep tightly closed.

Why should this supplement not be used?
If you have any serious chronic medical conditions check with your doctor before starting on a multivitamin supplement. You may have special requirements.

If your multivitamin supplement contains fluoride, check with your doctor. You should not use it if your drinking water contains more than 0.7 parts per million of fluoride.

Special warnings about this supplement
Do not take more of a multivitamin supplement than suggested on the packaging, or directed by your doctor. Very high doses of some vitamins and minerals can be harmful or even dangerous.

Possible food and drug interactions when taking this supplement
When taken as suggested on the packagin there are no known supplement interac

Special information
if you are pregnant or breastfeeding

Ask your doctor whether you should take a multivitamin supplement while you are pregnant or breastfeeding. Taking too much of any supplement may be harmful to you or your unborn child.

Recommended dosage

ADULTS

The usual dose is 1 tablet, teaspoonful, or tablespoonful daily according to package instructions, or as directed by your doctor.

CHILDREN

The usual dose of children's formulations is 1 tablet, teaspoonful, or dropperful daily or as directed by your doctor. Younger children may require only half this dose. Check the instructions on the package.

Overdosage

Megadoses of some vitamins and minerals can be harmful when taken for extended periods. If you have unexplained symptoms and suspect an overdose, check with your doctor.

Generic name:

MYLANTA

See Antacids, page 600.

Brand name:

NATALINS

See Stuartnatal Plus, page 684.

Generic Name:

NIACIN

Pronounced: NIE-uh-sin
Brand names: Nicolar, Nicobid

Why is this supplement prescribed?

Niacin is one of the B-complex vitamins. A severe deficiency can lead to the condition known as pellagra (diarrhea, stomach problems, skin problems, sores in the mouth, anemia, and mental problems).

Niacin is available in two forms. As niacinamide, it is found in many vitamin supplements. The other form, nicotinic acid, is also used as a supplement, but has the additional advantage of lowering the levels of fats and cholesterol circulating in the blood.

As a vitamin supplement, nicotinic acid is available over-the-counter under the brand name Nicobid. For lowering cholesterol and fats, a prescription form is available under the brand name Nicolar.

Nicolar is prescribed along with diet and other cholesterol-lowering drugs to reduce the high cholesterol levels that can clog the arteries and lead to heart disease.

Most important fact about this supplement

Before starting therapy with Nicolar, your doctor will try to control your cholesterol and triglyceride (fat) levels with a specific diet low in cholesterol and saturated fat as well as a program of exercise, and weight reduction if necessary. Nicolar is effective only when you follow your prescribed diet and continue to exercise.

How should you take this medication?

Take this medication exactly as prescribed by your doctor. To minimize the "flushing" effect of niacin, your doctor may ask you to take aspirin or nonsteroidal anti-inflammatory medications (NSAIDs) such as Motrin or Alleve before you begin niacin therapy. Do not take niacin on an empty stomach.

■ *If you miss a dose...*
Take it as soon as you remember. However, if it is almost time for your next dose, skip the one you missed and go back to your regular schedule. Do not take double doses.

■ *Storage instructions...*
Store at room temperature.

What side effects may occur?
The nicotinic acid form of niacin may cause side effects; niacinamide does not. When taking Nicolar or Nicobid, check with your doctor if you experience any of the following problems.

■ *Side effects of nicotinic acid may include:*
Allergies, darkening of the skin or urine, diarrhea, dry skin, eye disorders, gout (swollen joints), headache, indigestion, irregular heartbeat, itching, liver problems, low blood pressure, low urine output, mild-to-severe flushing, muscle pain or weakness, peptic ulcer, tingling, vomiting, warts in the armpits or genital area, yellow skin and eyes

Why should this drug not be prescribed?
Do not take niacin if you have ever had an allergic reaction to it. Make sure your doctor is aware of any drug reactions you have experienced. Also avoid niacin if you have liver disease, active peptic ulcer, or arterial bleeding. Check with your doctor before taking niacin if you have diabetes, heart problems, or have had problems with gout. In addition, you should avoid the Nicobid form of Niacin if you have gallbladder disease or the eye condition known as glaucoma.

Special warnings about this medication
Do not substitute any slowly released or timed-release form of niacin such as Nicobid if you are taking the regular (immediate-release) medication. Because the slowly released medication stays in your body longer, it is more likely to cause severe problems if your liver is weak. Before you start taking any form of niacin, your doctor may order a blood test to check your liver. Blood tests will probably be done at 6 and 12 weeks after you start niacin therapy and periodically after that. While you are taking niacin, your doctor will monitor you very closely if you have even had liver disease or if you are, or have even been, a heavy drinker. Do not drink alcohol or hot beverages with niacin as they may intensify the flushing and itching effects of the medication.

Possible food and drug interactions when taking this supplement
If you take niacin with certain other drugs, the effect of either could be increased, decreased, or altered. When combined with certain other cholesterol-lowering drugs, Nicolar sometimes can cause muscle damage. It is especially important to check with your doctor before combining niacin with the following:

Aspirin
Blood pressure drugs such as Procardia, Calan, Minipress and Hytrin
Cholesterol-lowering drugs such as Questran, Mevacor and Zocor

Special information if you are pregnant or breastfeeding
Niacin is needed during pregnancy. However, the effects of the nicotinic acid form of niacin have not been adequately studied. If you are pregnant or plan to become pregnant, notify your doctor. It is not known whether nicotinic acid appears in

breast milk. If this medication is essential to your health, your doctor may advise you to discontinue breast feeding until your treatment is finished.

Recommended dosage

ADULTS

Nicolar

Start with 1/2 tablet (250 milligrams) as a single daily dose following the evening meal. Your doctor may increase your dosage every 4 to 7 days, depending on your individual response in achieving the desired cholesterol or triglyceride level. The maximum dose is 2 to 4 tablets 2 to 3 times a day.

Nicobid

125-milligram or 250-milligram capsules: Take 1 capsule in the morning and a second in the evening. 500-milligram capsules: Take 1 capsule a day, in either the morning or evening.

Before taking 500 milligrams or more a day, consult your doctor.

CHILDREN

The safety and effectiveness of this medication in children and adolescents have not been established.

Overdosage

Any medication taken in excess can have serious consequences. If you suspect an overdose of niacin, seek medical attention immediately.

Generic name:

NICOBID

See Niacin, page 656.

Generic name:

NICOLAR

See Niacin, page 656.

Brand name:

NICOTINIC ACID

See Niacin, page 656.

Generic name:

NIZATIDINE

See Axid, page 602.

Brand name:

NOVOLIN

See Insulin, page 629.

Generic name:

OBY-CAP

See Fastin, page 624.

Generic name:

OMEPRAZOLE

See Prilosec, page 671.

Brand name:

ORINASE

Pronounced: OR-in-aze
Generic name: Tolbutamide

Why is this drug prescribed?

Orinase is an oral antidiabetic medication used to treat Type II (non-insulin-dependent) diabetes. Diabetes occurs when the body does not make enough insulin, or when the insulin that is produced no longer works properly. Insulin works by helping sugar get inside the body's cells, where it is then used for energy.

There are two forms of diabetes: Type I (insulin-dependent) and Type II (non-insulin-dependent). Type I diabetes usually requires taking insulin injections for life, while Type II diabetes can usually be treated by dietary changes, exercise, and/or oral antidiabetic medications such as Orinase. Orinase controls diabetes by stimulating the pancreas to secrete more insulin and by helping insulin work better.

Occasionally, Type II diabetics must take insulin injections temporarily during stressful periods or times of illness. When diet, exercise, and an oral antidiabetic medication fail to reduce symptoms and/or blood sugar levels, a person with Type II diabetes may require long-term insulin injections.

Most important fact about this drug

Always remember that Orinase is an aid to, not a substitute for, good diet and exercise. Failure to follow a sound diet and exercise plan can lead to serious complications, such as dangerously high or low blood sugar levels. Remember, too, that Orinase is *not* an oral form of insulin, and cannot be used in place of insulin.

How should you take this medication?

In general, Orinase should be taken 30 minutes before a meal to achieve the best control over blood sugar levels. However, the exact dosing schedule, as well as the dosage amount, must be determined by your physician. Ask your doctor when it is best for you to take this medication.

To help prevent low blood sugar levels (hypoglycemia) you should:

Understand the symptoms of hypoglycemia.
Know how exercise affects your blood sugar levels.
Maintain an adequate diet.
Keep a product containing quick-acting sugar with you at all times.
Limit alcohol intake. If you drink alcohol, it may cause breathlessness and facial flushing.

■ *If you miss a dose...*
Take it as soon as you remember. If it is almost time for the next dose, skip the one you missed and go back to your regular schedule. Do not take 2 doses at the same time.

■ *Storage instructions...*
Store at room temperature.

What side effects may occur?

Side effects cannot be anticipated. If any develop or change in intensity, inform your doctor as soon as possible. Only your doctor can determine if it is safe for you to continue taking Orinase.

Side effects from Orinase are rare and seldom require discontinuation of the medication.

■ *More common side effects may include:*
Bloating
Heartburn
Nausea

■ *Less common or rare side effects may include:*
Anemia and other blood disorders, blistering, changes in taste, headache, hepatic porphyria (a condition frequently characterized by sensitivity to light, stomach pain, and nerve damage, caused by excessive levels of a substance called porphyrin in the liver), hives, itching, redness of the skin, skin eruptions, skin rash

Orinase, like all oral antidiabetics, may cause hypoglycemia (low blood sugar). The risk of hypoglycemia can be increased by missed meals, alcohol, other medications, fever, trauma, infection, surgery, or excessive exercise. To avoid hypoglycemia, you should closely follow the dietary and exercise plan suggested by your physician.

■ *Symptoms of mild hypoglycemia may include:*
Cold sweat, drowsiness, fast heartbeat, headache, nausea, nervousness.

■ *Symptoms of more severe hypoglycemia may include:*
Coma, pale skin, seizures, shallow breathing.

Contact your doctor immediately if these symptoms of severe low blood sugar occur.

Ask your doctor what you should do if you experience mild hypoglycemia. Severe hypoglycemia should be considered a medical emergency, and prompt medical attention is essential.

Why should this drug not be prescribed?
You should not take Orinase if you have had an allergic reaction to it.

Orinase should not be taken if you are suffering from diabetic ketoacidosis (a life-threatening medical emergency caused by insufficient insulin and marked by excessive thirst, nausea, fatigue, pain below the breastbone, and fruity breath).

In addition, Orinase should not be used as the sole therapy in treating Type I (insulin-dependent) diabetes.

Special warnings about this medication
It's possible that drugs such as Orinase may lead to more heart problems than diet treatment alone, or diet plus insulin. If you have a heart condition, you may want to discuss this with your doctor.

If you are taking Orinase, you should check your blood or urine periodically for abnormal sugar (glucose) levels.

It is important that you closely follow the diet and exercise plan recommended by your doctor.

Even people with well-controlled diabetes may find that stress, illness, surgery, or fever results in a loss of control over their diabetes. In these cases, your physician may recommend that you temporarily stop taking Orinase and use injected insulin instead.

In addition, the effectiveness of any oral antidiabetic, including Orinase, may decrease with time. This may occur because of either a diminished responsiveness to the medication or a worsening of the diabetes.

Like other antidiabetic drugs, Orinase may produce severe low blood sugar if the dosage is wrong. While taking Orinase, you are particularly susceptible to episodes of low blood sugar if:

You suffer from a kidney or liver problem;

You have a lack of adrenal or pituitary hormone;

You are elderly, run-down, malnourished, hungry, exercising heavily, drinking alcohol, or using more than one glucose-lowering drug.

Possible food and drug interactions when taking this medication

If Orinase is taken with certain other drugs, the effects of either could be increased, decreased, or altered. It is especially important to check with your doctor before combining Orinase with the following:

Adrenal corticosteroids such as prednisone (Deltasone) and cortisone (Cortone)
Airway-opening drugs such as Proventil and Ventolin
Anabolic steroids such as testosterone
Barbiturates such as Amytal, Seconal, and phenobarbital
Beta blockers such as Inderal and Tenormin
Blood-thinning drugs such as Coumadin
Calcium channel blockers such as Cardizem and Procardia
Chloramphenicol (Chloromycetin)
Cinetidine (Tagamet)
Clofibrate (Atromid-S)
Colestipol (Colestid)
Epinephrine (Epipen)
Estrogens (Premarin)
Fluconazole (Diflucan)
Furosemide (Lasix)
Isoniazid (Laniazid, Rifamate)
Itracanazole (Sporanox)
Major tranquilizers such as Stelazine and Mellaril
MAO inhibitors such as Nardil and Parnate
Methyldopa (Aldomet)
Miconazole (Monistat)
Niacin (Nicobid, Nicolar)
Nonsteroidal anti-inflammatory agents such as Advil, aspirin, Motrin, Naprosyn, and Voltaren
Oral contraceptives
Phenytoin (Dilantin)
Probenecid (Benemid)

Rifampin (Rifadin)
Sulfa drugs such as Bactrim and Septra
Thiazide and other diuretics such as Diuril and HydroDIURIL
Thyroid medications such as Synthroid

Be cautious about drinking alcohol, since excessive alcohol can cause low blood sugar.

Special information if you are pregnant or breastfeeding

The effects of Orinase during pregnancy have not been adequately established in humans. Since Orinase has caused birth defects in rats, it is not recommended for use by pregnant women. Therefore, if you are pregnant or planning to become pregnant, you should take Orinase only on the advice of your physician. Since studies suggest the importance of maintaining normal blood sugar (glucose) levels during pregnancy, your physician may prescribe injected insulin during your pregnancy. While it is not known if Orinase enters breast milk, other similar medications do. Therefore, you should discuss with your doctor whether to discontinue the medication or to stop breastfeeding. If the medication is discontinued, and if diet alone does not control glucose levels, your doctor will consider giving you insulin injections.

Recommended dosage

Dosage levels are based on individual needs.

ADULTS

Usually an initial daily dose of 1 to 2 grams is recommended. Maintenance therapy usually ranges from 0.25 to 3 grams daily. Daily doses greater than 3 grams are not recommended.

CHILDREN

Safety and effectiveness have not been established in children.

ELDERLY

Elderly, malnourished, or debilitated people, or those with impaired kidney or liver function, are usually prescribed lower initial and maintenance doses to minimize the risk of low blood sugar (hypoglycemia).

Overdosage

Any medication taken in excess can have serious consequences. An overdose of Orinase can cause low blood sugar (see "Special warnings about this medication"). Eating sugar or a sugar-based product will often correct mild hypoglycemia. If you suspect an overdose, seek medical attention immediately.

Brand name:

OS-CAL 500

See Caltrate 600, page 608.

Brand name:

OYSTERCAL 500

See Caltrate 600, page 608.

Generic name:

PAROXETINE

See Paxil, page 662.

Brand name:

PAXIL

Pronounced: PACKS-ill
Generic name: Paroxetine hydrochloride

Why is this drug prescribed?

Paxil is prescribed for a serious, continuing depression that interferes with your ability to function. Symptoms of this type of depression often include changes in appetite and sleep patterns, a persistent low mood, loss of interest in people and activities, decreased sex drive, feelings of guilt or worthlessness, suicidal thoughts, difficulty concentrating, and slowed thinking.

Most important fact about this drug

Your depression may seem to improve within 1 to 4 weeks after beginning treatment with Paxil. Even if you feel better, continue to take the medication as long as your doctor tells you to do so.

How should you take this medication?

Take this medication exactly as prescribed by your doctor. Inform your doctor if you are taking or plan to take any prescription or over-the-counter drugs, since they may interact unfavorably with Paxil.

■ *If you miss a dose...*
  Skip the forgotten dose and go back to your regular schedule with the next dose. Do not take a double dose to make up for the one you missed.

■ *Storage instructions...*
  Paxil can be stored at room temperature.

What side effects may occur?

Side effects cannot be anticipated. If any develop or change in intensity, inform your doctor as soon as possible. Only your doctor can determine whether it is safe for you to continue taking this medication.

Over a 4 to 6 week period, you may find some side effects less troublesome (nausea and dizziness, for example) than others (dry mouth, drowsiness, and weakness).

■ *More common side effects may include:* Constipation, decreased appetite, diarrhea, dizziness, drowsiness, dry mouth, gas, male genital disorders, nausea, nervousness, sleeplessness, sweating, tremor, weakness

■ *Less common side effects may include:* Agitation, altered taste sensation, anxiety, blurred vision, burning or tingling sensation, decreased sex drive, drugged feeling, increased appetite, muscle tenderness or weakness, pounding heartbeat, rash, tightness in throat, twitching, upset stomach, urinary disorders, vomiting, yawning

Why should this drug not be prescribed?

Do not take Paxil if you are also taking an MAO inhibitor antidepressant or within 14 days after you discontinue treatment with this type of medication.

Special warnings about this medication

Paxil should be used cautiously by people with a history of manic disorders.

If you have a history of seizures, make sure your doctor knows about it. Paxil should be used with caution in this situation. If you develop seizures once therapy has begun, the drug should be discontinued.

If you have a disease or condition that affects your metabolism or blood circulation, make sure your doctor is aware of it. Paxil should be used cautiously in this situation.

Paxil may impair your judgment, thinking, or motor skills. Do not drive, operate dangerous machinery, or participate in any hazardous activity that requires full mental alertness until you are sure the medication is not affecting you in this way.

Possible food and drug interactions when taking this medication

Do not drink alcohol during your treatment with Paxil.

If Paxil is taken with certain other drugs, the effects of either could be increased, decreased, or altered. It is especially important to check with your doctor before combining Paxil with any of the following:

Antidepressants such as Elavil, Tofranil, Norpramin, Pamelor, Prozac, Nardil, Marplan, and Parnate
Cimetidine (Tagamet)
Diazepam (Valium)
Digoxin (Lanoxin)
Flecainide (Tambocor)
Lithium (Lithonate)
Phenobarbital
Phenytoin (Dilantin)
Procyclidine (Kemadrin)
Propafenone (Rythmol)
Propranolol (Inderal, Inderide)
Quinidine (Quinaglute)
Thioridazine (Mellaril)
Tryptophan
Warfarin (Coumadin)

Special information if you are pregnant or breastfeeding

The effects of Paxil during pregnancy have not been adequately studied. If you are pregnant or plan to become pregnant, inform your doctor immediately. Paxil appears in breast milk and could affect a nursing infant. If this medication is essential to your health, your doctor may advise you to discontinue breastfeeding until your treatment with Paxil is finished.

Recommended dosage

ADULTS

The usual starting dose is 20 milligrams a day, taken as a single dose, usually in the morning. Your physician may increase your dosage by 10 milligrams a day, up to a maximum of 50 milligrams a day.

CHILDREN

The safety and effectiveness of this drug in children have not been established.

ELDERLY

The recommended initial dose for elderly or weak individuals or those with severe kidney or liver disease is 10 milligrams a day. Your doctor may increase the dosage if needed, but it should not exceed 40 milligrams a day.

Overdosage

Any medication taken in excess can have serious consequences. If you suspect an overdose, seek medical attention immediately.

■ *The symptoms of Paxil overdose may include:*
Drowsiness
Enlarged pupils
Nausea
Rapid heartbeat
Vomiting

Brand name:

PENTASA

See Rowasa, page 681.

Brand name:

PEPCID

Pronounced: PEP-sid
Generic name: Famotidine

Why is this drug prescribed?

Pepcid is prescribed for the short-term treatment of active duodenal ulcer (in the upper intestine) for 4 to 8 weeks and for active, benign gastric ulcer (in the stomach) for 6 to 8 weeks. It is prescribed for maintenance therapy, at reduced dosage, after a duodenal ulcer has healed. It is also used for short-term treatment of GERD, a condition in which the acid contents of the stomach flow back into the esophagus, and for resulting inflammation of the esophagus. And it is prescribed for certain diseases that cause the stomach to produce excessive quantities of acid, such as Zollinger-Ellison syndrome. Pepcid belongs to a class of drugs known as histamine H_2 blockers.

Most important fact about this drug

To cure your ulcer, you need to take Pepcid for the full time of treatment your doctor prescribes. Keep taking the drug even if you begin to feel better.

How should you take this medication?

It may take several days for Pepcid to begin relieving stomach pain. You can use antacids for the pain, but should avoid taking them within 1 hour of a dose of Pepcid.

If you are taking Pepcid suspension, shake it vigorously for 5 to 10 seconds before use. ·

■ *If you miss a dose...*
Take it as soon as you remember. If it is almost time for your next dose, skip the one you missed and go back to your regular schedule. Do not take 2 doses at once.

■ *Storage instructions...*
Store at room temperature. Protect the suspension from freezing. Discard any unused portion after 30 days.

What side effects may occur?
Side effects cannot be anticipated. If any develop or change in intensity, inform your doctor as soon as possible. Only your doctor can determine if it is safe for you to continue taking Pepcid.

The most common side effect is headache.

■ *Less common or rare side effects may include:*
Abdominal discomfort, acne, agitation, altered taste, anxiety, breast development in males, changes in behavior, confusion, constipation, decreased sex drive, depression, diarrhea, difficulty sleeping, dizziness, dry mouth, dry skin, facial swelling due to fluid retention, fatigue, fever, flushing, grand mal seizures, hair loss, hallucinations, hives, impotence, irregular heartbeat, itching, loss of appetite, muscle, bone, or joint pain, nausea, pounding heartbeat, prickling, tingling, or pins and needles, rash, ringing in ears, severe allergic reation, sleepiness, vomiting, weakness, wheezing, yellow eyes and skin

Why should this drug not be prescribed?
If you are sensitive to or have ever had an allergic reaction to Pepcid, you should not take this medication. Make sure your doctor is aware of any drug reactions you have experienced.

Special warnings about this medication
If you have stomach cancer, Pepcid may relieve the symptoms without curing the disease. Your doctor will be careful to rule out this possibility.

Use Pepcid with caution if you have severe kidney disease.

Possible food and drug interactions when taking this medication
If Pepcid is taken with certain other drugs, the effects of either can be increased, decreased, or altered. It is especially important that you check with your doctor before combining Pepcid with the following:

Itraconazole (Sporanox)
Ketoconazole (Nizoral)

Special information if you are pregnant or breastfeeding
The effects of Pepcid during pregnancy have not been adequately studied. If you are pregnant or plan to become pregnant, inform your doctor immediately. Pepcid may appear in breast milk and could affect a nursing infant. If this medication is essential to your health, your doctor may advise you to discontinue breastfeeding until your treatment with this medication is finished.

Recommended dosage
ADULTS

For Duodenal Ulcer
The usual starting dose is 40 milligrams or 5 milliliters (1 teaspoonful) once a day at bedtime. Results should be seen within 4 weeks, and this medication should not be used at full dosage longer than 6 to 8 weeks. Your doctor may have you take 20 milligrams or 2.5 milliliters (one-half teaspoonful) twice a day. The normal maintenance dose after your ulcer has healed is 20 milligrams or 2.5 milliliters (one-half teaspoonful) once a day at bedtime.

Benign Gastric Ulcer
The usual dose is 40 milligrams or 5 milliliters (1 teaspoonful) once a day at bedtime.

Gastroesophageal Reflux Disease (GERD)
The usual dose is 20 milligrams or 2.5 milliliters (one-half teaspoonful) twice a day for up to 6 weeks. For inflammation of the esophagus due to GERD, the dose is 20 or 40 milligrams or 2.5 to 5 milliliters twice a day for up to 12 weeks.

Excess Acid Conditions (such as Zollinger-Ellison Syndrome)
The usual starting dose is 20 milligrams every 6 hours, although some people need a higher dose.

If your kidneys are not functioning properly, your doctor will adjust the dosage.

CHILDREN

The safety and effectiveness of Pepcid have not been established in children.

Overdosage
Any medication taken in excess can have serious consequences. If you suspect an overdose, seek medical attention immediately.

Brand name:

PERDIEM FIBER

See Metamucil, page 646.

Generic name:

PHENOBARBITAL, HYOSCYAMINE, ATROPINE, AND SCOPOLAMINE

See Donnatal, page 621.

Generic name:

PHENTERMINE

See Fastin, page 624.

Generic name:

PHENYLPROPANOLAMINE

See Acutrim, page 599.

Brand name:

POLY-VI-FLOR

Pronounced: pol-ee-VIE-floor
Generic ingredients: Vitamins, Fluoride

Why is this drug prescribed?
Poly-Vi-Flor is a multivitamin and fluoride supplement with 10 essential vitamins plus the mineral fluoride. It is prescribed for children aged 2 and older to provide fluoride where the drinking water contains less than the amount recommended by the American Dental Association to build strong teeth and prevent cavities. Poly-Vi-Flor supplies significant amounts of other vitamins to avoid deficiencies. The American Academy of Pediatrics recommends that children up to age 16 take a fluoride supplement if they live in areas where the drinking water contains less than the recommended amount of fluoride.

Most important fact about this drug
Do not give your child more than the recommended dose. Too much fluoride can cause discoloration and pitting of teeth.

How should you take this medication?
Do not give your child more than your doctor prescribes.

Poly-Vi-Flor should be chewed or crushed before swallowing.

- *If you miss a dose...*
  Take it as soon as you remember. If it is almost time for the next dose, skip the one you missed and go back to your regular schedule. Do not take 2 doses at once.

- *Storage instructions...*
  Store away from heat, light, and moisture.

What side effects may occur?
Rarely, an allergic rash has occurred.

Why should this drug not be prescribed?
Children should not take Poly-Vi-Flor if they are getting significant amounts of fluoride from other medications or sources.

Special warnings about this medication
Do not give your child more than the recommended dosage. Your child's teeth should be checked periodically for discoloration or pitting. Notify your doctor if white, brown, or black spots appear on your child's teeth.

The fluoride level of your drinking water should be determined before Poly-Vi-Flor is prescribed.

Let your doctor know if you change drinking water or filtering systems.

Fluoride does not replace proper dental habits, such as brushing, flossing, and having dental checkups.

Recommended dosage
The usual dose is 1 tablet every day as prescribed by the doctor.

Overdosage
Although overdose is unlikely, any medication taken in excess can have serious consequences. If you suspect an overdose, seek medical treatment immediately.

Brand name:

PONDIMIN

Pronounced: PON-di-min
Generic name: Fenfluramine hydrochloride

Why is this drug prescribed?
Pondimin is an appetite suppressant for short-term use in weight-loss programs. Pondimin is used in conjunction with a diet and exercise plan designed to help change eating habits and promote a healthier lifestyle. It is available only by prescription.

Most important fact about this drug
Do not take more of this medication than prescribed by your doctor. If you find that you are regaining your appetite, you may be building up a tolerance to the medication. Do not increase the dose to renew the effect. Too much Pondimin for too long a period can become habit-forming. Check with your doctor before you increase your dose.

How should you take this medication?
Take Pondimin 3 times a day, before meals.

- *If you miss a dose...*
  Take it as soon as you remember if it is within an hour or so of your scheduled time. If you do not remember until later, skip the dose you missed and go back to your regular schedule. Do not take 2 doses at once.

- *Storage instructions...*
  Store at room temperature. Keep tightly closed.

What side effects may occur?
Side effects cannot be anticipated. If any develop or change in intensity, tell your

doctor as soon as possible. Only your doctor can determine whether it is safe for you to continue taking Pondimin.

■ *More common side effects may include:*
Diarrhea
Drowsiness
Dry mouth

■ *Less common side effects may include:*
Anxiety, blurred vision, changes in sexual drive, chest pain, chills, clumsiness or unsteadiness, confusion, constipation, depression, difficulty in talking, dizziness, eye irritation, fainting, false sense of well being, fevers, headache, heart palpitations, hives, insomnia, low and high blood pressure, muscle pain, nausea, nervousness or tenseness, painful and frequent urination, rash, restlessness, stomach cramps, sweating, unpleasant taste, weakness or fatigue

Why should this drug not be prescribed?
If you are sensitive to or have ever had an allergic reaction to Pondimin or drugs of this type such as pseudoephedrine (Sudafed), phenylpropanolamine (Acutrim), ephedrine (Mudrane), phenylephrine (Entex), or terbutaline (Brethine), do not take Pondimin. You should also avoid taking Pondimin within 14 days of taking a monoamine oxidase (MAO) inhibitor, such as Nardil or Parnate, for depression.

Do not take Pondimin if you have a history of alcohol or drug abuse, or mental illness.

Special warnings about this medication
If you have very high blood pressure or heart disease, including problems with irregular heartbeat, Pondimin is not recommended. Make sure your doctor is aware of the problem. He may want to monitor your blood pressure while you are taking Pondimin.

Do not suddenly stop taking Pondimin without checking with your doctor.

Pondimin may cause you to become drowsy or less alert. Until you know how you react to this medication, do not drive or operate dangerous machinery or participate in any activity requiring mental alertness.

If you have to undergo emergency or elective surgery of any kind, tell your doctor or dentist that you are taking Pondimin. It can affect your response to anesthesia. Also tell your doctor if you notice any changes in your ability to exercise or perform physical tasks while on Pondimin.

If you have a history of depressive illness, be sure to tell your doctor, since this medication may increase depressive moods.

Possible food and drug interactions when taking this medication
If Pondimin is taken with certain other drugs, the effects of either could be increased, decreased, or altered. It is especially important to consult your doctor before taking Pondimin with any of the following:

Alcohol
Barbiturates such as phenobarbital and pentobarbital (Nembutal)
Antidepressants classified as MAO inhibitors, such as Nardil and Parnate
Blood pressure drugs such as Esimil, Aldomet and Reserpine
Chlordiazepoxide (Librium)
Reserpine
Temazepam (Restoril)

Special Information if you are pregnant or breastfeeding
The effects of Pondimin during pregnancy have not been adequately studied. If you are pregnant or plan to become pregnant, tell your doctor immediately. It is not known

whether this drug passes into breast milk and may affect a nursing infant. If the medication is essential to your health, your doctor may advise you to discontinue breastfeeding until your treatment with the drug is finished.

Recommended dosage

ADULTS

Your doctor will monitor your response to this medication carefully and will gradually increase or decrease the dose to suit your needs.

The usual starting dose is 20 milligrams 3 times a day, taken before meals. Your doctor may increase the dose each week by 20 milligrams per day to a maximum dose of 2 tablets 3 times per day. You should not take more than a total of 120 milligrams per day.

CHILDREN

Safety and effectiveness in children below the age of 12 have not been established.

Overdosage

Any medication taken in excess can have symptoms of overdose. If you suspect an overdose, seek medical attention immediately.

■ *The most frequent symptoms of Pondimin overdose include:*
Abdominal pain, agitation, confusion, dilated pupils, drowsiness, fever, flushing, hyperventilation (rapid breathing), irregular heartbeat, sweating, trembling or shaking

Massive overdose can lead to coma, convulsions, and cardiac arrest.

Generic name:

POTASSIUM CHLORIDE

See Micro-K, page 650.

Brand name:

PRAVACHOL

Pronounced: PRAV-a-coll
Generic name: Pravastatin sodium

Why is this drug prescribed?

Pravachol is a cholesterol-lowering drug. Your doctor may prescribe it along with a cholesterol-lowering diet if your blood cholesterol level is dangerously high, and if you have not been able to lower it by diet alone.

The drug works by helping to clear harmful low-density lipoprotein (LDL) cholesterol out of the blood and by limiting the body's ability to form new LDL cholesterol.

Most important fact about this drug

Pravachol is usually prescribed only if diet, exercise, and weight-loss fail to bring your cholesterol levels under control. It's important to remember that Pravachol is a supplement—not a substitute—for those other measures. To get the full benefit of the medication, you need to stick to the diet and exercise program prescribed by your doctor. All these efforts to keep your cholesterol levels normal are important because together they may lower your risk of heart disease.

How should you take this medication?

For an even greater cholesterol-lowering effect, your doctor may prescribe Pravachol along with a different kind of lipid-lowering drug such as Questran or Colestid. However, you must not take Pravachol at the same time of day as the other cholesterol-lowering drug. Take Pravachol at least 1 hour before or 4 hours after taking the other drug.

Pravachol should be taken once daily at bedtime. You may take it with or without food.

Your doctor will probably do blood tests for cholesterol levels every 4 weeks to determine the effectiveness of the dose.

■ *If you miss a dose...*
Take the forgotten dose as soon as you remember. If it is almost time for your next dose, skip the one you missed and go back to your regular schedule. Do not take a double dose.

■ *Storage instructions...*
Store at room temperature, in a tightly closed container away from moisture and light.

What side effects may occur?
Side effects from Pravachol cannot be anticipated. If any develop or change in intensity, inform your doctor as soon as possible. Only your doctor can determine if it is safe for you to continue taking Pravachol.

■ *Side effects may include:*
Abdominal pain, chest pain, cold, constipation, cough, diarrhea, dizziness, fatigue, flu, gas, headache, heartburn, inflammation of nasal passages, muscle aching or weakness, nausea, rash, urinary problems, vomiting

Why should this drug not be prescribed?
Do not take Pravachol if you are sensitive or have ever had an allergic reaction to it.

Do not take Pravachol if you have liver disease.

Special warnings about this medication
Pravachol should not be used to try to lower high cholesterol that stems from a medical condition such as alcoholism, poorly controlled diabetes, an underactive thyroid gland, or a kidney or liver problem.

Because Pravachol may cause damage to the liver, your doctor will do blood tests regularly. Your doctor should monitor you especially closely if you have ever had liver disease or if you are or have ever been a heavy drinker.

Since Pravachol may cause damage to muscle tissue, promptly report to your doctor any unexplained muscle pain, tenderness, or weakness, especially if you also have a fever or you just generally do not feel well.

Possible food and drug interactions when taking this medication
If Pravachol is taken with certain other drugs, the effects of either could be increased, decreased, or altered. It is especially important to check with your doctor before combining Pravachol with the following:

Cholestyramine (Questran)
Cimetidine (Tagamet)
Colestipol (Colestid)
Erythromycin (E.E.S., Erythrocin, others)
Gemfibrozil (Lopid)
Immunosuppressive drugs such as
    Sandimmune
Niacin
Warfarin (Coumadin)

Special information
if you are pregnant or breastfeeding
You must not become pregnant while taking Pravachol. Because this drug lowers cholesterol, and cholesterol is necessary for the proper development of an unborn baby, there is some suspicion that Pravachol might cause birth defects. Your doctor will

prescribe Pravachol only if you are highly unlikely to become pregnant while taking the drug. If you do become pregnant while taking Pravachol, inform your doctor immediately.

Because Pravachol appears in breast milk, and because its cholesterol-lowering effects might prove harmful to a nursing baby, you should not take Pravachol while you are breastfeeding.

Recommended dosage

ADULTS

The usual starting dose is 10 to 20 milligrams once a day at bedtime.

For ongoing therapy, the recommended dose is 10 to 40 milligrams, once a day at bedtime.

ELDERLY

The usual starting dose is 10 milligrams a day at bedtime; for ongoing therapy, the dose is 20 milligrams per day or less.

Overdosage

Although no specific information is available, any medication taken in excess can have serious consequences. If you suspect an overdose of Pravachol, seek medical attention immediately.

Generic name:

PRAVASTATIN

See Pravachol, page 669.

Generic name:

PRENATAL VITAMINS AND MINERALS

See Stuartnatal Plus, page 684.

Brand name:

PRILOSEC

Pronounced: PRILL-oh-sek
Generic name: Omeprazole

Why is this drug prescribed?

Prilosec is prescribed for the short-term treatment (4 to 8 weeks) of active duodenal ulcer, gastroesophageal reflux disease (backflow of acid stomach contents), and severe erosive esophagitis (inflammation of the esophagus). It is also used for the long-term treatment of conditions in which too much stomach acid is secreted such as Zollinger-Ellison syndrome, multiple endocrine adenomas (benign tumors), and systemic mastocytosis (cancerous cells).

Most important fact about this drug

Prilosec is not intended for long-term therapy after an ulcer has healed.

How should you take this medication?

Prilosec works best when taken before meals. It can be taken with an antacid.

The capsule should be swallowed whole. It should not be opened, chewed, or crushed.

Avoid excessive amounts of caffeine while taking this drug.

It may take several days for Prilosec to begin relieving stomach pain. Be sure to continue taking the drug exactly as prescribed even if it seems to have no affect.

■ *If you miss a dose...*
Take it as soon as you remember. If it is almost time for your next dose, skip the one you missed and go back to your regular schedule. Do not take 2 doses at once.

■ *Storage information...*
Store at room temperature in a tightly closed container, away from light and moisture.

What side effects may occur?
Side effects cannot be anticipated. If any develop or change in intensity, inform your doctor as soon as possible. Only your doctor can determine if it is safe for you to continue taking Prilosec.

■ *More common side effects may include:*
Abdominal pain
Diarrhea
Headache
Nausea
Vomiting

■ *Less common or rare side effects may include:*
Abdominal swelling, abnormal dreams, aggression, anemia, anxiety, apathy, back pain, breast development in males, blood in urine, changes in liver function, chest pain, confusion, constipation, cough, depression, difficulty sleeping, discolored feces, dizziness, dry mouth, dry skin, fatigue, fever, fluid retention and swelling, fluttery heartbeat, frequent urination, gas, general feeling of illness, hair loss, hallucinations, hepatitis, high blood pressure, hives, irritable colon, itching, joint and leg pain, loss of appetite, low blood sugar, muscle cramps and pain, nervousness, nosebleeds, pain, pain in testicles, rapid heartbeat, rash, ringing in ears, skin inflammation, sleepiness, slow heartbeat, taste distortion, tingling or pins and needles, throat pain, tremors, upper respiratory infection, urinary tract infection, vertigo, weakness, weight gain, yellow eyes and skin

Why should this drug not be prescribed?
If you are sensitive to or have ever had an allergic reaction to Prilosec or any of its ingredients, you should not take this medication. Make sure your doctor is aware of any drug reactions you have experienced.

Special warnings about this medication
The safety of long-term use of this drug has not been established.

Possible food and drug interactions when taking this medication
If Prilosec is taken with certain other drugs, the effects of either could be increased, decreased, or altered. It is especially important to check with your doctor before combining Prilosec with the following:

Ampicillin-containing drugs such as
   Spectrobid
Cyclosporine (Sandimmune)
Diazepam (Valium)
Disulfiram (Antabuse)
Iron
Ketoconazole (Nizoral)
Phenytoin (Dilantin)
Warfarin (Coumadin)

Special information if you are pregnant or breastfeeding
The effects of Prilosec during pregnancy have not been adequately studied. If you are pregnant or plan to become pregnant, inform your doctor immediately. Prilosec may appear in breast milk and could affect a nursing infant. If this medication is essential to your health, your doctor may advise you to discontinue breastfeeding until your treatment with this medication is finished.

Recommended dosage

ADULTS

Short-term Treatment of Active Duodenal Ulcer
The usual dose is 20 milligrams once a day. Most people heal within 4 weeks.

Severe Erosive Esophagitis or Poorly Responsive Gastroesophageal Reflux Disease (GERD)
The usual dose is 20 milligrams daily for 4 to 8 weeks.

Pathological Hypersecretory Conditions
The usual starting dose is 60 milligrams once a day. If you take more than 80 milligrams a day, your doctor will divide the total into smaller doses. The dosing will be based on your needs.

CHILDREN

The safety and effectiveness of Prilosec in children have not been established.

Overdosage

No specific symptoms of Prilosec overdose are known, but any medication taken in excess can have serious consequences. If you suspect an overdose of Prilosec, seek medical attention immediately.

Generic name:

PROBENECID WITH COLCHICINE

See ColBENEMID, page 613.

Generic name:

PROBUCOL

See Lorelco, page 642.

Brand name:

PROPULSID

Pronounced: pro-PUHL-sid
Generic name: Cisapride

Why is this drug prescribed?

Propulsid is prescribed to treat nighttime heartburn caused by gastroesophageal reflux disease, a condition in which the valve between the esophagus and the stomach opens or leaks, allowing stomach acid to back up and cause burning or "heartburn."

Most important fact about this drug

Propulsid by itself rarely causes drowsiness. However, it may speed up the effects of alcoholic beverages and tranquilizers.

How should you take this medication?

Take your medication 15 minutes before meals and at bedtime. Take Propulsid exactly as prescribed, even if your symptoms disappear.

■ *If you miss a dose...*
Take the forgotten dose as soon as you remember. If it is almost time for your next dose, skip the one you missed and go back to your regular schedule. Do not take 2 doses at once.

■ *Storage instructions...*
Store at room temperature. Protect from moisture.

What side effects may occur?

Side effects cannot be anticipated. If any develop or change in intensity, tell your doctor as soon as possible. Only your doctor can determine if it is safe for you to continue taking Propulsid.

■ *More common side effects may include:*
Abdominal pain
Bloating/gas
Constipation

Diarrhea
Headache
Inflamed nasal passages and sinuses
Nausea
Pain
Upper respiratory and viral infections

■ *Less common side effects may include:*
Abnormal vision, anxiety, back pain, chest
pain, coughing, depression, dehydration,
dizziness, fever, fatigue, frequent urination,
indigestion, insomnia, itching, inflammation
of the vagina, joint pain, muscle pain,
nervousness, rash, sore throat, urinary
tract infection, vomiting

Why should this drug not be prescribed?
You should not use Propulsid if you have
bleeding, blockage, or leakage in the
stomach or intestines. Do not take this drug
at the same time as Nizoral, Sporanox,
Monistat IV, or TAO. Also avoid Propulsid
if you are sensitive to or have ever had an
allergic reaction to it.

Special warnings about this medication
Propulsid is used only for nighttime
heartburn. It has not been shown to be
effective for daytime heartburn.

Rare, but serious, irregular heartbeats have
occurred in some people taking Propulsid;
tell your doctor if you have had any heart
trouble.

**Possible food and drug interactions
when taking this medication**
If Propulsid is taken with certain other
drugs, the effects of either could be
increased, decreased, or altered. It is
especially important to check with your
doctor before combining Propulsid with the
following:

Alcohol
Antispasmodic drugs such as Bentyl and
Cogentin

Cimetidine (Tagamet)
Itraconazole (Sporanox)
Ketoconazole (Nizoral)
Miconazole (Monistat IV)
Ranitidine (Zantac)
Tranquilizers such as Librium, Valium, and
Xanax
Troleandomycin (TAO)
Warfarin (Coumadin)

Remember that Propulsid may increase the
effects of alcohol. If you are taking blood
thinners (Warfarin), your doctor will give
you a blood test 1 week after you start on
Propulsid and after your therapy is
completed. Your blood-thinning medication
may need to be adjusted.

**Special information
if you are pregnant or breastfeeding**
The effects of Propulsid during pregnancy
have not been adequately studied. If you are
pregnant or plan to become pregnant, tell
your doctor immediately. The drug appears
in breast milk and could affect a nursing
infant. If this medication is essential to your
health, your doctor may advise you to
discontinue breastfeeding until your
treatment is finished.

Recommended dosage
ADULTS

The usual starting dose is 10 milligrams of
Propulsid 4 times daily, taken at least 15
minutes before meals and at bedtime.

Your doctor may need to adjust your
dosage to 20 milligrams 4 times daily,
depending on how well the drug works for
you.

CHILDREN

The safety and effectiveness of Propulsid in
children have not been established.

Overdosage

Any medication taken in excess can have serious consequences. If you suspect an overdose, seek medical attention immediately.

■ *Symptoms of Propulsid overdose may include:*
Frequent urination or bowel movements
Gas
Gurgling and rumbling in the stomach
Retching

Brand name:

PROZAC

Pronounced: PRO-zak
Generic name: Fluoxetine hydrochloride

Why is this drug prescribed?

Prozac is prescribed for the treatment of depression, that is, a continuing depression that interferes with daily functioning. The symptoms of major depression often include changes in appetite, sleep habits, and mind/body coordination; decreased sex drive; increased fatigue; feelings of guilt or worthlessness; difficulty concentrating; slowed thinking; and suicidal thoughts.

Prozac is also prescribed to treat obsessive-compulsive disorder. An obsession is a thought that won't go away; a compulsion is an action done over and over to relieve anxiety.

Prozac is thought to work by adjusting the balance of the brain's natural chemical messengers. It has also been used to treat obesity and eating disorders.

Most important fact about this drug

Serious, sometimes fatal, reactions have been known to occur when Prozac is used in combination with other antidepressant drugs known as MAO inhibitors, including Nardil, Parnate, and Marplan; and when Prozac is discontinued and an MAO inhibitor is started. Never take Prozac with one of these drugs or within 14 days of discontinuing therapy with one of them; and allow 5 weeks or more between stopping Prozac and starting an MAO inhibitor. Be especially cautious if you have been taking Prozac in high doses or for a long time.

If you are taking any prescription or nonprescription drugs, notify your doctor before taking Prozac.

How should you take this medication?

Prozac should be taken exactly as prescribed by your doctor.

Prozac usually is taken once or twice a day. To be effective, it should be taken regularly. Make a habit of taking it at the same time you do some other daily activity.

■ *If you miss a dose...*
Take the forgotten dose as soon as you remember. If several hours have passed, skip the dose. Never try to "catch up" by doubling the dose.

■ *Storage instructions...*
Store at room temperature.

What side effects may occur?

Side effects cannot be anticipated. If any develop or change in intensity, inform your doctor as soon as possible. Only your doctor can determine if it is safe for you to continue taking Prozac.

■ *More common side effects may include:*
Abnormal dreams, abnormal thinking, agitation, allergic reaction, anxiety, bronchitis, chest pain, chills, cough, diarrhea, dizziness, drowsiness and fatigue, dry mouth, flu symptoms, frequent urination, hay fever, headache, inability to

fall or stay asleep, increased appetite, indigestion, itching, joint pain, lack or loss of appetite, light-headedness, limb pain, muscle pain, nausea, nervousness, sinus inflammation, sore throat, stomach/intestinal disorder, sweating, tremors, weakness, weight loss, yawning

■ *Less common side effects may include:*
Abnormal ejaculation, abnormal gait, abnormal stoppage of menstrual flow, acne, altered sense of taste, amnesia, apathy, arthritis, asthma, bone pain, breast cysts, breast pain, brief loss of consciousness, bursitis, chills and fever, confusion, conjunctivitis, convulsions, dark, tarry stool, decreased sex drive, difficulty in swallowing, dilation of pupils, dry skin, ear pain, eye pain, exaggerated feeling of well-being, excessive bleeding, facial swelling due to fluid retention, fever, fluid retention, fluttery heartbeat, gas, hair loss, hallucinations, hangover effect, hiccups, high or low blood pressure, hives, hostility, impotence, infection, inflammation of the esophagus, inflammation of the gums, inflammation of the stomach lining, inflammation of the tongue, inflammation of the vagina, intolerance of light, involuntary movement, irrational ideas, irregular heartbeat, jaw or neck pain, lack of muscle coordination, low blood pressure upon standing, low blood sugar, migraine headach e, mouth inflammation, muscle spasm, neck pain and rigidity, nosebleed, ovarian disorders, paranoid reaction, pelvic pain, pneumonia, rapid breathing, rapid heartbeat, ringing in the ears, severe chest pain, skin inflammation, skin rash, thirst, tooth problems, twitching, uncoordinated movements, urinary disorders, vague feeling of bodily discomfort, vertigo, vision disturbances, vomiting, weight gain

■ *Rare side effects may include:*
Antisocial behavior, blood in urine, bloody diarrhea, bone disease, breast enlargement, cataracts, colitis, coma, deafness, decreased reflexes, dehydration, double vision, drooping of eyelids, duodenal ulcer, enlarged abdomen, enlargement of liver, enlargement or increased activity of thyroid gland, excess growth of coarse hair on face, chest, etc., excess uterine or vaginal bleeding, extreme muscle tension, eye bleeding, female milk production, fluid accumulation and swelling in the head, fluid buildup in larynx and lungs, gallstones, glaucoma, gout, heart attack, hepatitis, high blood sugar, hysteria, inability to control bowel movements, increased salivation, inflammation of eyes and eyelids, inflammation of fallopian tubes, inflammation of testes, inflammation of the gallbladder, inflammation of the small intestine, inflammation of tissue below skin, kidney disorders, lung inflammation, menstrual disorders, miscarriage, mouth sores, muscle inflammation or bleeding, muscle spasms, pai nful sexual intercourse for women, psoriasis, rashes, reddish or purplish spots on the skin, reduction of body temperature, rheumatoid arthritis, seborrhea, shingles, skin discoloration, skin inflammation and disorders, slowing of heart rate, slurred speech, spitting blood, stomach ulcer, stupor, suicidal thoughts, taste loss, temporary cessation of breathing, tingling sensation around the mouth, tongue discoloration and swelling, urinary tract disorders, vomiting blood, yellow eyes and skin

Why should this drug not be prescribed?
If you are sensitive to or have ever had an allergic reaction to Prozac or similar drugs, you should not take this medication. Make

sure that your doctor is aware of any drug reactions that you have experienced.

Do not take this drug while using an MAO inhibitor. (See "Most important fact about this drug.")

Special warnings about this medication
Unless you are directed to do so by your doctor, do not take this medication if you are recovering from a heart attack or if you have kidney or liver disease or diabetes.

Prozac may cause you to become drowsy or less alert and may affect your judgment. Therefore, driving or operating dangerous machinery or participating in any hazardous activity that requires full mental alertness is not recommended.

While taking this medication, you may feel dizzy or light-headed or actually faint when getting up from a lying or sitting position. If getting up slowly doesn't help or if this problem continues, notify your doctor.

If you develop a skin rash or hives while taking Prozac, discontinue use of the medication and notify your doctor immediately.

Prozac should be used with caution if you have a history of seizures. You should discuss all of your medical conditions with your doctor before taking this medication.

The safety and effectiveness of Prozac have not been established in children.

Possible food and drug interactions when taking this medication
Combining Prozac with MAO inhibitors is dangerous.

Do not drink alcohol while taking this medication.

If Prozac is taken with certain other drugs, the effects of either could be increased, decreased, or altered. It is especially important to check with your doctor before combining Prozac with the following:

Carbamazepine (Tegretol)
Diazepam (Valium)
Digitoxin (Crystodigin)
Drugs that act on the central nervous system (brain and spinal cord) such as Xanax
Flecainide (Tambocor)
Lithium (Eskalith)
Other antidepressants (Elavil)
Phenytoin (Dilantin)
Tryptophan
Vinblastine (Velban)
Warfarin (Coumadin)

**Special information
if you are pregnant or breastfeeding**
The effects of Prozac during pregnancy have not been adequately studied. If you are pregnant or plan to become pregnant, inform your doctor immediately. This medication appears in breast milk, and breastfeeding is not recommended while you are taking Prozac.

Recommended dosage

ADULTS

The usual starting dose is 20 milligrams per day, taken in the morning. Your doctor may increase your dose after several weeks if no improvement is observed. Patients with kidney or liver disease, the elderly, and those taking other drugs may have their dosages adjusted by their doctor.

Dosages above 20 milligrams daily should be taken once a day in the morning or in 2 smaller doses taken in the morning and at noon.

The usual daily dose for depression ranges from 20 to 60 milligrams. For obsessive-compulsive disorder the customary range is 20 to 60 milligrams, though 80 milligrams is sometimes prescribed.

Overdosage

Any medication taken in excess or in combination with other drugs can cause symptoms of overdose. If you suspect an overdose, seek medical attention immediately.

■ *Symptoms of Prozac overdose include:*
Agitation
Nausea
Restlessness
Vomiting

Generic name:

PSYLLIUM

See Metamucil, page 646.

Brand name:

QUESTRAN

Pronounced: KWEST-ran
Generic name: Cholestyramine
Other brand name: Questran Light

Why is this drug prescribed?

Questran is used to lower cholesterol levels in the blood of people with primary hypercholesterolemia (too much LDL cholesterol). Hypercholesterolemia is a genetic condition characterized by a lack of the LDL receptors that remove cholesterol from the bloodstream.

This drug is also prescribed for people with hypertriglyceridemia, a condition in which an excess of fat is stored in the body.

However, Questran is usually prescribed only when a low-fat, low-sugar, and low-cholesterol diet does not lower cholesterol levels enough.

This drug may also be prescribed to relieve itching associated with gallbladder obstruction.

It is available in two forms: Questran and Questran Light. The same instructions apply to both.

Most important fact about this drug

Questran is usually prescribed only if diet, exercise, and weight-loss fail to bring your cholesterol levels under control. It's important to remember that Questran is a supplement—not a substitute—for these other measures. To get the full benefit of the medication, you need to stick to the diet and exercise program prescribed by your doctor. All these efforts to keep your cholesterol levels normal are important because together they may lower your risk of heart disease.

How should you take this medication?

Never take Questran in its dry form. Always mix it with water or other liquids *before* taking it. For Questran, use 2 to 6 ounces of liquid per packet or level scoopful; for Questran Light, use 2 to 3 ounces. Soups or fruits with a high moisture content, such as applesauce or crushed pineapple, can be used in place of beverages.

■ *If you miss a dose...*
Take the forgotten dose as soon as you remember. If it is almost time for the next dose, skip the one you missed and go back to your regular schedule. Never try to "catch up" by doubling the dose.

■ *Storage instructions...*
Store at room temperature. Protect from moisture and high humidity.

What side effects may occur?

Side effects cannot be anticipated. If any develop or change in intensity, inform your doctor as soon as possible. Only your doctor can determine if it is safe for you to continue taking Questran.

The most common side effect of Questran is constipation.

■ *Less common or rare side effects may include:*
Abdominal discomfort, anemia, anxiety, arthritis, asthma, backache, belching, black stools, bleeding around the teeth, blood in the urine, brittle bones, burnt odor to urine, dental cavities, diarrhea, difficulty swallowing, dizziness, drowsiness, fainting, fatigue, fluid retention, gas, headache, heartburn, hiccups, hives, increased sex drive, increased tendency to bleed due to vitamin K deficiency, indigestion, inflammation of the eye, inflammation of the pancreas, irritation around the anal area, irritation of the skin and tongue, joint pain, lack or loss of appetite, muscle pain, nausea, night blindness due to vitamin A deficiency, painful or difficult urination, rash, rectal bleeding and/or pain, ringing in the ears, shortness of breath, sour taste, swollen glands, tingling sensation, ulcer attack, vertigo, vitamin D deficiency, vomiting, weight gain or loss, wheezing

Why should this drug not be prescribed?

If you are sensitive to or have ever had an allergic reaction to Questran or similar drugs such as Colestid, you should not take this medication. Make sure that your doctor is aware of any drug reactions that you have experienced.

Unless you are directed to do so by your doctor, do not take this medication if you are being treated for gallbladder obstruction.

Special warnings about this medication

If you have phenylketonuria, a genetic disorder, check with your doctor before taking Questran because this product contains phenylalanine.

If you are being treated for any disease that contributes to increased blood cholesterol, such as hypothyroidism (reduced thyroid function), diabetes, nephrotic syndrome (kidney and blood vessel disorder), dysproteinemia, or obstructive liver disease, consult with your doctor before taking this medication.

Questran should begin to reduce cholesterol levels during the first month of therapy. If adequate reduction of cholesterol is not obtained, this medication should be discontinued. Therefore, it is important that your doctor check your progress regularly.

The use of this medication may produce or worsen constipation and aggravate hemorrhoids. If this happens, inform your doctor. Only your doctor can determine if your dose needs to be reduced or discontinued.

The prolonged use of Questran may change acidity in the bloodstream, especially in younger and smaller individuals in whom the doses are relatively higher. Again, it is important that you or your child be checked by your doctor on a regular basis.

Possible food and drug interactions when taking this medication

If Questran is taken with certain other drugs, the effects of either could be increased, decreased, or altered. It is especially important to check with your doctor before taking Questran with the following:

Chlorothiazide (Diuril)
Digitalis (Lanoxin, Crystodigin)

Oral diabetes drugs such as DiaBeta and
Diabinese
Penicillin G (Pentids, others)
Phenobarbital
Phenylbutazone (Butazolidin)
Propranolol (Inderal)
Tetracycline (Achromycin V)
Thyroid medication such as Synthroid
Warfarin (Coumadin)

Your doctor may recommend that you take
other medications at least 1 hour before or
4 to 6 hours after you take Questran.

If you are taking a drug such as digitalis
(Lanoxin), stopping Questran could be
hazardous, since you might experience
exaggerated effects of the other drug.
Consult your doctor before discontinuing
Questran.

This drug may interfere with normal
digestion and absorption of fats, including
fat-soluble vitamins such as A, D, and K. If
supplements of vitamins A, D, and K are
essential to your health, your doctor may
prescribe an alternative form of these
vitamins.

There are no special considerations regarding
alcohol use with this medication.

Special information
if you are pregnant or breastfeeding

The effects of Questran during pregnancy
have not been adequately studied. If you are
pregnant or plan to become pregnant,
inform your doctor immediately. Because
this medication can interfere with vitamin
absorption, it may have an effect on nursing
infants. If this drug is essential to your
health, your doctor may advise you to
discontinue breastfeeding until your
treatment is finished.

Recommended dosage

ADULTS

The recommended starting dose is 1 single-
dose packet or 1 level scoopful, 1 to 2
times daily. The usual maintenance dosage is
a total of 2 to 4 packets or scoopfuls daily
divided into 2 doses preferably at mealtime
(usually before meals). The maximum daily
dose is 6 packets or scoopfuls. Although the
recommended dosing schedule is 2 times
daily, your doctor may ask you to take
Questran in up to 6 smaller doses per day.

CHILDREN

Experience with the use of Questran in
infants and children is limited. If this
medication is essential to your child's health,
follow your doctor's recommended dosing
schedule.

Overdosage

No ill effects from an overdose have been
reported. The main potential harm of an
overdose would be obstruction of the
stomach and intestines. If you suspect an
overdose, seek medical attention
immediately.

Generic name:

RANITIDINE

See Zantac, page 693.

Brand name:

REGULOID

See Metamucil, page 646.

Generic name:

ROLAIDS

See Antacids, page 600.

Brand name:

ROWASA

Pronounced: ROH-ace-ah
Generic name: Mesalamine
Other brand name: Pentasa, Asacol

Why is this drug prescribed?

Rowasa Suspension Enema, Pentasa, and
Asacol are used to treat mild to moderate
ulcerative colitis (inflammation of the large
intestine and rectum). Rowasa Suspension
Enema is also prescribed for inflammation
of the lower colon, and inflammation of the
rectum.

Rowasa Suppositories are used to treat
inflammation of the rectum.

Most important fact about this drug

Mesalamine, the active ingredient in these
products, has been known to cause side
effects such as:

Bloody diarrhea
Cramping
Fever
Rash
Severe headache
Sudden, severe stomach pain

If you develop any of these symptoms, stop
taking this medication and consult your
doctor.

How should you use this medication?

To Use Rowasa Suspension Enema
1. Rowasa Suspension Enema comes in
   boxes of 7 bottles each. After the foil on
   the box has been unwrapped, all Rowasa

Suspension Enemas should be used
promptly, following your doctor's
instructions. The Suspension Enema is
normally off-white to tan in color, but
may darken over time once its foil cover
is unwrapped. You may still use the
enema if it is slightly discolored, but do
not use Rowasa Suspension Enema if it is
dark brown. If you have any questions
about using Rowasa Suspension Enema,
contact your doctor.
2. Use Rowasa Suspension Enema at
   bedtime.
3. Shake the bottle thoroughly.
4. Uncover the applicator tip.
5. You may find it easier to use Rowasa
   Suspension Enema if you lie down on
   your left side, extending your left leg and
   bending your right leg forward for a
   comfortable balance. An alternative
   position is to squat with your knees to
   your chest.
6. Pointing the applicator tip up, gently
   insert the tip into the rectum.
7. Squeeze the bottle steadily to discharge
   the contents.
8. The enema should be retained all night (8
   hours) for best results.

To Use Rowasa Suppositories
1. Rowasa Suppositories should be used
   twice a day.
2. You should handle the suppositories as
   little as possible, because they are
   designed to melt at body temperature.
3. Remove one suppository from the strip
   of suppositories.
4. While holding the suppository upright,
   carefully remove the foil wrapper.
5. Using gentle pressure, insert the
   suppository (with the pointed end first)
   completely into the rectum.
6. The suppository should be retained for 1
   to 3 hours or longer for best results.

To take Pentasa or Asacol
Swallow the capsule or tablet whole. Do not break, crush, or chew it before swallowing.

You may notice what looks like small beads in your stool. These are just empty shells that are left after the medication has been absorbed into your body. However, if this continues, check with your doctor.

■ *If you miss a dose...*
Take it as soon as you remember. If it is almost time for your next dose, skip the one you missed and go back to your regular schedule. Never take 2 doses at the same time.

■ *Storage instructions...*
Store these products at room temperature.

What side effects may occur?
Side effects cannot be anticipated. If any side effects develop or change in intensity, tell your doctor immediately. Only your doctor can determine whether it is safe to continue using this medication.

■ *More common side effects of Rowasa Suspension Enema may include:*
Flu-like symptoms
Gas
Headache
Nausea
Stomach pain/cramps

■ *Less common side effects of Rowasa Suspension Enema may include:*
Back pain, bloating, diarrhea, dizziness, fever, hemorrhoids, itching, leg/joint pain, pain on insertion of enema tip, rash, rectal pain, sore throat, tiredness, weakness

■ *Rare side effects of Rowasa Suspension Enema may include:*
Constipation, hair loss, insomnia, swelling of the arms or legs, urinary burning

■ *More common side effects of Rowasa Suppositories may include:*
Diarrhea
Dizziness
Gas
Headache
Stomach pain

■ *Less common side effects of Rowasa Suppositories may include:*
Acne, cold symptoms, fever, inflammation of the colon, nausea, rash, rectal pain, swelling, weakness

■ *More common side effects of Pentasa and Asacol may include:*
Diarrhea
Headache
Nausea

■ *Less common or rare side effects of Pentasa and Asacol may include:*
Abdominal pain, abdominal swelling, acne, belching, blood in the urine, bloody diarrhea, breast pain, bruising, conjunctivitis, constipation, depression, difficulty sleeping, difficulty swallowing, dizziness, dry skin, duodenal ulcer, eczema, fever, fluid retention, general feeling of illness, hair loss, hives, inflammation of the pancreas, itching, joint pain, Kawasaki-like syndrome (rash, swollen glands, fever, mouth inflammation, strawberry tongue), lack or loss of appetite, leg cramps, menstrual irregularities, mouth sores and infections, muscle pain, nail problems, palpitations (rapid, fluttery heartbeat), rash, rectal bleeding, sensitivity to light, skin eruptions, sleepiness, stomach and intestinal bleeding, stool changes, sweating, thirst, tingling or pins and needles, ulcer of the esophagus, uncontrollable bowel movements, urinary frequency, weakness, worsening of ulcerative colitis, vomiting

Why should this drug not be prescribed?

These products should not be used by anyone who is allergic or sensitive to mesalamine or their other ingredients.

Pentasa and Asacol should not be used if you are allergic or sensitive to salicylates (aspirin).

Special warnings about this medication

Your doctor should check your kidney function while you are taking mesalamine, especially if you have a history of kidney disease or you are using other anti-inflammatory drugs such as Dipentum.

You should use mesalamine cautiously if you are allergic to sulfasalazine (Azulfidine). If you develop a rash or fever, you should stop using the medication and notify your doctor.

Some people using mesalamine have developed flare-ups of their colitis.

Rare cases of pericarditis, in which the membrane surrounding the heart becomes inflamed, have been reported with products containing mesalamine. Symptoms may include chest, neck, and shoulder pain, and shortness of breath.

Rowasa Suspension Enema contains a sulfite that may cause allergic reactions in some people. These reactions may include shock and severe, possibly fatal asthma attacks. Most people aren't sensitive to sulfites. However, some people with asthma might be sensitive and should take any medication containing sulfites cautiously.

Rowasa Suspension Enema may stain clothes and fabrics.

Possible food and drug interactions when taking this medication

If these products are taken with certain other drugs, the effects of either could be increased, decreased, or altered. It is especially important to check with your doctor before combining Rowasa Suspension Enema or Rowasa Suppositories with Sulfasalazine (Azulfidine).

Special information if you are pregnant or breastfeeding

Pregnant women should use mesalamine only if clearly needed. Mesalamine has been found in breast milk. If this medication is essential to your health your doctor may advise you to discontinue breastfeeding until your treatment is finished.

Recommended dosage

ADULTS

Rowasa Suspension Enema
The usual dose is 1 rectal enema (60 milliliters) per day, preferably used at bedtime and retained for about 8 hours. Treatment time usually lasts from 3 to 6 weeks, although improvement may be seen within 3 to 21 days.

Rowasa Suppositories
The usual dose is one rectal suppository (500 milligrams) 2 times a day. To get the most benefit from a Rowasa Suppository, it should be retained for 1 to 3 hours or longer. Treatment time usually lasts from 3 to 6 weeks, although improvement may be seen within 3 to 21 days.

Pentasa Capsules
The usual dose is 4 capsules taken 4 times a day for a total of 16 capsules daily.

Asacol Tablets
The recommended dose is 2 tablets 3 times a day for 6 weeks.

CHILDREN

Safety and effectiveness in children have not been established.

Overdosage

There have been no proven reports of serious effects resulting from overdoses of Rowasa. An overdose of Pantasa or Asacol could cause any of the following symptoms:

Confusion
Diarrhea
Drowsiness
Headache
Hyperventilation
Ringing in the ears
Sweating
Vomiting

Any medication taken in excess can have serious consequences. If you suspect an overdose, seek medical attention immediately.

Brand name:

SERUTAN

See Metamucil, page 646.

Generic name:

SIMVASTATIN

See Zocor, page 695.

Brand name:

SLOW-K

See Micro-K, page 650.

Generic name:

SODIUM FLUORIDE

See Luride, page 644.

Brand name:

STUARTNATAL PLUS

Pronounced: STU-art NAY-tal plus
Generic ingredients: Prenatal vitamins and minerals
Other brand names: Materna, Natalins Rx

Why is this drug prescribed?

Stuartnatal Plus contains vitamins and minerals including iron, calcium, zinc, and folic acid. The tablets are given during pregnancy and after childbirth to ensure an adequate supply of these critical nutrients. They may also be prescribed to improve a woman's nutritional status before she becomes pregnant.

Most important fact about this drug

Nutritional supplementation is especially important during pregnancy. Be sure to take Stuartnatal Plus regularly as prescribed.

How should you take this medication?

Take Stuartnatal Plus exactly as prescribed. The usual dosage is 1 tablet per day with or without food.

■ *If you miss a dose...*
Take it as soon as you remember, then return to your regular schedule.

■ *Storage instructions...*
Store at room temperature, away from excessive heat.

Why should this drug not be prescribed?

There are no known reasons to avoid this preparation.

Special information if you are pregnant or breastfeeding

Pregnancy and breastfeeding impose special nutritional demands on the mother. A vitamin and mineral supplement can help ensure that there are enough nutrients for both you and your baby.

Recommended dosage

ADULTS

Before, during, and after pregnancy, take 1 tablet daily, or as directed by your doctor.

Overdosage

Although no specific overdose information is available, even a nutritional supplement in extremely large amounts can have serious consequences. If you suspect an overdose of Stuartnatal Plus, seek medical attention immediately.

Generic name:

SUCRALFATE

See Carafate, page 609.

Generic name:

SULFASALAZINE

See Azulfidine, page 604.

Brand name:

SYLLACT

See Metamucil, page 646.

Brand name:

TAGAMET

Pronounced: TAG-ah-met
Generic name: Cimetidine

Why is this drug prescribed?

Tagamet is prescribed for the treatment of certain kinds of stomach and intestinal ulcers and related conditions. These include: active duodenal (upper intestinal) ulcers; active benign stomach ulcers; erosive gastroesophageal reflux disease (backflow of acid stomach contents); prevention of upper abdominal bleeding in those who are critically ill; and excess-acid conditions such as Zollinger-Ellison syndrome (a form of peptic ulcer with too much acid). It is also used for maintenance therapy of duodenal ulcer following the healing of active ulcers. Tagamet is known as a histamine blocker.

Some doctors also use Tagamet to treat acne and to prevent stress-induced ulcers. It may also be used to treat chronic hives, herpes virus infections (including shingles), abnormal hair growth in women, and overactivity of the parathyroid gland.

Most important fact about this drug

Short-term treatment with Tagamet can result in complete healing of a duodenal ulcer. However, there can be a recurrence of the ulcer after Tagamet has been discontinued. The rate of ulcer recurrence may be slightly higher in people healed with Tagamet rather than other forms of therapy. However, Tagamet is usually prescribed for more severe cases.

How should you take this medication?

You can take Tagamet with or between meals. Do not take antacids within 1 to 2 hours of a dose of Tagamet. Avoid excessive amounts of caffeine while taking this drug.

It may take several days for Tagamet to begin relieving stomach pain. Be sure to continue taking the drug exactly as prescribed even if it seems to have no affect.

■ *If you miss a dose...*
Take it as soon as you remember. If it is almost time for your next dose, skip the one you missed and go back to your regular schedule. Do not take 2 doses a once.

■ *Storage instructions...*
Store at room temperature in a tightly closed container, away from light.

What side effects may occur?

Side effects cannot be anticipated. If any develop or change in intensity, inform your doctor as soon as possible. Only your doctor can determine if it is safe for you to continue taking Tagamet.

■ *More common side effects may include:*
Breast development in men, headache

Less common side effects—agitation, anxiety, confusion, depression, disorientation, and hallucinations—may appear in severely ill individuals who have been treated for 1 month or longer. However, these reactions are not permanent and have cleared up within 3 to 4 days of discontinuation of the drug.

■ *Rare side effects may include:*
Allergic reactions, anemia, blood disorders, diarrhea, dizziness, fever, hair loss, impotence, inability to urinate, joint pain, kidney disorders, liver disorders, mild rash, muscle pain, pancreas inflammation, rapid heartbeat, skin inflammation or peeling, sleepiness, slow heartbeat

Why should this drug not be prescribed?

If you have ever had an allergic reaction to Tagamet, do not take this medication.

Special warnings about this medication

Ulcers may be more difficult to heal if you smoke cigarettes.

If you are being treated for a liver or kidney disorder, make sure the doctor is aware if it.

If you are over 50 years old, have liver or kidney disease, or are severely ill, you may experience temporary mental confusion while taking Tagamet. Notify your doctor.

Possible food and drug interactions when taking this medication

If Tagamet is taken with certain other drugs, the effects of either can be increased, decreased, or altered. It is especially important that you check with your doctor before combining Tagamet with the following:

Antiarrhythmic heart medications such as Cordarone, Tonocard, Quinidex, and Procan
Antidiabetic drugs such as Micronase and Glucotrol
Antifungal drugs such as Diflucan and Nizoral
Aspirin
Augmentin
Benzodiazepine tranquilizers such as Valium and Librium
Beta-blocking blood pressure drugs such as Inderal and Lopressor
Calcium-blocking blood pressure drugs such as Cardizem, Calan, and Procardia
Chlorpromazine (Thorazine)
Cisapride (Propulsid)
Cyclosporine (Sandimmune)
Digoxin (Lanoxin)
Narcotic pain relievers such as Demerol and Morphine

Metoclopramide (Reglan)
Metronidazole (Flagyl)
Nicotine (Nicoderm)
Paroxetine (Paxil)
Pentoxifylline (Trental)
Phenytoin (Dilantin)
Quinine (Quinamm)
Sucralfate (Carafate)
Theophylline (Theo-Dur, others)
Warfarin (Coumadin)

Avoid alcoholic beverages while taking Tagamet. This medication increases the effects of alcohol.

Antacids can reduce the effect of Tagamet when taken at the same time. If you take an antacid to relieve the pain of an ulcer, the doses should be separated by 1 to 2 hours.

Special information
if you are pregnant or breastfeeding

The effects of Tagamet during pregnancy have not been adequately studied. If you are pregnant or plan to become pregnant, notify your doctor immediately. Tagamet appears in breast milk and could affect a nursing infant. If this medication is essential to your health, your doctor may advise you to discontinue breastfeeding until treatment with this drug is finished.

Recommended dosage

ADULTS

Active Duodenal Ulcer
The usual dose is 800 milligrams once daily at bedtime. However, other doses shown to be effective are:

300 milligrams 4 times a day with meals and at bedtime

400 milligrams twice a day, in the morning and at bedtime

Most people heal in 4 weeks.

If you require maintenance therapy, the usual dose is 400 milligrams at bedtime.

Active Benign Gastric Ulcer
The usual dose is 800 milligrams once a day at bedtime or 300 milligrams taken 4 times a day with meals and at bedtime.

Erosive Gastroesophageal Reflux Disease
The usual dosage is a total of 1,600 milligrams daily divided into doses of 800 milligrams twice a day or 400 milligrams 4 times a day for 12 weeks. The beneficial use of Tagamet beyond 12 weeks has not been firmly established.

Pathological Hypersecretory Condition
The usual dosage is 300 milligrams 4 times a day with meals and at bedtime. Your doctor may adjust your dosage based on your needs, but you should take no more than 2,400 milligrams per day.

CHILDREN

Safety and effectiveness have not been established in children under 16 years old. However, your doctor may decide that the potential benefits of Tagamet use outweigh the potential risks. Doses of 20 to 40 milligrams per 2.2 pounds of body weight have been used.

ELDERLY

Dosage in the elderly is generally the same as that for other adults. However, many elderly people require reduced doses of a variety of drugs. Your doctor will decide if any dosage adjustment of Tagamet is needed due to your age or other existing medical condition.

Overdosage

Information concerning overdosage is limited. However, respiratory failure, an increased heartbeat, exaggerated side effect symptoms or reactions such as unresponsiveness may be signs of Tagamet overdose. If you experience any of these symptoms, notify your doctor immediately.

Brand name:

TEN-K

See Micro-K, page 650.

Brand name:

TENUATE

Pronounced: TEN-you-ate
Generic name: Diethylpropion hydrochloride

Why is this drug prescribed?

Tenuate, an appetite suppressant, is prescribed for short-term use (a few weeks) as part of an overall diet plan for weight reduction. It is available in two forms: immediate-release tablets (Tenuate) and controlled-release tablets (Tenuate Dospan). Tenuate should be used with a behavior modification program.

Most important fact about this drug

Tenuate will lose its effectiveness within a few weeks. When this begins to happen, you should discontinue the medicine rather than increase the dosage.

How should you take this medication?

Take this medication exactly as prescribed. Tenuate may be habit-forming and can be addicting.

If you are taking Tenuate Dospan (the controlled release formulation), do not crush or chew the tablets. Swallow the medication whole.

■ *If you miss a dose...*
If you are taking the immediate-release form of Tenuate, go back to your regular schedule at the next meal.

If you are taking Tenuate Dospan, take the missed dose as soon as you remember. If you do not remember until the next day, skip the dose. Never take 2 doses at once.

■ *Storage instructions...*
Store at room temperature in a tightly closed container. Protect from excessive heat.

What side effects may occur?

Side effects cannot be anticipated. If any develop or change in intensity, inform your doctor as soon as possible. Only your doctor can determine if it is safe for you to continue using Tenuate.

■ *Side effects may include:*
Abdominal discomfort, abnormal redness of the skin, anxiety, blood pressure elevation, blurred vision, breast development in males, bruising, changes in sex drive, chest pain, constipation, depression, diarrhea, difficulty with voluntary movements, dizziness, drowsiness, dryness of the mouth, feelings of discomfort, feelings of elation, feeling of illness, hair loss, headache, hives, impotence, inability to fall or stay asleep, increased heart rate, increased seizures in epileptics, increased sweating, increased volume of diluted urine, irregular heartbeat, jitteriness, menstrual upset, muscle pain, nausea, nervousness, overstimulation, painful urination, palpitations, pupil dilation, rash, restlessness, shortness of breath or labored breathing, stomach and intestinal disturbances, tremors, unpleasant taste, vomiting

Why should this drug not be prescribed?

If you are sensitive to or have ever had an allergic reaction to Tenuate or other appetite suppressants, you should not take this medication. Make sure your doctor is aware of any drug reactions you have experienced.

Do not take this drug if you have severe hardening of the arteries, an overactive thyroid, glaucoma, or severe high blood pressure, or if you are agitated, have a history of drug abuse or are taking an MAO inhibitor (antidepressant drug such as Nardil) or have taken one within the last 14 days.

Special warnings about this medication

Tenuate or Tenuate Dospan may impair your ability to engage in potentially hazardous activities. Therefore, make sure you know how you react to this medication before you drive, operate dangerous machinery, or do anything else that requires alertness or concentration.

If you have heart disease or high blood pressure, use caution when taking this medication.

This drug may increase convulsions in some epileptics. Your doctor should monitor you carefully if you have epilepsy.

Psychological dependence has occurred while taking this drug. Talk with your doctor if you find you are relying on this drug to maintain a state of well-being.

The abrupt withdrawal of this medication following prolonged use at high doses may result in extreme fatigue, mental depression, and sleep disturbances.

Possible food and drug interactions when taking this medication

Tenuate or Tenuate Dospan may interact with alcohol unfavorably. Do not drink alcohol while taking this medication.

If Tenuate or Tenuate Dospan is taken with certain other drugs, the effects of either could be increased, decreased, or altered. It is especially important that you consult your doctor before combining Tenuate with the following:

Blood pressure medications such as Ismelin
Insulin
Phenothiazine drugs such as the major
   tranquilizer Thorazine

Special information if you are pregnant or breastfeeding

The effects of Tenuate or Tenuate Dospan during pregnancy have not been adequately studied. If you are pregnant or plan to become pregnant, inform your doctor immediately. This drug appears in breast milk. If the medication is essential to your health, your doctor may advise you to discontinue breastfeeding until your treatment is finished.

Recommended dosage

ADULTS

Tenuate Immediate-Release
The usual dosage is one 25-milligram tablet taken 3 times a day, 1 hour before meals; you may take 1 tablet in the middle of the evening, if you want, to overcome night hunger.

Tenuate Dospan Controlled-Release
The usual dosage is one 75-milligram tablet taken once daily, swallowed whole, in midmorning.

CHILDREN

Safety and effectiveness have not been established in children below 12 years of age.

Overdosage

Any medication taken in excess can have serious consequences. If you suspect an overdose, seek emergency medical treatment immediately.

■ *Symptoms of Tenuate overdose may include:*
Abdominal cramps, assaultiveness, confusion, depression, diarrhea, elevated blood pressure, fatigue, hallucinations, irregular heartbeat, lowered blood pressure, nausea, overreactive reflexes, panic state, rapid breathing, restlessness, tremors, vomiting

Generic name:

THERAGRAN

See Multivitamins, page 655.

Generic name:

TOLAZAMIDE

See Tolinase, page 690.

Generic name:

TOLBUTAMIDE

See Orinase, page 659.

Brand name:

TOLINASE

Pronounced: TAHL-in-ace
Generic name: Tolazamide

Why is this drug prescribed?

Tolinase is an oral antidiabetic drug available in tablet form. It lowers the blood sugar level by stimulating the pancreas to release insulin. Tolinase may be given as a supplement to diet therapy to help control Type II (non-insulin-dependent) diabetes.

There are two type of diabetes: Type I (insulin-dependent) and Type II (non-insulin dependent). Type I diabetes usually requires insulin injection for life; Type II can usually be controlled by dietary changes, exercise, and oral diabetes medications. Occasionally—during stressful periods or times of illness, or if oral medications fail to work—a Type II diabetic may need insulin injections.

Most important fact about this drug

Always remember that Tolinase is an aid to, not a substitute for, good diet and exercise. Failure to follow a sound diet and exercise plan can lead to serious complications, such as dangerously low blood sugar levels. Remember, too, that Tolinase is *not* an oral form of insulin, and cannot be used in place of insulin.

How should you take this medication?

Remember that if you are diligent about diet and exercise, you may need Tolinase for only a short period of time. Take it exactly as prescribed.

While taking Tolinase, your blood and urine glucose levels should be monitored regularly. Your doctor may also want you to have a periodic glycosylated hemoglobin blood test, which will show how well you have kept your blood sugar down during the weeks preceding the test.

■ *If you miss a dose...*
Take it as soon as you remember. If it is almost time for the next dose, skip the one you missed and go back to your regular schedule. Do not take 2 doses at the same time.

■ *Storage instructions...*
Store at room temperature.

What side effects may occur?

Side effects cannot be anticipated. If any appear or change in intensity, inform your doctor as soon as possible. Only your doctor can determine if it is safe for you to continue taking Tolinase. The most frequently encountered side effects from Tolinase—nausea, a full, bloated feeling, and heartburn—may disappear if the dosage is reduced.

Hives, itching, and rash may appear initially and then disappear as you continue to take the drug. If a skin reaction persists, you should stop taking Tolinase.

■ *Less common side effects may include:*
Blistering on sun-exposed skin, sensitivity to light

■ *Rare side effects may include:*
Dizziness, fatigue, general feeling of illness, headache, vertigo, weakness

Why should this drug not be prescribed?

Do not take Tolinase if you are sensitive to it or have ever had an allergic reaction to it; if you are suffering from diabetic ketoacidosis (a chemical imbalance leading to nausea, vomiting, confusion and coma); or if you have Type I (insulin-dependent) diabetes and are not taking insulin.

Special warnings about this medication

It's possible that drugs such as Tolinase may lead to more heart problems than diet treatment alone, or diet plus insulin. If you have a heart condition, you may want to discuss this with your doctor.

Like other oral antidiabetic drugs, Tolinase may produce severe low blood sugar (hypoglycemia) if the dosing is wrong. While taking Tolinase, you are particularly susceptible to episodes of low blood sugar if:

You suffer from a kidney or liver problem;
You have a lack of adrenal or pituitary hormones; or
You are elderly, run-down, or malnourished.

You are at increased risk for a low blood sugar episode if you are hungry, exercising heavily, drinking alcohol, or using more than one glucose-lowering drug.

Note that an episode of low blood sugar may be difficult to recognize if you are elderly or if you are taking a beta-blocker drug (Inderal, Lopressor, Tenormin, and others).

If switching to Tolinase from chlorpropamide (Diabinese), you should take special care to avoid an episode of low blood sugar.

Stress such as fever, trauma, infection, or surgery may increase blood sugar to the point that you require insulin injections.

Possible food and drug interactions when taking this medication

If Tolinase is taken with certain other drugs, the effects of either could be increased, decreased, or altered. It is especially important to check with your doctor before combining Tolinase with the following:

Airway-opening drugs such as Sudafed and Ventolin

Alcohol

Aspirin or related drugs

Beta-blocking blood pressure medications such as Inderal and Lopressor

Blood-thinning drugs such as Coumadin

Calcium channel blockers such as Calan and Isoptin

Chloramphenicol (Chloromycetin)

Corticosteroids such as Cortef, Decadron and Medrol

Diuretics such as Esidrix and Diuril

Estrogens such as Premarin and Estraderm

Isoniazid (Nydrazid)

MAO inhibitors (antidepressants such as Marplan, Nardil, and Parnate)

Miconazole (Monistat)

Nicotinic acid (Nicobid)

Nonsteroidal anti-inflammatory drugs such as Motrin and Naprosyn

Oral contraceptives

Phenothiazines (antipsychotic drugs such as Mellaril)

Phenytoin (Dilantin)

Probenecid (Benemid)

Rifampin (Rifadin)

Sulfa drugs such as Bactrim and Gantrisin

Thyroid drugs such as Synthroid

Special information if you are pregnant or breastfeeding

If you are pregnant or plan to become pregnant, inform your doctor immediately. Tolinase is not recommended for use during pregnancy, and should not be prescribed if you might become pregnant while taking it.

Control of diabetes during pregnancy is very important, but in most cases it should be accomplished with insulin injections rather than oral antidiabetic drugs.

Tolinase should not be used during breastfeeding because of possible harmful effects on the baby. If you are a new mother, you may need to choose between taking Tolinase and breastfeeding your baby.

Recommended dosage

Your doctor will determine the dosage level based on your needs.

ADULTS

The usual starting dose of Tolinase tablets for the mild to moderately severe Type II diabetic is 100 to 150 milligrams daily taken with breakfast or the first main meal.

ELDERLY

If you are malnourished, underweight, elderly, or not eating properly, the initial dose is usually 100 milligrams once a day. Failure to follow an appropriate dosage regimen may precipitate hypoglycemia (low blood sugar). If you do not stick to your prescribed dietary regimen, you are more likely to have an unsatisfactory response to this medication.

Overdosage

An overdose of Tolinase can cause an episode of low blood sugar. Mild low blood sugar without loss of consciousness should be treated with oral glucose, an adjusted meal pattern, and possibly a reduction in the Tolinase dosage. Severe low blood sugar, which may cause coma or seizures, is a medical emergency and must be treated in a hospital. If you suspect an overdose of Tolinase, seek medical attention immediately.

Generic name:

TUMS

See Antacids, page 600.

Brand name:

VELOSULIN

See Insulin, page 629.

Generic name:

VI-DAYLIN

See Multivitamins, page 655.

Generic name:

VITAMINS WITH FLUORIDE

See Poly-Vi-Flor, page 666.

Brand name:

ZANTAC

Pronounced: ZAN-tac
Generic name: Ranitidine hydrochloride

Why is this drug prescribed?

Zantac is prescribed for the short-term treatment (4 to 8 weeks) of active duodenal ulcer and active benign gastric ulcer, and as maintenance therapy for duodenal ulcer, at a reduced dosage, after the ulcer has healed. It is also used for the treatment of conditions in which the stomach produces too much acid, such as Zollinger-Ellison syndrome and systemic mastocytosis, for gastroesophageal reflux disease (backflow of acid stomach contents) and for healing erosive esophagitis (severe inflammation of the esophagus).

Some doctors prescribe Zantac to prevent damage to the stomach and duodenum from long-term use of nonsteroidal anti-inflammatory drugs such as Indocin and Motrin, and to treat bleeding of the stomach and intestine. Zantac is also sometimes prescribed for stress-induced ulcers.

Most important fact about this drug

Zantac helps to prevent the recurrence of duodenal ulcers and aids the healing of ulcers that do occur.

How should you take this medication?

Take this medication exactly as prescribed by your doctor. Make sure you follow the diet your doctor recommends.

Dissolve "Efferdose" tablets and granules in 6 to 8 ounces of water before taking them.

You can take an antacid for pain while you are taking Zantac.

■ *If you miss a dose...*
Take it as soon as you remember. If it is almost time for your next dose, skip the one you missed and go back to your regular schedule. Never take 2 doses at the same time.

■ *Storage instructions...*
Store this medication at room temperature in the container it came in, tightly closed and away from moist places and direct light. Keep Zantac Syrup from freezing.

What side effects may occur?

Side effects cannot be anticipated. If any develop or change in intensity, inform your doctor as soon as possible. Only your doctor can determine if it is safe for you to continue taking Zantac.

■ *More common side effects may include:*
Headache, sometimes severe

■ *Less common or rare side effects may include:*
Abdominal discomfort and pain, agitation, changes in blood count (anemia), changes in liver function, constipation, depression, diarrhea, difficulty sleeping, dizziness, hair

loss, hallucinations, heart block, hepatitis, hypersensitivity reactions, inflammation of the pancreas, involuntary movements, irregular heartbeat, joint pain, muscle pain, nausea and vomiting, rapid heartbeat, rash, reduced white blood cells, reversible mental confusion, sleepiness, slow heartbeat, vague feeling of bodily discomfort, vertigo, yellow eyes and skin

Why should this drug not be prescribed?
If you are sensitive to or have ever had an allergic reaction to Zantac or similar drugs such as Tagamet, you should not take this medication. Make sure that your doctor is aware of any drug reactions that you have experienced.

Special warnings about this medication
A stomach malignancy could be present, even if your symptoms have been relieved by Zantac.

If you have kidney or liver disease, this drug should be used with caution.

If you have phenylketonurea, you should be aware that the "Efferdose" granules contain phenylalamine.

Possible food and drug interactions when taking this medication
If Zantac is taken with certain other drugs, the effects of either could be increased, decreased, or altered. It is especially important to check with your doctor before combining Zantac with the following:

Alcohol
Blood-thinning drugs such as Coumadin
Glipizide (Glucotrol)
Glyburide (DiaBeta, Micronase)
Itraconazole (Sporanox)
Ketoconazole (Nizoral)
Metoprolol (Lopressor)
Midazolam (Versed)
Nifedipine (Procardia)

Phenytoin (Dilantin)
Procainamide (Procardia)
Sucralfate (Carafate)
Theophylline (Theo-Dur)

Special information if you are pregnant or breastfeeding
The effects of Zantac in pregnancy have not been adequately studied. If you are pregnant or plan to become pregnant, inform your doctor immediately. Zantac appears in breast milk and could affect a nursing infant. If this medication is essential to your health, your doctor may advise you to discontinue breastfeeding until your treatment with this medication is finished.

Recommended dosage

ADULTS

Active Duodenal Ulcer
The usual starting dose is 150 milligrams 2 times a day or 10 milliliters (2 teaspoonfuls) 2 times a day. Your doctor might also prescribe 300 milligrams or 20 milliliters (4 teaspoonfuls) once a day, after the evening meal or at bedtime, if necessary for your convenience. The dose should be the lowest effective dose. Long-term use should be reduced to a daily total of 150 milligrams or 10 milliliters (2 teaspoonfuls), taken at bedtime.

Other Excess Acid Conditions (such as Zollinger-Ellison Syndrome)
The usual dose is 150 milligrams or 10 milliliters (2 teaspoonfuls) 2 times a day. This dose can be adjusted upwards by your doctor.

Benign Gastric Ulcer and Gastroesophageal Reflux Disease (GERD)
The usual dose is 150 milligrams or 10 milliliters (2 teaspoonfuls) 2 times a day.

CHILDREN

The safety and effectiveness of Zantac have not been established in children.

ELDERLY

Dosage should be tailored to your particular needs.

Overdosage

Any medication taken in excess can have serious consequences. If you suspect an overdose, seek medical attention immediately.

Information concerning Zantac overdosage is limited. However, an abnormal manner of walking, low blood pressure, and exaggerated side effect symptoms may be signs of an overdose.

If you experience any of these symptoms, notify your doctor immediately.

Brand name:

ZOCOR

Pronounced: ZOH-core
Generic name: Simvastatin

Why is this drug prescribed?

Zocor is a cholesterol-lowering drug. Your doctor may prescribe Zocor in addition to a cholesterol-lowering diet if your blood cholesterol level is too high, and if you have been unable to lower it by diet alone.

Most important fact about this drug

Zocor is usually prescribed only if diet, exercise, and weight-loss fail to bring your cholesterol level under control. It's important to remember that Zocor is a supplement to—not a substitute for—those other measures. To get the full benefit of the medication, you need to stick to the diet and exercise program prescribed by your doctor. All these efforts to keep your cholesterol levels normal are important because together they may lower your risk of heart disease.

How should you take this medication?

Take Zocor exactly as prescribed.

■ *If you miss a dose...*
Take it as soon as you remember. If it is almost time for your next dose, skip the one you missed and go back to your regular schedule. Do not take 2 doses at once.

■ *Storage instructions...*
Store at room temperature.

What side effects may occur?

Side effects cannot be anticipated. If any develop or change in intensity, inform your doctor as soon as possible. Only your doctor can determine whether it is safe for you to continue taking Zocor.

■ *More common side effects may include:*
Abdominal pain
Headache

■ *Less common side effects may include:*
Constipation, diarrhea, gas, nausea, upper respiratory infection, upset stomach, weakness

Why should this drug not be prescribed?

Do not take Zocor if you have ever had an allergic reaction to it or are sensitive to it.

Do not take Zocor if you have active liver disease.

Do not take Zocor if you are pregnant or plan to become pregnant.

Special warnings about this medication

Because Zocor may damage the liver, your doctor may order a blood test to check your liver enzyme levels before you start taking the drug. Blood tests will probably be done every 6 weeks for the first 3 months of treatment, every 8 weeks for the rest of the first year, and about every 6 months after that. If your liver enzyme levels rise too high, your doctor may tell you to stop taking Zocor.

Since Zocor may cause damage to muscle tissue, be sure to tell your doctor of any unexplained muscle tenderness, weakness, or pain right away, especially if you also have a fever or feel sick. Your doctor may want to do a blood test to check for signs of muscle damage.

Possible food and drug interactions when taking this medication

If you take Zocor with certain other drugs, the effects of either could be increased, decreased, or altered. It is especially important to check with your doctor before combining Zocor with any of the following:

Blood-thinning drugs such as Coumadin and
    Dicumarol
Cimetidine (Tagamet)
Clofibrate (Atromid-S)
Cyclosporine (Sandimmune)
Digoxin (Lanoxin, Lanoxicaps)
Erythromycin (PCE and others)
Gemfibrozil (Lopid)
Itraconazole (Sporanox)
Ketoconazole (Nizoral)
Nicotinic acid
Spironolactone (Aldactone, Aldactazide)

Special information
if you are pregnant or breastfeeding

You must not become pregnant while taking Zocor. This drug lowers cholesterol, and cholesterol is needed for a baby to develop properly. If you do become pregnant while taking Zocor, notify your doctor right away. Based on studies of other cholesterol-lowering drugs, it is assumed that Zocor could appear in breast milk and could cause severe adverse effects in a nursing baby. Do not take Zocor while breastfeeding your baby.

Recommended dosage

You will have to follow a standard cholesterol-lowering diet before starting treatment with Zocor and continue this diet while using Zocor.

All doses should be adjusted to your individual needs.

ADULTS

The usual starting dose is 5 to 10 milligrams per day, taken as a single dose in the evening. The maximum recommended dose is 40 milligrams per day. Dosage adjustments may be made every 4 weeks, and dose levels should be reduced as cholesterol levels come down.

Those who have severe kidney disease should use Zocor with caution. The recommended dose is 5 milligrams per day.

Zocor may be used with other drugs. Your doctor will determine the proper dose based on your individual needs.

ELDERLY

Reduction of cholesterol in the elderly may be achieved with doses of 20 milligrams per day or less.

Overdosage

Although no specific information about Zocor overdose is available, any medication taken in excess can have serious consequences. If you suspect an overdose of Zocor, seek medical attention immediately.

Brand name:

ZYLOPRIM

Pronounced: ZYE-loe-prim
Generic name: Allopurinol
Other brand name: Lopurin

Why is this drug prescribed?

Zyloprim is used in the treatment of many symptoms of gout, including acute attacks, tophi (collection of uric acid crystals in the tissues, especially around joints), joint destruction, and uric acid stones. Gout is a form of arthritis characterized by increased blood levels of uric acid. Zyloprim works by reducing uric acid production in the body, thus preventing crystals from forming.

Zyloprim is also used to manage the increased uric acid levels in the blood of patients with certain cancers, such as leukemia. It is also prescribed to manage some types of kidney stones.

Most important fact about this drug

Zyloprim will not stop a gout attack that is already underway. However, when taken over a period of several months, this drug will begin to reduce your symptoms. It's important to keep taking it regularly, even if it seems to have no immediate effect.

How should you take this medication?

Take Zyloprim exactly as prescribed. Your doctor will probably start you on a low dosage, increasing it gradually each week until you reach the dosage that is best for you.

A typical starting dose is one 100-milligram tablet per day. You may want to take Zyloprim immediately after a meal to minimize the risk of stomach irritation.

You should avoid taking large doses of vitamin C because of the increased possibility of kidney stone formation.

While taking Zyloprim you should drink plenty of liquids—10 to 12 glasses (8 ounces each per day) unless otherwise prescribed by your doctor.

To help prevent attacks of gout, you should also avoid beer, wine, and purine-rich foods such as anchovies, sardines, liver, kidneys, lentils, and sweetbreads.

If you have been taking colchicine and/or an anti-inflammatory drug, such as Anaprox, Indocin, and others, to relieve your gout, your doctor will probably want you to continue taking this medication while your Zyloprim dosage is being adjusted. Later, when you have had no attacks of gout for several months, you may be able to stop taking these other medications.

If you have been taking a drug that promotes the excretion of uric acid in the urine, such as probenecid (Benemid) or sulfinpyrazone (Anturane), to try to prevent attacks of gout, your doctor will probably want to reduce or stop your dosage of this drug while increasing your dosage of Zyloprim.

■ *If you miss a dose...*
Take it as soon as you remember. If it is almost time for your next dose, skip the one you missed and go back to your regular schedule. Do not take 2 doses at once.

■ *Storage instructions...*
Store at room temperatures in a cool, dry place, away from light.

What side effects may occur?

Side effects cannot be anticipated. If any develop or change in intensity, inform your doctor as soon as possible. Only your doctor can determine if it is safe for you to continue taking Zyloprim.

Because a skin reaction, the most common side effect of Zyloprim, may occasionally become severe or even fatal, you should stop taking Zyloprim if you notice even the beginnings of a rash. Such a rash may be itchy or scaly or may make your skin peel off in sheets; it may be accompanied by chills and fever, aching joints, or jaundice.

■ *More common side effects may include:*
Acute attack of gout
Diarrhea
Nausea
Rash

■ *Less common or rare side effects may include:*
Abdominal pain, bruising, chills, fever, hair loss, headache, hepatitis, hives, indigestion, itching, joint pain, kidney failure, loosening of nails, muscle disease, nosebleed, rare skin condition characterized by severe blisters and bleeding on the lips, eyes, or nose, reddish-brown or purplish spots on skin, skin inflammation or peeling, sleepiness, stomach inflammation, taste loss or change, tingling or pins and needles, unusual bleeding, vomiting, yellowing of skin and eyes

Why should this drug not be prescribed?
Do not take Zyloprim if you have ever had a severe reaction to it in the past.

Special warnings about this medication
If you notice a rash or other signs of an allergic reaction, stop taking Zyloprim immediately and consult your doctor. In some people, a Zyloprim-induced rash may lead to a serious skin disease, generalized inflammation of a blood or lymph vessel, irreversible liver damage, or even death.

You may experience acute attacks of gout more often in the early stages of Zyloprim therapy, even when normal uric acid levels have been attained. These attacks will become shorter and less severe after several months of therapy.

A kidney problem may turn a normal dose of Zyloprim into an overdose. If you have a kidney disease, or a condition such as diabetes or high blood pressure that may affect your kidneys, your doctor should prescribe Zyloprim cautiously and order periodic blood and urine tests to assess your kidney function.

Because Zyloprim may make you drowsy, do not drive or perform hazardous tasks until you know how the medication affects you.

It may be 2 to 6 weeks before you see any results from this medication.

Possible food and drug interactions when taking this medication
If Zyloprim is taken with certain other drugs, the effects of either could be increased, decreased, or altered. It is especially important to check with your doctor before combining Zyloprim with the following:

Amoxicillin (Amoxil, Larotid, Polymox)
Ampicillin (Amcill, Omnipen, Polycillin, Principen)
Azathioprine (Imuran)
Blood thinners such as Coumadin
Drugs for diabetes, such as Diabinese and Orinase
Mercaptopurine (Purinethol)
Probenecid (Benemid, ColBENEMID)
Sulfinpyrazone (Anturane)
Theophylline (Theo-Dur, Slo-Phyllin, and others)
Thiazide diuretics such as HydroDIURIL,

Diuril, and others
Vitamin C

Special information
if you are pregnant or breastfeeding

The effects of Zyloprim during pregnancy have not been adequately studied. If you are pregnant or plan to become pregnant, notify your doctor immediately. Zyloprim should be taken during pregnancy only if it is clearly needed.

Zyloprim appears in breast milk; what effect it may have on a nursing baby is unknown. Caution is advised when Zyloprim is taken during breastfeeding.

Recommended dosage

ADULTS

Your doctor will tailor the dosage of Zyloprim individually to control the severity of symptoms and to bring the uric acid levels to normal or near normal.

Gout
The usual starting dose is 100 milligrams once daily. Your doctor may increase your dose by 100 milligrams per day at 1-week intervals until desired results are attained. The average dose is 200 to 300 milligrams per day for mild gout and 400 to 600 milligrams daily for moderate to severe gout. The most you should take in a day is 800 milligrams.

Recurrent Kidney Stones
The usual dose is 200 to 300 milligrams daily, divided into smaller doses or taken as one dose.

Management of Uric Acid Levels in Certain Cancers
The usual dose is 600 to 800 milligrams daily for 2 to 3 days, together with a high fluid intake.

CHILDREN

The usual recommended dose for children 6 to 10 years of age is 300 milligrams daily for the management of uric acid levels in certain types of cancer. Children under 6 years of age are generally given 150 milligrams daily.

Overdosage

Although no specific information is available regarding Zyloprim overdosage, any medication taken in excess can have serious consequences. If you suspect an overdose of Zyloprim, seek medical attention immediately.

Lists, Tables, and Guides

Fat, Cholesterol, and Calorie Counter

Two of the most important rules of thumb for healthy eating are:

- Keep your daily intake of cholesterol under 300 milligrams
- Keep the calories you get from fat under 30 percent

That doesn't mean that everything you eat must be low in fat. But if you choose a dish that delivers more than 30 percent of its calories in the form of fat, you should try to compensate with other selections rated at less than 30 percent. This table helps to keep your fat intake in balance by listing the total calories in many popular dietary choices and, in the right-most column, the percentage of those calories derived from fat. Any food that exceeds the 30 percent target is marked with a blue square at its left.

Another way of controlling your fat intake is to add up the number of grams of fat in your daily diet. If you average 2,200 calories per day, you should keep total fat intake below 73 grams. If you're limiting yourself to 1,800 calories daily, the ceiling on fat falls to 60 grams. The formula for figuring your fat allowance, plus a table giving the allowance at typical calorie levels, can be found in Chapter 10, "What to Do About Fat."

Food	Portion	Cholesterol (milligrams)	Fat (grams)	Calories	% Fat Calories
Acorn Squash, baked	1 cup	0	0.2	114	2%
Alfalfa Sprouts	1 cup	0	0.2	10	18%
■ Almonds dried, blanched	1 oz.	0	15.0	167	81%
■ Almond Butter	1 Tb.	0	9.5	100	85%
■ Anchovy, canned, in oil	5 med.	0	1.9	42	41%
Apple, raw	1 med.	0	0.5	80	6%
Apple, cooked	1 cup	0	0.6	91	6%
Apple Butter	1 Tb.	0	0	33	—
■ Apple Pie	4 1/4 in. wedge	0	18.0	405	40%
Applesauce, unsweetened	1/2 cup	0	trace	53	—
Apricot, canned, in juice	1/2 cup	0	trace	60	—
Apricot, dried	1/2 cup	0	0.6	155	4%
Apricot, fresh, raw	3	0	0.5	51	9%
Arrowroot Flour	1 cup	0	trace	457	—
Artichoke, fresh, cooked	1 med.	0	trace	55	—
Artichoke Hearts, cooked	1 cup	0	0.2	84	2%
■ Arugula	1 cup	0	0.2	4	45%
Asparagus, fresh, cooked	4 spears	0	trace	15	—
Asparagus, cuts, tips	1 cup	0	0	44	—
■ Avocado (Florida)	1 med.	0	27.0	340	72%
■ American Cheese (processed)	1 oz.	16	6.0	82	66%
Angel Food Cake	2 1/2 in.wedge	0	trace	125	—
■ Bacon, fried	3 oz.	72.9	42.2	494	77%
■ Bacon, Canadian, grilled	1-oz. slice	13.5	2.0	43	42%
Bagel, plain	(3 1/2 in.)	0	2.0	200	9%
Bamboo Shoots, canned	1 cup	0	0.6	26	21%
Banana	1 med.	0	1.0	105	9%
Barbecue Sauce	1/2 cup	0	2.3	94	22%
Barley, Pearled, dry	1/2 cup	0	1.0	350	3%
Bass, Freshwater, baked/broiled	3 oz.	74.3	4.1	125	30%
Bass, Sea, baked/broiled	3 oz.	45	2.2	106	19%
Bass, Striped, baked/broiled	3 oz.	87.8	2.6	106	22%
Bean Sprouts, Mung, cooked	1 cup	0	0.2	26	7%
■ Bean Sprouts, Soy, cooked	1 cup	0	4.2	76	50%
■ Bearnaise Sauce	1/2 cup	99	34.1	351	87%
■ Beechnuts, dried	1 oz.	0	14.0	164	77%
■ Beef, Bottom Round, trimmed, braised	3 oz.	82.3	8.3	190	39%
■ Beef, Brisket, trimmed, braised	3 oz.	79.7	11.0	207	48%
■ Beef, Chuck, Arm, trimmed, braised	3 oz.	86.6	8.6	198	39%
■ Beef, Chuck, Blade, trimmed, braised	3 oz.	90.9	13.1	231	51%
■ Beef, Flank, trimmed, braised	3 oz.	60.9	11.8	209	51%
■ Beef, Ground, lean, broiled	3 oz.	74.6	15.9	233	61%
■ Beef, T-Bone Steak, trimmed, broiled	3 oz.	68.6	8.9	183	44%
Beef, Top Round, trimmed, broiled	3 oz.	72	5.3	164	29%
Beef, Broth/Bouillon	1 cup	0	0	31	—

■ *Exceeds Target*

Food	Portion	Cholesterol (milligrams)	Fat (grams)	Calories	% Fat Calories
Beef Heart, braised	3 oz.	164.2	4.8	149	29%
Beef Kidney, braised	3 oz.	331.7	2.9	123	21%
Beef Liver, braised	3 oz.	333.4	4.2	138	27%
■ Beef Pot Pie, 9-in. diam.	1/3 pie	42	30.0	515	52%
■ Beef Tongue	3 oz.	90.8	17.6	241	66%
Beets, fresh, sliced, cooked	1 cup	0	0.4	76	5%
■ Biscuits, 2-in. diam.	1	trace	5.0	100	45%
Black Beans, dry, cooked	1/2 cup	0	0.5	113	4%
Black Turtle Bean Soup	1 cup	0	0.6	240	2%
Blackberries/Boysenberries, fresh, raw	1 cup	0	0.6	74	7%
Black-Eyed Peas, dry, cooked	1/2 cup	0	0.6	100	5.4%
■ Blue Cheese	1 oz.	21	8.2	100	74%
Blueberries, fresh, raw	1 cup	0	0.6	82	7%
■ Blueberry Pie	4 3/4-in. wedge	0	17.0	380	40%
■ Bluefish, baked/broiled	3 oz.	64.5	4.7	135	31%
■ Bologna, beef	1 slice	16.6	8.1	89	82%
■ Bologna, chicken	1-oz. slice	31	5.0	64	70%
■ Bologna, pork	1 slice	15	8.0	89	81%
■ Bologna, turkey	1 slice	33	5.1	67	69%
Boston Brown Bread, canned	1/2-in. slice	3	1.0	95	10%
■ Bratwurst	1 oz.	17.1	7.4	86	77%
■ Braunschweiger	1-oz. slice	45	9.0	103	79%
■ Brazil Nuts	1 oz.	0	18.8	186	91%
Bread, French	1-in. slice	0	1.0	100	9%
Bread, Italian	3/4-in. slice	0	trace	85	—
Bread, Pita, 6 1/2 in. diam.	1	0	1.0	165	6%
Bread, Pumpernickel	1 slice	0	1.0	80	11%
Bread, White/Rye	1 slice	0	1.0	65	14%
Bread, Whole Wheat	1 slice	0	1.0	70	13%
Bread Crumbs	1/2 cup	0	2.5	195	12%
Bread Pudding with raisins	1/2 cup	85	8.1	248	29%
Broad Beans (Fava), dry, cooked	1/2 cup	0	0.3	93	3%
Broad Beans (Fava) young, cooked	1 cup	0	1.2	128	8%
Broccoli, cooked	1 spear	0	0.6	51	11%
Broccoli, chopped, cooked	1 cup	0	0.4	44	8%
■ Brownie frosted	1 1/2 x 1 3/4 x 7/8-in.	14	4.0	100	36%
Brussels Sprouts, fresh, cooked	1 cup	0	0.8	60	12%
Buckwheat Flour, (sifted), light	1 cup	0	1.0	340	3%
Buckwheat Groats, (Kasha), cooked	1 cup	0	1.2	182	6%
Bulgur, (Parboiled Wheat), dry	1/2 cup	0	1.5	300	5%
■ Butter, regular	1 Tb.	31	11.0	100	100%
Butter Beans, fresh, cooked	1 cup	0	0.6	208	3%
■ Butterfish, baked/broiled	3 oz.	70.5	8.8	159	50%
Buttermilk	8 fl. oz.	9	2.2	99	20%
Butternut Squash, cooked	1 cup	0	0.2	82	2%

Exceeds Target ■

Food	Portion	Cholesterol (milligrams)	Fat (grams)	Calories	% Fat Calories
Cabbage, raw	1 cup	0	0.2	18	10%
Cabbage, cooked	1 cup	0	0.6	34	16%
Cabbage, Chinese, cooked	1 cup	0	0.2	20	9%
Cake/Pastry Flour	1 cup	0	1.0	350	3%
Calf (see Veal)					
■ Camembert Cheese	1 oz.	20	6.9	85	73%
Candy, Hard	1/2 oz.	0	0	50	—
Candy Corn	1/2 oz.	0	0	55	—
Cantaloupe, cubed	1 cup	0	0.4	58	6%
■ Capon with skin, roasted	3 oz.	73.4	9.9	195	46%
■ Carp, baked/broiled	3 oz.	71.3	6.1	138	40%
Carrot, raw	1	0	trace	31	—
Carrot, sliced, cooked	1 cup	0	0.2	70	3%
■ Carrot Cake (cream cheese frosting)	3-in. wedge	74	21.0	385	49%
Casaba Melon, cubed	1 cup	0	0.2	46	4%
■ Cashew Butter	1 oz.	0	14.0	167	75%
■ Cashew Nuts	1 oz.	0	13.2	163	73%
Catfish, baked/broiled	3 oz.	61.5	2.4	89	24%
Cauliflower, cooked	1 cup	0	0.6	28	19%
Celeriac, cooked	1 cup	0	0.4	56	6%
Celery, raw, diced	1 cup	0	0.2	20	9%
■ Cheddar Cheese	1 oz.	30	9.4	114	74%
■ Cheese Sauce	1/2 cup	26	8.6	154	50%
■ Cheese Souffle (Cheddar)	1/2 cup	80	8.1	104	70%
■ Cheese Spread (American, processed)	1 oz.	16	6.0	80	68%
■ Cheesecake	2 1/3-in. wedge	170	18.0	280	58%
Cherries, Sweet, fresh	10	0	1.0	50	18%
■ Cherry Pie	4 3/4-in. wedge	0	18.0	410	40%
Chestnuts	1 oz.	0	1.1	105	9%
■ Chicken, fried (breaded), breast	1/2 (5.6 oz.)	119	18.0	365	44%
■ Chicken, fried (breaded), drumstick	1 (3.4 oz.)	62	11.0	195	51%
■ Chicken, roasted, with skin	3 oz.	75	11.6	203	51%
■ Chicken, roasted, without skin	3 oz.	75.8	6.3	161	35%
■ Chicken, Roaster, roasted with skin	3 oz.	64.5	11.4	190	54%
■ Chicken, Stewing, with skin	3 oz.	67.5	16.1	242	60%
■ Chicken, Stewing, without skin	3 oz.	70.5	10.1	202	45%
■ Chicken Ala King	1 cup	221	34.0	470	65%
Chicken Broth	1 cup	0	trace	22	—
Chicken Noodle Soup	1 cup	7	2.0	75	24%
■ Chicken Roll (light meat)	1-oz. slice	14	2.0	45	40%
■ Chicken Soup, Cream of	1 cup	27	11.0	190	52%
Chickpeas (Garbanzos), dried, cooked	1/2 cup	0	2.2	135	15%
Chicory, chopped	1 cup	0	0.6	42	13%
■ Chili with beans	1/2 cup	14	8.0	170	42%
Chili Sauce	1 Tb.	0	0	15	—

■ *Exceeds Target*

Food	Portion	Cholesterol (milligrams)	Fat (grams)	Calories	% Fat Calories
■ Chocolate, baking	1 oz.	0	15.0	145	93%
■ Chocolate, dark, sweet	1 oz.	0	10.0	150	60%
■ Chocolate, milk	1 oz.	6	9.0	145	56%
■ Chocolate Milk	8 fl. oz.	31	8.0	210	34%
Chocolate Pudding	1/2 cup	15	4.0	150	24%
Chocolate Syrup	1 Tb.	0	trace	43	—
Clams, steamed	3 oz.	57	1.7	126	12%
Clams, raw	2 large/5 small	60	1.0	41	22%
Clam Chowder, Manhattan	1 cup	0	2.5	81	28%
■ Clam Chowder, New England	1 cup	22	7.0	165	38%
Cocktail Sauce	1 Tb.	0	0	20	—
Cocoa	8 fl. oz.	1.3	1.3	133	9%
■ Coconut, raw, shredded	1/2 cup	0	13.5	143	85%
■ Coconut, dried, sweetened	1/2 cup	0	16.5	235	63%
■ Coconut Milk	8 fl. oz.	0	51.2	480	96%
Cod, baked/broiled	3 oz.	42.8	0.8	89	8%
Cod, dried	3 oz.	126	2.1	243	8%
■ Cod Liver Oil	1 tsp.	26	4.5	41	99%
Coffee	8 fl. oz.	0	0	5	—
Collard Greens, fresh, boiled	1 cup	0	0.2	34	5%
Collard Greens, frozen, boiled	1 cup	0	0.8	62	12%
■ Cookies, chocolate chip	1 (2 1/4 in.)	4.5	2.8	46	55%
Cookies, fig bar	1	6.8	1.0	53	17%
Cookies, gingersnaps	1	0	0.5	30	15%
Cookies, graham crackers	1 (2 1/2-in.)	0	0.5	30	15%
■ Cookies, oatmeal	1 (2 5/8 in.)	0.5	2.5	61	37%
■ Cookies, oatmeal-raisin	1 (2 5/8 in.)	0.5	2.5	61	37%
■ Cookies, peanut butter	1 (2 5/8 in.)	5.5	3.5	61	52%
■ Cookies, sandwich	1 (1 3/4 in.)	0	2.0	49	37%
■ Cookies, shortbread	1 sm.	6.8	2.0	39	46%
■ Cookies, sugar	1 (2 1/2 in.)	7.3	3.0	59	46%
■ Cookies, vanilla wafers	1 (1 3/4 in.)	2.4	0.7	19	33%
Corn, fresh, cooked	1 cup	0	2.2	178	11%
Corn, fresh, cooked	1 ear	0	1.0	89	10%
Corn, canned, creamed	1 cup	0	1.0	186	5%
■ Corn Chips	1 oz.	0	9.0	155	52%
Corn Grits, cooked	1 cup	0	0.5	146	3%
■ Corn Oil	1 Tb.	0	14	120	100%
■ Cornbread	2-in. square	30	3.2	93	31%
■ Corned Beef, brisket	3 oz.	84	16.3	215	68%
■ Corned Beef, canned	3 oz.	80	10.0	185	49%
■ Cornish Game Hen, dark meat	3 oz.	87	9.9	147	61%
■ Cornish Game Hen, light meat	3 oz.	75	6.9	123	51%
Cornmeal, whole-ground	1 cup	0	5.0	435	10%
■ Cottage Cheese, creamed	1/2 cup	17	5.1	117	39%

Food	Portion	Cholesterol (milligrams)	Fat (grams)	Calories	% Fat Calories
Cottage Cheese, low-fat	1/2 cup	5	1.2	82	13%
Crab, Alaska King, boiled	3 oz.	45	1.3	83	14%
Crabapple, sliced	1 cup	0	0.4	84	4%
■ Crackers, butter	1 oz.	0	8.0	140	51%
■ Crackers, cheese, plain	10 (1-in. sq.)	6	3.0	50	54%
■ Crackers, cheese/peanut butter	1	1	2.0	40	45%
Crackers, matzoh, egg	1 oz.	50	4.0	264	14%
Crackers, saltines	4	4	1.0	50	18%
Crackers, wheat thins	4	0	1.0	35	26%
Cranberries, fresh chopped	1 cup	0	0.2	54	3%
Cranberry Sauce	1 cup	0	0.4	418	1%
■ Cream, light	1/4 cup	40	11.6	116	90%
■ Cream, whipping, heavy	1/4 cup	84	22.4	208	97%
■ Cream Cheese	1 oz.	31	9.9	99	90%
■ Creamer, Nondairy	1 tsp.	0	1.0	10	90%
■ Creole Sauce	1/2 cup	0	2.8	76	33%
■ Croissant	1	13	12.0	235	46%
Crookneck Squash, cooked	1 cup	0	0.6	36	15%
Cucumber	1 med.	0	trace	29	—
Cupcake, chocolate	1	5	6.0	180	30%
Currants, dried	1/4 cup	0	trace	102	—
■ Custard, Baked	1/2 cup	139	7.5	153	44%
■ Custard Pie	4 3/4-in. wedge	169	17.0	330	46%
Dates	1	0	trace	23	—
■ Devil's Food Cake, (chocolate icing)	1 3/4-in. wedge	37	8.0	235	31%
■ Doughnut, plain 3 1/4-in.	1	20	12.0	210	51%
■ Doughnut, glazed 3 3/4-in.	1	21	13.0	235	50%
■ Duck with skin	3 oz.	71.3	24.1	287	76%
■ Egg (chicken), boiled/poached	1 egg	274	6.0	80	68%
■ Egg (chicken), fried	1 egg	278	7.0	95	66%
■ Egg (chicken), scrambled/omelet	1 egg	282	8.0	110	66%
■ Eggnog	8 fl. oz.	150	19.0	340	50%
Eggplant, cubed, cooked	1 cup	0	0.2	26	7%
■ Enchilada	1	19	16.0	235	61%
English Muffin	1	0	1.0	140	6%
Escarole, chopped	1 cup	0	0.2	8	23%
Farina, cooked	1 cup	0	0	116	—
Fennel, sliced	1 cup	0	0.4	54	7%
Figs, dried	1	0	0.2	47	4%
Figs, fresh	1	0	0.2	48	4%
■ Filberts, (Hazelnuts), dry-roasted	1 oz.	0	17.8	179	90%
Finnan Haddie (Smoked Haddock)	3 oz.	65.3	0.8	99	7%
Flounder, baked/broiled	3 oz.	57.8	1.3	100	12%
■ Frankfurter, beef	1	30.5	14.3	158	82%
■ Frankfurter, chicken	1	45	9.0	115	70%

■ *Exceeds Target*

Food	Portion	Cholesterol (milligrams)	Fat (grams)	Calories	% Fat Calories
■ Frankfurter, pork	1	23	13.0	145	81%
■ Frankfurter, turkey	1	54	8.9	113	71%
■ French Toast	1 slice	112	7.0	155	41%
Fruit, Mixed, canned, in juice	1 cup	0	0	112	—
■ Fruitcake (tube cake)	2/3-in. wedge	20	7.0	165	38%
Fudge (Chocolate)	1 oz.	1	3.0	115	24%
■ Fudge Topping	1 Tb.	0	2.5	63	36%
Garlic	1 clove	0	trace	4	—
■ Gazpacho	1 cup	0	2.2	57	35%
Ginger, fresh, sliced	1 Tb.	0	trace	4	—
Gingerbread	2 1/2 in.-square	1	4.0	175	21%
Gooseberries fresh	1 cup	0	0.8	68	11%
■ Granola	1/2 cup	0	16.6	298	50%
Grapefruit	1/2 med.	0	trace	38	—
Grapes, Concord	1 cup	0	1.6	66	22%
Grapes, seedless	1 cup	0	1.0	114	8%
Gravy, canned, au jus	1/4 cup	0.5	0.2	40	5%
■ Gravy, canned, beef	1/4 cup	2	1.4	31	41%
■ Gravy, canned, chicken	1/4 cup	1.5	3.4	48	64%
■ Gravy, canned, turkey	1/4 cup	1.5	1.3	31	38%
Great Northern Beans, dry, cooked	1/2 cup	0	0.5	105	4%
Gum Drops	1 oz.	0	trace	100	—
Haddock, baked/broiled	3 oz.	63	0.8	95	7%
■ Haddock, fried (breaded)	3 oz.	75	9.0	175	46%
■ Halibut, baked/broiled	3 oz.	62	6.0	140	39%
■ Halvah	1 oz.	0	11.0	160	62%
■ Ham, boiled	1-oz. slice	16	3.0	53	51%
■ Ham, canned, spiced	3 x 2 x 1/2-in.	13	6.5	70	84%
■ Ham, chopped	1-oz.	14	4.7	64	66%
■ Ham, cured, roasted	3 oz.	50.6	7.7	153	45%
■ Ham, cured, picnic, lean, roasted	3 oz.	41.1	6.0	146	37%
■ Ham, cured steak, extra lean	3 oz.	38.6	3.6	105	31%
■ Ham, fresh, shank, roasted lean	3 oz.	78.9	9.0	184	44%
■ Ham, minced	1 oz.	20	5.9	75	71%
■ Herring, Atlantic, baked/broiled	3 oz.	65.3	9.8	173	51%
■ Herring, Atlantic, kippered	3 oz.	69.8	10.5	185	51%
■ Herring, Atlantic, pickled	3 oz.	85	13.0	140	84%
■ Hickory Nuts, dried, shelled	1 oz.	0	18.3	187	88%
Hake, baked/broiled	3 oz.	57	1.1	93	11%
■ Hollandaise Sauce	1/2 cup	94	34.1	353	87%
Honey	1 Tb.	0	0	64	—
Honeydew Melon, fresh, cubed	1 cup	0	0.2	60	3%
Hubbard Squash, cubed	1 cup	0	1.2	100	11%
■ Ice Cream, vanilla	1/2 cup	30	7.2	135	48%
■ Ice Milk, vanilla	1/2 cup	9	2.8	72	35%

Exceeds Target ■

Food	Portion	Cholesterol (milligrams)	Fat (grams)	Calories	% Fat Calories
■ Italian Sausage	3 oz.	66.9	22.0	277	72%
Jelly Beans	1 oz.	0	0	100	—
Jerusalem Artichoke, sliced	1 cup	0	trace	114	—
Kale, cooked	1 cup	0	0.6	42	13%
Ketchup	1 Tb.	0	0	15	—
Kidney Beans, dry, cooked	1/2 cup	0	0.5	113	4%
Kiwi Fruit, fresh	1 med.	0	trace	45	—
Kohlrabi, cooked	1 cup	0	0.2	48	4%
Kumquat, fresh	1 med.	0	trace	12	—
■ Lamb, Chops, arm, braised, lean	3 oz.	104.6	12.5	239	47%
■ Lamb, Chops, loin, broiled, lean	3 oz.	80.6	8.1	184	40%
■ Lamb, Heart, braised	3 oz.	211.5	6.8	158	39%
Lamb, Kidney, braised	3 oz.	480.8	3.1	116	24%
■ Lamb, Leg, roasted, lean	3 oz.	76.3	7.0	164	38%
Lamb, Liver	3 oz.	255.2	3.7	116	29%
■ Lamb, Rib, roasted, lean	3 oz.	75.4	10.5	199	48%
■ Lamb, Tongue, braised	3 oz.	160.5	17.3	234	67%
■ Lard	1 Tb.	12	12.8	115	100%
Leek, cooked	1 cup	0	0.2	32	6%
Lemon	1 lge.	0	trace	15	—
■ Lemon Meringue Pie	4 3/4-in. wedge	143	14.0	355	36%
Lentils dry, cooked	1/2 cup	0	0.5	108	4%
Lettuce, Iceberg	large head	0	1.0	70	13%
Licorice	1 oz.	0	1.0	100	9%
Lima Beans, fresh, cooked	1 cup	0	0.8	218	3%
Lime	1 med.	0	trace	20	—
Linguine, cooked	1 cup	0	0.9	197	4%
■ Liverwurst/Liver Sausage	1 oz.	45.1	8.1	93	78%
Lobster, Northern, boiled	3 oz.	61.5	0.5	83	5%
■ Lox	3 oz.	19.5	3.7	100	33%
■ Macadamia Nuts	1 oz.	0	20.9	199	95%
Macaroni, Elbow, cooked	1 cup	0	1.0	155	6%
■ Macaroni and Cheese	1 cup	44	22.0	430	46%
■ Mackerel, Atlantic, baked/broiled	3 oz.	63.8	15.2	223	61%
■ Mackerel, Jack, canned	3 oz.	67.5	5.3	133	36%
■ Malted Milk, chocolate	8 fl. oz.	34	9.0	235	35%
■ Malted Milk, plain	8 fl. oz.	37	10.0	235	38%
Mango	1 med.	0	1.0	135	7%
Maple Syrup	1 Tb.	0	0	50	—
■ Margarine	1 Tb.	0	11.0	100	99%
Marshmallow	1	0	0	25	—
■ Mayonnaise	1 Tb.	8	11.0	100	99%
■ Milk, whole	8 fl. oz.	33	8.2	150	49%
■ Milk, 2%	8 fl. oz.	18	4.7	121	35%
Milk, 1%	8 fl. oz.	10	2.6	102	23%

■ *Exceeds Target*

Food	Portion	Cholesterol (milligrams)	Fat (grams)	Calories	% Fat Calories
Milk, skim	8 fl. oz.	4	0.4	86	4%
Milk, Condensed, canned, sweetened	4 fl. oz.	52	13.6	490	25%
■ Milk, Evaporated, canned	4 fl. oz.	37	9.6	170	51%
Milkshake, chocolate	8 fl. oz.	29.6	8.4	288	26%
Milkshake, vanilla	8 fl. oz.	26.4	7.2	252	26%
Millet, cooked	1 cup	0	2.0	287	6%
Minestrone	1 cup	0	3.4	105	29%
Miso	1/4 cup	0	4.2	142	27%
Molasses, Barbados	1 Tb.	0	0	54	—
■ Mozzarella, part-skim	1 oz.	15	5.0	80	56%
■ Mozzarella, whole-milk	1 oz.	22	6.0	80	67%
■ Muffins, blueberry	1 avg.	19	5.0	135	33%
■ Muffins, bran	1 avg.	24	6.0	125	43%
■ Muffins, corn	1 avg.	23	5.0	145	31%
Mullet, baked/broiled	3 oz.	53.3	4.1	128	29%
Mushrooms, raw	1 cup	0	0.4	18	20%
■ Mushroom Soup, (with milk)	1 cup	20	14.0	205	62%
Mussels, raw	1/2 cup	21	1.7	65	24%
Mustard Greens, cooked	1 cup	0	0.4	22	16%
Navy Beans, dry, cooked	1/2 cup	0	0.5	113	4%
Nectarine, fresh	1 med.	0	0.7	67	9%
■ Noodles, Chow Mein	1 cup	5	11.0	220	45%
Noodles, Egg, cooked	1 cup	50	2.0	200	9%
Oatmeal, cooked	1 cup	0	2.4	145	15%
Ocean Perch, baked/broiled	3 oz.	45.8	1.8	103	16%
■ Ocean Perch, fried	1 fillet	66	11.0	185	54%
■ Okra fresh, cooked	1 cup	0	0.2	50	4%
■ Olive Oil	1 Tb.	0	14.0	120	100%
■ Olives, Green	4 med.	0	1.5	15	90%
Onion, raw, chopped	1 cup	0	0.2	60	3%
Onion, cooked, chopped	1 cup	0	0.4	94	4%
■ Onion Soup	1 cup	0	2.4	65	33%
Orange	1 med.	0	0	62	—
Oysters, raw	1 cup	120	4.0	160	23%
■ Oysters, fried (breaded)	1	35	5.0	90	50%
Pancakes	1 (4-in. diam.)	16	2.0	60	30%
Papaya, fresh	1 med.	0	0.5	117	4%
■ Parmesan Cheese, grated	1 Tb.	4	2.0	25	72%
Parsley fresh, chopped	1/4 cup	0	trace	5	—
Parsnips, sliced, cooked	1 cup	0	0.4	126	3%
Peach, canned, in juice	1/2 cup	0	trace	55	—
Peach, dried	5 halves	0	0.5	156	3%
Peach, fresh	1	0	trace	37	—
■ Peach Pie	4 3/4-in. wedge	0	17.0	405	38%
■ Peanut Brittle	1/2 oz.	0	2.5	65	35%

Exceeds Target ■

Food	Portion	Cholesterol (milligrams)	Fat (grams)	Calories	% Fat Calories
■ Peanut Butter	1 Tb.	0	8.0	94	77%
■ Peanut Flour, low fat	1 cup	0	13.1	257	46%
■ Peanut Oil	1 Tb.	0	14.0	120	100%
■ Peanuts	1 oz.	0	14.0	164	77%
Pea Pods, Chinese, cooked	1 cup	0	0.4	65	6%
Pear, Bartlett, fresh	1 med.	0	1.0	100	9%
Pears, canned, in juice	1/2 cup	0	trace	62	—
Pears, canned, dried	1/4 cup	0	0.3	118	2%
Pea Soup, with water	1 cup	0	2.9	164	16%
Peas, Green, fresh, cooked	1 cup	0	0.4	134	3%
Pecan Flour	4 oz.	0	1.6	372	4%
■ Pecans	1 oz.	0	18.4	187	87%
Pepper, raw, chili	1	0	trace	18	—
Pepper, raw, sweet, green/red	1	0	trace	20	—
Perch, baked/broiled	3 oz.	97.5	1.0	100	9%
Persimmon	1 med.	0	trace	32	—
Pickle, Dill	1 3-3/4-in.	0	trace	5	—
Pickle, Sweet (Gherkin)	1 2-1/2-in.	0	trace	20	—
■ Pie Crust, 9-in. diam.	1	0	60	900	60%
■ Pecan Pie	4 3/4-in. wedge	95	32.0	575	50%
■ Pig's Feet, pickled	3 oz.	78	13.8	174	71%
Pike, Walleye, baked/broiled	3 oz.	93.8	1.4	101	13%
Pimiento, canned	1	0	0	11	—
■ Pine Nuts, (Pignolia)	1 oz.	0	14.4	146	89%
Pineapple, canned, in juice	1/2 cup	0	0.3	75	4%
Pineapple, fresh	1 cup	0	0.6	78	7%
Pinto Beans, dry, cooked	1/2 cup	0	0.5	133	3%
■ Pistachio Nuts	1 oz.	0	13.7	164	75%
Pizza, Cheese	1/8 lge.	56	9.0	290	28%
Plantain, sliced, cooked	1 cup	0	0.2	178	1%
Plum, canned, in juice	1/2 cup	0	trace	73	—
Plum, fresh	1	0	0.4	36	10%
Pollock, Atlantic, baked/broiled	3 oz.	77.3	1.1	101	9%
■ Pompano, baked/broiled	3 oz.	54.8	10.4	179	52%
Popcorn, air-popped	1 cup	0	trace	30	—
■ Popcorn, oil-popped	1 cup	0	3.0	55	49%
■ Pork, Chitterlings, simmered	3 oz.	122.6	24.7	260	86%
■ Pork, Chop, loin, lean, broiled	3 oz.	85.2	9.6	198	44%
Pork, Kidney, braised	3 oz.	411.4	4.0	129	28%
Pork, Liver, braised	3 oz.	304.3	3.8	141	24%
■ Pork, Loin, sirloin, roasted, lean	3 oz.	77.1	11.3	202	50%
■ Pork, Loin, top-loin, roasted, lean	3 oz.	153.4	11.8	210	51%
■ Pork, Shoulder, blade, roasted, lean	3 oz.	84	14.4	219	59%
■ Pork, Spareribs, braised	3 oz.	103.7	26.0	340	69%
Pork, Tenderloin, roasted	3 oz.	78.8	4.1	141	26%

■ *Exceeds Target*

Food	Portion	Cholesterol (milligrams)	Fat (grams)	Calories	% Fat Calories
■ Potato Chips	10	0	7.0	105	60%
■ Potato Salad	1/2 cup	170	10.5	180	53%
■ Potatoes, Au Gratin	1/2 cup	28	9.5	163	53%
Potatoes, Baked in skin	1 med.	0	trace	220	—
Potatoes, Boiled	1 med.	0	trace	120	—
■ Potatoes, French-Fried in oil	10 pieces	0	8.0	160	45%
■ Potatoes, Hash-Browned	1/2 cup	0	9.0	170	48%
■ Potatoes, Mashed	1/2 cup	2	4.5	113	36%
■ Potatoes, Scalloped	1/2 cup	14.5	4.5	105	39%
■ Pound Cake	1/2-in. slice	64	5.0	110	41%
Pretzels, 2 1/4-in. sticks	10	0	trace	10	—
■ Provolone Cheese	1 oz.	20	7.6	100	68%
Prunes, dried	5 lge	0	trace	115	—
Prunes, dried, stewed	1/2 cup	0	trace	113	—
Puffed Cereal	1 cup	0	0	50	—
Pumpkin, canned	1 can	0	0.6	82	7%
Pumpkin, fresh, cooked, mashed	1 cup	0	0.2	48	4%
■ Pumpkin Pie	4 3/4-in. wedge	109	17.0	320	48%
■ Pumpkin Seeds (Pepitas)	1 oz.	0	12.0	148	73%
■ Quiche Lorraine	3-in. wedge	285	48.0	600	72%
Quince	1 med.	0	trace	53	—
Radicchio, shredded	1 cup	0	0.2	10	18%
Radish	4	0	trace	5	—
Raisin Bread	1 slice	0	1.0	65	14%
Raisins, loosely packed	1/2 cup	0	0.5	218	2%
Raspberries, fresh, black	1 cup	0	2.0	100	18%
Raspberries, fresh, red	1 cup	0	0.7	61	10%
Red Snapper, baked/broiled	3 oz.	39.8	1.5	109	12%
Refried Beans	1/2 cup	0	1.5	148	9%
Relish, Sweet	1 Tb.	0	trace	19	—
Rhubarb, cooked, sweetened	1/2 cup	0	trace	140	—
Rice, Brown, long-grain, cooked	1 cup	0	1.0	230	4%
Rice, White, long-grained, cooked	1 cup	0	0.6	226	2%
Rice, Wild, cooked	1 cup	0	0.6	166	3%
Rice, Sweet, cooked	1 cup	0	0.6	234	2%
Rice Pudding	1/2 cup	15	4.0	155	23%
■ Ricotta Cheese, part-skim	1/2 cup	25	9.0	156	52%
■ Ricotta Cheese, whole-milk	1/2 cup	58	14.7	197	67%
Roll, Dinner	2-1/2-in. diam.	12	3.0	120	23%
Roll, Hard	3-3/4-in. diam.	trace	2.0	155	12%
Roll, Submarine (Hoagie)	1	trace	8.0	400	18%
■ Romano Cheese	1 oz.	29	7.6	110	62%
Rutabaga, cooked	1 cup	0	0.4	66	6%
Rye Flour, medium	1 cup	0	1.8	360	5%
Rye Grain, dry	1/2 cup	0	2.1	284	7%

Food	Portion	Cholesterol (milligrams)	Fat (grams)	Calories	% Fat Calories
■ Salad Dressing, Blue Cheese	1 Tb.	3	8.0	75	96%
■ Salad Dressing, French	1 Tb.	0	9.0	85	95%
■ Salad Dressing, Italian	1 Tb.	0	7.1	69	93%
■ Salad Dressing, Oil and Vinegar	1 Tb.	0	8.0	70	100%
■ Salad Dressing, Russian	1 Tb.	0	7.8	76	92%
■ Salad Dressing, Thousand Island	1 Tb.	4	5.6	60	84%
■ Safflower Oil	1 Tb.	0	14.0	120	100%
■ Salami, Beef	1 slice	18.6	5.9	75	71%
■ Salami, Cooked	1-oz. slice	18.5	5.5	73	68%
■ Salami, Hard (dry), Pork	1 slice	8	3.5	43	73%
■ Salmon, Atlantic, baked/broiled	3 oz.	60.8	6.9	155	40%
■ Salmon, Pink, canned	3 oz.	34	5.0	120	38%
■ Salt Pork, raw	3 oz.	75	68.4	636	97%
Salt Water Taffy	1/2 oz.	0	0.5	50	9%
■ Sardines, canned	3 oz.	85	9.0	175	46%
Sauerkraut	1 cup	0	0.4	44	8%
■ Sausage, Beef	2 links	67	26.9	312	78%
■ Sausage, Fresh, cooked	3 oz.	66	25.2	300	76%
■ Sausage, Smoked, grilled	3 oz.	58.3	27.3	333	74%
Scallions, chopped	1/4 cup	0	trace	8	—
■ Scallops, fried (breaded)	6 lge.	70	10.0	195	46%
Scallops, raw	4 lge.	20	0.4	52	7%
Sea Bass, baked/broiled	3 oz.	45	2.2	106	19%
■ Sea Trout, baked/broiled	3 oz.	90	4.0	113	32%
Semolina, dry	1/2 cup	0	0.9	301	3%
■ Sesame Oil	1 Tb.	0	14.0	120	100%
■ Sesame Seeds, toasted	1 oz.	0	13.6	160	77%
■ Sesame Tahini	1 Tb.	0	8.1	90	81%
Sheet Cake (frosted)	3-in.	70	14.0	445	28%
Sherbet, Orange	1/2 cup	7	1.9	135	13%
■ Shortening, Vegetable	1 Tb.	0	12.8	115	100%
Shrimp, boiled/steamed	1 lge.	10.8	trace	6	—
Smelts, baked/broiled	3 oz.	76.5	2.6	106	22%
■ Smelts, fried (breaded)	3 oz.	168	10.0	200	45%
Sole, baked/broiled	3 oz.	43	1.0	80	11%
■ Sour Cream	1/4 cup	20	12.0	100	100%
■ Sour Cream, Nondairy	1/4 cup	4	8.0	80	90%
■ Sour Cream Sauce (with milk)	1/2 cup	45	15.1	255	53%
■ Soy Flour, Full-Fat	1 cup	0	17.6	371	43%
■ Soy Milk	8 fl. oz.	0	4.6	79	52%
■ Soy Oil	1 Tb.	0	14.0	120	100%
■ Soybean Kernels, toasted	1/2 cup	0	13.0	245	48%
■ Soybeans, Dry, cooked	1/2 cup	0	5.0	118	38%
Spaghetti, cooked firm	1 cup	0	1.0	155	6%
■ Spaghetti and Meatballs	1 cup	89	12.0	330	33%

■ *Exceeds Target*

Food	Portion	Cholesterol (milligrams)	Fat (grams)	Calories	% Fat Calories
Spaghetti Squash, cooked	1 cup	0	0.4	46	8%
Spinach, fresh, chopped, raw	1 cup	0	0.2	12	15%
Spinach, cooked	1 cup	0	0.4	42	9%
■ Spinach Souffle	1/2 cup	92	9.0	110	74%
Split Peas, cooked	1/2 cup	0	0.4	115	3%
Split Pea Soup	1 cup	0	3.2	145	20%
Squid, raw	3 oz.	198.8	1.2	78	14%
Strawberries, fresh	1 cup	0	0.6	46	12%
String Beans, cooked	1 cup	0	0.4	44	8%
■ Stuffing, dry	1 cup	0	31.0	500	56%
■ Stuffing, moist	1 cup	67	26.0	420	56%
Succotash, fresh, cooked	1 cup	0	1.6	222	7%
Sugar, white	1 Tb.	0	0	46	—
Summer Squash, cooked	1 cup	0	0	36	—
■ Sunflower Butter	1 Tb.	0	8.0	92	78%
■ Sunflower Oil	1 Tb.	0	14.0	120	100%
■ Sunflower Seeds	1 oz.	0	14.0	165	76%
Sweet and Sour Sauce	1/2 cup	0	trace	147	—
Sweet Potato, baked	1 med.	0	trace	115	—
Sweet Potato, boiled	1/2 cup	0	trace	160	—
Sweet Potato, candied	2 1/2 x 2-in.	8	3.0	145	19%
Swiss Chard, cooked	1 cup	0	0.2	36	5%
■ Swiss Cheese	1 oz.	26	7.8	107	66%
Swordfish, baked/broiled	3 oz.	42.8	4.4	132	30%
■ Taco	1	21	11.0	195	51%
Taffy	1/2 oz.	0	0.5	50	9%
Tangelo	1	0	0	39	—
Tangerine	1 med.	0	trace	35	—
Tapioca Pudding	1/2 cup	15	4.0	145	25%
■ Tartar Sauce	1 Tb.	4	8.0	75	96%
Tea	8 fl. oz.	0	0	3	—
■ Tempeh	4 oz.	0	8.8	224	35%
■ Toffee	1/2 oz.	0	3.3	68	44%
■ Tofu raw, firm	4 oz.	0	10.0	164	55%
Tomato, raw	1 med.	0	trace	25	—
Tomato, stewed	1 cup	0	2.0	60	30%
Tomato, Paste. canned	2 oz.	0	0.6	48	11%
Tomato, Puree. canned	1 cup	0	0.2	105	2%
Tomato, Sauce, canned	1 cup	0	0.4	75	5%
Tomato Soup	1 cup	0	2.5	88	26%
Tortillas, Corn	1	0	1.0	65	14%
Triticale, dry	1/2 cup	0	2.0	323	6%
■ Trout, broiled	3 oz.	71	9.0	175	46%
Tuna, baked/broiled	3 oz.	42	5.3	157	30%
■ Tuna, canned, chunk light, oil	3 oz.	55	7.0	165	38%

Exceeds Target ■

Food	Portion	Cholesterol (milligrams)	Fat (grams)	Calories	% Fat Calories
Tuna, canned, solid white, water	3 oz.	48	1.0	135	7%
■ Tuna Salad	1/2 cup	40	9.5	188	46%
■ Turkey, dark meat, with skin	3 oz.	100.3	6.1	156	35%
Turkey, light meat, with skin	3 oz.	81.4	3.9	141	25%
■ Turkey, Ground, cooked	3 oz.	87	11.1	201	50%
Turkey Giblets, simmered	3 oz.	355.5	4.4	142	28%
Turkey Loaf	3/4-oz. slice	8.5	0.5	23	20%
■ Turkey Roll	3 oz.	47.1	6.0	128	42%
Turnip, fresh, cooked	1 cup	0	0.2	28	6%
Turnip Greens, fresh, cooked	1 cup	0	0.4	30	12%
Veal, Arm Steak, lean	3 oz.	77.1	4.5	171	24%
■ Veal, Blade, lean	3 oz.	77.1	6.7	181	33%
■ Veal, Brains, fried	3 oz.	1,803	14.3	182	71%
Veal, Chop, loin, lean	3 oz.	77.1	5.7	177	29%
Veal, Cubed, stewed	3 oz.	123	3.7	160	21%
■ Veal, Cutlet	3 oz.	109.7	9.4	232	37%
■ Veal, Heart, braised	3 oz.	150	5.8	158	33%
■ Veal, Kidney, braised	3 oz.	672.8	4.8	139	31%
■ Veal, Liver, braised	3 oz.	477	5.9	140	38%
Veal, Rump Roast, lean	3 oz.	109.7	1.9	134	13%
Veal, Sirloin, lean, roasted	3 oz.	109.7	2.7	131	19%
Vanilla Pudding	1/2 cup	15	4.0	145	25%
■ Vegetable Oil	1 Tb.	0	14.0	120	100%
Vegetable Soup	1 cup	0	2.0	78	23%
Venison, roasted	3 oz.	95.3	2.7	134	18%
■ Vienna Sausage	2-in. link	8	4.0	45	80%
Vinegar, Distilled	1 Tb.	0	0	2	—
■ Waffles, 7-in. diam.	1	102	13.0	245	48%
■ Walnuts, English	1 oz.	0	17.6	182	87%
Water Chestnuts, canned, sliced	1/2 cup	0	trace	35	—
Watercress, chopped	1/2 cup	0	trace	2	—
Watermelon	1 cup	0	1	50	18%
Wheat, Durum, dry	1/2 cup	0	2.4	325	7%
Wheat Bran, raw	1/4 cup	0	0.6	24	23%
Wheat Germ, raw	1 oz.	0	3.4	103	30%
■ Whipped Topping, frozen	1 Tb.	0	1.0	15	60%
■ Whipped Topping, pressurized	1 Tb.	0	1.0	10	90%
■ White Cake, white frosting	1 3/4-in. wedge	3	9.0	260	31%
White Flour, all-purpose, (sifted)	1 cup	0	1.0	420	2%
■ White Sauce, medium	1/2 cup	16	15.0	198	68%
■ Whitefish, baked/broiled	3 oz.	65.3	6.4	146	40%
Whitefish, smoked	3 oz.	27.8	0.8	92	8%
Whiting, baked/broiled	3 oz.	71.3	1.4	98	13%
Whole Wheat Flour	1 cup	0	2.0	400	5%
Worcestershire Sauce	1 Tb.	0	0	10	—

■ *Exceeds Target*

Food	Portion	Cholesterol (milligrams)	Fat (grams)	Calories	% Fat Calories
Yam, baked/boiled	1 cup	0	0.2	158	1%
Yeast, baker's	1 oz.	0	0.5	80	6%
Yeast, brewer's	1 Tb.	0	trace	25	—
■ Yellow Cake, chocolate frosting	1 3/4-in. wedge	36	8.0	235	31%
Yogurt, low-fat, fruit	1/2 cup	5	1.3	113	10%
Yogurt, low fat, plain	1/2 cup	2	0.2	63	3%
■ Yogurt, regular	1/2 cup	14	3.7	70	48%
Zucchini, fresh, raw	1 cup	0	0.2	18	10%
Zucchini, fresh, cooked	1 cup	0	0.2	28	6%

How to Read the "Nutrition Facts" Label

The new label has been carefully crafted to make healthy choices easier. It not only gives the amount of each major nutrient supplied in a serving, but tells you how far that amount goes towards fulfilling your daily allowance. For instance, if a product lists a "% Daily Value" of 60 percent for fat, you can be sure it presents a problem. The percentage may not exactly reflect your unique dietary requirements, but it's generally close enough to allow a quick assessment of the product's impact on your diet.

AMOUNT PER SERVING

The calorie counts listed here give you the information you need to keep your "fat quotient" in line. The target for good health is to get no more than 30 percent of your total calories from fat. In the example seen here, 33 percent (30 divided by 90) of the calories are derived from fat—slightly more than the ideal, but an excess that can easily be counterbalanced by other, lower-fat selections

VITAMINS AND MINERALS

All manufacturers are required to provide information on the four nutrients found here. They can add more if they wish. The percentages show how much of the official Recommended Dietary Allowance (RDA) a serving supplies. These figures can give you a fairly good idea of how important the product is in meeting your requirements. Remember, however, that some people may need more of these nutrients than called for by the basic RDA.

SERVING SIZE

These sizes are now somewhat standardized, and reflect a realistic portion. Caution is still in order, however. Your idea of a serving may be different from the average.

% DAILY VALUE

These figures show what part of your key nutritional allowances a serving of the product supplies.

*Allowances for **fat, carbohydrates**, and **fiber** depend on the total number of calories you take in each day; and the figures here assume a 2,000-calorie diet. If you eat more than that on a daily basis, you're allowance for each nutrient will be higher, and a serving of the product will provide less than the share listed here. Still, even if the figures don't exactly coincide with your diet, they can give you a rough idea of the way the product will fit into your daily nutritional budget.*

*The allowances for **cholesterol** and **sodium** are the same no matter how many calories you eat, so you can use these percentages without any adjustment.*

*No percentages are listed for **sugars** and **protein**. Both are vital; but because almost all Americans get more than they need, the allowances usually aren't listed.*

Depending on the size of the label and the content of the food, figures for some of these nutrients may not be listed.

DAILY VALUES TABLE

This table lists the ideal allowances currently recommended by nutritional experts for two typical calorie levels. The "% Daily Values" figures further up the label are based on the numbers in the 2,000 calorie column. The table is often omitted due to lack of space.

Ideal Allowances

Use this table to get a closer estimate of the allowances justified by your actual calorie intake. All allowances are listed in grams.

Nutrition Facts

Serving Size 1 cup (228g)
Servings Per Container 2

Amount Per Serving
Calories 90   Calories from Fat 30

	%**Daily Value***
Total Fat 3g	**5%**
Saturated Fat 0g	**0%**
Cholesterol 0mg	**0%**
Sodium 300 mg	**13%**
Total Carbohydrate 13g	**4%**
Dietary Fiber 3g	**12%**
Sugars 3g	
Protein 3g	

Vitamin A 80%	•	Vitamin C 60%
Calcium 4%	•	Iron 4%

*Percent Daily Values are based on a 2,000 calorie diet. Your daily values may be higher or lower depending on your calorie needs:

		Calories:	2,000	2,500
Total Fat	Less than		65g	80g
Sat Fat	Less than		20g	25g
Cholesterol	Less than		300mg	300mg
Sodium	Less than		2,400mg	2,400mg
Total Carbohydrate			300g	375g
Dietary Fiber			25g	30g

Calories per gram:
Fat 9 • Carbohydrate 4 • Protein 4

NUTRIENT	DAILY CALORIE INTAKE					
	1,600	**2,000**	**2,200**	**2,500**	**2,800**	**3,200**
Total Fat	53	65	73	80	93	107
Saturated Fat	18	20	24	25	31	36
Total Carbohydrates	240	300	330	375	420	480
Dietary Fiber	20	25	25	30	32	37

How To Keep Your Food Safe

The 500 people who became ill from eating undercooked hamburgers at fast food establishments in the Northwest in 1993 bear witness that food can cause infection as well as fight it. Health experts estimate that food-borne illnesses affect somewhere between 33 to 81 million Americans each year and cost as much as $23 billion in health care bills and lost productivity.

Years ago, food-related infections merely caused a few hours or days of nausea and vomiting, diarrhea, and abdominal pain. But changes in production methods, such as giving animals antibiotics to increase their growth, have led to the development of more dangerous organisms in food. Some of these newer bugs are now causing more serious illness, even death. Children, the elderly, and those with chronic diseases are especially vulnerable. Unfortunately, because some of these disease-causing bacteria do not produce easily detectable changes in food or animals, infected food may pass the government's—and your—inspection.

Leaving contaminated foods unrefrigerated, or not cooking them thoroughly enough, allows bacteria to multiply to levels sufficient to cause illness. (Remember that refrigerated convenience foods generally are not sterile; you need to keep them cold at all times.) The most common bugs, and the foods they favor, are listed in the table on the following pages.

All meat, fish, poultry, and dairy products—and dishes containing them—may contain the seeds of serious contamination, so careful storage and handling is the key to avoiding some very nasty surprises. You can't control what happens in the ocean, the barn, or the restaurant, but you can take precautions once the food is in your kitchen. Ideally, you should follow all of the guidelines listed below.

- Clean food—and everything it touches—scrupulously. This includes washing food, utensils, counters, sinks, and bowls.
- Always wash your hands before preparing food and after using the bathroom, blowing your nose, or touching a pet. Make sure your apron, clothing, dish towel, and

anything else on which you wipe your hands is clean.

- Keep cuts, scrapes, sores, and other hand injuries away from contact with food. They are a breeding ground for infections which could be passed to the food.
- Keep meat, fish, poultry, and dairy products refrigerated or frozen. If you expect a delay between the supermarket and your refrigerator, put the food in a cooler for the trip home. Refrigerate leftovers promptly.
- Never thaw frozen food at room temperature. Use the refrigerator or microwave.
- Keep your refrigerator at 40 degrees or colder and the freezer at zero or colder. Store raw meat, poultry, and seafood in the coldest parts.
- Refrigerate milk and soft cheeses and use them promptly. (Eating moldy cheese is safe, however.)
- Keep uncooked meat, poultry, and fish in leakproof containers. Never put other food on the same surface as uncooked animal products. Wash cutting boards and knives immediately.
- Never taste or eat raw, rare, or even pink *ground* meat or poultry. Cook hamburgers, meat loaf, turkey, and chicken until the juices run clear. (You don't need to worry about rare steaks and chops.)

- The only 100 percent sure way to avoid contaminated raw oysters or clams is to never eat them, even in an expensive restaurant. No one can be certain about the pollution levels in the water in which the shellfish grew. Avoid raw fish, such as sushi, unless you have confidence in the vendor.
- Buy only clean, uncracked eggs. Use them within 5 weeks of purchase. Never eat raw or uncooked eggs; do not even taste cake or cookie batter. Use only pasteurized eggs or an egg substitute in Caesar salad or any other recipe calling for raw eggs. In restaurants, ask how such foods are prepared and don't order them if they include uncooked eggs.
- Wash all fruits and vegetables thoroughly, even if you plan to peel them before eating them. If possible, use a separate cutting board to prepare foods that will be eaten raw.

FAVORITE HIDE-OUTS OF FOOD-BORNE INFECTIONS . . .

FOOD UNDER SUSPICION	POSSIBLE INFECTION
Egg yolks and dishes that contain them	Salmonella
Raw eggs	Listeria
Custards	Salmonella
	Staphylococcus
Milk	Shigella
	Listeria
Unpasteurized milk	Campylobacter jejuni Salmonella Escherichia coli
Salad dressings	Salmonella
Chicken, potato, ham, and egg salads	Staphylococcus
Sandwich fillings	Salmonella
Seafood	Salmonella (especially in shellfish)
	Listeria
Shellfish and smoked and salted fish	*Clostridium botulinum* (infection also known as botulism)
Uncooked tofu salad	Shigella
Shredded lettuce and cabbage packaged for restaurants and retail sale	Shigella
Poultry	Campylobacter jejuni Listeria Salmonella
Meat and meat products	Clostridium botulinum (ham, sausage) Escherichia coli (undercooked ground meat) Listeria Staphylococcus (processed meats)
Cheeses	Staphylococcus
Unpasteurized cheese	Salmonella
Soft-surface ripened cheeses	Listeria
Sauces	Staphylococcus
Cream-filled baked goods	Staphylococcus
Improperly home-canned foods	Clostridium botulinum (botulism)
Apple cider	Escherichia coli
Fruits and vegetables	Salmonella

... AND WHAT TO EXPECT FROM EACH

INFECTION	SYMPTOMS	TREATMENT
Campylobacter jejuni	Diarrhea; fever; discomfort; headache; chills. Symptoms start within 2 to 11 days of exposure; last 7 to 14 days. Can lead to life-threatening Guillain-Barre syndrome.	If diarrhea and fever last longer than 5 or 6 days, give replacement fluids: 1 teaspoon salt and 4 heaping teaspoons sugar in 1 quart water. The doctor may prescribe Cipro or erythromycin.
Clostridium botulinum	Symptoms range from mild discomfort to death within 24 hours. Initial symptoms are nausea, vomiting, weakness, and dizziness. This can progress to paralysis, including inability to breathe.	Hospitalization is required; mechanical breathing assistance may be needed.
Escherichia coli	Watery diarrhea within 1 to 8 days of exposure; diarrhea becomes bloody; abdominal pain, nausea, occasional vomiting, sometimes fever. In children, can lead to life-threatening kidney damage. Lasts 5 to 8 days.	Give replacement fluids (see above). Do not use antidiarrheal medications. Antibiotics are usually not needed.
Listeria	Especially in the elderly, pregnant women, infants, and people with suppressed immune systems; severe diarrhea; flu-like fever and headache; pneumonia; and infections of the membranes around the brain (meningitis) or heart (endocarditis)	The doctor will prescribe antibiotics (Bactrim, Cotrim, Septra, ampicillin, or penicillin G).
Salmonella	Symptoms range from mild diarrhea to severe pain and diarrhea: also watery stools, nausea, vomiting, fever exceeding 101 degrees Fahrenheit. Illness develops 6 to 72 hours after eating contaminated food.	Give replacement fluids (see above). Antibiotics may be prescribed.
Shigella	Symptoms range from mild diarrhea to fatal dysentery. Severe cases are more likely in children.	Give replacement fluids (see above). For severe cases, the doctor may prescribe Bactrim, Cotrim, or Septra.
Staphylococcus	Severe cramping and abdominal pain; vomiting; watery diarrhea; perspiration; headache; and, rarely, fever. Symptoms start abruptly within 1 to 6 hours of exposure and last 24 to 48 hours.	Give replacement fluids (see above).

Sources: Williams SR, Anderson SL. *Nutrition and Diet Therapy.* St. Louis, Missouri: Mosby-Year Book; 1993:308.
Brody JE. Why the food you eat may be hazardous to your health. *The New York Times.* October 5, 1994:C11.

Safe Medication Use

Using medications safely is largely a matter of common sense and caution. Remember that the effects of a drug can vary from one person to another, so don't rely on others for drug information. Seek the advice of trained professionals such as your doctor or pharmacist before making any changes in the way you take a medication. The following are general guidelines for most situations:

You and your doctor

■ Always tell your doctor everything about your medical history, including reactions to medications you've used in the past. In fact, it may be a good idea to keep a family medication log to help your doctor.

■ Tell the doctor about any medications you are using now, even if they are over-the-counter drugs like antacids or cold medications. They may contain ingredients that could cause a reaction with the drugs your doctor prescribes.

■ Keep track of your reactions to a medication—both positive and negative—and report them to your doctor at a follow-up visit.

■ Ask your doctor what you can or cannot do when given a new drug. For example, are there any foods to avoid when taking the drug? Should you avoid alcohol? Is it safe to drive a car? Is it alright to go out in bright sunlight?

■ Never change your dose schedule unless your doctor tells you to do so.

■ Ask about the addiction or dependence potential of any new drug.

■ Don't be shy—ask your doctor ANY question you may have in mind and report any side effect, even if it seems trivial or embarrassing.

You and your pharmacist

■ Your pharmacist is a medication specialist. Don't be afraid to ask questions you might have forgotten to ask your doctor. See if there are any written instructions that you can take with you.

■ Ask the pharmacist to explain clearly when and how to take the drug, or to translate into plain English any information you don't understand, such as "milliliters" or "kilograms."

■ Check the ingredients of over-the-counter drugs you may be taking to ensure that your prescription doesn't interact with them.

■ If you are starting a new medication, ask your pharmacist to fill only half the prescription in case you have an adverse reaction and the drug is stopped.

■ Ask how long the medication remains effective. Don't take it after its expiration date.

■ If you are going on a vacation, make sure your drug can be used in different climates.

You and your medications

■ Never take someone else's medication; and don't share your own medicines with anyone else.

■ Check the label each time you take a drug. Don't take a drug in the dark.

■ Keep your medications in a dry, safe spot.

■ Avoid confusion: If the label falls off, tape it back on or replace it. Keep each medicine in the bottle from the drug store. Don't mix medicines together in a single bottle.

■ If you think you are pregnant or plan to become pregnant, consult with your doctor before using any medication.

■ Destroy any unused portions of a drug and throw out the bottle.

■ If you need a certain medicine (for instance, insulin) in case of emergency, carry the information with you or obtain a special bracelet from an organization such as Medic Alert. This will help a paramedic or emergency room doctor treat you properly.

Your medicines and your children

■ Keep all medications in a locked cabinet or in a spot that is well out of the reach of children.

■ Ask the pharmacist to use child-proof safety bottles.

■ To ensure that you're giving the proper dose, be alert and awake when giving a child medication.

■ Make sure that children know medications are only to be taken when sick and can be dangerous if misused.

■ Keep antidotes such as Syrup of Ipecac on hand.

■ Keep the numbers of your EMS and poison control centers handy.

Your medicines and the elderly

■ The elderly are no different than anyone else when it comes to safe medication use. They are, however, more likely to suffer a side effect or adverse reaction if proper dosing is not followed. The elderly should always be aware of any potential side effects from a medication and should report them to a doctor or family member whenever they occur. □

Special Terms in Nutrition and Health

Additive (AD-i-tiv): Substance added to food in small amounts to change it in some way, such as improving color or taste, or increasing shelf-life.

Aerobic exercise (a-RO-bik EK-ser-size): Exercise that strengthens the cardiovascular and respiratory systems. "Aerobic" means "in the presence of oxygen."

Allergen (AL-er-jen): Any substance that causes an allergic reaction.

Allergenic (al-er-JEN-ik): Capable of causing an allergic reaction.

Allergy (AL-er-jee): An abnormal immune response to an ordinarily harmless substance.

Amenorrhea (a-men-o-REE-a): Absence of menstruation.

Anabolic steroids (An-a-BOL-ik ste-roydz): Drugs used illegally by athletes to build muscle tissue. Can be very harmful.

Anorexia Nervosa (an-or-REK-see-a ner-VO-suh): Emotional illness characterized by abnormal fear of becoming overweight accompanied by a distorted self-image, a persistent aversion to food, prolonged fasting, excessive exercise, and severe weight loss.

Antibody (AN-tee-bah-dee): A protein produced by the body in response to a specific foreign substance. Antibodies provoke the immune system into destroying the invader.

Antigens (AN-tee-jens): Toxins, bacteria, and other foreign substances that, when introduced to the body, stimulate the production of antibodies to fight them.

Antimutagens (an-tee-MYOO-tuh-jens): Substances that can prevent healthy cells from mutating into cancerous cells.

Antioxidants (AN-te-OK-si-dance): Substances (including certain vitamins) that help inhibit the destructive oxidation process within the body by preventing molecules called free radicals from damaging healthy cells.

Arthritis (ar-THRI-tis): A disease that typically involves inflammation of the joints, but can also affect connective tissue, ligaments, and cartilage.

Atherosclerosis (ath-eh-ro-skler-RO-sis): Condition caused by build-up of plaque and debris that narrows and stiffens the arteries.

Basal metabolic rate (BAY-zul met-uh-BOL-ik rate): Minimum number of calories you need per day to maintain normal physical functions. You need additional calories to supply energy for daily activities.

Binge-eating disorder (BINJ-ee-ting dis-or-der): Newly categorized illness, characterized by excessive overeating and subsequent feelings of guilt, depression, and self-condemnation; also known as compulsive overeating.

Botulin spores (BOCH-u-lin sporz): Bacteria-causing spores that, if ingested, can cause a severe, sometimes fatal case of food poisoning.

Bulimia Nervosa (boo-LEEM-ee-uh ner-VO-suh): Emotional illness characterized by episodic binge-eating followed by efforts to prevent weight-gain by purging.

Carcinogen (car-SIN-o-jen): Cancer-causing substance.

Cellular allergy (SEL-yuh-ler-AL-er-jee): Type of allergic reaction in which immune cells called lymphocytes become sensitized over time to certain chemicals and proteins in food. Eventually, the lymphocytes reject a food they view as a foreign substance.

Cellulose (SEL-u-loce): The most prevalent of the four major types of fiber. It softens stools, prevents constipation, and absorbs bile acids in the bowel.

Chemoprevention (KEE-mo-pree-VEN-shun): Term coined to describe the possible use of concentrated supplements to cut the odds of developing a specific cancer.

Cholesterol (Ko-LES-ter-ol): A substance that is both manufactured in the liver and supplied by animal food products. It is involved in a number of functions in the body including hormone production and building protective cell membranes. Cholesterol levels can influence the development of certain diseases such as coronary artery disease. There are both "good" (HDL) and "bad" (LDL) types of cholesterol. Your cholesterol level can be measured by a simple blood test.

Coincidental allergies ko-IN-si-DEN-tl al-er-jeez): Allergies to foods in unrelated food families.

Collagen KOL-uh-jen): Fiber that reinforces blood vessel walls and other parts of the body.

Colostrum (Kuh-LOS-trum): Yellowish fluid produced by the breast after childbirth. The fluid is high in protein, antibodies, and minerals, and low in fat and carbohydrates.

Depression (dee-PRESH-en): Emotional illness with a set of specific symptoms, such as feelings of despondency or worthlessness, that affect one's body, behavior, and emotions. Sometimes seen in patients with eating disorders.

Diabetes (di-uh-BEE-tees): Disability characterized by the inability to produce or properly use insulin. Insulin-dependent diabetes requires insulin; non-insulin dependent diabetes, which typically appears in adulthood, is usually treated with changes in diet and exercise.

Diastolic pressure (di--uh-STAHL-ik PRESH-er): The second (and lower) of the two blood pressure measures, taken between beats when the heart is resting.

Diuretic (di-yoo-RET-ik): Prescription medication that helps the body eliminate excess fluid. Diuretics are often prescribed to help lower high blood pressure by reducing the fluid volume of blood in the vessels. Often abused by bulimics as a method of purging.

Diverticulitis (DI-ver-tik-u-LIE-tis): Inflammation of a bulging or out-pouching in the intestinal wall. Can cause constipation, diarrhea, pain and tenderness in the bowel, and gas.

Elimination diet (ee-lim-uh-NA-shun di-it): Diet that requires you to stop eating certain foods, then reintroduce them one at a time to determine each food's effect on the body.

Emetic (eh-ME-tic): Agent used to cause vomiting.

Electrolytes (eh-LEK-troh-lites): Minerals such as sodium, magnesium, calcium, and potassium that are often added to sports drinks. Electrolytes play an important role in maintaining the body's fluid balance.

Enzyme deficiency (EN-zime dee-FISH-en-cee): Lack of one of the numerous proteins that cause biochemical reactions to take place in the body. One of the most common examples is a lack of lactase, an intestinal enzyme used to break down a natural sugar in dairy foods during digestion.

Estrogen (ES-tro-jen): Hormone produced by the ovaries. Supplies are sometimes affected by anorexic and bulimic behavior.

False-positive (fawls POS-it-iv): Test that incorrectly yields a positive result.

Free radicals (free RAD-i-kulz): Unstable molecules that damage other molecules in the body's cells. Some of this cell damage is believed to lead to heart disease and cancer.

Gestational diabetes (Jeh-STAY-shun-ul di-uh-BEE-tees): Type of diabetes that can occur during pregnancy.

Glucose tolerance test (GLOO-kose TAHL-uh-rents test): Test given to determine if you have diabetes.

Gluten intolerance (GLOO-ten in-TAHL-uh-rents): Inability to digest gluten, a major component of wheat, rye, oats, and barley.

Gums (Gumz): Sticky fibers derived from plants. Often used as thickeners in processed foods. Gums are believed to lower cholesterol and have anti-cancer effects.

HCAs or heterocyclic amines (heh-ter-o-SIK-lik A-meenz): Chemical substances created in the process of grilling food that are believed to be associated with various cancers.

HDL: High density lipoproteins -- the "good" form of cholesterol that helps keep arteries clean.

Histamine (HIS-ta-meen): Chemical released in abnormal quantities during an allergic reaction.

Hydrogenation (hi-droj-e-NA-shun): Process used to solidify unsaturated liquid fats; used to create margarines and shortenings for deep-fat frying. Transfatty acids created by this process can increase levels of bad cholesterol.

Hypersensitivity (Hi-per-sen-suh-TIV-i-tee): Excessive sensitivity to a substance. Similar to, but not a true allergy.

Hypertension HI-per-ten-shun): High blood pressure.

Insomnia (in-SOM-nee-uh): Sleeplessness; inability to sleep during normal nighttime hours.

Insulin (IN-suh-lin): A hormone that governs the body's use of sugar and other carbohydrates. Important in the regulation of blood sugar levels.

Intolerance (in-TAHL-uh-rents): Inability to properly process a drug, food, or other substance.

Irradiation (ih-RAY-dee-a-shun): Process that treats food with gamma rays to kill salmonella bacteria and other organisms, kill insects in spices and produce, and delay ripening and sprouting in fruits and vegetables.

Lactation (Lak-TAY-shun): Secretion of milk from the mammary glands.

LDL: Low density lipoproteins -- the "bad" cholesterol that can leave fatty deposits on the arterial walls.

Leukotriene (LOO-ko-TREE-en): A chemical related to prostaglandin; promotes inflammation.

Lignin (LIG-nin): One of the four major types of fiber. It acts as a binder for cellulose.

Lipogenesis (lip-o-GEN-uh-sis): Process by which fat cells store calories for future use.

Lipolysis (li-POL-uh-sis): Process by which fat cells release fat when you need it.

Lipoproteins (LIP-o-pro-teenz): Compounds made of fats (lipids), proteins, and triglycerides (another kind of fat) that are categorized by weight: VLDL—very low density; LDL—low density; HDL—high density; and VHDL—very high density. Cholesterol travels through the bloodstream attached to lipoproteins.

Lymphocytes (LIM-foh-sites): Infection-fighting white blood cells that play a role in making antibodies.

Macrophages (MAK-ro-fajez): Cells that kill bacteria by surrounding, and in effect, eating them.

Metabolism (meh-TAB-oh-liz-m): The physical and chemical processes, occurring within every cell, that are necessary for maintaining life. During metabolism, some substances are broken down for energy, while other needed substances are synthesized.

Monounsaturated fat (MAH-no-un-SACH-uh-ray-tid fat): Type of fat found in some fowl, almonds, pecans, cashews, peanuts, olive oil, canola oil, avocados, and certain fish. May help lower cholesterol.

Neutrophil (NOO-truh-fil): Type of white blood. Accounting for about 75 percent of circulating white blood cells, neutrophils, along with macrophages, are considered natural killer cells that fight germs.

Nitrosamines (Ni-TRO-suh-meenz): Compounds, naturally present in some foods, and also derived from preservatives such as nitrates and nitrites, that are suspected of causing cancer.

Osteoporosis (OS-tee-o-po-RO-sis): Severe loss of bone mass, resulting in brittle bones.

Osteoarthritis (OS-tee-o-ar-THRI-tis): Form of arthritis that causes chronic degeneration of the joints, particularly in the hands and knees.

PAHs or polycyclic aromatic hydrocarbons (pol-ee-SIK-lik a-roh-MA-tik HI-dro-car-benz): Chemical substances, believed to cause cancer, that develop on food surfaces during smoking or grilling. After grilling, PAHs can be scraped from the charred surface.

Pectin (PEK-tin): One of the four major types of fiber. Pectin is a gelatinous substance that absorbs bile acids and complements the function of cellulose.

Perimenopause (PER-ee-men-oh-pawz): Time before menopause when a woman's reproductive system prepares to retire. Usually begins four to ten years before menopause.

Pharmacologic reaction (Far-muh-ko-LOJ-ik ree-AK-shun): Reaction to a specific chemical in a food or drink, rather than a reaction to the food itself.

Phytochemical (FI-to-kem-i-kul): Name given to a wide range of chemicals found in plants. These compounds may prove to have far-reaching health benefits.

Phytoestrogen (FI-to-ESS-tro-jen): Estrogen-like compounds found in plants. By taking over the role of more harmful human estrogen, phytoestrogens may cut the risk of estrogen-based tumors.

Placebo (pluh-SEE-bo): An inactive substance used for comparison when testing an experimental compound.

Placebo effect (pluh-SEE-bo eh-FEKT): A beneficial response to a substance caused by the patient's desire to improve rather than the substance itself.

Prostaglandins (pross-ta-GLAN-dinz): Hormone-like substances that play a role in a wide range of physiological functions such as expansion and constriction of blood vessels.

Polyunsaturated fat (pol-ee-un-SACH-uh-ray-tid fat): Type of fat found in corn, soybean, safflower, sunflower, and sesame oils, and in certain fish, such as salmon and mackerel. May help lower cholesterol.

Preservative (Pri-ZER-vuh-tiv): Chemical used to inhibit food spoilage.

Relapsing condition (Ree-LAP-sing kon-DISH-un): A disorder that goes from improvement to regression after partial or apparently full recovery.

Saturated fat (SACH-uh-ray-tid fat): Fat filled with hydrogen atoms, making it more solid and more dangerous to your health.

Includes animal fat (beef, veal, pork, lamb, and fowl); fat from dairy products (whole milk products, butter, most cheeses); and palm, palm kernel and coconut oils, and cocoa butter.

Serotonin (sehr-o-TOE-nin): One of the brain's major chemical regulators. Governs the feeling of being full after eating, among other things.

Sleep apnea (sleep AP-ne-uh): Condition characterized by temporary interruptions of breathing during sleep; often linked to obesity.

Systolic pressure (sis-TOL-ik PRESH-er): The first (and higher) of the two blood pressure measures. Systolic pressure is taken as the heart contracts, forcing blood into the arteries.

Supplementation diet (sup-luh-men-TA-shun di-it): Diet characterized by the addition of vitamin and mineral supplements, sometimes in mega-doses.

T-Cell (TEE sel): Type of lymphocyte attacked by the HIV virus.

Target Heart Rate (THR) (TAR-git hart rate): The number of heartbeats per minute (heart rate) at which the heart is being safely but effectively stressed. THR is used as guide when exercising.

Thymus (THI-mus): The gland where cells mature lymphocytes.

Triglycerides (tri-GLIS-uh-rides): Major component of fats and oils.

Unsaturated fat (un-SACH-uh-ray-tid fat): Term used to describe fats with a relatively high number of hydrogen atoms. These fats are believed to be less dangerous to your health.

Nutrition Directory

The organizations listed below can provide you with nutritional recommendations and other information about the medical conditions in which they specialize. Only national headquarters are listed. Many can put you in touch with local chapters or provide referrals to nearby specialists.

Agency for Health Care Policy and Research
U.S. Public Health Service
P.O. Box 8547
Silver Spring, MD 20907
Phone: 800-358-9295

American Academy of Allergy and Immunology
611 East Wells Street
Milwaukee, WI 53202
Phone: 414-272-6071
Physicians' Referral and
Information Line: 800-822-ASMA

American Anorexia/Bulimia Association
c/o Regent Hospital
425 East 61 Street
New York, NY 10021
Phone: 212-891-8686

American Cancer Society
1599 Clifton Road, N.E.
Atlanta, GA 30329
Phone: 800-ACS-2345

American Dietetic Association
216 West Jackson Boulevard, Suite 800
Chicago, IL 60606
Phone: 312-899-0040
Nutrition Hot Line
(and referrals): 800-366-1655

American Heart Association
National Center
7272 Greenville Avenue
Dallas, TX 75321
Phone: 800-634-1242

Anorexia Nervosa and Related Eating Disorders, Inc.
P.O. Box 5102
Eugene, OR 97405
Phone: 503-344-1144

Arthritis Foundation
P.O. Box 19000
Atlanta, GA 30326
Phone: 800-283-7800

Center for Science in the Public Interest
1875 Connecticut Avenue, N.W., Suite 300
Washington, DC 20009
Phone: 202-332-9110

Food Allergy Network
4744 Holly Avenue
Fairfax, VA 22030
Phone: 800-929-4040

La Leche League International
1400 North Meacham Road
Schaumberg, IL 60173
Phone: 800-LA LECHE

National Association of Anorexia and Associated Disorders
Box 7
Highland Park, IL 60035
Phone: 701-831-3438

National Cancer Institute
Cancer Information Service (CIS)
Building 31, Room 10A24
Bethesda, MD 20892
Phone: 800-4-CANCER

National Eating Disorders Association
445 East Granville Road
Worthington, OH 43085
Phone: 614-436-1112

Weight Watchers International
The Jericho Atrium
500 North Broadway
Jericho, NY 11753
Phone: 516-939-0400

Poison Control Centers

I f there is one phone number that no home should be without, it is the nearest poison control center.

Some of the centers listed in this section are regional centers that are certified members of the American Association of Poison Control Centers. (They are marked with an asterisk.) To be certified, they must be supervised by a medical director; have pharmacists and nurses available to answer questions; be open 24-hours a day; and be accessible by direct dialing or a toll-free number.

The Centers are listed alphabetically by state and city. TTY and TDD phone numbers are for use by the hearing inpaired.

ALABAMA

BIRMINGHAM
Regional Poison Control Center
Children's Hospital of Alabama(*)
1600 7th Ave. South
Birmingham, AL 35233-1711
Business: 205-939-9720
Emergency: 205-933-4050
                      205-939-9201
                      800-292-6678 (AL)
Fax: 205-939-9245

TUSCALOOSA
Alabama Poison Control System, Inc.
408 A. Paul Bryant Dr. East
Tuscaloosa, AL 35401
Business: 205-345-0600
Emergency: 205-345-0600
                      800-462-0800
                      (AL)
Fax: 205-759-7994

ALASKA

ANCHORAGE
Anchorage Poison Center
Providence Hospital
P.O. Box 196604
3200 Providence Dr.
Anchorage, AK 99519-6604
Business: 907-562-2211 ext. 3633
Emergency: 907-261-3193
                      800-478-3193 (AK)
Fax: 907-261-3645

FAIRBANKS
Fairbanks Poison Control Center
1650 Cowles St.
Fairbanks, AK 99701
Business and
Emergency: 907-456-7182
Fax: 907-452-5776

ARIZONA

PHOENIX
Samaritan Regional Poison Center(*)
Good Samaritan Medical Center
1111 E. McDowell Rd.
Phoenix, AZ 85006
Emergency: 602-253-3334
Fax: 602-495-4881

TUCSON
Arizona Poison and Drug
Information Center(*)
University of Arizona
Arizona Health Sciences Center
Room 1156
1501 N. Campbell Ave.
Tucson, AZ 85724
Emergency: 602-626-6016
                      800-362-0101 (AZ)
Fax: 602-626-4063

ARKANSAS

LITTLE ROCK
Arkansas Poison and Drug
Information Center
College of Pharmacy — UAMS
4301 West Markham St.
Slot 522
Little Rock, AR 72205
Business: 501-661-6161
Emergency: 800-376-4766 (AR)

CALIFORNIA

FRESNO
Fresno Regional Poison Control
Center(*) Valley Children's
Hospital
3151 N. Millbrook
Fresno, CA 93703
Emergency: 209-445-1222
                   800-346-5922 (Central CA)
Fax: 209-442-6483

LOS ANGELES
Los Angeles County Regional Drug
and Poison Information Center
LAC and USC Medical Center
1200 N. State St.
Room 1107 A and B
Los Angeles, CA 90033
Business: 213-226-7741
Emergency: 213-222-3212
                   800-777-6476
Fax: 213-226-4194

SACRAMENTO
UC Davis Medical Center
Regional Poison Control Center(*)
2315 Stockton Blvd.
Sacramento, CA 95817
Emergency: 916-734-3692
                   800-342-9293 (N. CA)
Fax: 916-734-7796

SAN DIEGO
San Diego Regional
Poison Center(*)
UCSD Medical Center
200 W. Arbor Dr.
San Diego, CA 92103-8925
Emergency: 619-543-6000
                   800-876-4766
                   (San Diego and Imperial
                   Counties only)
Fax: 619-692-1867

SAN FRANCISCO
San Francisco Bay Area
Regional Poison Control Center(*)
SF General Hospital
1001 Potrero Ave.
Bldg. 80, Room 230
San Francisco, CA 94110
Business: 415-821-5524
Emergency: 415-476-6600
                   800-523-2222
Fax: 415-821-8513

COLORADO

DENVER
Rocky Mountain Poison
and Drug Center(*)
645 Bannock St.
Denver, CO 80204
Emergency: 303-629-1123
Fax: 303-623-1119

CONNECTICUT

FARMINGTON
Connecticut Poison
Control Center
University of Connecticut
Health Center
263 Farmington Ave.
Farmington, CT 06032
Business: 203-679-3473
Emergency: 203-679-3456
                   800-343-2722 (CT)
TDD: 203-679-4346
Fax: 203-679-1250

DISTRICT OF COLUMBIA

WASHINGTON, DC
National Capital
Poison Center(*)
3201 New Mexico Ave., NW
Suite 310
Washington, DC 20016
Emergency: 202-625-3333
TTY: 202-362-8536
Fax: 202-784-2530

FLORIDA

TAMPA
Florida Poison Information
and Toxicology Resource Center(*)
Tampa General Hospital
P.O. Box 1289
Tampa, FL 33601
Emergency: 813-253-4444
                   800-282-3171(FL)
Fax: 813-253-4443

GEORGIA

ATHENS
Georgia Animal Poison Information
Center College of Veterinary
Medicine
University of Georgia
Athens, GA 30602
706-542-4979
 (9AM to 5PM)

ATLANTA
Georgia Poison Center(*)
Grady Memorial Hospital
80 Butler St. SE
P.O. Box 26066
Atlanta, GA 30335-3801
Emergency: 404-616-9000
                   800-282-5846 (GA)
Fax: 404-616-9288

MACON
Regional Poison Control Center
Medical Center of Central Georgia
777 Hemlock St.
Macon, GA 31208
Poison Ctr: 912-633-1427
Fax: 912-633-1538

HAWAII

HONOLULU
Hawaii Poison Center
Kapiolani Women's and Children's
Medical Center
1319 Punahou St.
Honolulu, HI 96826
Emergency: 808-941-4411
                   800-362-3585 (HI)
Fax: 808-973-3173

ILLINOIS

CHICAGO
Chicago and NE Illinois
Regional Poison Control Center
Rush-Presbyterian-St. Luke's
Medical Center
1653 West Congress Pkwy.
Chicago, IL 60612
Business: 312-942-7064
Emergency: 312-942-5969
              800-942-5969 (IL)
Fax: 312-942-4260

NORMAL
Bro Menn Poison Control Center
Bro Menn Regional Medical Center
Virginia at Franklin
Normal, IL 61761
Business: 309-454-0738
Emergency: 309-454-6666
Fax: 309-888-0902

URBANA
Animal Poison Control Center
University of Illinois College of
Veterinary Medicine
Vet Med Basic
  Sciences Bldg.
2001 South Lincoln, Rm 1220
Urbana, IL 61801
Business: 217-333-2053
              800-548-2423
              (24 hr subscribers)
Fax: 217-244-1580

INDIANA

INDIANAPOLIS
Indiana Poison Center(*)
Methodist Hospital of Indiana
1701 North Senate Blvd.
P.O. Box 1367
Indianapolis, IN 46206-1367
Emergency: 317-929-2323
              800-382-9097 (IN)
Fax: 317-929-2337

IOWA

DES MOINES
Mid-Iowa Poison and Drug
Information Center
Iowa Methodist Medical Center
1200 Pleasant St.
Des Moines, IA 50309
              515-241-6254
              800-362-2327 (IA)
Fax: 515-241-5085 (or 4407)

IOWA CITY
Poison Control Center
University of Iowa
Hospital and Clinics
200 Hawkins Dr.
Iowa City, IA 52242
Business: 319-356-2577
Emergency: 800-272-6477 (IA)

SIOUX CITY
Poison Control Center St. Lukes
Regional Medical Center
2720 Stone Park Blvd.
Sioux City, IA 51104
Business: 712-279-3710
Emergency: 712-277-2222
              800-352-2222
              (IA, NE, SD)
Fax: 712-279-1852

KANSAS

KANSAS CITY
Mid-America Poison Control Center
University of Kansas
Medical Center
3901 Rainbow Blvd.,Rm B-400
Kansas City, KS 66160-7231
Business and
Emergency: 913-588-6633
              800-332-6633
              (KS)
Fax: 913-588-2350

TOPEKA
Stormont-Vail Regional Medical
Center Emergency Department
1500 West 10th
Topeka, KS 66604
Business: 913-354-6100
Emergency: 913-354-6106
Fax: 913-354-5004

WICHITA
Poison Control Center
Wesley Medical Center
550 North Hillside Ave.
Wichita, KS 67214
Business: 316-688-2277
Emergency: 316-688-2222
Fax: 316-688-2668

KENTUCKY

LOUISVILLE
Kentucky Regional Poison Center
of Kosair Children's Hospital
Medical Towers South, Suite 572
P.O. Box 35070
Louisville, KY 40232-5070
Business: 502-629-7264
Emergency: 502-629-7275
              502-589-8222
              800-722-5725 (KY)
Fax: 502-629-7277

LOUISIANA

HOUMA
Terrebonne General Medical
Center Drug and Poison
Information Center
936 East Main St.
Houma, LA 70360
Business: 504-873-4067
Emergency: 504-873-4069
Fax: 504-873-4573

MONROE
Louisiana Drug and Poison
Information Center
Northeast Louisiana University
School of Pharmacy
Monroe, LA 71209-6430
Business: 318-342-1699
Emergency: 800-256-9822 (LA)
Fax: 318-342-1744

MAINE

PORTLAND
Maine Poison Center Maine
Medical Center
22 Bramhall St.
Portland, ME 04102
Business: 207-871-2950
Emergency: 800-442-6305 (ME)
Fax: 207-871-6226

MARYLAND

BALTIMORE
Maryland Poison Center(*)
University of Maryland
School of Pharmacy
20 North Pine St.
Baltimore, MD 21201
Emergency: 410-528-7701
              800-492-2414 (MD)
Fax: 410-706-7184

MASSACHUSETTS

BOSTON
Massachusetts Poison Control System(*)
The Children's Hospital
300 Longwood Ave.
Boston, MA 02115
Emergency: 617-232-2120
              800-682-9211

MICHIGAN

DETROIT
Poison Control Center(*)
Children's Hospital of Michigan
3901 Beaubien Blvd.
Detroit, MI 48201
Emergency: 313-745-5711

GRAND RAPIDS
Blodgett Regional
Poison Center(*)
Blodgett Memorial
Medical Center
1840 Wealthy St. SE
Grand Rapids, MI 49506
Business: 616-774-7851
Emergency: 800-764-7661 (MI)
TTY: 800-356-3232
Fax: 616-774-7204

KALAMAZOO
Bronson Poison Information Center Bronson Methodist Hospital
252 East Lovell St.
Kalamazoo, MI 49007
Business: 616-341-6409
Emergency: 616-341-6409
              800-442-4112 (MI)
Fax: 616-341-7861

MINNESOTA

MINNEAPOLIS
Hennepin Regional Poison Center(*) Hennepin County Medical Center
701 Park Ave.
Minneapolis, MN 55415
Emergency: 612-347-3141
TDD: 612-337-7474
Petline: 612-337-7387
Fax: 612-347-3968

ST. PAUL
Minnesota Regional Poison Center(*) St. Paul-Ramsey Medical Center
640 Jackson St.
St. Paul, MN 55101
Emergency: 612-221-2113
              (Telephone and TTY
              access)
Fax: 612-221-2877

MISSISSIPPI

HATTIESBURG
Poison Center
Forrest General Hospital
400 South 28th Ave.
Hattiesburg, MS 39401
Business: 601-288-4221
Emergency: 601-288-4235

JACKSON
Regional Poison Control Center University of Mississippi Medical Center
2500 North State St.
Jackson, MS 39216
Business: 601-984-1675
Emergency: 601-354-7660
Fax: 601-984-1676

MISSOURI

KANSAS CITY
Poison Control Center
Children's Mercy Hospital
2401 Gillham Rd.
Kansas City, MO 64108
Business: 816-234-3053
Emergency: 816-234-3430
              816-234-3000
Fax: 816-234-3039

ST. LOUIS
Cardinal Glennon Children's Hospital(*) Regional Poison Center
1465 South Grand Blvd.
St. Louis, MO 63104
Emergency: 314-772-5200
              800-366-8888
Fax: 314-577-5355

MONTANA

DENVER, CO
Rocky Mountain Poison and Drug Center(*)
645 Bannock St.
Denver, CO 80204
Emergency: 303-629-1123
              800-525-5042 (MT)
Fax: 303-623-1119

NEBRASKA

OMAHA
The Poison Center(*)
Children's Memorial Hospital
8301 Dodge St.
Omaha, NE 68114
Emergency: 402-390-5555
              (Omaha)
              800-955-9119 (NE, WY)

NEVADA

LAS VEGAS
Poison Center
Humana Hospital Sunrise
3186 Maryland Pkwy.
Las Vegas, NV 89109
Emergency: 800-446-6179 (NV)

RENO
Poison Center
Washoe Medical Center
77 Pringle Way
Reno, NV 89520
Business: 702-328-4100
Emergency: 702-328-4144

NEW HAMPSHIRE

LEBANON
New Hampshire Poison Information Center Dartmouth-Hitchcock Memorial Hospital
1 Medical Center Dr.
Lebanon, NH 03756
Emergency: 603-650-5000
              800-562-8236 (NH)

NEW JERSEY

NEWARK
New Jersey Poison Information and Education System(*)
Newark Beth Israel Medical Center
201 Lyons Ave.
Newark, NJ 07112
Emergency: 800-962-1253
Fax: 201-926-0013

PHILLIPSBURG
Warren Hospital Poison Control Center
185 Roseberry St.
Phillipsburg, NJ 08865
Business: 908-859-6768
Emergency: 908-859-6768
           800-962-1253

NEW MEXICO

ALBUQUERQUE
New Mexico Poison and Drug Information Center(*)
University of New Mexico
Albuquerque, NM 87131-1076
Emergency: 505-843-2551
           800-432-6866 (NM)

NEW YORK

BUFFALO
Western New York Regional Poison Control Center
Children's Hospital of Buffalo
219 Bryant St.
Buffalo, NY 14222
Business: 716-878-7657
Emergency: 716-878-7654
           800-888-7655 (NY and
                    Western PA only)

MINEOLA
L.I. Regional Poison Control Center(*)
Winthrop University Hospital
259 First St.
Mineola, NY 11501
Emergency: 516-542-2323
           516-542-2324
           516-542-2325
           516-542-3813

NEW YORK
New York City Poison Control Center(*)
NYC Dept. of Health
455 First Ave., Rm 123
New York, NY 10016
Emergency: 212-340-4494
           212-POISONS
TDD: 212-689-9014

NYACK
Hudson Valley Poison Center(*)
Nyack Hospital
160 North Midland Ave.
Nyack, NY 10960
Emergency: 914-353-1000
           800-336-6997
Fax: 914-353-1050

ROCHESTER
Life Line/Finger Lakes Regional Poison Control Center
University of Rochester at Strong Memorial Hospital
601 Elmwood Ave.
Rochester, NY 14642
Business: 716-423-9490
           716-275-5151
           800-333-0542 (NY)
TTY: 716-275-2700
Fax: 716-244-6129

SYRACUSE
Central New York Poison Control Center
SUNY Health Science Center
750 East Adams St.
Syracuse, NY 13210
Business: 315-464-7073
Emergency: 315-476-4766
           800-252-5655 (NY)
Fax: 315-464-7077

NORTH CAROLINA

ASHVILLE
Western North Carolina Poison Control Center
Memorial Mission Hospital
509 Biltmore Ave.
Ashville, NC 28801
Emergency: 704-255-4490
           800-542-4225 (NC)

DURHAM
Duke University Regional Poison Control Center
Duke University Medical Center
P.O. Box 3007
Durham, NC 27710
Business: 919-684-4438
Emergency: 919-684-8111
           800-672-1697 (NC)

HICKORY
Catawba Memorial Hospital Poison Control Center
810 Fairgrove Church Rd. SE
Hickory, NC 28602
Business: 704-326-3385
Emergency: 704-322-6649
Fax: 704-326-3324

NORTH DAKOTA

FARGO
North Dakota Poison Information Center
Meritcare Medical Center
720 North 4th St.
Fargo, ND 58122
Business: 701-234-6062
Emergency: 701-234-5575
           800-732-2200 (ND)
Fax: 701-234-5090

OHIO

AKRON
Akron Regional Poison Control Center
Children's Hospital Medical Center
1 Perkins Square
Akron, OH 44308
Business: 216-258-3066
Emergency: 216-379-8562
           800-362-9922 (OH)
TTY: 216-379-8446
Fax: 216-379-8447

CINCINNATI
Regional Poison Control System and Cincinnati Drug and Poison Information Center(*)
Univ. of Cincinnati College of Medicine
P.O. Box 670144
Cincinnati, OH 45267-0144
Emergency: 513-558-5111
           800-872-5111 (OH)
Fax: 513-558-5301

CLEVELAND
Greater Cleveland Poison
Control Center
2101 Adelbert Rd.
Cleveland, OH 44106
Emergency: 216-231-4455

COLUMBUS
Central Ohio Poison Center(*)
Columbus Children's Hospital
700 Children's Dr.
Columbus, OH 43205-2696
Emergency: 614-228-1323
614-461-2012
800-682-7625
TTY: 614-228-2272
Fax: 614-221-2672

DAYTON
Western Ohio Regional Poison and
Drug Information Center
Children's Medical Center
1 Children's Plaza
Dayton, OH 45404-1815
Business: 513-226-8300 ext. 8718
Emergency: 513-222-2227
800-762-0727 (OH)
Fax: 513-223-5004

TOLEDO
Poison Information Center
of Northwest Ohio
Medical College of Ohio Hospital
3000 Arlington Ave.
Toledo, OH 43614
Business: 419-381-3898
Emergency: 419-381-3897
800-589-3897 (OH)
TTY: 216-746-5510

YOUNGSTOWN
Mahoning Valley Poison Center
St. Elizabeth Hospital Medical
Center
1044 Belmont Ave.
Youngstown, OH 44501
Business: 216-746-7211 ext. 3540
Emergency: 216-746-2222
800-426-2348 (OH)
TTY: 216-746-5510

ZANESVILLE
Drug Information/Poison
Control Center
Bethesda Hospital
2951 Maple Ave.
Zaneville, OH 43701
Business: 614-454-4246
Emergency: 614-454-4221
614-454-4000
800-686-4221 (OH)
Fax: 614-454-4059

OKLAHOMA

OKLAHOMA CITY
Oklahoma Poison Control Center
Children's Memorial Hospital
940 Northeast 13th St.
Oklahoma City, OK 73104
Business: 405-271-5120
800-522-4611 (OK)
405-271-5454

OREGON

PORTLAND
Oregon Poison Center(*)
Oregon Health Sciences University
3181 SW Sam Jackson Park Rd.
Portland, OR 97201
Emergency: 503-494-8968
800-452-7165 (OR)

PENNSYLVANIA

HERSHEY
Central Pennsylvania Poison Center(*)
University Hospital
Milton S. Hershey Medical Center
P.O. Box 850
Hershey, PA 17033
Emergency: 800-521-6110

LANCASTER
Poison Control Center
St. Joseph Hospital and
Health Care Center
250 College Ave.
Lancaster, PA 17604
Business: 717-291-8485
Emergency: 717-291-8111

PHILADELPHIA
Delaware Valley Regional Poison
Control Center(*)
3600 Market St., Rm. 220
Philadelphia, PA 19104
Emergency: 215-386-2100
Fax: 215-590-4419

PITTSBURGH
Pittsburgh Poison Center(*)
Children's Hospital of Pittsburgh
3705 Fifth Ave.
Pittsburgh, PA 15213
Emergency: 412-681-6669
Fax: 412-692-7497

RHODE ISLAND

PROVIDENCE
Rhode Island Poison Center(*)
Rhode Island Hospital
593 Eddy St.
Providence, RI 02903
Emergency: 401-444-5727
Fax: 401-277-8062

SOUTH CAROLINA

COLUMBIA
Palmetto Poison Center
College of Pharmacy
University of South Carolina
Columbia, SC 29208
Business: 803-777-7909
Emergency: 803-777-1117
800-922-1117 (SC)
Fax: 803-777-6127

SOUTH DAKOTA

ABERDEEN
Poison Control Center
St. Luke's Midland
Regional Medical Center
305 South State St.
Aberdeen, SD 57401
Business: 605-622-5000
Emergency: 605-622-5100
605-622-5678
800-592-1889
(SD, MN, ND, WY)

RAPID CITY
Rapid City Regional Poison Center
835 Fairmont Blvd.
P.O. Box 6000
Rapid City, SD 57709
Business: 605-341-3333
Emergency: 605-341-3333

SIOUX FALLS
McKennan Poison Center
McKennan Hospital
800 East 21st St.
P.O. Box 5045
Sioux Falls, SD 57117-5045
Business: 605-339-7873
Emergency: 605-336-3894
800-952-0123 (SD)
800-843-0505
(IA, MN, NE, ND)
Fax: 605-333-8206

TENNESSEE

MEMPHIS
Southern Poison Center
847 Monroe Ave., Suite 230
Memphis, TN 38163
Emergency: 901-528-6048
   800-288-9999 (S. TN)

NASHVILLE
Middle Tennessee Center
501 Oxford House
1161 21st Ave. S.
Nashville, TN 37232-4632
Business: 615-936-0760
Emergency: 615-322-6435
   800-288-9999 (TN)
Fax: 615-343-7082

TEXAS

DALLAS
North Texas Poison Center(*)
Parkland Memorial Hospital
5201 Harry Hines Blvd.
P.O. Box 35926
Dallas, TX 75235
Emergency: 800-764-7661
Fax: 214-590-5008

EL PASO
El Paso Poison Control Center
Thomason General Hospital
4815 Alameda Ave.
El Paso, TX 79905
Emergency: 915-533-1244

GALVESTON
Texas State Poison Center(*)
University of Texas Trauma Center
Room 3-112
Galveston, TX 77555-1175
Emergency: 409-765-1420
Fax: 409-761-3917

UTAH

LAYTON
Poison Control Center
Columbia/HCA Davis Hospital
and Medical Center
1600 West Antelope Dr.
Layton, UT 84041
Emergency: 801-825-4357

SALT LAKE CITY
Utah Poison Control Center(*)
University of Utah Hospital
410 Chipeta Way,
Suite 230
Salt Lake City, UT 84108
Emergency: 801-581-2151
   800-456-7707 (UT)
Fax: 801-581-4199

VERMONT

BURLINGTON
Vermont Poison Center
Medical Center Hospital of
Vermont
111 Colchester Ave.
Burlington, VT 05401
Business: 802-656-2439
Emergency: 802-658-3456

VIRGINIA

CHARLOTTESVILLE
Blue Ridge Poison Center(*)
Blue Ridge Hospital
Box 67
Charlottesville, VA 22901
Emergency: 804-924-5543
   800-451-1428

RICHMOND
Virginia Poison Center
Virginia Commonwealth University
MCV Station, Box 522
Richmond, VA 23298-0522
Business: 804-786-4780
Emergency: 804-786-9123
   800-552-6337 (VA)
Fax: 804-225-3299

WASHINGTON

SEATTLE
Washington Poison Center
P.O. Box 5371
Seattle, WA 98105
Emergency: 206-526-2121
   800-732-6985 (WA)
Fax: 206-526-8490

WEST VIRGINIA

CHARLESTON
West Virginia Poison Center(*)
West Virginia University
3110 MacCorkle Ave. SE
Charleston, WV 25304
Emergency: 304-348-4211
   800-642-3625 (WV)
Fax: 304-348-9560

PARKERSBURG
Poison Center
St. Josephs Hospital Center
19th St. and Murdoch Ave.
Parkersburg, WV 26101
Emergency: 304-424-4222

WISCONSIN

MADISON
Regional Poison Control Center
University of Wisconsin
Hospital and Clinics
600 Highland Ave., ES/238
Madison, WI 53792
Emergency: 608-262-3702
   800-815-8855 (WI)

MILWAUKEE
Milwaukee Poison Center
Children's Hospital of Wisconsin
9000 W. Wisconsin Ave.
P.O. Box 1997
Milwaukee, WI 53201
Business: 414-266-2000
Emergency: 414-266-2222
   800-815-8855 (WI)

*Source: Red Book and POISINDEX®
System, MICROMEDEX, INC.*

Sources

What's Really Important in Nutrition?

Applegate L. Label logic: the FDA trims the fat from food labeling. *Runner's World*. 1993; 28(11): 26.

Benson S. Has sugar taken too many lumps? *Health*. 1991; 5:20.

Briley M. Choosing wellness in a land of plenty. *Arthritis Today*. 1989; 3:26.

Brownlee S. A loaf of bread, a glass of wine: the new Mediterranean diet is causing both heartburn and the 'aahs' of contentment. *US News and World Report*. 1994; 117: 62.

Consumers more familiar with pyramid, food labels. *Milling & Baking News*. 1994; 73: 1.

Decoding menus for hidden fat. *Environmental Nutrition*. 1992; 15: 8.

Enforcement Policy Statement on Food Advertising. May 1994; Federal Trade Commission, Washington, DC.

FDA Consumer. Focus on Food Labeling. May 1993; Food and Drug Administration, Rockville, MD.

The Food Guide Pyramid . . . Beyond the Basic 4. US Department of Agriculture Human Nutrition Information Service and the Food Marketing Institute; Washington, DC.

Gershoff S, Whitney C. *The Tufts University Guide to Total Nutrition*. New York, NY: Harper & Row; 1990.

How much fat in your diet? *Consumer Reports on Health*. 1994; 6: 104.

Hudnall M. Are the dangers of salt overstated? *Environmental Nutrition*. 1990; 13: 1.

Hudnall M. Should everyone cut salt? A third opinion checks in. *Environmental Nutrition*. 1991; 14: 1.

Just what is a balanced diet, anyway? *Tufts University Diet & Nutrition Letter*. 1992; 9: 3.

Korn W. Defending nutritional villains. *Weight Watchers Magazine*. 1993; 26: 20.

Landman B. Too good to be true. *New York*. 1994; 27: 34.

Liebman B. Just the fiber facts. *Nutrition Action Healthletter*. September 1994; 10-11.

Liebman B. Non-trivial pursuit. Playing the research game. *Nutrition Action Healthletter*. 1994; 21: 1.

Liebman B. The salt shakeout. *Nutrition Action Healthletter*. 1994; 21: 1.

Mahan KL, Arlin MT. *Krause's Food, Nutrition & Diet Therapy*, 8th ed. Philadelphia, PA: WB Saunders Company; 1992.

Mason M. The man who has a beef with your diet. *Health*. 1994; 8: 52.

Maximizing your minerals. *The University of Berkeley Wellness Letter*. 1992; 8: 4.

The Mediterranean diet: a better way to eat? *Consumer Reports on Health*. 1994; 6: 121.

Nelson JK, Moxness KE, Jensen MD, Gastineau CF. *Mayo Clinic Diet Manual*. A Handbook of Nutrition Practices. 7th ed. Mosby, St. Louis.

New RDAs call for more calcium, less sodium. *Tufts University Diet & Nutrition Letter*. 1990; 7: 1.

And now we have trans fat to worry about! *Medical Update*. 1993; 17: 2.

Nutrition and Your Health: Dietary Guidelines for Americans. 3rd ed., 1990: US Department of Agriculture and US Department of Health and Human Services; Home and Garden Bulletin no. 232.

Phillips P. Salt intake leads lifestyle links to hypertension in global study [sic]. *Medical World News*. 1988; 29: 10.

Read the label, set a healthy table. Department of Health and Human Services, Public Health Service, Food and Drug Administration; US Department of Agriculture Food Safety and Inspection Service. November 1994; DHHS Publication No. (FDA) 94-2273.

Recommended Dietary Allowances. 10th ed. Washington, DC: National Research Council. National Academy Press; 1989.

Schardt D. The problem with protein. *Nutrition Action Healthletter*. 1993; 20: 1.

Schardt D. Vitamins 101. How to buy them. *Nutrition Action Healthletter*. 1993; 20: 1.

Sharp D. The all-you-can-eat diet. *Health*. 1993; 7: 59.

Shils ME, Olson JA, Shike M. *Modern Nutrition in Health and Disease*. 8th ed., Philadelphia, Penn: Lea & Febiger; 1994.

Small change, big effect. *University of California Berkeley Wellness Letter*. October 1994; 3.

Spleen T. Mediterranean diet touted by specialists. *Supermarket News.* 1994; 44: 15.

Townsend CE. *Nutrition and Diet Therapy.* 6th ed. Albany, N. Y.: Delmar Publishers Inc.; 1994.

Williams SR, Anderson SL. *Nutrition and Diet Therapy.* 7th ed., St. Louis, MO: Mosby-Year Book, Inc.; 1993.

Williams SR. *Basic Nutrition and Diet Therapy.* 9th ed., St. Louis, MO: Mosby-Year Book, Inc.; 1992.

Weinberg L. Low-fat, low-calorie foods: key to health or green light for gluttony? *Environmental Nutrition.* 1993; 16: 1.

Zoler M. RDA revision ends vitamin row. *Medical World News.* 1989; 30: 28.

Basics Questions:
Vitamins, Minerals, Fiber, and More

Are you eating right? *Consumer Reports.* 1992; 57: 644.

Be Your Best: Nutrition After Fifty. Washington, DC: American Institute for Cancer Research; 1988.

Begley S. Beyond vitamins. *Newsweek.* April 25, 1994: 45.

Buying vitamins: What's worth the price? *Consumer Reports.* 1994; 59: 565.

Carper J. *Food—Your Miracle Medicine.* New York, NY: HarperCollins; 1993.

Cooper KH. *Dr. Kenneth H. Cooper's Antioxidant Revolution.* Nashville, Tenn: Thomas Nelson Publishers; 1994.

Eades MD. *The Doctor's Complete Guide to Vitamins and Minerals.* New York, NY: Dell; 1994.

Galton L. *The Truth About Fiber in Your Food.* New York, NY: Crown; 1976.

Garrison RH, Somer E. *The Nutrition Desk Reference.* New Canaan, Conn: Keats; 1990.

Hall SS. The power of garlic. *Health.* 1994; 8: 83.

Hausman P, Hurley JB. *The Healing Foods.* New York, NY: Dell; 1992.

Herbert V. What you should know about vitamins: The case against supplements. *Bottom Line Personal.* 1994; 15: 13.

Hunter BT. How safe are nutritional supplements? *Consumers' Res.* 1994; 77: 21.

Husten L. A new reason to B. *Harvard Health Letter.* 1994; 19: 1.

Husten L. Second thoughts about antioxidants. *Harvard Health Letter.* 1995; 20: 4.

Kolata G. Vitamin supplements are seen as no guard against diseases. *The New York Times.* April 14, 1994; A1.

Liebman B. Antioxidants: surprise, surprise. *Nutrition Action Healthletter.* 1994; 21: 4.

Liebman B. Fiber: separating fact from fiction. *Nutrition Action Healthletter.* 1994; 21: 1.

O'Neill M. So it may be true after all: eating pasta makes you fat. *The New York Times.* Feb. 8, 1995; A1,C6.

Ornish D. *Eat More, Weigh Less.* New York, NY: HarperCollins; 1993.

Passwater RA. *Cancer Prevention and Nutritional Therapies.* New Canaan, Conn: Keats Publishing; 1993.

Ramirez A. A crackdown on phone marketing. *The New York Times.* Feb. 10, 1995; D1.

Scala J. *Prescription for Longevity: Eating Right for a Long Life.* New York, NY: Plume/Dutton Signet/Penguin; 1994.

Schardt D. Grading vitamin C. *Nutrition Action Healthletter.* 1994; 21: 10.

Schardt D. Phytochemicals: plants against cancer. *Nutrition Action Healthletter.* 1994; 21: 1.

Schardt D. The supplement-takers guide to the universe. *Nutrition Action Healthletter.* 1993; 20: 1.

Shapiro L. The skinny on fat. *Newsweek.* Dec. 5, 1994; 52–60.

Shuchman M, Wilkes M. The vitamin uprising. *The New York Times Magazine.* Oct. 2, 1994; 79.

Sicca-Cohen R. What you should know about vitamins: The case for supplements. *Bottom Line Personal.* 1994; 15: 13.

Women's Knowledge and Behavior Regarding Health and Fitness. Princeton, N.J.: The Gallup Organization; June 1993.

Health or Hype?
The Lowdown on Natural Foods

Back to nature: organic food use grows as consumers seek healthier products. *Research Alert.* Dec. 3, 1993; 11.

Berkowitz KF. Is milk safe? Bringing biotechnology to the table. *Environmental Nutrition.* July 1991; 14: 1.

The brave new world of food irradiation. *The University of California, Berkeley Wellness Letter.* May 1992; 8: 1.

BST given green light, no labels required. *Environmental Nutrition.* March 1994.

Castleman M. What should you do? MSG reactions. *Medical SelfCare.* March-April 1989; 51: 10.

Cioffi JA, Wagner TE. Application of biotechnology and trangenic animals toward the study of growth hormone. *American Journal of Clinical Nutrition:* August 1993; 58: 296S.

Consumer advocates or organic food promoters (Center for Science in the Public Interest). *NCAHF Newsletter.* January-February 1989; 12: 2.

Edlow J. The case of the unhealthy health food. *Ladies Home Journal.* February 1993; 110: 76.

Enforcement Policy Statement on Food Advertising. Federal Trade Commission. Washington, DC; May 1994: 9.

FDA approves hormones for cows, but safety questions remain. *Environmental Nutrition.* Dec. 1993; 16: p3.

Finally, FDA gives green light to Monsanto's BST. *Successful Farming.* January 1994; 92: 48.

Food industry avoids labeling of MSG, activist says. *Food Labeling News.* July 28, 1994; vol. 2.

Food irradiation: how safe? *Health News.* October 1993; 11: 7.

Food irradiation: the controversy heats up. *Tufts University Diet & Nutrition Letter.* March 1992; 10: 4.

Gibbons A. FDA publishes bovine growth hormone data. *Science.* August 24, 1990; 249: 852.

Going with the grain(s). *Tufts University Diet & Nutrition Letter.* March 1994; 12: 7.

Hadfield, LC. A walk through a health food store. *Current Health.* November 2, 1991; 18: 10.

Haidet, JM. Health food store probe yields poor advice plus doubletalk. *Nutrition Forum.* January-February 1992; 9: 6

Harris M. Cloudy judgment? *Vegetarian Times.* July 1994; 16.

Hearn W. Is it safe to drink milk? *American Medical News.* March 7, 1994; 37: 25.

Is holier more wholesome? *Tufts University Diet & Nutrition Letter.* August 1993; 11: 1.

Jacobson MF. *Safe food. Eating wisely in a risky world,* Los Angeles, Calif: Living Planet Press; 1991.

Juskevich J, Guyer CG. Bovine growth hormone: human food safety evaluation. *Science.* August 1990; 249: 875.

Just the fiber facts. *Nutrition Action Healthletter.* September 1994: 10–11.

Katzenstein L. Food irradiation: the story behind the scare. *American Health: Fitness of Body and Mind.* Dec. 1992; 11: 60.

Kleiner S. Healthy health food shopping. *Executive Health Report.* July 1990; 26: p. 7.

Kleiner SM. Health food stores: are they really more healthful? *The Physician and Sportsmedicine.* Feb. 1991; 19: 15.

Larkin M. Organic foods get government "blessing" despite claims that aren't kosher. *Nutrition Forum.* July-August 1991; 8: 25.

Mahan KL, Arlin MT. *Krause's Food, Nutrition & Diet Therapy.* Philadelphia, Penn: WB Saunders Company; 1992.

Messinger L. *Turn Your Supermarket into a Health Food Store.* New York, N. Y.: Pharos Books; 1991.

Milner I. Supermarket or health food store: which carries the most clout? *Environmental Nutrition.* May 1993; 16: 1.

Organic food retail sales. *Research Alert.* Dec. 3, 1993; vol. 11.

Organic food update. *Green MarketAlert.* January 1994; vol. 5.

Organic goes mainstream. *Research Alert.* December 1993; vol. 11.

Papazian R. Food irradiation: a hot issue. *Harvard Health Letter.* August 1992; 17: 1.

Roberts M. Keeping yogurt honest: its reputation as a "health food" may not always be deserved. *US News and World Report.* November 1990; 109: 76.

Schardt D. Diving into the gene pool. *Nutrition Action Healthletter.* July-August 1994; 8–9.

Schardt D. Food sensitivity: nothing to sneeze at. *Nutrition Action Healthletter.* May 1994; 12–13.

Shils ME, Olson JA, Shike M. *Modern Nutrition in Health and Disease.* 8th ed. Philadelphia, Penn: Lea & Febiger; 1994.

Stolzenburg W. Hormone-boosted milk passes FDA review. *Science News.* August 1990; 138: 116.

Survey finds "staggering" selection of organic grocery items. *Food Labeling News.* July 1994; vol. 2.

Tartrazine and eczema. *Nutrition Research Newsletter.* July-August 1992; 11: 85.

Townsend CE. *Nutrition and Diet Therapy.* 6th ed. Albany, New York: Delmar Publishers Inc.; 1994.

Trojan cow; an embattled hormone raises social questions. *Scientific American.* November 1990; 263: 26.

Waltz M. A shopper's guide to natural food stores. *Vegetarian Times.* December 1991; 58.

What drives the critics? *American Health: Fitness of Body and Mind.* December 1992; 11: 64.

Williams SR, Anderson SL. *Nutrition and Diet Therapy.* 7th ed. St. Louis, MO: Mosby-Year Book, Inc.; 1993.

Williams SR. *Basic Nutrition and Diet Therapy.* 9th ed. St. Louis, MO: Mosby-Year Book, Inc.; 1992.

Weinberg L. Low-fat, low-calorie foods: key to health or green light for gluttony? *Environmental Nutrition.* February 1993; 16: 1.

How to Pick a Nutritional Plan

American Heart Association. *An Eating Plan for Healthy Americans.* Dallas, Tex: American Heart Association; 1991.

American Heart Association. *Cholesterol and Your Heart.* Dallas, Tex: American Heart Association; 1993.

American Heart Association. *Dietary Guidelines for Healthy American Adults.* Dallas, Tex: American Heart Association; January 1994.

Berstein S. Jewish food and health: Es, mamele; it's good for you. *North Jersey Jewish Standard.* October 14, 1994; 64: 14–15.

Brody J. *Jane Brody's Nutrition Book.* New York, NY: Bantam Books; 1988.

DeBakey M, et al. *The Living Heart Diet.* New York, NY: Raven Press; 1984.

Gershoff S, et al. *The Tufts University Guide to Total Nutrition*. New York, NY: HarperPerennial; 1991.

Hamilton M, et al. *The Duke University Medical Center Book of Diet and Fitness*. New York, NY: Fawcett Columbine; 1990.

Heindendry C. *Making the Transition to Macrobiotic Diet*. Wayne, NJ: Avery Publishing Group Inc.; 1987.

Jenkins NH. *The Mediterranean Diet Cookbook*. New York: Bantam Books; 1994.

Kushi M, Kushi A. *Macrobiotic Diet*. Tokyo and New York: Japan Publications, Inc.; 1993.

Mazel J. *The Beverly Hills Diet*. New York, NY: Macmillan Publishing Co., Inc.; 1981.

Null G. *The Complete Guide to Health and Nutrition*. New York, NY: Dell Publishing; 1986.

Pritikin N, McGrady P Jr. *The Pritikin Program for Diet and Exercise*. New York, NY: Grosset & Dunlap; 1979.

Scala J. *The Arthritis Relief Diet*. New York: Plume; 1987.

Sharon M. *Complete Nutrition, How to Live in Total Health*. London: Prion; 1994.

Simone CB. *Cancer and Nutrition*. Garden City Park, NY: Avery Publishing Group Inc.; 1992.

Smith L. *Dr. Lendon Smith's Low Stress Diet*. New York, NY: McGraw-Hill Book Company; 1985.

Wurtman JJ. *The Carbohydrate Craver's Diet*. Boston, Mass: Houghton Mifflin Company; 1983.

How Much Weight is Too Much: Setting a Healthy Goal

Abernathy RP, Black DR. Is adipose tissue oversold as a health risk? *Journal of the American Dietetic Association*. June 1994; 94: 641–644.

The American Heart Association Diet: An Eating plan for Healthy Americans. Dallas, Texas: American Heart Association; 1993.

Bailey C. *Fit or Fat?* Boston, Mass: Houghton Mifflin Company; 1978.

Bailey C. *The Fit-or-Fat Target Diet*. Boston, Mass: Houghton Mifflin Company; 1984.

Bean A. Live thin and prosper. *Runner's World*. April 1994; 29: 18–20.

Black R. Attention, baby boomers . . . you're in your fat-gaining years! *Redbook*. March 1991; 176: 164–166.

Body fat percentage: more important than weight? *USA Today*. September 1993; 122: 9.

Controlling Your Risk Factors for Heart Attack. Dallas, Tex: American Heart Association; 1994.

Diet: Cholesterol blues. *Newsweek*. November 28, 1994; 124: 63.

Dietary Guidelines for Healthy American Adults: A Statement for Physicians and Health Professionals. Dallas, Tex: American Heart Association; 1988.

Delaney L. Your customized weigh-loss kit. *Prevention*. October 1992; 44: 49–62.

Easy Food Tips for Heart-Healthy Eating. Dallas, Tex: American Heart Association; 1994.

Eat Well, But Wisely. Dallas, Tex: American Heart Association; 1992.

Fackelmann KA. Warning about those very-low-cal diets. *Science News*. January 30, 1993; 143: 78.

Feeding the heart. *Time*. February 1, 1993; 141: 22–23.

The Food Guide Pyramid. Hyattsville, Md: Human Nutrition Information Service, U.S. Department of Agriculture; August 1992.

Garner DM, Wooley SC. Confronting the failure of behavioral and dietary treatments for obesity. *Clinical Psychology Review*. 1991; 11: 729–780.

Guidelines for Weight Management Program for Healthy Adults. Dallas, Tex: American Heart Association; 1994.

Heart and Stroke Facts. Dallas, Tex: American Heart Association; 1993.

Heart and Stroke Facts: 1994 Statistical Supplement. Dallas, Tex: American Heart Association; 1993.

Lafavore M. Letter from the editor. *Men's Health*. May 1994; 9: 45.

Lee I, Paffenbager RS Jr. Change in body weight and longevity. *JAMA, The Journal of the American Medical Association*. October 21, 1992; 268: 2045–2049.

Long P. The great weight debate. *Health*. February-March 1992; 6: 42–47.

Lutter JM. Does big mean bad? Large Women may be healthier and happier than their thin friends. *Women's Sports and Fitness*. March 1991; 13: 16–17.

Marwick C. Obesity experts say less weight is still best. *JAMA, The Journal of the American Medical Association*. May 26, 1993; 269: 2617–2619.

1983 Metropolitan Height and Weight Tables for Men and Women. New York, Metropolitan Life Insurance Company, reprint from *Statistical Bulletin*. January-June 1983; 64.

Nutrition and Your Health: Dietary Guidelines for Americans, ed. 3. Hyattsville, Md: U.S. Department of Agriculture, U.S. Department of Health and Human Services; 1990.

Obesity: waist not, but okay behind. *Science News*. May 26, 1990; 137: 334.

Pi-Sunyer FX. The fattening of America. *JAMA, The Journal of the American Medical Association*. July 20, 1994; 272: 238–240.

Pritikin R. *The New Pritikin Program*. New York: Pocket Books; 1991.

Rubin R. Fat and fit? *U.S. News & World Report.* May 16, 1994; 116: 64–69.

Sandmaier M. If you think you weigh too much, read this. *McCall's.* October 1994; 122: 134–139.

Sifton D, ed. *The PDR Family Guide to Women's Health and Prescription Drugs.* Montvale, NJ: Medical Economics Data; 1994.

Silent Epidemic: The Truth About Women and Heart Disease. Dallas, Tex: American Heart Association; 1992.

Stunkard AJ, Foch TT, Hrubec Z. A twin study of human obesity. *JAMA, The Journal of the American Medical Association.* July 4, 1986; 256: 51–54.

Stunkard AJ, Sørensen TIA, Hanis C, et al. An adoption study of human obesity. *The New England Journal of Medicine.* January 23, 1986; 314: 193–198.

Best Strategies for Losing Extra Pounds

Bailey C. *The New Fit or Fat.* New York, NY: Houghton Mifflin; 1991.

Barish EB. "Dieting may be a losing proposition." *Harvard Health Letter.* August 1994; 19: 4.

Bergman Y, Eller D. *Food Cop.* New York: NY: Bantam Books; 1991.

Blake JS. *Eat Right the E.A.S.Y. Way!* New York, NY: Prentice Hall Press; 1991.

Carlson S, Sonnenberg LM, Cummings S. "Dieting readiness test predicts completion in a short-term weight loss program. *Journal of the American Dietetic Association.* 1994; 94: 552.

Carper J. *Food Your Miracle Medicine.* New York, NY: HarperCollins; 1993.

Daley R. *In the Kitchen with Rosie: Oprah's Favorite Recipes.* New York, NY: Alfred A. Knopf; 1994.

Diamond H. *Fit For Life.* New York, NY: Warner Books; 1987.

Ferguson S. *The Diet Center Program.* Boston, Mass: Little, Brown; 1990.

Finn S. *The Real Life Nutrition Book.* New York, NY: Penguin Books; 1992.

Fuller K. Sizing up a weight–loss plan. *Better Homes and Gardens.* 1994; 72: 54.

Gershoff S. *The Tufts University Guide to Total Nutrition.* New York, NY: HarperPerennial; 1990.

Haus G, Hoerr, SL, Mavis B, Robison J. Key modifiable factors in weight maintenance: fat intake, exercise, and weight cycling. *Journal of the American Dietetic Association.* 1994; 94: 409.

Jacobson MF. *The Completely Revised and Updated Fast-Food Guide,* 2nd ed. New York, NY: Workman; 1991.

Katahn M. *One Meal At A Time.* New York, NY: Warner Books; 1989.

Kusinitz M. To eat or not to eat; the dieter's dilemma. *Science World.* 1994; 50: 18.

Losing weight: what works. What doesn't. *Consumer Reports.* 1993; 58: 347.

Margolis D. Do you need to lose weight? *American Health.* 1994; 13: 36.

Medical update: the heavy toll of dieting and eating disorders. *Health News.* 1994; 12: 8.

Nash JM. Is a lowfat diet risky: a controversial new study suggests that making meals too lean could be dangerous to your health. *Time.* 1994; 144: 62.

Podell RN. *The G-Index Diet.* New York, NY: Warner Books; 1993.

Rader WC. Why some diets don't work. *Total Health.* 1994; 16: 12.

Rating the diets. *Consumer Reports.* 1993; 58: 353.

Scanlon D. *Diets That Work: For Weight Control or Medical Needs.* Los Angeles, Calif: Lowell House; 1993.

Serdula MK, Williamson DF, Anda RF, Levy A, Heaton A, Byers T. Weight control practices in adults: results of a multistate telephone survey. *The American Journal of Public Health.* 1994; 84: 1821.

Seven bad diet ideas: and why they can be so dangerous. *Better Homes and Gardens.* 1992; 70: 46.

Shulman MR. *Mediterranean Light: Delicious Recipes from the World's Healthiest Cuisine.* New York, NY: Bantam; 1989.

The Wellness Encyclopedia. University of California, Berkeley. Boston, Mass: Houghton Mifflin; 1991.

To diet or not? The experts battle it out. *Tufts University Diet & Nutrition Letter.* 1994; 12: 3.

How to Keep the Lost Pounds Off

Barish EB. Dieting may be a losing proposition. *Harvard Health Letter.* 1994; 19: 4.

Blackburn GL. Comparison of medically supervised and unsupervised approaches to weight loss and control. *Annals of Internal Medicine.* 1993; 119: 714.

Blake JS. Eat Right the E.A.S.Y. Way. New York, NY: Prentice Hall Press; 1991.

Brody JE. Gaining health benefits without working up a sweat. *The New York Times.* Feb. 8, 1995; C11.

Brody JE. Why bad health habits drive out the good ones. *The New York Times.* Feb 1, 1995.

Carper J. Food Your Miracle Medicine. New York, NY: HarperPerennial; 1994.

The carrot diet: what's up, Doc? *The Edell Health Letter.* 1991; 10: 1.

Conference statement: voluntary weight loss and control. *Nutrition Research Newsletter.* 1992; 11: 100.

Cousens G. Consciously eating toward the Sacred. *Body Mind Spirit*. March 1995; 6–11.

Forbes GB, Brown M. Energy need for weight maintenance in human beings: effect of body size and composition. *Journal of the American Dietetic Association*. 1989; 89: 499.

Hart J, Einav C, Weingarten MA, Stein M. The importance of family support in a behavior modification weight loss program. *Journal of the American Dietetic Association*. 1990; 90: 1270.

Haus G, Hoerr SL, Mavis B, Robison J. Key modifiable factors in weight maintenance: fat intake, exercise, and weight cycling. *Journal of the American Dietetic Association*. 1994; 94: 409.

In Control: A Video Weight Loss and Maintenance Program, 2nd ed. *Journal of the American Dietetic Association*. 1994; 94: 801.

Jeffery RW. Methods for voluntary weight loss and control. *Annals of Internal Medicine*. 1993; 119: 764.

Kayman S, Bruvold W, Stern JS. Behavioral aspects of weight-loss maintenance. *Nutrition Research Newsletter*. 1991; 10: 2.

Kayman S, Bruvold W, Stern JS. Maintenance and relapse after weight loss in women: behavioral aspects. *American Journal of Clinical Nutrition*. 1990; 52: 800.

Kirk Constance. Think and shrink: mental imagery can be an effective tool to shape your body. *American Fitness*. 1994; 12: 22.

Medich R. Drop That Cheese Ball-It's a New Year, Baby. *Men's Health*. Jan-Feb 1995; 92–95.

Meyer B. Sex and the slimming woman. *Weight Watchers Magazine*. 1994; 27: 36.

Roman M. Know When to Quit. *Men's Health*. Apr: 1994; 36–37.

Scanlon D. Diets That Work: For Weight Control or Medical Needs. Los Angeles, Calif: Lowell House; 1991.

Summary: weighing the options—criteria for evaluating weight-management programs. *Journal of the American Dietetic Association*. 1995; 95: 96.

Undieting. *Nutrition Research Newsletter*. 1992; 11: 75.

Weight maintenance in males. *Nutrition Research Newsletter*. 1990; 9: 19.

Weight maintenance: should you diet or exercise? *Executive Health Report*. 1990; 26: 8.

Wood ER. Weight loss maintenance 1 year after individual counseling. *Journal of the American Dietetic Association*. 1990; 90: 1256.

Exercise: The Other Half of Weight Control

Bjorklund D, Bjorklund B. Physically Fit Families. *Parent's Magazine*. 1989; 64: 215.

Body Fat Percentage: More Important than Weight? *USA Today Magazine*. 1993; 122: 9.

Cooper KH. *The Antioxidant Revolution*. Herbert M. Katz, Inc; 1994.

Doing the Circuit. *Weight Watchers Magazine*. 1994; 27: 28.

Fabricant F. How Sad, How True. . . . *New York Times*. October 19, 1994.

Fitness Tip of the Month: Stationary Bike Form. *Men's Health*. 1994; 9: 34.

Flippin R. Doing the Circuit. . . . *American Health*. 1994; 13: 50–53.

Glover B, Shepherd J. *The Family Fitness Handbook*. New York, NY: Penguin; 1989.

Gurin J. Leaner, Not Lighter. *Psychology Today*. 1989; 23: 32–4.

Hamilton M, et al. *The Duke University Medical Center Book of Diet and Fitness*. New York, NY: Fawcett Columbine; 1990.

Larson DE, ed. *The Mayo Clinic Family Health Book*. New York, NY: William Morrow & Co., Inc; 1990.

Hanc J. Calisthenics Reconsidered. *Men's Health*. 1990; 5: 18.

Heyneman CA, Premo DE. A Water Walkers' Exercise Program. . . . *Public Health Reports*. 1992; 107: 213–5.

Higdon D. Stretch! The Best Strategy for Staying Young. *Longevity/America OnLine*. September 1994.

Howard P. *Execu-cize*. New York, NY: Cornerstone Library, 1979.

Hulet D. The New Gurus of Fitness. *Los Angeles Magazine*. 1993; 38: 92–7.

Johnson S. Playin' Jane. *Entertainment Weekly*. February 4, 1994; 22.

Jordan P. A Weight Full of Water? *American Fitness*. 1994; 12: 65.

Liparulo R. How to Choose a Health Club. *Consumers Digest*. 1992; 31: 26.

Little T, Dranov P. *Technique*. Time Warner; 1994

Long P. Fat Chance. *Hippocrates*. 1989; 3: 38.

McCleary K. The No-Gimmick Weight-Loss Plan. *In Health*. 1991; 5: 82.

Medicine Ball Bounces Back. *The University of California, Berkeley Wellness Letter*. 1991; 8: 6.

Meyers C. *Walking*. New York, NY: Random House; 1992.

New York Times Magazine. October 30, 1994; p. 23.

Nieman DC. *Fitness and Your Health*. Palo Alto, Calif: Bull Publishing; 1993

Pinckney C. *Callanetics*. Avon Books; 1994.

Rama SS. *Exercise Without Movement, Manual One*. Honesdale, Penn: The Himalayan International Institute; 1984.

Recommendations: Home Gyms. *Consumer Reports*. November 1993.

Rippe JM, Amend P. *The Exercise Exchange Program.* New York, NY: Simon & Schuster; 1992.

Robinson A. Take the Plunge. *American Health.* 1994; 13: 42–3.

Schaeffer C, Chapman C. Is Your Health Club Healthy? *Changing Times.* 1989; 43: 116.

Schroeder CR. *Taking the Work Out of Work-Out.* Minn: Chronimed Publishing; 1994.

Smith K. *Kathy Smith's WalkFit™ for a Better Body.* Warner Books; 1994.

Stetson B, et al. The Effects of Aerobic Exercise on Psychological Adjustment. *Women & Health.* 1992; 19: 1–14.

Sykes D. Everybody Into the Pool. . . . *American Fitness.* 1993; 11: 28.

Turning Points: Anatomy of a Fitness Start-up. *Inc.* 1990; 12: 72S.

Veit K. Best Exercise Videos. *Consumers Digest.* 1993; 32: 67.

Video Review '91. *Good Housekeeping.* 1991; 212: 114.

Want to Lose Weight? Don't Diet. *HeartCorps.* 1989; 2: 10–11.

What You Should Look for in an Exerciser. *Sunset.* 1987; 178: 74.

Winters C. Fit & Fun: Fitness Strategies for the Kids. . . . *Working Woman.* 1987; 12: 159.

Wood PD. New Research: Eat Well & Lose Weight. *Executive Health's Good Health Report.* 1991; 28: 1–4.

Going Too Far:
Anorexia, Bulimia, and Bingeing

Anorexia nervosa and bulimia. Bethesda, MD: National Institute of Mental Health; 1987.

APA issues practice guidelines for eating disorders. *American Family Physician.* 1993; 47: 1290–1.

Avoidance of treatment for eating disorders. *American Family Physician.* 1993; 48: 663–664.

Bailey L. Managing eating disorders. *Drug Topics.* 1991; 135: 76–84.

Balentine M, et al. Self-reported eating disorders of black, low-income adolescents: behavior, body weight perceptions, and methods of dieting. *Journal of School Health.* 1991; 61: 392–396.

Blinder BJ. Eating disorders in psychiatric illness. *The Western Journal of Medicine.* 1991; 155: 519.

CATOR study displays benefits of eating disorder treatment. *The Addiction Letter.* 1992; 8: 1–2.

Christopher FS, Johnston CS. Multivariate analysis of the eating disorders inventory: examination of basic statistical assumptions. *Journal of the American Dietetic Association.* 1992; 92: 605–607.

Chronic dieting in adolescence. *Nutrition Research Newsletter.* 1991; 10: 117–118.

Clark N. Beyond hunger: the truth and consequences of eating sprees. *American Fitness.* 1993; 11: 58.

Clark N. Counseling the athlete with an eating disorder: a case study. *Journal of the American Dietetic Association.* 1994; 94: 656–658.

Diagnostic and Statistical Manual of Mental Disorders, Fourth Edition. Washington, DC: American Psychiatric Association; 1994.

Eckstein-Harmon M. Eating disorders: the changing role of nutrition intervention with anorexic and bulimic patients during psychiatric hospitalization. *Journal of the American Dietetic Association.* 1993; 93: 1039–1040.

Emmons L. Dieting and purging behavior in black and white high school students. *Journal of the American Dietetic Association.* 1992; 92: 306–312.

Ending negative thinking patterns in concurrent treatment of eating disorder and chemical dependence. *The Addiction Letter.* 1991; 7: 3.

Facts about anorexia nervosa. Bethesda, MD: National Institute of Child Health and Human Development; 1990.

Fairburn CG. Psychotherapy and bulimia nervosa: longer-term effects of interpersonal psychotherapy, behavior therapy, and cognitive behavior therapy. *The Journal of the American Medical Association.* 1994; 271: 106.

Farley D. Eating disorders require medical attention. *FDA Consumer.* 1992; 26: 27–29.

Garner DM, et al. Comparison of cognitive-behavioral and supportive-expressive therapy for bulimia nervosa. *American Journal of Psychiatry.* 1993; 150: 37–46.

Haller E. Eating disorders: a review and update. *The Western Journal of Medicine.* 1992; 157: 658–662.

Halmi KA, et al. Anorexia and bulimia: You can help. *Patient Care.* 1993; 27: 24–52.

Hawkins WE. Depression and maladaptive eating practices in college students. *Women & Health.* 1992; 18: 55–67.

Henderson R. Anorectics and the cult of being thin. *The Baltimore Sun.* February 25, 1982; C1.

Hudson JI, et al. Eating disorders in hospitalized substance abusers. *American Journal of Drug and Alcohol Abuse.* 1992; 18: 75–85.

Hsu LKG, Lee S. Is weight phobia always necessary for a diagnosis of anorexia nervosa? *American Journal of Psychiatry.* 1993; 150:1466–1471.

Kendler KS, et al. The genetic epidemiology of bulimia nervosa. *American Journal of Psychiatry.* 1991; 148: 1627–1637.

Krizmanic J. Perfection, obsession: can vegetarianism cover up an eating disorder? *Vegetarian Times.* June 1992; 52–59.

Larson BJ. Relationship of family communication patterns to eating disorder inventory scores in adolescent girls. *Journal of the American Dietetic Association.* 1991; 91: 1065–1067.

Luppino T. Yo-yo dieting: early education is the key in the potentially fatal gain-lose weight cycle. *American Fitness.* 1992; 10: 60.

Mallozzi M. Food for thought. *American Fitness.* 1993; 11: 40–43.

Marano HE. Chemistry & craving: not the same old diet story. *Psychology Today.* 1993; 26: 30–35.

Marcus MD. Beating eating disorders. *Diabetes Forecast.* August 1991; 44: 62–3.

Medical update: the heavy toll of dieting and eating disorders. *Health News.* 1994; 12: 8.

Miller C. *My Name is Caroline.* New York: Doubleday; 1988.

Models 'r us. *Psychology Today.* 1992; 25: 11.

Newman MM, Gold MS. Preliminary findings of patterns of substance abuse in eating disorder patients. *American Journal of Drug and Alcohol Abuse.* June 1992; 18: 207–211.

Othersen M. My body, my self. *Runner's World.* 1993; 28: 68.

Pigott TA, et al. Symptoms of eating disorders in patients with obsessive-compulsive disorder. *American Journal of Psychiatry.* 1991; 148: 1552–1557.

Reinstein N, et al. Prevalence of eating disorders among dietetics students: does nutrition education make a difference? *Journal of the American Dietetic Association.* 1992; 92: 949–953.

Robertson L. She wanted to be perfect; instead Christy Henrich is dead. *Knight-Ridder/Tribune News Service.* August 4, 1994.

Rosen M. Eating disorders: a Hollywood history. *People Weekly.* 1992; 37: 96–98.

Schneiderman H. What's your diagnosis? *Consultant.* 1991; 31: 57–58.

Sifton DW, ed. *The PDR Family Guide to Women's Health and Prescription Drugs.* Montvale, NJ: Medical Economics Data; 1994.

Skolnick AA. 'Female athlete triad' risk for women. *Journal of the American Medical Association.* 1993; 270: 921–923.

Smith LH. The rigid family's road to eating disorders. *Health News & Review.* 1992; 2: 6.

Williams K. Deadly dieting: eating disorders among women can devastate more than athletic performances. *Women's Sports and Fitness.* 1991; 13: 22–23.

Yager J. Bulimia nervosa. *The Western Journal of Medicine.* 1991; 155: 523–524.

Yanovski SZ. Bulimia nervosa: the role of the family physician. *American Family Physician.* 1991; 44: 1231–1238.

Yanovski, SZ, et al. Association of binge eating disorder and psychiatric comorbidity in obese subjects. *American Journal of Psychiatry.* 1993; 150: 1472–1479.

What to Do About Fat

The American Heart Association Diet: An Eating plan for Healthy Americans. Dallas, Tex: American Heart Association; 1993.

Bailey C. *Fit or Fat?* Boston, Mass: Houghton Mifflin Company; 1978.

Bailey C. *The Fit-or-Fat Target Diet.* Boston, Mass: Houghton Mifflin Company; 1984.

Bellerson KJ. *The Complete & Up-to-Date Fat Book: A Guide to the Fat, Calories, and Fat Percentages in Your Food.* Garden City Park, NY: Avery Publishing Group; 1993.

Brody JE. *Jane Brody's Good Food Book.* New York, NY: W. W. Norton & Company; 1985.

Cholesterol and Your Heart. Dallas, Tex: American Heart Association; 1993.

Cholesterol Facts: A Joint Statement by the American Heart Association and the National Heart, Lung, and Blood Institute. Dallas, Tex: American Heart Association; 1990.

A consumer's guide to your local cholesterol factory. *Fortune Magazine.* December 18, 1989; 104.

Controlling Your Risk Factors for Heart Attack. Dallas, Tex: American Heart Association; 1994.

Dietary Guidelines for Healthy American Adults: A Statement for Physicians and Health Professionals. Dallas, Tex: American Heart Association; 1988.

Dietary Treatment of Hypercholesterolemia: A Handbook for Counselors. Dallas, Tex: American Heart Association; 1988.

Easy Food Tips for Heart-Healthy Eating. Dallas, Tex: American Heart Association; 1994.

Eat Well, But Wisely. Dallas, Tex: American Heart Association; 1992.

Facts About the New Food Label. Dallas, Tex: American Heart Association; 1993.

Feeding the heart. *Time.* 1993; 141: 22–23.

Findlay S, Silberner J. The truth about cholesterol. *U.S. News & World Report.* 1989; 107: 82–88.

The Food Guide Pyramid. Hyattsville, Md: Human Nutrition Information Service, U.S. Department of Agriculture; 1992.

Gannes S. Behind the battle over cholesterol. *Fortune Magazine.* December 18, 1989; 101.

Grouse L. Taking on the fat of the land: cholesterol and health. *JAMA, The Journal of the American Medical Association.* 1986; 256: 2873–2874.

Guidelines for Weight Management Program for Healthy Adults. Dallas, Tex: American Heart Association; 1994.

Heart and Stroke Facts. Dallas, Tex: American Heart Association; 1993.

Heart and Stroke Facts: 1994 Statistical Supplement. Dallas, Tex: American Heart Association, November 1993.

Highlights of the Report of the Expert Panel on Blood Cholesterol Levels in Children and Adolescents: A Reprint of the Pediatric Panel Report by the National Heart, Lung, and Blood Institute. Dallas, Tex: American Heart Association; 1991.

How To Have Your Cake and Eat It Too. Dallas, Tex: American Heart Association; 1994.

How to pig out but avoid fat. *Time International:* Hong Kong ed. February 12, 1990; 48.

Jaroff L. A crusader from the heartland. *Time Magazine.* March 25, 1991; 56.

Kelly RB, Hazey JA, McMahon SH. Patients' knowledge about fats and cholesterol in the community cholesterol survey project. *Archives of Family Medicine.* September 1992; 75.

Michaels E. The fat and cholesterol debate. *Chatelaine.* 1994; 67: 24.

Napier K. Taking fat to heart. *Weight Watchers Magazine.* 1993; 26: 24–25.

Nash JM. Is a low-fat diet risky? *Time Magazine.* September 5, 1994; 62.

Netzer CT. *The Complete Book of Food Counts.* New York, NY: Dell Publishing; 1988.

Newman J. The sat fat rap. *American Health: Fitness of Body and Mind.* 1990; 9: 106–107.

Nutrition and Your Health: Dietary Guidelines for Americans. 3rd ed. Hyattsville, Md: U.S. Department of Agriculture, U.S. Department of Health and Human Services; 1990.

Nutritious Nibbles: A Guide to Healthy Snacking. Dallas, Tex: American Heart Association; 1984.

Pritikin R. *The New Pritikin Program.* New York, NY: Pocket Books; 1991.

Rationale of the Diet-Heart Statement of the American Heart Association. Dallas, Tex: The Nutrition Committee, American Heart Association; 1993.

Sacks FM, Willett WW. More on chewing the fat: the good fat and the good cholesterol. *The New England Journal of Medicine.* 1992; 325: 1740–1742.

Saturated fat and cholesterol blunt benefits of reducing fat intake. *Executive Health's Good Health Report.* 1994; 30: 7.

Say it ain't so, oleo! *Time Magazine.* August 27, 1990; 53.

Sifton DW, ed. *The PDR Family Guide to Prescription Drugs.* Montvale, NJ: Medical Economics Data; 1993.

Sifton DW, ed. *The PDR Family Guide to Women's Health and Prescription Drugs.* Montvale, NJ: Medical Economics Data; 1994.

Silent Epidemic: The Truth About Women and Heart Disease. Dallas, Tex: American Heart Association; 1992.

Thompson D. A how-to guide on cholesterol. *Time Magazine.* October 19, 1987; 45.

Toufexis A. The food you eat may kill you. *Time Magazine.* August 8, 1988; 66.

Toufexis A. Watch what you eat, kid. *Time Magazine.* April 22, 1991; 76.

Your Heart and Cholesterol. Dallas, Tex: American Heart Association; 1992.

Heart Healthy Ways to Perk up Your Diet

Alcohol and coronary mortality. *Nutrition Research Newsletter.* 1993; 12: 59.

Alcohol and heart disease: reviewing the evidence. *The Brown University Digest of Addiction Theory and Application.* 1994; 13: 6–7.

Alcohol use and mortality from coronary heart disease. *American Family Physician.* December 1992; 46: 1796.

Antioxidant vitamins and coronary mortality. *Nutrition Research Newsletter.* 1994; 8: 88–89.

Barker DJP, et al. Why Londoners have low death rates from ischaemic heart disease and stroke. *British Medical Journal.* 1992; 305: 1551–1553.

A clove a day: healthy hearts. *The Economist.* 1994; 331: 92–3.

Coate D. Moderate drinking and coronary heart disease mortality: evidence from National Health and Nutrition Examination Survey I and the NHANES I Follow-up. *The American Journal of Public Health.* 1993; 83: 888–890.

Cox J. Garlic Power. *Men's Health.* 1992; 7: 34–35.

de Lorgeril M, et al. Mediterranean alpha-linolenic acid-rich diet in secondary prevention of coronary heart disease. *The Lancet.* 1994; 343: 1454–1459.

Diet and heart disease: the French paradox. *Nutrition Research Newsletter.* 1992; 11: 86.

Does alcohol really prevent heart disease? *Berkeley Wellness Letter.* 1991; 8: 1.

Duffy J. Drinking to your health. *New Statesman & Society.* 1993; 6: 30–31.

Eating for Life. *National Cancer Institute.* June 1988; 1–23.

Fairchild M, Utermohlen V. Your live-longer eating guide. *Woman's Day.* 1992; 55: 101–104.

Fish intake and coronary mortality: effect of glucose tolerance. *Nutrition Research Newsletter.* 1993; 12: 106A.

Folic acid: preventing birth defects. *Johns Hopkins Women'sHealth.* 1993; 1: 5.

For your heart's sake, more B vitamins. *Tufts University Diet & Nutrition Letter*. 1994; 11: 1–2.

Garlic as a lipid-lowering agent. *Nutrition Research Newsletter*. 1994; 13: 57.

Hein HO, et al. Alcohol consumption, Lewis phenotypes, and risk of ischaemic heart disease. *The Lancet*. 1993; 341: 392–396.

Hertog MGL, et al. Dietary antioxidant flavonoids and risk of coronary heart disease: the Zutphen Elderly Study. *The Lancet*. 1993; 342: 1007–1011.

Hettinger ME. Vitamin E pioneers were right: E fights heart disease and more. *Health News & Review*. 1993; 3: 1–2.

Hrabak D. A fish oil story: omega-3's return to fight heart disease, cancer. *Environmental Nutrition*. 1994; 17: 1–2.

Hunter BT. Glutathione: an unheralded antioxidant. *Consumers' Research Magazine*. 1993; 76: 8–9.

Kemm J. Alcohol and heart disease: the implications of the U-shaped curve. *British Medical Journal*. 1993; 307: 1373–1374.

Laliberte R. Your body: an owner's manual. *Men's Health*. 1994; 9: 72–78.

Liebman B. Fiber: separating fact from fiction. *Nutrition Action Healthletter*. 1994; 21: 1–4.

Light-to-moderate alcohol intake may protect against heart disease. *Medical World News*. 1992; 33: 31.

Lorente CW. The skinny on fat. *Vegetarian Times*. December 1993; 4.

Marcus E. Undoing the damage: can we reverse the ill effects of a lifetime of eating a meat-based diet? *Vegetarian Times*. December 1993; 58–63.

McCaleb R. Garlic: heart herb. *Better Nutrition for Today's Living*. 1993; 55: 58–61.

McKeigue P. Diets for secondary prevention of coronary heart disease: can linolenic acid substitute for oily fish? *The Lancet*. 1994; 343: 1445.

Moderate alcohol intake, HDL levels, and heart disease. *Nutrition Research Newsletter*. 1994; 13: 9.

More on vitamin E and heart disease. *Nutrition Research Newsletter*. 1994; 13: 29–30.

Mori TA, et al. Effects of varying dietary fat, fish, and fish oils on blood lipids in a randomized controlled trial in men at risk of heart disease. *American Journal of Clinical Nutrition*. 1994; 59: 1060–1068.

Napier K. Should you take vitamin E? *American Health*, September 1993; 12: 86–87

Nutritional aspects of ambulatory practice: oxidized LDL, antioxidant nutrients and CAD. *Journal of the American Dietetic Association*. 1994; 94: 371–372.

Our vitamin prescription: the big four. *Berkeley Wellness Letter*. 1994; 10: 1–2.

Posner BM, et al. Healthy People 2000; the rationale and potential efficacy of preventive nutrition in heart disease: the Framingham Offspring-Spouse Study. *Archives of Internal Medicine*. 1993; 153: 1549–1556.

Pressing garlic for possible health benefits. *Tufts University Diet & Nutrition Letter*. 1994; 12: 3–6.

Protective effect of fiber. *Nutrition Research Newsletter*. 1994; 13: 16.

Rath M. How vitamin C and other nutrients can help nip heart disease in the bud. *Executive Health's Good Health Report*. 1993; 30: 1–3.

Relation of vitamin C to cardiovascular risk factors. *Nutrition Research Newsletter*. 1992; 11: 47.

Renaud S, de Lorgeril M. Wine, alcohol, platelets, and the French paradox. *The Lancet*. 1992; 339: 1523–1526.

Review: antioxidant vitamins and cardiovascular disease. *Nutrition Research Newsletter*. 1992; 11: 47.

Schardt D. Do or diet: treating disease with food. *Nutrition Action Healthletter*. 1993; 20: 1–4.

Scharffenberg J. Living a longer, healthier, and happier life. *Vibrant Life*. 1992; 8: 16–18.

Shapiro L. A Food Lover's Guide to Fat. *Newsweek*. December 5, 1994; 52–60.

Sherwood B. Wine and poses. *Washington Monthly*. 1993; 25: 22–26.

Smart JM. Antioxidants for the uninitiated: nutrition's latest buzzword may actually deserve the hype. *Vegetarian Times*. April 1994; 26–27.

Steinberg D. Antioxidant vitamins and coronary heart disease. *The New England Journal of Medicine*. 1993; 328: 1487–1489.

Thomas P. A toast to the heart. *Harvard Health Letter*. 1994; 19: 4–5.

To take antioxidant pills or not? The debate heats up. *Tufts University Diet and Nutrition Newsletter*. 1994; 12: 3–6.

Tyson S. Fishing for better health? *Health News & Review*. 1992; 2: 1–2.

Vitamin E and heart attacks. *Nutrition Research Newsletter*. 1994; 13: 29.

Vitamin E cuts risk of coronary heart disease. *Better Nutrition for Today's Living*. 1993; 55: 16–18.

Wisner P. Rx for the heart; more and more studies are showing that drinking wine in moderation—white as well as red—can be good for your health. *House Beautiful*. 1994; 136: 76–77.

The Dietary Approach to High Blood Pressure

Nutritional factors and prevention of hypertension. *Amer Fam Physician*. 1993; 47: 1866.

Ahern DA, Kaley LA. Electrolyte content of salt-replacement seasonings. *J Amer Dietetic Assn*. 1989; 89: 935.

Altura BM, Brodsky MA, et al. Magnesium: growing in clinical importance. *Patient Care*. 1994; 28: 130–150.

American Heart Association Nutrition Committee. Dietary guidelines for healthy American adults. *Circulation.* 1988; 77.

Geleijnse JM, Witteman JC, et al. Reduction in blood pressure with a low sodium, high potassium, high magnesium salt in older subjects with mild to moderate hypertension. *Brit Med J.* 1994; 309: 436.

Heart and stroke facts: 1995 statistical supplement. Dallas, Tex: American Heart Association; 1994.

Kurtzweil P. Scouting for sodium: and other nutrients important to blood pressure. *FDA Consumer.* 1994; 28: 18.

Moser M. *Lower your blood pressure and live longer.* New York, NY: *Villard;* 1989.

Moser M. Update on the management of hypertension. *Prim Cardiol.* 1990; 16: 31–45.

Moser M, Becker B. *Week by week to a strong heart.* Emmaus, Pa: Rodale Press; 1992.

Smith R. The shake out on sodium: an interview with David A. McCarron. *Total Health.* 1994; 16: 46.

Starke RD, Winston M. *American Heart Association low-salt cookbook: A complete guide to reducing sodium and fat in the diet.* New York, NY: *Times Books;* 1990.

Swales JD. Salt substitutes and potassium intake. *Br Med J.* 1991; 303: 1084.

Taylor KB, Anthony LE. *Clinical nutrition.* New York, NY: McGraw-Hill; 1983.

Wylie-Rosett J, Wassertheil-Smoller S, et al. Trial of antihypertensive intervention and management: greater efficacy with weight reduction than with a sodium-potassium intervention. *J Amer Dietetic Assn.* 1993; 93: 408.

Cut Back on These Foods to Cut Your Cancer Risk

Alcohol and breast cancer. *Nutrition Research Newsletter.* 1993; 12: 60.

Alcohol and lung cancer in Uruguay. *Nutrition Research Newsletter.* 1993; 12: 44–45.

The alcohol/breast cancer connection. *The University of California, Berkeley Wellness Letter.* 1994; 10: 1–2.

Alcohol consumption and breast cancer. *Nutrition Research Newsletter.* 1991; 10: 112–113.

Alcohol intake and breast cancer. *Nutrition Research Newsletter.* 1994; 13: 54–55.

Alar, UDMH shown not to be carcinogenic. *Cancer Weekly.* 1992; 10–11.

Austoker J. Reducing alcohol intake. *British Medical Journal.* 1994; 308: 1549–1552.

Beer may increase risk of rectal cancer. *Executive Health's Good Health Report.* 1992; 28: 8.

Birth control pills, cigarettes, alcohol linked to liver cancer. *Cancer Weekly.* December 23, 1991; 8–9.

Blocking skin cancer through diet. *Tufts University Diet & Nutrition Letter.* 1994; 12: 8.

Brown LM. Are racial differences in squamous cell esophageal cancer explained by alcohol and tobacco use? [abstract]. *Journal of the National Cancer Institute.* 1994; 86: 1340.

Butrum R, et al. NCI dietary guidelines: rationale. *American Journal of Clinical Nursing.* 1988; 48: 888–95.

Can drinking beer lead to colon cancer? [abstract]. *Mayo Clinic Health Letter.* 1993; 11: 3.

Chow WH, et al. Protein intake and risk of renal cell cancer [abstract]. *Journal of the National Cancer Institute.* 1994; 86: 1131.

Cody RP, et al. Hematologic effects of benzene: job-specific trends during the first year of employment among a cohort of benzene-exposed rubber workers [abstract]. *Journal of Occupational Medicine.* 1993; 35: 776.

Colgan M. *Prevent Cancer Now.* San Diego, Calif: C.I. Publications; 1990.

Comparing possible cancer hazards from natural and man-made substances. *Journal of the American Dietetic Association.* 1992; 92: 597.

Conkling W. Pesticide perspectives; are pesticides poisoning your food? *American Health.* 1994; 13: 46–48.

Court broadens pesticide ban to include all carcinogens concentrated in food. *Milling & Baking News.* 1992; 71: 21.

Delaney's folly. *National Review.* 1993; 45: 18–19.

Diet and stomach cancer in Spain. *Nutrition Research Newsletter.* 1994; 13: 53–54.

Diet, Nutrition & Cancer Prevention: A Guide to Food Choices. *National Institutes of Health, NIH Publication No. 87-2878.* May 1987.

Dietary factors and the risk of endometrial cancer. *Cancer Research Weekly.* July 19, 1993; 26.

Effects of coffee, alcohol, and tobacco: two studies. *Nutrition Research Newsletter.* 1993; 12: 92–93.

Findings suggest alcohol use raises estrogen levels and breast cancer risk. *Cancer Research Weekly.* May 10, 1993; 2.

Freedman LS, et al. Dietary fat and breast cancer: where we are. *Journal of the National Cancer Institute.* 1993; 85: 764–765.

Fried JJ. Pesticides, other chemicals increase breast cancer, researchers think. *Knight-Ridder/Tribune News Service.* December 8, 1993; 1208K0784.

Garlic fights nitrosamine formation . . . as do tomatoes and other produce. *Science News.* 1994; 145: 190.

Garro AJ, et al. Alcohol and cancer. *Alcohol Health & Research World.* 1992; 16: 81–86.

Goldin BR, et al. The effect of dietary fat and fiber on serum estrogen concentrations in premenopausal women under controlled dietary conditions [abstract]. *Cancer.* 1994; 74: 1125.

Greenwald P. Statement before Committee on Government Operations, Subcommittee on Human Resources and Intergovernmental Relations, U.S. Congress. September 13, 1993.

Henig RM. 10 ways to lower cancer risks. *Woman's Day.* 1992; 56: 70–72.

Henkel J. From shampoo to cereal: seeing to the safety of color additives. *FDA Consumer.* 1993; 27: 14–21.

Hope J. DDT's revenge—and other sobering news. *Good Housekeeping.* 1994; 219: 86.

Howe GR. Dietary fat and breast cancer risks: an epidemiologic perspective [abstract]. *Cancer.* 1994; 74: 1078.

Hsia CC, et al. Mutations of p53 gene in hepatocellular carcinoma: roles of hepatitis B virus and aflatoxin contamination in the diet [abstract]. *Journal of the National Cancer Institute.* 1992; 84: 1638.

Hunter BT. The diet-cancer connection. *Consumers' Research Magazine.* 1994; 77: 8.

Hunter BT. Dietary recommendations for certain health conditions. *Consumers' Research Magazine.* 1993; 76: 8–9.

Hunter BT. Some unanticipated interactions. *Consumers' Research Magazine.* 1993; 76: 8–9.

Jacobs MM. Diet, nutrition, and cancer research: an overview. *Nutrition Today.* 1993; 28: 19–23.

Jakobsson R, et al. Acute myeloid leukemia among petro station attendants. *Archives of Environmental Health.* 1993; 48: 255–259.

Joint announcement about emergency pesticide use. *FDA Consumer.* 1993; 27: 4–5.

Keough C, ed. *The Complete Book of Cancer Prevention.* Emmaus, Pa: Rodale Press; 1988.

Link between saccharin and human cancer questioned. *Cancer Weekly.* May 11, 1992; 6.

Lippman SM, et al. Cancer Chemoprevention. *Journal of Clinical Oncology.* 1994; 12: 851–873.

Livermore Lab studies cancer agents in diet. *Cancer Weekly.* October 26, 1992; 5–6.

Longnecker MP. Alcohol consumption in relation to risk of cancers of the breast and large bowel. *Alcohol Health & Research World.* 1992; 16: 223–229.

Mason M. The man who has a beef with your diet. *Health.* 1994; 8: 52–57.

Mead N. Does sugar make you old before your time? *Natural Health.* 1993; 23: 96–98.

Mettlin C. Dietary cancer prevention in children [abstract]. *Cancer.* 1993; 71: 3367.

Meyerhoff A. We must get rid of pesticides in the food supply: exposure to these deadly chemicals can cause cancer, birth defects, and neurological damage. *USA Today Magazine.* 1993; 122: 51–53.

Micronutrients and gastric cancer in Northern Italy. *Nutrition Research Newsletter.* 1994; 8: 86.

Nagao M, et al. Dietary carcinogens and mammary carcinogenesis: induction of rat mammary carcinomas by administration of heterocyclic amines in cooked foods [abstract]. *Cancer.* 1994; 74: 1063.

National Cancer Institute 1996 Estimated Budget for Scientific Opportunities. September 1994.

National Cancer Institute Division of Cancer Prevention and Control. *94 Annual Report.*

Ozturk M. p53 mutation in hepatocellular carcinoma after aflatoxin exposure. *The Lancet.* 1991; 338: 1356–1359.

Papazian R. Food irradiation: a hot issue. *Harvard Health Letter.* 1992; 17: 1–3.

Potter JF. *How to Improve Your Odds Against Cancer.* Hollywood, FL: Compact Books; 1988.

Prentice RL, et al. Breast cancer risk from diet, tobacco, and alcohol. *The Journal of the American Medical Association.* 1993; 269: 1790–1792.

Rademacher JJ, et al. Gastric cancer mortality and nitrate levels in Wisconsin drinking water. *Archives of Environmental Health.* 1992; 47: 292–294.

Raloff J. Sorting out cancer IQs in browned meat. *Science News.* 1994; 145: 22.

Raloff JA. Coffee: Key to cooked-meat vulnerability? *Science News.* 1994; 145: 265.

Raloff JA. Not so hot hot dogs? Fleshing out risks associated with how we treat meat. *Science News.* 1994; 145: 264–266.

Ravage B. A battlefield called cancer. *Current Health.* 1994; 20: 6–11.

Review: alcohol consumption and colorectal cancer. *Nutrition Research Newsletter.* 1993; 12: 8.

Risk factors for colorectal adenomas: three reports. *Nutrition Research Newsletter.* 1993; 12: 89–90.

Ross RK, et al. Urinary aflatoxin biomarkers and risk of hepatocellular carcinoma. *The Lancet.* 1992; 339: 943–946.

Saccharin-caused cancer may be limited to rats. *Cancer Weekly.* April 20, 1992; 9–10.

Sachs JS. Hidden dangers in your food and water. *McCalls.* 1994; 121: 40–41.

Simone CB. *Cancer & Nutrition.* Garden City Park, NY: Avery Publishing Group, Inc.; 1992.

Snyderwine EG. Some perspectives on the nutritional aspects of breast cancer research: food-derived heterocyclic amines as etiologic agents in human mammary cancer [abstract]. *Cancer.* 1994; 74: 1070.

Study finds suspect digestive by-product of cooked meat does not cause gene mutation or cancer. *Cancer Research Weekly.* January 10, 1994; 2–3.

Study finds women beer-drinkers have greater cancer risk. *Cancer Weekly*. October 28, 1991; 6–7.

Study links pesticides to cancer. *Cancer Research Weekly*. October 17, 1994; 3.

Styrene in foods: what does it mean? *Science News*. 1994; 146: 191.

A tomato a day keeps nitrosamines at bay. *Better Nutrition for Today's Living*. 1994; 56: 18–19.

Tyson S. What causes cancer? *Health News & Review*. Summer 1992; 2: B.

Van Itallie TB. Cancer. (The Basics of Good Nutrition). In *The Columbia University College of Physicians & Surgeons Complete Home Medical Guide*. 2nd Edition. Crown Publishers; 1989; 332–334.

Vrazo F. Studies find lumpectomy safe, no link between breast cancer and pesticides. *Knight-Ridder/Tribune News Service*. April 19, 1994; 0419K8708.

Weisburger JH. Heterocyclic amines, carcinogens formed during cooking of meats. *Cancer Research Weekly*. January 31, 1994; 20.

Welsch C. Interrelationship between dietary lipids and calories and experimental mammary gland tumorigenesis [abstract]. *Cancer*. 1994; 74: 1055–1062.

Whelan E. Restore scientific focus to EPA policy. *Insight on the News*. 1993; 9: 20–21.

Whittemore AS, Henderson BE. Dietary fat and breast cancer: where are we? *Journal of the National Cancer Institute*. 1993; 85:762–763.

Food That Fights Cancer: What Science Knows Today

Alpha-tocopherol, beta-carotene cancer prevention study: vitamin E and beta-carotene supplements did not prevent lung cancer in male smokers. *National Cancer Institute press release*. April 13, 1994.

Antioxidants and oral cancer. *Nutrition Research Newsletter*. 1993; 12: 39–40.

Beecher CWW. Cancer preventive properties of varieties of Brassica oleracea: a review [abstract]. *American Journal of Clinical Nutrition*. 1994; 59: 1166S.

Beta carotene's extended family. *University of California Berkeley Wellness Letter*. 1994; 10: 2.

Beta-carotene, vitamin E, and lung cancer: results of a major intervention trial. *Nutrition Research Newsletter*. 1994; 13: 39–41.

Blot WJ, et al. Nutrition intervention trials in Linxian, China: supplementation with specific vitamin/mineral combinations, cancer incidence, and disease-specific mortality in the general population. *Journal of the National Cancer Institute* [abstract]. 1993; 85: 1483–1492.

Broccoli key supplier of cancer-fighting agents. *Better Nutrition for Today's Living*. 1994; 56: 22.

Butrum R, et al. NCI dietary guidelines: rationale. *American Journal of Clinical Nursing*. 1988; 48: 888–95.

Byers T. Dietary trends in the United States: relevance to cancer prevention [abstract]. *Cancer*. 1993; 72: 1015.

Cabbage cuts cancer risk. *Organic Gardening*. 41:24; 24.

Calcium and colorectal epithelial cell proliferation: a preliminary randomized double-blinded placebo-controlled clinical trial. *Cancer Weekly*. February 8, 1993; 21–22.

Calcium, bile acids, and colon cancer. *Nutrition Research Newsletter*. 1994; 13: 10.

Calcium protective against colon cancer. *Cancer Weekly*. May 11, 1992; 4.

Carotenoids found to inhibit tumor growth. *Cancer Researcher Weekly*. October 11, 1993; 8.

Carroll M. "Meet the crucifers: cruciferous vegetables have earned their reputation as disease-fighters. *Vegetarian Times*. July 1994; 30–32.

Chollar S, Macht HA. Should you take vitamins? *McCall's*. 1994; 121: 102–104.

Chug-Ahuja JK, et al. The development and application of a carotenoid database for fruits, vegetables, and selected multicomponent foods. *Journal of the American Dietetic Association*. 1993; 93: 318–323.

Cichoke AJ. Designer foods: nutrients of the future. *Total Health*. 1994; 16: 34–36.

Common garlic powder blocks potent carcinogens in cells. *Cancer Researcher Weekly*. March 14, 1994; 7.

"Cruciferous = splendiferous. *University of California Berkeley Wellness Letter*. 1994; 10: 7.

Designer' foods: tomorrow's answer to breast cancer prevention? *Nutrition Health Review*. Spring 1993; 15.

Dicken CH, et al. Retinoids: what role in your practice? *Patient Care*. 1992; 26: 18–34.

Diet and stomach cancer in Spain. *Nutrition Research Newsletter*. 1994; 13: 53–54.

Dwyer JT, et al. Tofu and soy drinks contain phytoestrogens. *Journal of the American Dietetic Association*. 1994; 94: 739–743.

Fish oil capsules vs. fish. *University of California Berkeley Wellness Letter*. 1994; 10: 4.

Frentzel-Beyme R, Chang-Claude J. Vegetarian diets and colon cancer: the German experience [abstract]. *American Journal of Clinical Nutrition*. 1994; 59: 1143S.

Fruit, vegetable intake protects against disease. *Better Nutrition for Today's Living*. 1993; 55: 18.

Fuller CJ, et al. Carotenoid-depletion diet for use in long-term studies. *Journal of the American Dietetic Association*. 1993; 93: 812–814.

Garlic alters and even kills human cancer cells. *Cancer Researcher Weekly*. May 9, 1994; 7.

Garlic as an anti-carcinogen in breast cancer. *Cancer Researcher Weekly*. January 17, 1994; 3–4.

Garlic inhibits germs, cholesterol and cancer. *Better Nutrition for Today's Living*. 1994; 56: 10.

Garlic, the food-aceutical. *University of California Berkeley Wellness Letter*. 1992; 8: 1–2.

Garlic: the healing herb. *Total Health*. 1992; 14: 41–42.

Gemperlein J. Broccoli gets healthier all the time. *Knight-Ridder/Tribune News Service*. April 18, 1994; 0418K7979.

Genistein, a dietary derived inhibitor of in vitro angiogenesis. *Cancer Researcher*. May 17, 1993; 23–24.

Greenwald, Peter. Statement before Committee on Government Operations, Subcommittee on Human Resources and Intergovernmental Relations, U.S. Congress. September 13, 1993.

Grubbs CJ. Carotenoids, vitamin A and breast cancer. *Cancer Researcher Weekly*. June 7, 1993; 21–22.

Hankin JH. Role of nutrition in women's health: diet and breast cancer. *Journal of the American Dietetic Association*. 1993; 93: 994–999.

Hathcock JN. Safety and regulatory issues for phytochemical sources: designer foods. *Nutrition Today*. 1993; 28: 23–25.

Havas S, et al. 5 a day for better health: a new research initiative. *Journal of the American Dietetic Association*. 1994; 94: 32–36.

Hrabak D. A fish oil story: omega-3's return to fight heart disease, cancer. *Environmental Nutrition*. 1994; 17: 1–2.

Hunter BT. The diet-cancer connection. *Consumers' Research Magazine*. June 1994; 77:8.

Hunter DJ, et al. A prospective study of the intake of vitamins C, E, and A and the risk of breast cancer [abstract]. *The New England Journal of Medicine*. July 22, 1993; 329: 234.

Ip C, et al. Conjugated linoleic acid suppressed mammary carcinogenesis and proliferative activity of the mammary gland in the rat. *Cancer Research*. 1994; 54: 1212.

Ip C, et al. Conjugated linoleic acid: a powerful anticarcinogen from animal fat sources. *Cancer*. 1994; 74: 1050.

Jacobs MM. Diet, nutrition, and cancer research: an overview. *Nutrition Today*. 1993; 28: 19–23.

Kennedy B. Breast cancer prevention: garlic, estrogen and Pacific yew. *Total Health*. 1992; 14: 32–33.

Kennedy B. Green food energy. *Total Health*. 1993; 15: 30–32.

Keough C, ed. *The Complete Book of Cancer Prevention*. Emmaus, Pa: Rodale Press; 1988.

Kleiner SM. Yogurt: tasty disease preventive. *Executive Health's Good Health Report*. 1993; 29: 6–7.

Langer S. Immune boosters. *Better Nutrition for Today's Living*. 1993; 55: 30–32.

Lin RI. Cancer protective effects of garlic. *Total Health*. 1993; 15: 20–23.

Lindner L, Hordern BB. The new ABCs of vitamins: a nutrient-by-nutrient rundown of the latest research. *Working Woman*. 1994; 19: 76–81.

Lippman SM, et al. Cancer Chemoprevention. *Journal of Clinical Oncology*. 1994; 12: 851–873.

Lustgarden S. Holy mackerel! Protective fats from plants, not fish. *Vegetarian Times*. October 1994; 20.

Mancini L. From research to responsibility. *Chilton's Food Engineering*. 1993; 65: 65–67.

Mangels AR, et al. Carotenoid content of fruit and vegetables: an evaluation of analytic data. *Journal of the American Dietetic Association*. 1993; 93: 284–296.

Martin D. Folklore, old wives were right: garlic stimulates the immune system, fights free radicals, inhibits tumors. *Health News & Review*. 1991; 1: 1–2.

Micozzi MS. Plant flavonoids—can they heal us? *Executive Health's Good Health Report*. 1993; 29: 1–3.

Micronutrients and gastric cancer in Northern Italy. *Nutrition Research Newsletter*. 1994; 8: 86.

Milk isn't just for kids anymore. *Medical Update*. 1992; 15: 2–3.

Morse DE. Vitamin A, retinoids, and beta-carotene as oral cancer chemopreventive agents: findings from human intervention trials. *Cancer Researcher Weekly*. July 11, 1994; 20.

Murray F. Garlic: cancer's freshest enemy. *Better Nutrition for Today's Living*. 1994; 56: 56–58.

Murray F. Selenium offers hope in cancer prevention. *Better Nutrition for Today's Living*. 1991; 53: 10–11.

Narisawa T, et al. Effect of different levels of w-3 polyunsaturated fatty acid (PUFA) alpha-linolenic acid in a medium-fat diet on colon carcinogenesis in F344 rats. *Cancer Researcher Weekly*. January 31, 1994; 20.

National Cancer Institute 1996 Estimated Budget for Scientific Opportunities. September 1994.

National Cancer Institute Division of Cancer Prevention and Control. *94 Annual Report*.

Passwater RA. A day without vitamin C is a day without cancer protection: C helps prevent and treat cancers of the breast, kidney, and cervix. *Health News & Review*. 1993; 3: 12.

A plate of protection: nutrients may lower stomach cancer risk. *Prevention*. 1994; 46: 10–11.

Pressing garlic for possible health benefits. *Tufts University Diet & Nutrition Letter*. September 1994; 12: 3–6.

Raloff JA. Not so hot hot dogs? Fleshing out risks associated with how we treat meat. *Science News*. 1994; 145: 264–266.

Raloff J. This fat may fight cancer several ways. *Science News*. 1994; 145: 182–183.

Ravage B. A battlefield called cancer. *Current Health*. 1994; 20: 6–11.

Retinoid/interferon-alpha combination shows efficacy in squamous cell carcinomas. *Cancer Weekly*. February 24, 1992; 11–12.

Review: oral cancer inhibition by micronutrients. *Nutrition Research Newsletter*. 1993; 12: 87–88.

Role of nutrition in preventing and treating cancer. *Cancer Researcher Weekly*. August 22, 1994; 14.

Schardt D. Yogurt: bacteria to basics. *Nutrition Action Healthletter*. 1993; 20: 8–9.

Scheer James F. Green foods: beneficial nourishments, protectors. *Better Nutrition for Today's Living*. 1993; 55: 36–40.

Scheer JF. Selenium: cancer fighter. *Better Nutrition for Today's Living*. 1992; 54: 15–17.

Scientists discover new hormone. *Cancer Weekly*. February 3, 1992; 2.

Sifton DW, ed. *The PDR Family Guide to Women's Health and Prescription Drugs*. Montvale, NJ: Medical Economics Data; 1994.

Simone CB. *Cancer & Nutrition*. Garden City Park, NY: Avery Publishing Group, Inc.; 1992.

Skerrett PJ. Low selenium linked to precancerous colon polyps. *Medical World News*. April 1993; 16.

Sources of provitamin A carotenoids. *Nutrition Research Newsletter*. 1994; 13: 58–59.

Spicing up your isoflavones and phytoesterols. *University of California Berkeley Wellness Letter*. 1993; 10: 1–2.

Substance in some vegetables may fight cancer in pancreas. *Cancer Researcher Weekly*. October 4, 1993; 11–12.

Supplements reduce deaths in a high-risk population in China. *National Cancer Institute press release*. September 14, 1993.

Ternus M. Don't count out 'other' carotenoids; they may offer big health bonus. *Environmental Nutrition*. 1994; 17: 1–2.

Tiwari RK, et al. Selective responsiveness of human breast cancer cells to indole-3-carbinol, a chemopreventive agent [abstract]. *Journal of the National Cancer Institute*. 1994; 86: 126–131.

To guard against cancer, don't forget carotenoids. *Better Nutrition for Today's Living*. September 1994; 56: 16.

A tomato a day keeps nitrosamines at bay. *Better Nutrition for Today's Living*. 1994; 56: 18–19.

Van Itallie TB. Cancer. (The Basics of Good Nutrition). In *The Columbia University College of Physicians & Surgeons Complete Home Medical Guide*, 2nd ed. Crown Publishers: 1989; 332–334.

Vandenbrandt RA, et al. A prospective cohort study on selenium status and the risk of lung cancer [abstract]. *Cancer Research*. 1993; 53(20): 4860.

Vitamin C, fiber may prevent breast cancer. *Better Nutrition for Today's Living*. 1993; 55: 16.

Vitamins and selenium reduce cancer deaths. *Better Nutrition for Today's Living*. 1993; 55: 10–11.

Vitamins, fiber may deter breast cancer. *Better Nutrition for Today's Living*. 1994; 56: 12–13.

Wein DA. Do calcium's disease-fighting roles go beyond bone building? *Environmental Nutrition*. 1994; 17: 1–2.

Weinberg L. Research hints garlic may be wonder bulb against disease. *Environmental Nutrition*. 1994; 17: 1–2.

Willett WC. Micronutrients and cancer risk [abstract]. *American Journal of Clinical Nutrition*. 1994; 59: 1162S.

Yogurt and the immune system. *The Edell Health Letter*. 1992; 11: 1.

Yogurt: folklore and fact. *University of California Berkeley Wellness Letter*. 1993; 9: 3.

Targeting Specific Cancer Risks

Alabaster O. *What You Can Do To Prevent Cancer*. New York, NY: Simon & Schuster; 1985.

American Cancer Society. *Nutrition and Cancer: Cause and Prevention: An American Cancer Society Special Report*. New York, NY: American Cancer Society; 1984.

Carper J. *Food—Your Miracle Medicine*. New York, NY: HarperCollins; 1993.

Colbin A. *Food and Healing*. New York, NY: Ballantine Books; 1986.

Cooper KH. *Dr. Kenneth H. Cooper's Antioxidant Revolution*. Nashville, Tenn: Thomas Nelson Publishers; 1994.

Dreher H. *Your Defense Against Cancer: The Complete Guide to Cancer Prevention*. New York, NY: Harper & Row; 1988.

Eades MD. *The Doctor's Complete Guide to Vitamins and Minerals*. New York, NY: Dell; 1994.

Editors of Prevention Magazine Health Books. *The Complete Book of Cancer Prevention: Foods, Lifestyles & Medical Care to Keep You Healthy*. Emmaus, Pa: Rodale Press; 1988.

Gorbach SL, Zimmerman DR, Woods M. *The Doctors' Anti-Breast Cancer Diet*. New York, NY: Simon and Schuster; 1984.

Hall SS. The power of garlic. *Health*. 8:83.

Hausman P, Hurley JB. *The Healing Foods*. New York, NY: Dell; 1992.

Henderson BE, Ross RK, Pike MC. Toward the primary prevention of cancer. *Science*. 1991; 254: 1131.

Hilts PJ. U.S. breast cancer deaths fell nearly 5 percent in three years. *The New York Times*. Jan. 13, 1995; A17.

Holleb AI, ed. *The American Cancer Society Cancer Book: Prevention, Detection, Diagnosis, Treatment, Rehabilitation, Cure*. New York, NY: Doubleday; 1986.

Kemeny MM, Dranov P. *Breast Cancer & Ovarian Cancer: Beating the Odds*. Reading, Mass: Addison-Wesley; 1992.

Lerner M. *Choices in Healing: Integrating the Best of Conventional and Complementary Approaches to Cancer*. Cambridge, Mass: MIT Press; 1994.

Liebman B. Fiber: separating fact from fiction. *Nutrition Action Healthletter*. 21: 1.

Liebman B. The salt shakeout. *Nutrition Action Healthletter*. 21:1.

McAllister RM, Horowitz ST, Gilden RV. *Cancer*. New York, NY: HarperCollins; 1993.

Michnovicz JJ, Klein DS. *How to Reduce Your Risk of Breast Cancer*. New York, NY: Warner; 1994.

National Institutes of Health. NCI's 5 A Day Program (press release). NCI Press Office; July 1, 1992.

Nixon DW. *The Cancer Recovery Eating Plan*. New York, NY: Times Books; 1994.

Passwater RA. *Cancer Prevention and Nutritional Therapies*. New Canaan, Conn: Keats Publishing; 1993.

Potter JF. *How to Improve Your Odds Against Cancer*. Hollywood, Fla: Frederick Fell Publishers; 1988.

Quillen P. *Beating Cancer with Nutrition*. Tulsa, Okla: Nutrition Times Press; 1994.

Schardt D. Phytochemicals: plants against cancer. *Nutrition Action Healthletter*. 21: 1.

Seltzer VL. *Every Woman's Guide to Breast Cancer: Prevention, Treatment, Recovery*. New York, NY: Viking; 1987.

Shapiro L. The skinny on fat. *Newsweek*. Dec. 5, 1994; 52–60.

Simone CB. *Cancer & Nutrition: A Ten-Point Plan to Reduce Your Risk of Getting Cancer*. Garden City Park, NY: Avery Publishing Group; 1992.

The Changes to Make When You're Pregnant

American College of Obstetricians and Gynecologists. *Nutition During Pregnancy*. Washington, DC: American College of Obstetricians and Gynecologists; April 1992.

American College of Obstetricians and Gynecologists. *Nutition During Pregnancy*. ACOG Technical Bulletin No. 179. Washington, DC: American College of Obstetricians and Gynecologists; April 1993.

American College of Obstetricians and Gynecologists. *Planning for Pregnancy, Birth, and Beyond*. New York, NY: Dutton; 1992.

American Dietetic Association. *Blue Ribbon Babies: Eating Well During Pregnancy*. Chicago, Ill: American Dietetic Association; 1989.

American Dietetic Association. *Caffeine: How Little, How Much for You and Your Family?* Chicago, Ill: American Dietetic Association; 1988.

American Dietetic Association. *How to Have a Healthier Baby: Tips for Pregnant Teens*. Chicago, Ill: American Dietetic Association; 1989.

Behan E. *Eat Well, Lose Weight While Breastfeeding*. New York, NY: Villard Books; 1993.

Brewer GS, Brewer T. *What Every Pregnant Woman Should Know: The Truth About Diets and Drugs in Pregnancy*. New York, NY: Random House; 1977.

Brown JE. *Nutrition for Your Pregnancy: The University of Minnesota Guide*. Minneapolis, Minn: University of Minnesota Press; 1983.

Committee on Nutritional Status During Pregnancy and Lactation, Food and Nutrition Board, Institute of Medicine, Natinal Academy of Sciences. *Nutrition During Pregnancy and Lactation: An Implementation Guide*. Washington, DC: National Academy Press; 1992.

Eisenberg A, Murkoff HE, Hathaway SE. *What to Eat When You're Expecting*. New York, NY: Workman Publishing; 1986.

Henry AK, Feldhausen J. *Drugs, Vitamins, Minerals, Pregnancy*. Tucson, Ariz: Fisher Books; 1989.

Hess MA, Hunt AE. *Eating for Two: The Complete Guide to Nutrition During Pregnancy*. New York, NY: Macmillan; 1992.

Institute of Human Nutrition, Columbia University College of Physicians and Surgeons. *The Columbia Encyclopedia of Nutrition*. New York, NY: GP Putnam's Sons; 1988: 252–263.

Jonaitis MA. Nutrition during pregnancy. In Todd WD, Tapley DF, eds. *The Columbia University College of Physicians and Surgeons Complete Guide to Pregnancy*. New York, NY: Crown Publishers, Inc; 1988.

Kamen K, Kamen S. *Total Nutrition for Breast-Feeding Mothers*. Boston, Mass: Little, Brown; 1986.

Kitzinger S. *The Complete Book of Pregnancy and Childbirth*. New York, NY: Knopf; 1989.

La Leche League International. *Nutrition and Breastfeeding*. Franklin Park, Ill: La Leche League International; 1987

Morales K, Inlander CB. *Take This Book to the Obstetrician with You: A Consumer's Guide to Pregnancy and Childbirth*. Reading, Mass: Addison-Wesley; 1991.

Placksin S. *Mothering the New Mother: Your Postpartum Resource Companion*. New York, NY: Newmarket Press; 1994.

Reuben C. *The Healthy Baby Book: A Parent's Guide to Preventing Birth Defects and Other Long-Term Medical Problems Before, During, and After Pregnancy*. Los Angeles, Calif: Jeremy P. Tarcher (Putnam); 1994.

Stoppard M. *Dr. Miriam Stoppard's Pregnancy and Birth Book*. New York, NY: Ballantine Books; 1985.

Swinney B. *Eating Expectantly: The Essential Eating Guide and Cookbook for Pregnancy*. Colorado Springs, Colo: Fall River Press; 1993.

Todd L. *You and Your Newborn Baby: A Guide to the First Months After Birth*. Boston, Mass: Harvard Common Press, 1993.

Worth C. *Health and Beauty During Pregnancy*. New York, NY: McGraw-Hill; 1984.

Worthington-Roberts B, Williams SR. *Nutrition in Pregnancy and Lactation*. 5th ed. St. Louis, Mo: Mosby-Year Book; 1993.

Yntema S. *Vegetarian Pregnancy: The Definitive Nutritional Guide to Having a Healthy Baby*. Ithaca, NY: McBooks Press; 1994.

Giving Your Baby an Ideal Diet

Baker S, Henry R. *Parents' Guide to Nutrition*. Boston Children's Hospital. Reading, Mass: Addison-Wesley; 1986.

Barnes, LA, ed. Committee on Nutrition. *Pediatric Nutrition Handbook*. Elk Grove Village, Ill: American Academy of Pediatrics; 1993.

Calvo EB, Galindo AC, Aspres NB. Iron status in exclusively breast-fed infants. *Pediatrics*. 1992; 90: 375–79.

Chandra R. Food allergy: 1992 and beyond. *Nutrition Research 1992*. 12: 93–99.

Dewey KG, Heinig MJ. Nommesen LA, Peerson JM; Lonnerdal B. Growth of breast-fed and formula-fed infants from 0 to 18 months: the DARLING study. *Pediatrics*. 1992; 89: 1035–41.

Duncan B; et al. Exclusive breast-feeding for at least four months protects against otitis media. *Pediatrics*. 1993; 91: 867–72.

Eisenberg A, Murkoff HE, Hathaway SE. *What To Expect The First Year*. New York: Workman Publishing; 1989.

Krebs NF, Hambidge, KM. Zinc requirements and zinc intakes of breast-fed infants. *American Journal of Clinical Nutrition*. 1985; 4: 571–77.

Kimmel M, Kimmel D. *Mommy Made and Daddy Too! Home Cooking for a Healthy Baby & Toddler*. New York, NY: Bantam Books; 1990.

La Leche League International. *The Womanly Art of Breastfeeding*. Franklin Park, Ill: La Leche League International; 1991.

Mohrbacher N, Stock J. *The Breastfeeding Answer Book*. Franklin Park, Ill: La Leche League International; 1991.

Renfrew M, Fisher C, Arms S. *Bestfeeding: Getting Breastfeeding Right for You*. Berkeley, Calif: Celestial Arts; 1990.

Satter E. *Child of Mine, Feeding With Love and Good Sense*. Palo Alto, Calif: Bull Publishing; 1986.

Shannon MW, Graef VR. Lead intoxication in infancy. *Pediatrics*. 1992; 89: 87–90.

Food and Nutrition Service. *Infant Nutrition and Feeding*. Washington, DC: U.S Department of Agriculture; 1993.

Young ME, Young MW. *The Right Start: Guidelines for Your Baby's Nutrition and Lifelong Health*. New York, NY: Walker and Company; 1987.

Ziegler EE. Milk and formulas for older infants. *Journal of Pediatrics*. 1990; 116: 11–18.

Ziegler EE, et al. Cow's milk feeding in infancy: further observations on blood loss from the gastrointestinal tract. *Journal of Pediatrics*. 1990; 117: 576–579.

What's Right—and Wrong—for the Kids

Ames LB, et al. *Your Ten-to-Fourteen Year Old*. Dell; 1988.

Alster N. Pass the sugar. *Forbes*. Apr. 13, 1992; 149.

Attwood CR. *Low-Fat Prescription for Kids*. Viking; 1995.

Brabin B, Brabin L. The cost of successful adolescent growth and development in girls. . . . *American Journal of Clinical Nutrition*. May 1992; 55.

Burger SE, et al. Testing the effects of nutrient deficiencies on behavioral performance. *American Journal of Clinical Nutrition*. Feb. 1993; 57.

Crombie IK, et al. Effect of vitamin and mineral supplementation on verbal & non-verbal reasoning of schoolchildren. *The Lancet*. Mar. 31, 1990; 335.

Davis WJ. Food Allergies. In: *The Columbia University College of Physicians & Surgeons Complete Home Medical Guide*. 2nd ed. 1989.

Feingold B, Feingold, H. *The Feingold Cookbook for Hyperactive Children*. Random House; 1979.

Food allergies linked to ear infections. *Science News*. Oct. 8, 1994; 146.

Jacobson MF. *What Are We Feeding Our Kids?* Workman Publishing; 1994.

Kleinman RE, Jellinek MS. *Let Them Eat Cake!* Villard Books; 1994.

Knox AJ. Salt & asthma: A high salt diet may make asthma worse. *British Medical Journal*. Nov. 6, 1993; 307.

Lack of effect of sucrose & aspartame on children's behavior. *Nutrition Research Newsletter*. Feb. 1994; 13.

Lansky V. *Feed Me! I'm Yours*. Rev ed. Meadowbrook (Simon & Schuster); 1986.

Marks A. Sexual Development. In *The Columbia University College of Physicians & Surgeons Complete Home Medical Guide*. 2nd ed. 1989.

Mayo Clinic Family HealthBook. IVI Publishing; 1993.

McNicol J. *Your Child's Food Allergies*. John Wiley & Sons; 1992.

Miller PM. *The Hilton Head Diet for Children & Teenagers*. Warner; 1993.

Murray F. Don't neglect kid's supplement needs. *Today's Living*. Mar 1990; 21.

Ridder CM, et al. Dietary habits, sexual maturation and plasma hormones in pubertal girls. *American Journal of*

Clinical Nutrition. Nov. 1991; 54.

Satter E. *Child of Mine: Feeding with Love & Good Sense.* Bull Publishing Co; 1991.

Satter E. *How to Get Your Kid to Eat. . . . But Not Too Much.* Bull Publishing Co; 1978.

Schauss A, et. al. *Eating for A's.* Pocket Books; 1991.

Springen K. Living with food allergies. *Vegetarian Times.* Apr 1994; 98.

Wender EH. Effects of sugar on aggressive and inattentive behavior. . . . *Pediatrics.* Nov. 1991; 88.

Changes to Make at Menopause

Diet and Cancer. New York: American Council on Science and Health; 1993.

Gittleman A. Are you burning up all those carbohydrates? *Menopause News.* 1994; 2: 3.

Gleason S. Menopause: It's not a disease. *Good Medicine.* 1994; 3: 8–10.

Greenwood S. *Menopause Naturally: Preparing for the Second Half of Life.* Volcano, Calif: Volcano Press; 1989.

Herman P. You can sail through mennopause with these natural remedies. *Health News & Review.* Winter 1993.

Lee JR. Osteoporosis reversal: The role of progesterone. *International Clinical Nutrition Review.* 1990; 10: 384–91.

Lissner L, Odell P, D'Agostino R, et al. Variability of body weight and health outcomes in the Framingam population. *New England Journal of Medicine.* 1991; 324: 1839–44.

Menopause. Bethesda, Md: National Institutes of Health; 1992.

Menopause. Washington, DC: National Women's Health Resource Center; 1993.

The Menopause Years. Washington, DC: American College of Obstetricians and Gynecologists; 1992.

Trien SF. *The Menopause Handbook.* New York, NY: Ballantine Books; 1986.

Dietary Targets for Your Senior Years

The Alpha-Tocopherol, Beta Carotene Cancer Prevention Study Group. The effect of vitamin E and beta carotene on the incidence of lung cancer and other cancers in male smokers. *N Engl J Med.* 1994; 330: 1029–35.

Be Sensible About Salt. *Age Page.* Bethesda, Md: National Institute on Aging; 1991.

Beers MK, Urice SK. *Aging in Good Health.* New York, NY: Pocket Books; 1992.

Constipation. *Age Page.* Bethesda, Md: National Institute on Aging; 1992.

Centers for Disease Control and Prevention. Daily dietary fat and total food-energy intakes—NHANES III, Phase I, 1988-91. *JAMA.* 1994; 271: 1309.

Detsky AS, Smalley PS, Chang J. Is this patient malnourished? *JAMA.* 1994; 271: 54–8.

Dietary Supplements: More Is Not Always Better. *Age Page.* Bethesda, Md: National Institute on Aging; 1993.

Digestive Do's and Don'ts. *Age Page.* Bethesda, Md: National Institute on Aging, 1992.

Fiatarone MA, et al. Exercise training and nutritional supplementation for physical frailty in very elderly people. *N Engl J Med.* 1994; 330: 1769–75.

Folson AR, et al. Body fat distribution and five-year risk of death in older women. *JAMA.* 1993; 269: 483–7.

Hints for Shopping, Cooking, and Enjoying Meals. *Age Page.* Bethesda, Md: National Institute on Aging, 1991.

Jenkins DJA, et al. Effect on blood lipids of very high intakes of fiber in diets low in saturated fat and cholesterol. *N Engl J Med.* 1993; 329: 21–6.

Johnson CL, et al. Declining serum total cholesterol levels among U.S. adults. *JAMA.* 1993; 269: 3002–8.

Krall LP, Beaser, RS. *Joslin Diabetes Manual* 12th ed. Philadelphia, Pa: Lea & Febiger; 1989.

Krumholz HM, et al. Lack of association between cholesterol and coronary heart disease mortality and morbidity and all-cause mortality in persons older than 70 years. *JAMA.* 1994; 272: 1335–40.

Lyder C. More life to your years: eating for a satisfying today and a healthier tomorrow. *Vibrant Life.* 1993; 9: 26.

Nature, Causes, and Consequences of Harmful Dietary Practices. *Clinics in Applied Nutrition.* 1991; 1: 32–59.

Nelson HD, et al. Smoking, alcohol, and neuromuscular and physical function of older women. *JAMA.* 1994; 272: 1825–31.

NIH Consensus Development Panel on Optimal Calcium Intake. Optimal calcium intake. *JAMA.* 1994; 272: 1942–7.

Nutrition: A Lifelong Concern. *Age Page.* Bethesda, Md: National Institute on Aging; 1991.

Roberts SB, et al. Control of food intake in older men. *JAMA.* 1994; 272: 1601–6.

Russell RM. Nutrition. *JAMA.* 1994; 271: 1687–9.

Scala J. *Prescription for Longevity.* New York, NY: Penguin Books, 1992.

Sempos CT, et al. Prevalence of high blood cholesterol among U.S. adults. *JAMA.* 1993; 269: 3009–14.

Voelker R. Recommendations for antioxidants: How much evidence is enough? *JAMA.* 1994; 271: 1148–9.

Weiss RJ, Subak-Sharpe, Genell J, eds. *The Columbia University School of Public Health Complete Guide to Health and Well-Being After 50.* New York, NY: Times Books; 1988.

Boosting Energy and Fitness: Which Foods Really Work?

Adams R. Carnitine: The Amino Acid with Muscle. *Better Nutrition for Today's Living.* 1990; 52: 16.

Alexander A. Juicy Details. *Bicycling.* 1992; 33: 72.

Applegate L. *Power Foods.* Emmaus, Penn: Rodale Press; 1991.

Applegate L. Carbo-Hydration. *Runner's World.* 1990; 25: 24.

Athletic Performance Aids. *NCAHF Newsletter.* 1993; 16: 2.

Beltz S.D. Efficacy of Nutritional Supplements Used by Athletes. *Clin-Pharm.* 1993; 12: 900–8.

Bowles WV. Three Important Minerals for a Healthy Body. *Total Health.* 1992; 14: 22.

Brody J. *Jane Brody's Nutrition Book.* Rev. ed. New York, NY: Bantam; 1987.

Burke LM. Dietary Supplements in Sports. *Sports-Med.* 1993; 15: 43–65

Caffeine as an Ergogenic Aid. *Nutrition Research Newsletter.* 1990; 9: 85.

Clark N. *Sports Nutrition Guidebook.* Il. Leisure Press; 1990.

Clark N. Fitness Foods. *American Fitness.* 1991; 9: 37.

Clift E. Do Vitamins Really Work? *Longevity.* Oct. 1993;

Colgan M. *Optimum Sports Nutrition.* New York: Advanced Research Press; 1993.

Connelly AS. *MET-Rx™ Owner's Manual.* Myosystems, Inc; 1993.

Cramer T. Firm Calls Them 'Health Foods.' *FDA Consumer.* Jan-Feb 1992. v26, n1, p41(2).

Eliason BC. Desiccated Thyroid. *Journal of Family Practice.* 1994; 38: 287–8.

Farley D. FDA Questions Safety of Dietary Supplements. *Consumers' Research Magazine.* 1994; 77: 15.

FDA Plans Tougher Rules. . . . *Chemical Marketing Reporter.* 1993; 243: 3.

For Losing Extra Weight, Try Chromium Picolinate. *Better Nutrition for Today's Living.* Sept. 1994.

Getting Classic with Arnold. *Saturday Evening Post.* 1993; 265: 36.

Haas R. *Eat To Succeed.* New York, NY: Penguin; 1991

Hadfield LC. Amino Acid Supplements: Health or Hype. *Current Health 2.* 1991; 18: 19.

Health Report. *Time.* 1994; 143: 20.

Higdon D. Fitness Hangovers. *Longevity.* August 1994.

Higgs Robert. FDA Rules for Labeling Could Shorten Our Lives. *Insight on the News.* 1994; 10: 18.

Hunter BT. How Safe Are Nutritional Supplements? *Consumers' Research.* 1994; 77: 21.

Kamen B. Fighting Stress With Ginseng. *Total Health.* 1992; 14: 51.

Kleiner SM, Bazzarre TL, Litchford MD. Metabolic Profiles, Diet and Health Practices of Bodybuilders. *Journal of the American Dietetic Assn.* 1990; 90: 962.

Kloss J. *Back to Eden.* Calif: Back to Eden® Publishing Co; 1994.

Kreider RB. Amino Acid Supplementation & Exercise Performance. *Sports Medicine.* Sept 1993; 16: 190–209.

Kronhausen E, Kronhausen P, Demopoulos, HB. *Formula for Life.* New York, NY: William Morrow; 1989.

Langer S. Mighty Metabolizers. *Better Nutrition for Today's Living.* 1991; 53: 12.

Martin S. The Banana. *Bicycling.* 1991; 32: 116.

McCarty MF. Homologous Physiological Effects of Phenformin & Chromium Picolinate. *Med-Hypotheses.* 1993; 41: 316–24.

Milner I. Health Food Industry Sells Supplements, Not Science. *Environmental Nutrition.* 1990; 13: 1.

Narcotic Educational Foundation of America. *Anabolic Steroids.* June 1991.

Nutritional Alternative to Pills & Potions. *Palaestra.* 1994; 10: 11.

Nutrition, Not Steroids, Accelerates Bodybuilding. *Better Nutrition for Today's Living.* 1993; 55: 20.

Peterson K, Peterson M. *Eat to Compete.* Yearbook Medical Publishers; 1988.

Pimholster G. Keeping Cool with Sports Drinks. *Total Health.* 1991; 13: 37.

Pipes TV. The Steroid Alternative. *American Fitness.* 1991; 9: 38.

Radical Protection for Athletes. *Science News.* 1992; 141: 398.

Resnick SK. Supplement Review: The Perils of Protein. *East West Natural Health.* 1992; 22: 49.

Scher SK. Botanical: Myth & Reality. *Cosmetics and Toiletries.* 1991; 106: 65.

Selling Sweat. *Consumer Reports.* 1993; 58: 491.

Sherman WM, et al. "Dietary Carbohydrates. . . ." *American Journal of Clinical Nutrition.* 1993; 57: 27.

Silverglade BA. Without Regulation, Charlatans Prosper. *Insight on the News.* 1994; 10: 20.

Smith DA, Perry PJ. The Efficacy of Ergogenic Agents. . . Part I & II *Ann Pharmocother.* 1992; 26: 520–8.

Somer E. Legal Aid. *Women's Sports & Fitness.* 1993; 15: 25.

Stifler J. Drink to Your Health. *Runner's World.* 1989; 24: 72.

Taking Vitamins. *Consumer Reports.* Sept. 1994.

Taylor DS. Sports Nutrition: Boost Your Performance Naturally. *Better Nutrition for Today's Living.* 1990; 52: 24.

Tessler G. Lose Weight Without Counting Calories. *Total Health.* 1989; 11: 15.

Too Many Building Blocks. *The University of California, Berkeley Wellness Letter.* 1990; 6: 6.

Weak Potions for Strong Muscles. *Tufts University Diet & Nutrition Letter.* 1992; 10: 7.

Williams MH. Nutritional Ergogenics: Help or Hype? *Journal of the American Dietetic Assn,* 1992; 92: 1213.

Williams MH. Nutritional Ergogenic Aids. . . . *Nutrition Today.* 1989; 24: 7.

Yesalis CE, et al. Anabolic-androgenic Steroid Use in the United States. *JAMA,* 1993; 270: 1217.

Zupke MP, Milner I. Bee Pollen, Shark Cartilage—The Truth About Ten Top Supplements. *Environmental Nutrition.* 1993; 16: 1.

Best Bets When You're Stressed Out

Bankhead CD. Caffeine-cortisol reaction seen. *Medical World News.* 1989; 30: 21.

Bloyd-Peshkin, Sharon. Counting on China. *Vegetarian Times.* 76: 42.

Bower B. High cadmium diet: Recipe for stress? *Science News.* 1987; 132: 101.

Brody J. *Jane Brody's Nutrition Book.* Rev ed. New York, NY: Bantam; 1987.

Clark Nancy. Fighting fatigue with food. *American Fitness.* 1990; 8: 32.

Coffee worsens stressful situations. *Edell Health Letter.* 1990; 9: 6.

FTC blasts 'stress vitamin' ads. *Nutrition Forum.* 1990; 11: 76.

Fischman B. Unsweetened stress. *Psychology Today.* 1989; 23: 72.

Healthy diet helps. *Environmental Nutrition.* 1993; 16: 7.

Hodgkin G. Stress & Nutrition. *Vibrant Life.* 1992; 8: 30.

Kipp D. Stress & nutrition. *ASDC J Dent Child.* 1985; 52: 68–71.

Kloss J. *Back to Eden.* Calif: Back to Eden® Publishing Co; 1994

Kronhausen E, Kronhausen P, Demopoulos HB. *Formula for Life.* New York, NY: William Morrow; 1989.

Langer S. Nutrients to combat stress. *Better Nutrition for Today's Living.* 1991; 53: 16.

Larson DE, ed. *The Mayo Clinic Family Health Book.* New York, NY: William Morrow & Co., Inc. 1990.

Murray F. Put the squeeze on stress. *Better Nutrition for Today's Living.* 1992; 54: 24.

Natelson EJ. Beating stress naturally with herbs. *Vegetarian Times.* 198: 86.

Newbold HL. Chronic Depression. *Health News & Review.* 1993; 3: 8.

OSHA lowers cadmium exposure limit. *Occupational Hazards.* 1992; 54: 10.

Perriseau JJ. Soothing foods. *Vegetarian Times.* Feb. 1994; 48.

Schauss A. Stress-caused zinc deficit. *Health News & Review.* 1989; 7: 5.

Scheer JF. Camomile. *Better Nutrition for Today's Living.* 1990; 52: 15.

Stressed out? Junk food won't help. *USA Today Magazine.* 1993; 123: 14.

Taylor DS. Handle Stress with Diet. *Better Nutrition for Today's Living.* 1989; 51: 14.

Turner EF. Ask the herbalist. *Nutrition Health Review.* Summer 1992; 16.

Unbalanced diets lead to stress and fatigue. *Better Nutrition for Today's Living.* 1994; 56: 16.

Vitamin E reduces cadmium toxicity. *Nutrition Research Newsletter.* 1992; 11: 76.

Wurtman JJ. *Managing Your Mind & Mood Through Food.* New York, NY: Harper & Row; 1988.

Coping with Diabetes:
The Basic Rules to Remember

American Diabetes Association. *Medical Management of Non-insulin-dependent (Type II) Diabetes.* 3rd ed. Alexandria, Va: 1994.

Bradstock M, et al. Evaluation of reactions to food additives: The aspartame experience. *American Journal of Clinical Nutrition.* 1986; 43: 464–469.

Davidson M, et al. Real-world management of type II diabetes. *Patient Care.* 1994; 28: 68–85.

The Diabetes Control and Complications Trial. Alexandria, Va: American Diabetes Association; 1993.

Franz MJ, et al. Nutrition principles for the management of diabetes and related complications. *Diabetes Care.* 1994; 17: 490–518.

Lebovitz H. Introduction: Goals of treatment. In Lebovitz H, et al. *Therapy for Diabetes Mellitus and Related Disorders.* 2nd ed. Alexandria, Va: American Diabetes Association; 1994: 1–3.

Leon A, Hunninghake D. Safety of chronic consumption of large doses of aspartame. *FASEB Journal.* 1988; 2: A633.

Olefsky J. Obesity. In Isselbacher, K, et al, eds. *Harrison's Principles of Internal Medicine.* 13th ed. New York, NY: McGraw-Hill, Inc; 1994: 449–452.

White J, Campbell R. Magnesium and diabetes: A review. *The Annual of Pharmacology.* 1993; 27: 775–780.

When Good Food Makes You Feel Bad: Living with Allergy

American Academy of Allergy and Immunology. *Adverse Reactions to Foods*. Milwaukee, Wisc: American Academy of Allergy and Immunology; 1994.

American Academy of Allergy and Immunology. *Understanding Food Allergy*. Milwaukee, Wisc: American Academy of Allergy and Immunology; 1993.

Astor S. *Hidden Food Allergies*. Garden City Park, NY: Avery Publishing Group; 1988.

Brostoff J, Gamlin L. *The Complete Guide to Food Allergy and Intolerance: Prevention, Identification, and Treatment of Common Illnesses and Allergies Caused by Food*. New York, NY: Crown; 1989.

Crook WG. *Detecting Your Hidden Allergies*. Jackson, Tenn: Professional Books; 1988.

Dobler ML. *Food Allergies*. Chicago, Ill: National Center for Nutrition and Dietetics of the American Dietetic Association; 1993.

Dobler ML. *Lactose Intolerance*. Chicago, Ill: National Center for Nutrition and Dietetics of the American Dietetic Association; 1992.

Feldman BR, Carroll D. *The Complete Book of Children's Allergies: A Guide for Parents*. New York, NY: Times Books; 1986.

Hass F, Haas SS. *The Essential Asthma Book: A Manual for Asthmatics of All Ages*. New York, NY: Charles Scribner's Sons; 1987.

Joneja JMV, Bielory L. *Understanding Allergy, Sensitivity and Immunity: A Comprehensive Guide*. New Brunswick, NJ: Rutgers University Press; 1990.

Meizel J. *Your Food-Allergic Child: A Parent's Guide*. Bedford, Mass: Mills & Sanderson; 1988.

Orenstein NS, Bingham SL. *Food Allergies: How to Tell if You Have Them, What to Do About Them if You Do*. New York, NY: Putnam; 1987.

Postley JE, Barton J. *The Allergy Discovery Diet: A Rotation Diet for Discovering Your Allergies to Food*. New York, NY: Doubleday; 1990.

Rapp D. *Is This Your Child? Discovering and Treating Unrecognized Allergies*. New York, NY: William Morrow, 1991.

Roth J. *The Allergic Gourmet*. Chicago, Ill: Contemporary Books; 1983.

Schardt D. Food sensitivity: Nothing to sneeze at. *Nutrition Action Healthletter*. May 1994; 12–13.

Weinstein AM. *Asthma: The Complete Guide to Self-Management of Asthma and Allergies for Patients and Their Families*. New York, NY: McGraw-Hill; 1987.

Young SH, Shulman SA, Shulman MD. *The Asthma Handbook: A Complete Guide for Patients and Their Families*. New York, NY: Bantam; 1985.

Dealing With Digestive Disorders

Breitenbach RA. Halloween diarrhea: An unexpected trick of sorbitol-containing candy. *Postgrad Med*. 1992; 92: 63–66.

Cerrato PL. The patient's eating—why is he losing weight? *RN*. April 1992; 77–80.

Donatele EP. Constipation: Pathophysiology and treatment. *Am Fam Physician*. 1990; 42: 1335–42.

Garrow JS, James WPT, Ralph A, eds. *Human Nutritional and Dietetics*. 9th ed. New York: Churchill Livingstone; 1993.

Hunter BT. Good news for gastric sufferers. *Consumer's Research*. October 1993; 8–9.

Hunter BT. Medications and the digestive tract. *Consumer's Research*. January 1994; 8–9.

Lambert JP, et al. The value of prescribed 'high-fibre' diets for the treatment of the irritable bowel syndrome. *Eur J Clin Nutr*. 1991; 45: 601–9.

Marieb EN, 2nd ed. *Human Anatomy and Physiology*. 2nd ed. Redwood City, Calif: The Benjamin/Cummings Publishing Co. Inc., 1991.

McLaren DS, Meguid MM, eds. *Nutrition and its Disorders*. 4th ed. New York, NY: Churchill Livingstone; 1988.

Oski FA. *Don't Drink Your Milk*. 9th ed. Brushton, NY: TEACH Services; 1983.

Polanco I. Current status of digestive intolerance to food protein. *J Pediatrics*. 1992; 121: S108–10.

Sleisenger MH, Fordtran JS, eds. *Gastrointestinal Disease: Pathophysiology, Diagnosis, Management, Volumes I & II*. 4th ed. Philadelphia, Penn: W.B. Saunders Co; 1989.

Suarez FL, Savaiano DA. Lactose digestion and tolerance in adult and elderly Asian-Americans. *Am J Clin Nutrition*. 1994; 59: 1021–4.

Tomlin J, Lewis C, Read NW. Investigation of normal flatus production in health volunteers. *Gut*. 1991; 32: 665–9.

Tomlin J, Read NW. The effect of resistant starch on colon function in humans. *British Journal of Nutrition*. 1990; 64: 589–595.

Wandycz K. The H. pylori factor. *Forbes*. August 2, 1994; 128.

Werbach M. *Healing Through Nutrition: A Natural Approach to Treating 50 Common Illnesses with Diet and Nutrients*. New York, NY: HarperCollins; 1993.

Willen JL. Peptic ulcers: Cause, treatment. *Nation's Business*. March 1994; 70.

Zim HS. *Your Stomach and Digestive Tract*. New York, NY: William Morrow & Co; 1973.

Arthritis Diet Remedies: Fact or Folklore?

The Arthritis Foundation. Arthritis on the rise. *Arthritis Today*. September/October, 1994; 13.

The Arthritis Foundation. *Basic Facts: Answers to Your Questions*. #4001.

The Arthritis Foundation. *Diet: Guidelines & Research*. #4280.

The Arthritis Foundation. *Services of the Arthritis Foundation*. #4010.

Centers for Disease Control and Prevention. Arthritis prevalence and activity limitations—United States, 1990. *MMWR*. 1994; 43: 433–438.

Darlington LG, Ramsey NW. Review of dietary therapy for rheumatoid arthritis. *Brit J Rheum*. 1993; 32: 507–514.

Denissov LN, Sharafetdinov KH, Samsonov MA. On the medicinal efficacy of dietetic therapy in patients with rheumatoid arthritis. *Int J Clin Pharm*. 1992; 12: 19–25.

Dunkin MA. The Food Factor in Arthritis. *Arthritis Today*. September/October 1991; 23–25.

Fries JF. *Arthritis: A Comprehensive Guide*. Reading, Mass: Addison-Wesley Publishing Company; 1987.

Kjeldsen-Kragh J, et al. Controlled trial of fasting and one-year vegetarian diet in rheumatoid arthritis. *Lancet*. 1991; 338: 899–902.

Kushner I, Forer A, McGuire AB, eds. *Understanding Arthritis*. New York, NY: Simon & Schuster; 1984.

Panush RS, ed. *Nutrition and Rheumatic Diseases. Rheumatic Disease Clinics of North America*. Philadelphia, Penn: W.B. Saunders Co; 1991; 1: 1991.

Peretz A, Neve J, Duchateau J, Famaey JP. Adjuvant treatment of recent onset rheumatoid arthritis by selenium supplementation: Preliminary observations. *Lancet*. 1992; 31: 281–282.

Sobel D, Klein AC. *Arthritis: What Works*. New York, NY: St. Martin's Press; 1989.

Steinman L. Autoimmune disease. *Scientific American*. 1993; 269: 107–114.

U.S. Department of Health and Human Services. *The Immune System—How It Works*. June 1992; NIH Publication No. 92-3229.

Wallace J. *Arthritis Relief*. Emmaus, Penn: Rodale Press Inc; 1989.

Watson J, Byars ML, McGill P, Kelman AW. Cytokine and prostaglandin production by monocytes of volunteers and rheumatoid arthritis patients treated with dietary supplements of blackcurrant seed oil. *Brit J Rheum*. 1993; 32: 1055–1058.

Latest Thinking on Diet and Immunity

Abrams B, Duncan D, Hertz-Picciotto I. A prospective study of dietary intake and acquired immune deficiency syndrome in HIV-seropositive homosexual men. *Journal of Acquired Immune Deficiency Syndromes*. 1993; 6: 949.

Blumberg J. Point of View. The RDA: Is the concept still valid? *Nutrition & the MD*. 1994; 20: 5.

Brody, JE. Why the food you eat may be hazardous to your health. *The New York Times*. October 5, 1994; C11.

Can good nutrition keep immunity strong? *Consumer Reports on Health*. 1992; 4: 84–86.

Cerrato PL. Vitamins, minerals, and the common cold. *RN*. December 1991; 71–73.

Chandra, RK. 1990 McCollum Award Lecture. Nutrition and immunity: lessons from the past and new insights into the future. *American Journal of Clinical Nutrition*. 1991; 53: 1087–1101.

Chicken soup for the common cold: folklore or fact? *Environmental Nutrition*. February 1994; 7

DeNoon DJ. Diet, immunity, and nutritional therapies. *CDC AIDS Weekly*. Jan. 29, 1990; 15.

Ellerhirst-Ryan JM. Infection. In: Groenwald SL, Frogge MH, Goodman M, Yarbo CH, eds. *Cancer Nursing: Principles and Practice*. 3d ed. Boston, Mass: Jones & Bartlett Publishers; 1993.

Ford ND. Nutritional support needed to prevent or shorten colds, flu; immune system responds to vitamins A, C, zinc; worldwide studies show major symptom reduction. *Health News & Review*. 1989; 7: 1–2.

Gershoff S, Whitney C. *The Tufts University Guide to Total Nutrition*. New York, NY: Harper Perennial; 1991.

Healthy elderly can improve immune response. *HealthFacts*. 1989; 14: 3.

Hilderly LJ. Radiotherapy. In: Groenwald SL, Frogge MH, Goodman M, Yarbo CH, eds. *Cancer Nursing: Principles and Practice*. 3d ed. Boston, Mass: Jones & Bartlett Publishers; 1993.

Koop, CE. *The Surgeon General's Report on Nutrition and Health*. Rocklin, Calif: Prima Publishing and Communications; 1988.

Liebman B. Antioxidants: surprise, surprise. *Nutrition Action Healthletter*. June 1994; 4.

Long P. The power of vitamin C. *Health*. October 1992; 67–72.

Mahan KL, Arlin MT. *Krause's Food, Nutrition and Diet Therapy*. 7th ed. Philadelphia, Penn: WB Saunders Co.; 1992.

Meydani, SN, Ribaya-Mercado, JD. Vitamin B-6 deficiency impairs interleukin 2 production and lymphocyte proliferation in elderly adults. *American Journal of Clinical Nutrition*. 1991; 53: 1275–1281.

Meydani SN, et al. Vitamin E supplementation enhances cell-mediated immunity in healthy elderly subjects. *American Journal of Clinical Nutrition*. 1990; 52: 557.

Newman CF. The role of nutritional assessments and nutritional plans in the management of HIV/AIDS. *Nutrition & HIV/AIDS*. Chicago, Ill: PAAC Publishing, Inc.; 1992; 1: 64.

Penn ND, et al. The effect of dietary supplementation with vitamins A, C and E on cell-mediated immune function in elderly long-stay patients: a randomized controlled trial. *Age and Ageing.* 1991; 20: 169–175.

Pumping immunity. (improving immunity through nutrition). *Nutrition Action Healthletter.* 1993; 20: 1–5.

Quick studies. *Nutrition Action Healthletter.* April 1994; 4.

Saltman P, Gurin J, Mothner I. *The University of California San Diego Nutrition Book.* Boston, Mass: Little, Brown and Company; 1993.

Shils, ME, Olson JA, Shike M. *Modern Nutrition in Health and Disease.* 8th ed., Philadelphia, Penn: Lea & Febiger; 1994.

Skipper A, Szeluga DJ, Groenwald SL. Nutritional disturbances. In: Groenwald SL, Frogge MH, Goodman M, Yarbo CH, eds. *Cancer Nursing: Principles and Practice.* 3d ed. Boston, Mass: Jones & Bartlett Publishers; 1993.

Soup's on, cold's off? *University of California at Berkeley Wellness Letter.* January 1994.

Vitamin E enhances immunity in elderly. *Nutrition Research Newsletter.* 1990; 9: 114

Williams SR, Anderson SL. *Nutrition and Diet Therapy.* 7th ed. St. Louis, MO: Mosby-Year Book, Inc.; 1993.

Sure-Fire Ways to Prevent Brittle Bones

Barrett-Connor E, Chang JC, Edelstein SL. Coffee-associated osteoporosis offset by daily milk consumption: The Rancho Bernardo Study. JAMA, *Journal of the American Medical Association.* 1994; 271: 280–283.

Bilezikian JP, Silverberg SJ. Osteoporosis: a practical approach to the perimenopausal woman. *Journal of Women's Health.* 1992; 1: 21–7.

Eaton SB, Nelson DA. Calcium in evolutionary perspective. *American Journal of Clinical Nutrition.* 1991; 54: 281–7.

Farley D. Look for 'Legit' health claims on foods. *FDA Consumer.* 1993; 27: 15–21.

Food labeling: Health claims; calcium and osteoporosis. *Federal Register.* 1993; 58: 2665–81.

Heaney RP. Calcium intake and bone health throughout life. *Journal of the American Medical Women's Association.* 1990; 45: 80–6.

Heaney RP. Protein intake and the calcium economy. *Journal of the American Dietetic Association.* 1993; 93: 1261–2.

Heaney RP. Thinking straight about calcium. *New England Journal of Medicine.* 1993; 328: 503–5.

Heaney RP, Weaver CM. Calcium Absorption from Kale. *American Journal of Clinical Nutrition.* 1990; 51: 646–57.

How Strong Are Your Bones? Washington, DC: National Osteoporosis Foundation; 1994.

Kurtzweil P. Good reading for good eating. *FDA Consumer.* 1993; 29: 7–9.

Lindsay R. Prevention and treatment of osteoporosis. *The Lancet.* 1993; 341: 801–5.

Nordin BEC, et al. Sodium, calcium and osteoporosis. In: Burckhardt, P, Heaney RP, eds. *Nutritional Aspects of Osteoporosis.* New York, NY: Raven Press; 1991.

Nordin BEC, et al. The nature and significance of the relationship between urinary sodium and urinary calcium in women. *Journal of Nutrition.* 1993; 123: 1615–22.

Osteoporosis. Medicine for the Layman. *Clinical Center Communications.* Bethesda, Md: National Institutes of Health; 1989.

Osteoporosis: The Bone Thinner. *Age Page.* Bethesda, Md: National Institutes of Health; 1983.

Padgett, YM, ed. Integrate new calcium guidelines into education. *Women's Health Center Management.* 1994; 2: 136–7.

Papazian R. Osteoporosis treatment advances. *FDA Consumer.* 1991; 3: 29–32.

Reid IR, et al. Effect of calcium supplementation on bone loss in postmenopausal women. *New England Journal of Medicine.* 1993; 328: 460–4.

Stand Up to Osteoporosis. Washington, DC: National Osteoporosis Foundation; 1992.

Wardlaw, GM. Putting osteoporosis in perspective. *Journal of the American Dietetic Association.* 1993; 93: 1000–6.

Weaver CM, et al. Human calcium absorption from whole-wheat products. *Journal of Nutrition.* 1991; 121: 1769–75.

Wyshak G. Dietary animal fat intake, calcium intake, and bone fractures in women 50 years and older. *Journal of Women's Health.* 1993; 2: 329–34.

Foods to Watch Out For When Taking Medication

House Officer's Pocket Drug Reference. Springhouse; 1990.

The Columbia University College of Physicians and Surgeons Complete Home Medical Guide. Crown; 1989.

The Over-50 Guide to Psychiatric Medications. American Psychiatric Association Council on Aging; 1989.

Anderson K, Harmon L. *The Prentice-Hall Dictionary of Nutrition & Health.* Prentice-Hall; 1985.

Hirsh J, Rodgers GM, Rubin RN. Fine-tuning anticoagulant therapy. *Patient Care.* 1992; 26: 69–87.

Solomon P. Medicine on the menu: When food and drugs interact. *HeartBeat.* Summer 1988; 2932.

Taylor KB, Anthony LE. *Clinical Nutrition.* McGraw-Hill; 1983.

What Smokers Need to Know About Diet

American Family Physician. Cigarette Smoking and Incidence of Cancer. 1992; 45: 278.

Austin H. Case Controlled Study of Endrometrial Cancer in Relation to Cigarette Smoking. *American Journal of Obstetrics and Gynecology*. 1993; 169: 1086.

Brooks AC. Study Links Smoking, Pancreatic Cancer. *Science News*. 1994; 146: 261.

Brown K., et al. Vitamin E Supplementation Suppresses Indexes of Lipid. *American Journal of Clinical Nutrition*. 1994; 60: 383.

Cigarette Smoking Linked to Colon Cancer. *Cancer Researcher Weekly*. 1994; 5.

Cooper M. Evidence of Smoking and Cervical Cancer. *NCI Cancer Weekly*. July 31, 1989; 3.

Daling, JR. Cigarette Smoking and the Risk of Anogenital Cancer. *JAMA*. 1992; 268: 188.

Diana JN, Pryor W, eds. *Tobacco Smoking and Nutrition*. New York, NY: York Academy of Sciences; 1993.

Fiore MC, et al. Methods Used to Quit Smoking in the US. *JAMA*. 1990; 263: 2760.

Gritz ER. Goals for Cigarette Smoking. *Cancer*. 1994; 74: 1423.

Hollenback KA, et al. Cigarette Smoking and Bone Mineral Density. *American Journal of Public Health*. 1993; 83: 1265.

Kronhausen E, Kronhausen P, Demopoulos HB. *Formula for Life*. New York, NY: William Morrow; 1989.

Larson DE, ed. *The Mayo Clinic Family Health Book*. New York, NY: William Morrow & Co.; 1990.

Matthews R. How one in five have given up smoking. *New Scientist*. 1992; 136: 6.

Olds DL. Intellectual impairment in children of women who smoke. *Pediatrics*. 1994; 93: 221.

Vegetables Can Shield Lungs of Smokers. *Better Nutrition for Today's Living*. 1994; 56: 24.

Fitting Health into Your Everyday Meals

Bergman Y, Bergman DE. *Food Cop*. New York, NY: Bantam Books; 1991.

Best D. Piecing together the nutrition puzzle. *Prepared Foods*. March 1993; 44–49.

Bovsun, M. The diet dilemma. *Medical World News*. May 1992; 17–22.

Carper J. *Food: Your Miracle Medicine*. New York, NY: HarperCollins; 1993.

Cooking Solo: Menus and Recipies for One or Two That Follow the Dietary Guidelines to Lower Cancer Risk. American Institute for Cancer Research.

Dahl L, Klodt L. On the right track. *Shape*. Jan. 1992; 30–31.

Dieting is Fruitless. *USA Today*. Aug. 1994; 5.

Dilks C. To your health: restyling your life to shed extra pounds. *Nation's Business*. Jan. 1988; 35.

Fabricant F. From mega-food, mega-girth. *The New York Times*. Oct. 19, 1994; C1, C8.

Foreyt JP. Diet, behavior modification, and obesity: Nine questions most often asked of physicians. *Consultant*. June 1990; 53–56.

Fredman C. Meals in minutes. *Working Woman*. Jan. 1992; 79.

Gershoff S. *The Tufts University Guide to Total Nutrition*. New York, NY: HarperCollins; 1990.

Getting slim. *U.S News & World Report*. May 14, 1990; 56–58.

Karmally W. What's a real serving? *Newsweek*. May 3 1993; S22–S25.

Katahn M. *One Meal At A Time*. New York, NY: Warner Books; 1989.

Kleiner S. Tricking the taste buds. *The Physician and Sportsmedicine*. July 1991; 19–21

Kort M. The eating plan. *Shape*. Jan. 1994; 65–72.

Kostas GG. Balance your act. *Shape*. Aug. 1994; 70–80.

Labell F. Taste: The partner in nutrition. *Prepared Foods*. Aug. 1993; 93–96.

Linder L. Type A diet traps. *Health*. Aug. 1989; 36–37.

Mothersbaugh DL, Herrmann RO, Warland RH. Perceived time pressure and recommended dietary practices: The moderating effect of knowledge of nutrition. *Journal of Consumer Affairs*. Summer 1993; 106–127.

Podolsky D. Eat your beans: It's time to start thinking of chicken, fish and meat as side dishes and legumes, grains and vegetables as the main course. *U.S. News & World Report*. May 20 1991; 70–72.

Rosenberg, M. How to hook your kids on healthy eating. *Chatelaine*. Mar 1994; 122–124.

Shapiro L. Feeding frenzy: Overwhelmed by conflicting advice, most Americans have thrown in the napkin on healthy eating. *Newsweek*. May 27, 1991; 46–52.

Sifton DW, ed. *The PDR Family Guide to Women's Health and Prescription Drugs*. Montvale, NJ: Medical Economics Data; 1994.

The University of California. The eye-mouth gap. *Berkeley Wellness Letter*. April 1993; 7

The University of California. Kids and parents and food. *Berkelely Wellness Letter*. Jan. 1994; 2–4.

U.S. Department of Agriculture. *The Food Guide Pyramid*. Human Nutrition Information Service.

Zarrow S. London C. The new diet priorities: Results of an exclusive prevention survey. *Prevention*. Sept. 1991; 33–40.

Improving Your Diet with International Flair

Apgar T. Food fight. *Vegetarian Times*. October 1994; 6.

Applegate L. Ethnic delights. *Runner's World*. 1990; 25: 23

Applegate L. Ethnic eats: For good health and great taste, eat ethnically for a change. *Runner's World.* 1993; 28: 26.

Broihier CA. How you can borrow from the global pantry and come up healthy. *Environmental Nutrition.* 1993; 16: 1.

Campbell TC, Junshi C. Diet and chronic degenerative diseases: Perspectives from China. *Am J Clin Nutr.* 1994; 59: 1153S.

Celli E. The world's 5 healthiest cuisines. *Mature Health.* April 1990; 37.

Cerrato PL. Suggest diets with a difference. *RN.* 1993; 56: 67–72.

Chinese food ordered by doctors. *The Edell Health Letter.* 1990; 9: 5.

Chinese food to stay. *The Edell Health Letter.* 1990; 9: 1.

Chinese food vindicated. *The University of California Berkeley Wellness Letter.* 1994; 11: 3.

Cooking wisdom from the Far East. *Tufts University Diet & Nutrition Letter.* 1994; 12: 7.

Cooper RM. Eating at ethnic restaurants can be an exciting experience. *Diabetes in the News.* 1991; 10: 24.

Diet and heart disease: The French paradox. *Nutrition Research Newsletter.* 1992; 11: 86.

Dolnick E. Le paradoxe Francais: how do the French eat all that rich food and skip the heart disease? *In Health.* 1990; 4: 40.

Gershoff S. *The Tufts University Guide to Total Nutrition.* New York, NY: HarperCollins Publishers; 1990; 161–166.

Green tea linked to less throat cancer. *Environmental Nutrition.* 1994; 17: 1.

Hirayama T. Nutrition: overview on possible role of diet and cancer. *Cancer Weekly.* April 8, 1991; 19.

Hurley J, Liebman B. When in Rome. . . . *Nutrition Action Healthletter.* 1994; 21: 1.

Hurley J, Schmidt S. A wok on the wild side. *Nutrition Action Healthletter.* 1993; 20: 10.

Hurley J, Schmidt S. Mexican food: oile. *Nutrition Action Healthletter.* 1994; 21: 1.

Mason M. The man who has a beef with your diet. *Health.* 1994; 8: 52–58.

Negotiating with Middle Eastern favorites. *The University of California Berkeley Wellness Letter.* 1994; 10: 3.

North of the border: the best of Mexican food. *The University of California Berkeley Wellness Letter.* 1990; 6: 3

Renaud S. De Lorgeril M. Wine, alcohol, platelets, and the French paradox for coronary heart disease. *Lancet.* 1992; 339: 1523–1526.

Robb B. Ethnic dining: a guide for making the right choices. *HeartCare.* 1990; 3: 27.

Robinson CH, Lawler MR, Chenoweth WL, Garwick AE. *Normal and Therapeutic Nutrition.* New York, NY: Macmillan Publishing Company; 1986: 235–239.

Saltman P, Gurin J, Mothner I. *The University of California San Diego Nutrition Book.* Boston, Mass: Little, Brown and Company; 1993: 127–130.

Schrambling R. Ethnic light. *Health.* 1993; 7: 39–50.

Schwab, K. A taste of the Orient, American style. *Environmental Nutrition.* 1992; 15: 4.

Should Americans be eating more Chinese food? *Tufts University Diet & Nutrition Letter.* 1990; 8: 3.

South of the border goes north. *Tufts University Diet & Nutrition Letter.* 1993; 11: 7.

Soy: the bean most likely to succeed in fending off cancer, heart disease. *Environmental Nutrition.* 1994; 17: 1.

Sweet CA. Rethinking eating out. *FDA Consumer.* 1989; 23: 8.

Warshaw H. Eating ethnic: Translating exotic cuisine into healthful dining. *Environmental Nutrition.* 1990; 13: 1.

Williams SR. *Nutrition and Diet Therapy.* St. Louis, MO: Mosby-Year Book; 1993: 316–319.

Herbs and Spices:
Your Allies For Healthier Meals

Balch JF, Balch, PA. *Prescription for Nutritional Healing.* Garden City Park, New York, NY: 1990.

Berkowitz KF. Herbs and spices may be barrier against cancer, heart disease. *Environmental Nutrition.* 1993; 16: 1–2.

Elliot R. *The Complete Vegetarian Cuisine.* New York, NY: Pantheon Books, 1988.

Furth P. Americans are getting spicier. *Frozen Food Digest.* 1993; 8: 12.

Hunter BT. The wisdom of moderation. *Consumers' Research Magazine.* 1993; 76: 8–9.

Murray F. Spice up your health with curcumin. *Better Nutrition.* 1989; 51: 8.

Nutrition craze adds dash to spice sales. *Chain Store Age Supermarkets.* 1983; 59: 104–105.

Pritikin R. *The New Pritikin Program.* New York: Pocket Books; 1991.

Red and black pepper affect transit time. *Nutrition Research Newsletter.* 1992; 11:52–53.

Rinzler CA. *The Complete Book of Herbs, Spices and Condiments.* New York, NY: Henry Holt and Company; 1991.

Toussaint-Samat M; Bell, A, trans. *History of Food.* Cambridge, Mass: Blackwell Publishers; 1994.

Trager J. *The Foodbook.* New York, NY: Grossman Publishers; 1970.

Turmeric as a cancer inhibitor. *Nutrition Research Newsletter.* 1992; 11: 53.

Zeigler J. A sweet spice for diabetics: cinnamon may boost the effects of insulin. *American Health: Fitness of Body and Mind.* 1989; 8: 96–97.

Junk Food:
How Much Can You Get Away With?

Bergman Y, Eller D. *Food Cop.* New York, NY: Bantam Books; 1991.

Blake JS. *Eat Right the E.A.S.Y. Way!* New York, NY: Prentice Hall Press; 1991

Can fast food be good food? *Consumer Reports; Buyers Guide.* Aug. 1994; 493–499.

Columbia University School of Public Health & Institute of Human Nutrition. Fifty sure-fire ways to cut calories. *Health & Nutrition Newsletter,* Mar 1987; 1–3.

Ferguson S. *The Diet Center Program.* Boston, Mass: Little Brown and Company; 1990

Gershoff S. *The Tufts University Guide to Total Nutrition.* New York, NY: HarperCollins; 1990.

Given a Choice, Students Pick Low-Fat Meals. *American Academy of Pediatrics: News Release.* June 8, 1993; 1.

Hamlin S. Eating in 1994: The year beef came back. *The New York Times.* Dec. 28, 1994; C6.

Harris J. I don't want good, I want fast. *Forbes.* Oct. 1, 1990; 186.

Hermann MG. The ABCs of children's nutrition. *McCall's.* Oct 1991; 75–82.

Jacobson MF, Fritschner S. *The Completely Revised and Updated Fast-Food Guide.* New York, NY: Workman Publishing Company, Inc; 1991.

Katahn M. *One Meal At A Time.* New York, NY: Warner Books; 1989.

Linder L. Type A Diet Traps. *Health.* Aug. 1989; 36–37.

Podell RN, Proctor W. *The G-Index Diet.* New York, NY: Warner Books; 1993.

Roberts M. Health food? Fast-food restaurants are rolling out new, lower-fat versions of their bestsellers. But they aren't always better for you. *U.S. News & World Report.* May 20, 1991.

Shapiro L. Feeding frenzy: Overwhelmed by conflicting advice, most Americans have thrown in the napkin on healthy eating. *Newsweek.* May 27 1991; 46–52.

Sifton DW, ed. *The PDR Family Guide to Women's Health and Prescription Drugs.* Montvale, NJ: Medical Economics Data; 1994.

Stressed Out? Junk food won't help. *USA Today.* Aug 1994; 14.

Wurtman JJ. *Managing Your Mind And Mood Through Food.* New York, NY: Rawson Associates; 1986.

Zarrow S. London C. The new diet priorities: Results of an exclusive prevention survey. *Prevention.* Sept. 1991; 33–40.

The Secret to Healthy Restaurant Dining

Bergman Y, Eller D. *Food Cop.* New York, NY: Bantam Books; 1991.

Blake JS. *Eat Right the E.A.S.Y. Way!* New York, NY: Prentice-Hall; 1991.

Carper J. *Food: Your Miracle Medicine.* New York, NY: HarperCollins; 1993.

Gershoff S. *The Tufts University Guide to Total Nutrition.* New York, NY: HarperPerennial; 1990.

Jacobson M. *The Completely Revised and Updated Fats— Food Guide.* 2nd ed. New York, NY: Workman Publishing Company; 1991.

Katahn M. *One Meal At A Time.* New York, NY: Warner Books; 1989.

National Cancer Institute. Insights into fruit and vegetable consumptions: a summary of recent findings for planning the 5-a-day program. Bethesda, MD: Office of Cancer Communications, NCI; 1992.

University of California at Berkeley. *The Wellness Encyclopedia.* Boston, Mass: Houghton Mifflin Company; 1991.

Fat, Cholesterol, and Calorie Counter

Bellerson, KJ. *The Complete & Up-To-Date Fat Book.* Garden City Park, NY: Avery Publishing Group; 1993.

Eating to Lower Your High Blood Cholesterol. U.S. Department of Health & Human Services, Public Health Service, National Institutes of Health; 1989.

Kirschmann, JD. *Nutrition Almanac.* New York, NY: McGraw-Hill Book Co.; 1979.

Netzer, CT. *The Complete Book of Food Counts.* New York, NY: Dell Publishing; 1994.

Nutritive Value of Foods. U.S. Department of Agriculture, Human Nutrition Information Service; Home & Garden Bulletin #72; 1981.

Disease and Disorder Index

U se this index to find out which drugs and supplements are available for a specific medical problem. Both brand and generic names are listed; the generic name is shown in italics. Only brands listed in the drug profiles are included in the index.

General Index

L isted in this index are all major subjects addressed in the book. Included are the page numbers of the vitamin, mineral, and medication profiles that appear in Parts 3 and 4, together with other references to these substances appearing elsewhere in the text.

bean scores, 48-49
grain scores, 46-47
Centrum. *See* Multivitamins
Cereal
  arthritis and, 375
  choosing, 450, 547
    for children, 271
  fat content, 45, 272
  fiber content, 41
  iron-fortified, 257
  nutritional comparison, 54-55
  recommended servings
    for adolescents and teens, 270
    for elementary school children, 268
    for preschoolers, 265
  serving sizes, 427
  shopping suggestions, 436
  sugar content, 45, 271-272
  television advertising, 281
Chaparral, hepatitis and, 50
Chayote, selection, storage, and preparation, 503
CHB (cyanohydroxybutene), anticancer effects, 213
Cheese
  chymosin in, 58
  fat and cholesterol content, 7
Chemoprevention, 207, 208
Child, Julia, and others *Mastering the Art of French Cooking, Volume 1*, 527
Child, Julia, *The Way to Cook*, 524
Child nutrition, 263-282
  See also Adolescent and teen nutrition; Infant nutrition
  calcium in, 397-398
  developing healthy eating habits, 264-267, 429, 542
  evaluating conflicting theories, 263-264
  junk food, 541-542
  meal planning, 429
    adolescents and teens, 270
    elementary school children, 268
    preschoolers, 265
Children
  cholesterol levels, 163
  exercise, 134-135, 277
  food allergies, 267, 277-279, 338, 339, 346
  food and drug interactions in, 411-412
  hyperactivity in, 351
  overweight, 275, 277
  snack foods, 429
  steroid use, 318
Chili peppers
  cooking with, 518
  healing properties, 510
  negative side effects, 515
Chin, Mary Lee, 551
Chinese cuisine
  cooking techniques, 476-477
  dining out, 473-477, 554-555
  foods to avoid, 555
  health benefits, 473-474, 476
  recipes and cooking techniques, 490-491

regional differences, 474, 490
  seasoning, 516
  staple items, 477
Chinese Restaurant Syndrome, 279
Chlordiazepoxide with clidinium. *See* Librax
Chloride, 562
Chlorogenic acid
  anticancer effects, 211
  food sources, 28
  inhibition of nitrosamine formation by, 203
Chlorophylls, anticancer effects, 212
Chlorpropamide. *See* Diabinese
Chocolate, pharmacologic reaction to, 343
Choking in infants, foods to avoid, 261
Cholecalciferol. *See* Vitamin D
Cholesterol
  See also High-density lipoproteins
  arterial deposition, 160
  blood levels
    chromium picolinate and, 308
    interpreting, 161
    recommended, 161
  in children, 163
  cigarette smoking and, 418
  content of common foods, 6-7
  dietary guidelines, 4
    older adults, 297
  exercise and, 89
  fat intake and, 4, 39
  fiber and, 39, 177
  on food labels, 18
  food sources, 4, 39, 160, 297
  health effects, 1-2
  heart disease and, 39, 159-160
  medication reducing, 4, 163
  oat bran and, 21, 45
  ratio of high-density lipoproteins to, 161
  reducing intake of, 15, 162-163
    diabetics, 333
    meal planning, 427
    at menopause, 289-290
    substituting soy products, 474
  in whole vs. skim milk, 22
Cholestyramine. *See* Questran
Choline, 562
  fitness claims, 310
  lecithin and, 572
Chromium, 563
  blood sugar with deficiency of, 334
  dietary sources, 26, 334, 564
  supplements, 309
Chromium picolinate, to reduce body fat, 308-309
Chronulac syrup, 611
Chutney, 481
  recipes, 447
Chy, Donal, *Plyometric Exercises*, 133
Chyme, 357
Chymosin, in cheese, 58

Cigarette smoking
  alcohol and, 418
  calcium absorption and, 403
  cancer and, 201, 224-225, 290, 415
    dietary prevention strategies, 224-225, 226
  dietary recommendations, 416-418
  diseases linked to, 414
  fetal effects, 236
  health risks, 414-416
    for women, 290, 415-416
  heart disease and, 415
  history of public reaction, 413-414
  hypertension and, 191
  obesity and, 82-83
  osteoporosis and, 396, 415
  during pregnancy, 415
  quitting, 419-420
    immediate benefits of, 420
    programs for, 419
  toxins in cigarettes, 415-416
  vitamin and mineral supplements and, 36, 417-418
Cimetidine. *See* Tagamet
Cinnamon
  cooking with, 517
  healing properties, 510
  negative side effects, 514
Circuit training, 128-129
Cirrhosis of the liver, liver cancer and, 227
Cisapride. *See* Propulid
CLA (conjugated linoleic acid)
  anticancer effects, 217
Claiborne, Craig, *The New York Times Cookbook*, 523
Clifford, Carolyn K., 31, 198, 200, 204, 208, 220
Clindex. *See* Librax
Clinical ecology, 351
Cloves
  cooking with, 517
  healing properties, 510
Cobalamin. *See* Vitamin B-12
Cobalt, 564
Coenzyme Q-10, therapeutic claims, 310
Colace, 612
ColBENEMID, 613
Colds, diet therapy, 390-391
Colestid, 616
Colestipol. *See* Colestid
Colic
  foods causing, 247
  remedies for, 347
Colitis, ulcerative, 357, 366
Collagen, vitamin C and production of, 171
Colon cancer
  alcohol consumption and, 202
  calcium and, 224
  diet and prevention of, 222
  fat intake and, 164
  fiber and, 208, 223-224
  at menopause, 287
  red meat and, 200
  risk factors, 223, 224
Colon, role in digestion, 357

Colorectal cancer, dietary prevention strategies, 223-224
Colostrum, 252-253
Col-PROBENECID. *See* Col-BENEMID
Comfrey-pepsin capsules, 49-50
Commonweal, 226
Complex carbohydrates, 37-38
  caloric value, 21
  dietary sources, 286, 294-295, 313
  function of, 312
  gas and, 364
  health benefits, 312
  recommended daily allowance, 312, 326
Condiments, selecting healthy, 434
Conjugated linoleic acid, anticancer effects, 217
Constipation
  causes of, 364
    dietary, 296
    medications, 363, 409
  nutritional therapy, 364-365
  during pregnancy, dietary remedies, 244
Consumer Reports on Health, 4
Contaminants
  avoiding during pregnancy, 235-236
  food-borne illnesses, 261
  in formula feeding, 256
Cookbooks
  arthritis, 373
  dessert, 520, 526
  evaluating, 520-521
  general, 520, 521-524
  gourmet, 520
  health recipes, 466
  low-fat, 520, 524-529
  nutritionists' rating of, 521-529
  snacks, 272
  specialty, 524-529
  vegetarian, 520
Cooking equipment, 437-438
Cooking for a New Earth (Jerome), 525
Cooking Light Cookbook, 1994, 525
Cooking techniques
  breakfast, 449-454
  Chinese, 476-477, 490
  cuisine fusion, 485
  desserts, 463, 465
  French, 486-487
  garlic, 512
  Greek, 472
  healthy substitutions, 442-445
  Indian, 495-496
  for infant meals, 259
  Italian, 471, 492
  legumes, 437
  lunches, 456-457
  main dishes, 457-461
  meat, 437
  Middle Eastern, 498
  nutritionally correct, 439-442
  parchment paper, 441-442
  pasta, 437
  reduced fat ingredients, 442

Nutmeg
  cooking with, 517
  negative side effects, 514-515
NutraSweet. *See* Aspartame
Nutri-System, 104-105
Nutrition
  common misconceptions,
    19-21
  controversies, 17, 19
  health and, 1, 62
  hype, 15
  promising theories in, 12-17
Nutrition Facts labels
  on breakfast cereal, 271
  sodium content, 300
Nutritional counseling for eat-
    ing disorders, 146, 150
Nuts, fiber content, 41

O

Oat bran, effect on choles-
    terol, 21, 45
Obesity
  binge-eating syndrome and,
    151
  in children, 275
  definition, 94
  diabetes and, 331, 332
  ethnic, religious, and class
    differences, 86
  gender differences, 83
  genetic factors, 93-94
  health effects, 6, 80-82
  vs. overweight, 79
  risk of cancer and, 199-200
  size acceptance, 94
  social stigma, 94
Oby-Cap. *See* Fastin
Oil of evening primrose. *See*
    Gamma-linolenic acid
Oils. *See* Vegetable oils
Older adults
  calcium requirements, 398-
    399
  carbohydrate and fiber rec-
    ommendations, 294-296
  digestive disorders, 296, 362
  exercise, 122
  hip fractures, 395
  nutritional needs, 293-301,
    429
    problems meeting, 292-293
    for protein, 294
  reducing fat and cholesterol
    intake, 296-298
  shopping and food prepara-
    tion suggestions, 300
  vitamin and mineral supple-
    ments, 298-300, 391-392
Oleic acid, anticancer effects,
    217
Olive oil
  anticancer effects, 217
  high-density lipoproteins
    and, 170
  in Mediterranean Diet, 13-
    14, 158
  processing and cooking dif-
    ferences, 493

Omega-3 fatty acids, 39, 158
  anticancer effects, 217, 221
  anti-inflammatory effects, 366
  in arthritis treatment, 376
  blood-thinning effect, 175-
    176, 177
  cardiovascular benefits, 176-
    177, 299
  definition, 579
  dietary sources, 217, 579
  effects of excess, 177, 377,
    579
  in fish, 170, 377
  function, 579
  nutritional claims, 299
  recommended daily al-
    lowance, 579
  for smokers, 418
  supplements, 176-177
  therapeutic effects, 19
Omega-6 fatty acids, 39
Omega-9 fatty acids, 39
  anticancer effects, 221
Omeprazole. *See* Prilosec
Onions
  anticancer effects, 215
  high blood pressure and, 408
Optifast, medical complica-
    tions, 107
"Optimum Diet for Optimum
    Health," 326
Oral contraceptives, vitamin B
    complex and, 386
Oregano, cooking with, 518
Organic Crop Improvement
    Association, 52
Organic farming, 52
Organic foods
  See also Health food; Nat-
    ural foods
  certification of, 52
  health food store vs. super-
    market products, 51
  lack of definition for, 43
  price issues, 52
Orinase, 659
Ornish, Dean, 22, 98
  Eat More, Weigh Less, 525
  Life Choice diet, 27
Os-Cal 500. *See* Caltrate 600
Osteoarthritis, 369
  See also Arthritis; Rheuma-
    toid arthritis
  calcium and, 379
  joint changes, 370
  obesity and, 80
  vitamin B deficiency and, 379
Osteomalacia, gluten intoler-
    ance and, 360
Osteoporosis
  alcohol and, 290
  anorexia-associated, 144, 145
  body weight and, 396
  calcium and, 20, 34, 192,
    286, 298, 397-401
  cigarette smoking and, 415
  common fracture sites, 395
  ethnic differences, 396
  exercise and, 122
  extent of problem, 395
  gender differences, 395-396

in postmenopausal women,
    286
  prevention of, 397, 403, 404
    foods to avoid, 286
  protein and, 20
  risk factors, 395-396
  sodium intake and, 10-11,
    280-281, 288-289
  treatment of, 404
Overeaters Anonymous, 88,
    146, 151
Overweight
  American incidence of, 79
  arthritis and, 383
  body fat and, 84
  body shape and, 84, 85
  causes of, 82-83, 92-94
  in children, 275, 277
  complications of pregnancy
    in, 239
  cultural factors, 92-93
  definition, 94
  gender differences, 83
  genetic factors, 93-94
  health consequences, 79-82
  lifestyle and, 93
  vs. obesity, 79
  osteoporosis and, 396
  prostate cancer and, 223
  self-assessment, 95
  social, economic, and psy-
    chological stresses, 81-82
Ovolactovegetarians, 63
Oystercal 500. *See* Caltrate 600

P

PABA, 579
PAHs. *See* Polycyclic aromatic
    hydrocarbons
Pakistani cuisine, 556
Pancreas, manufacture of in-
    sulin by, 330
Pancreatic cancer, cigarette
    smoking and, 226
Pantethine. *See* Pantothenic
    acid
Pantothenic acid, 580
  anticancer effects, 216-217
  in arthritis treatment, 379
Paprika, cooking with, 518
Parchment paper cooking,
    441-442
Parker, Kathryn A., 423, 548,
    551
Paroxetine. *See* Paxil
Parsley, healing properties, 512
Parsnips, selection, storage,
    and preparation, 505
Pasta
  cookbooks, 528-529
  cooking techniques, 438
  dining out, 552
  recipes, 459-460
  serving sizes, 427
  shopping suggestions, 436
Pauling, Linus, *Vitamin C and
    the Common Cold*, 30, 386,
    387
Paxil, 662

Pectin
  anticancer effects, 209
  dietary sources, 209
Pentamidine, low blood sugar
    and, 392
Pentasa. *See* Rowasa
Pepcid, 664
Perdiem fiber. *See* Metamucil
Perimenopause
  nutritional needs, 284
  symptoms, 283
  relief of, 288
Peristalsis, 357
Pernicious anemia
  cobalt and, 564
  vitamin B-12 and, 591
Personal trainers, 137
Pesticides in food, 52
  avoiding during pregnancy,
    235-236
  cancer and, 204-206
  removing, 235
  self-protective measures,
    205-206
Pharmacologic reactions
  to chemicals found naturally
    in foods, 343
  to food additives, 343, 344-
    346
Phenethyl isothiocyanate, can-
    cer and, 29
Phenobarbital. *See* Donnatal
Phenolics, cardiovascular ef-
    fects, 178
Phenolphthalein, pharmaco-
    logic reaction to, 346
Phentermine. *See* Fastin
Phenylalanine, 580
Phenylpropanolamine, in diet
    pills, 108
  See also Acutrim
Phosphorus, 581
  calcium absorption and,
    403, 404
  dietary sources, 26, 582
  function, 24, 581
  osteoporosis and, 286
  in protein-rich foods, 403
  side effects, 299
  in soft drinks, 286
Physical fitness, diet books,
    73-76
Phytochemicals
  cancer-fighting properties,
    28-29, 212-215
  food sources, 28
  health benefits, 28
Phytoestrogens
  cancer and, 214
  dietary sources, 214
Phytoestrols, estrogen produc-
    tion and, 214
*Pillbook: A Guide to Chil-
    dren's Medications*, The
    (Mitchell), 279
Pinckney, Callan, *Callanetics*,
    140
Pi-Sunyer, Xavier, 92, 93, 102,
    108, 110, 111
Plaque, 160
Plyometric Exercises (Chy), 133
Plyometrics, 133